I0065834

Clinical Pulmonology

Clinical Pulmonology

Edited by **Michael Glass**

hayle
medical

New York

Published by Hayle Medical,
30 West, 37th Street, Suite 612,
New York, NY 10018, USA
www.haylemedical.com

Clinical Pulmonology
Edited by Michael Glass

© 2016 Hayle Medical

International Standard Book Number: 978-1-63241-399-4 (Hardback)

This book contains information obtained from authentic and highly regarded sources. Copyright for all individual chapters remain with the respective authors as indicated. All chapters are published with permission under the Creative Commons Attribution License or equivalent. A wide variety of references are listed. Permission and sources are indicated; for detailed attributions, please refer to the permissions page and list of contributors. Reasonable efforts have been made to publish reliable data and information, but the authors, editors and publisher cannot assume any responsibility for the validity of all materials or the consequences of their use.

The publisher's policy is to use permanent paper from mills that operate a sustainable forestry policy. Furthermore, the publisher ensures that the text paper and cover boards used have met acceptable environmental accreditation standards.

Trademark Notice: Registered trademark of products or corporate names are used only for explanation and identification without intent to infringe.

Printed in the United States of America.

Contents

Preface   IX

Chapter 1   **Trends in Pulmonary Hypertension Mortality and Morbidity**   1
Alem Mehari, Orlando Valle and Richard F. Gillum

Chapter 2   **Fungal Exposure and Low Levels of IL-10 in Patients with Sarcoidosis**   6
Marjeta Terčelj, Sanja Stopinšek, Alojz Ihan, Barbara Salobir, Saša Simčič
and Ragnar Rylander

Chapter 3   **Association of Serum Magnesium Levels with Frequency of Acute Exacerbations
in Chronic Obstructive Pulmonary Disease: A Prospective Study**   10
Aziz Gumus, Muge Haziroglu and Yilmaz Gunes

Chapter 4   **Pleural Fluid Cholesterol in Differentiating Exudative and Transudative
Pleural Effusion**   15
A. B. Hamal, K. N. Yogi, N. Bam, S. K. Das and R. Karn

Chapter 5   **Comparison Study of Airway Reactivity Outcomes Due to a Pharmacologic
Challenge Test: Impulse Oscillometry versus Least Mean Squared Analysis
Techniques**   19
Elena Rodriguez, Charrell M. Bullard, Milena H. Armani, Thomas L. Miller and
Thomas H. Shaffer

Chapter 6   **Effects of Inactivated _Bordetella_ Pertussis on Phosphodiesterase in the Lung of
Ovalbumin Sensitized and Challenged Rats**   28
Ya-Juan Wang, Shun-De Song, Jun-Chun Chen, Xue-Feng Wang, Ya-Li Jiang,
Qiang-Min Xie, Ji-Qiang Chen, Zi-Gang Li and Hui-Fang Tang

Chapter 7   **Clinical Investigation of Benign Asbestos Pleural Effusion**   39
Nobukazu Fujimoto, Kenichi Gemba, Keisuke Aoe, Katsuya Kato,
Takako Yokoyama, Ikuji Usami, Kazuo Onishi, Keiichi Mizuhashi,
Toshikazu Yusa and Takumi Kishimoto

Chapter 8   **Retrospective Observations on the Ability to Diagnose and Manage Patients with
Asthma Through the Use of Impulse Oscillometry: Comparison with Spirometry
and Overview of the Literature**   45
Constantine Saadeh, Blake Cross, Charles Saadeh and Michael Gaylor

Chapter 9   **Markers of Myocardial Ischemia in Patients with Obstructive Sleep Apnea and
Coronary Artery Disease**   54
Misa Valo, Annette Wons, Albert Moeller and Claudius Teupe

Chapter 10   **The Pattern of Respiratory Disease Morbidity and Mortality in a Tertiary Hospital in Southern-Eastern Nigeria**   60
Victor Aniedi Umoh, Akaninyene Otu, Henry Okpa and Emmanuel Effa

Chapter 11   **The Immediate Pulmonary Disease Pattern Following Exposure to High Concentrations of Chlorine Gas**   66
Pallavi P. Balte, Kathleen A. Clark, Lawrence C. Mohr, Wilfried J. Karmaus, David Van Sickle and Erik R. Svendsen

Chapter 12   **Sarcoidosis Treatment with Antifungal Medication: A Follow-Up**   73
Marjeta Terčelj, Barbara Salobir, Mirjana Zupancic and Ragnar Rylander

Chapter 13   **The Role of the High-Sensitivity C-Reactive Protein in Patients with Stable Non-Cystic Fibrosis Bronchiectasis**   77
Meng-Heng Hsieh, Yueh-Fu Fang, Guan-Yuan Chen, Fu-Tsai Chung, Yuan-Chang Liu, Cheng-Hsien Wu, Yu-Chen Chang and Horng-Chyuan Lin

Chapter 14   **A Simple Clinical Measure of Quadriceps Muscle Strength Identifies Responders to Pulmonary Rehabilitation**   85
James R. Walsh, Norman R. Morris, Zoe J. McKeough, Stephanie T. Yerkovich and Jenny D. Paratz

Chapter 15   **Effects of Symptom Perception Interventions on Trigger Identification and Quality of Life in Children with Asthma**   93
Thomas Janssens and Andrew Harver

Chapter 16   **Factors Influencing Early Health Facility Contact and Low Default Rate Among New Sputum Smear Positive Tuberculosis Patients, India**   101
Ashok Kumar Bhardwaj, Surender Kashyap, Pradeep Bansal, Dinesh Kumar, Sunil Kumar Raina, Vishav Chander and Sushant Sharma

Chapter 17   **Evaluation of Anthropometric and Metabolic Parameters in Obstructive Sleep Apnea**   106
Yaşar Yildirim, Süreyya Yilmaz, Mehmet Güven, Faruk Kılınç, Ali Veysel Kara, Zülfükar Yilmaz, Gökhan Kırbaş, Alpaslan Kemal Tuzcu and Fatma Yılmaz Aydın

Chapter 18   **In Situ Thrombosis of Small Pulmonary Arteries in Pulmonary Hypertension Developing after Chemotherapy for Malignancy**   112
Kay Maeda, Yoshikatsu Saiki and Shigeo Yamaki

Chapter 19   **Sleep Disordered Breathing in Children with Mitochondrial Disease**   118
Ricardo A. Mosquera, Mary Kay Koenig, Rahmat B. Adejumo, Justyna Chevallier, S. Shahrukh Hashmi, Sarah E. Mitchell, Susan E. Pacheco and Cindy Jon

Chapter 20   **Carbon Ion Radiotherapy for Oligo-Recurrence in the Lung**   126
Naoyoshi Yamamoto, Mio Nakajima, Hirohiko Tsujii and Tadashi Kamada

Chapter 21   **Frequency and Intensive Care Related Risk Factors of Pneumothorax in Ventilated Neonates**   132
Ramesh Bhat Yellanthoor and Vidya Ramdas

Chapter 22   **Latex Hypersensitivity among Allergic Egyptian Children: Relation to Parental/Self Reports**   136
Zeinab A. El-Sayed, Shereen S. El-Sayed, Rehab M. Zaki and Mervat A. Salama

Chapter 23   **Knowledge Level of the Primary Healthcare Providers on Chronic Obstructive Pulmonary Disease and Pulmonary Rehabilitation**   142
Tuğba Göktalay, Ayşe Nur Tuncal, Seçil Sarı, Galip Köroğlu, Yavuz Havlucu and Arzu Yorgancıoğlu

Chapter 24   **The Role of Cardiopulmonary Exercise Test in IPF Prognosis**   149
Christina Triantafillidou, Effrosyni Manali, Panagiotis Lyberopoulos, Likourgos Kolilekas, Konstantinos Kagouridis, Sotirios Gyftopoulos, Konstantinos Vougas, Anastasia Kotanidou, Manos Alchanatis, Anna Karakatsani and Spyros A. Papiris

Chapter 25   **Intravenous Dexmedetomidine Provides Superior Patient Comfort and Tolerance Compared to Intravenous Midazolam in Patients Undergoing Flexible Bronchoscopy**   158
Umesh Goneppanavar, Rahul Magazine, Bhavya Periyadka Janardhana and Shreepathi Krishna Achar

Chapter 26   **Hemoglobin Variant (Hemoglobin Aalborg) Mimicking Interstitial Pulmonary Disease**   166
Vasiliki Panou, Peter-Diedrich Mathias Jensen, Jan Freddy Pedersen, Lars Pilegaard Thomsen and Ulla MøllerWeinreich

Chapter 27   **Higher Mobility Scores in Patients with Cystic Fibrosis are Associated with Better Lung Function**   172
Aneesha Thobani, Jessica A. Alvarez, Shaina Blair, Kaila Jackson, Eric R. Gottlieb, Seth Walker and Vin Tangpricha

Chapter 28   **Study of Exhaled Nitric Oxide in Subjects with Suspected Obstructive Sleep Apnea: A Pilot Study in Vietnam**   178
Sy Duong-Quy, Thong Hua-Huy, Huyen-Tran Tran-Mai-Thi, Nhat-Nam Le-Dong, Timothy J. Craig and Anh-Tuan Dinh-Xuan

Chapter 29   **The Epidemiology of Pulmonary Nontuberculous Mycobacteria: Data from a General Hospital in Athens, Greece, 2007–2013**   185
Marios Panagiotou, Andriana I. Papaioannou, Konstantinos Kostikas, Maria Paraskeua, Ekaterini Velentza, Maria Kanellopoulou, Vasiliki Filaditaki and Napoleon Karagiannidis

Chapter 30   **The Interpretation of Dyspnea in the Patient with Asthma**   194
Marc H. Lavietes

Chapter 31   **Accuracy of the Hospital Anxiety and Depression Scale for Identifying Depression in Chronic Obstructive Pulmonary Disease Patients**   198
Christoph Nowak, Noriane A. Sievi, Christian F. Clarenbach, Esther Irene Schwarz, Christian Schlatzer, Thomas Brack, Martin Brutsche, Martin Frey, Sarosh Irani, Jörg D. Leuppi, Jochen Rüdiger, Robert Thurnheer and Malcolm Kohler

Chapter 32   **Patients with MAC Lung Disease Have a Low Visceral Fat Area and Low Nutrient Intake**   205
Kentaro Wakamatsu, Nobuhiko Nagata, Sanae Maki, Hisamitsu Omori, Hiroyuki Kumazoe, Kayoko Ueno, Yuko Matsunaga, Makiko Hara, Koji Takakura, Nagisa Fukumoto, Nobuhisa Ando, Mami Morishige, Takashi Akasaki, Ichiro Inoshima, Shinji Ise, Miiru Izumi and Masayuki Kawasaki

Chapter 33   **Drug Resistance among Pulmonary Tuberculosis Patients in Calabar, Nigeria**   **210**
Akaninyene Otu, Victor Umoh, Abdulrazak Habib, Soter Ameh, Lovett Lawson
and Victor Ansa

Chapter 34   **Driving-Related Neuropsychological Performance in Stable COPD Patients**   **216**
Foteini Karakontaki, Sofia-Antiopi Gennimata, Anastasios F. Palamidas,
Theocharis Anagnostakos, Epaminondas N. Kosmas, Anastasios Stalikas,
Charalambos Papageorgiou and Nikolaos G. Koulouris

Chapter 35   **Differences between Risk Factors Associated with Tuberculosis Treatment
Abandonment and Mortality**   **226**
Nathália Mota de Faria Gomes, Meire Cardoso da Mota Bastos, Renata Magliano
Marins, Aline Alves Barbosa, Luiz Clóvis Parente Soares, Annelise Maria de
Oliveira Wilken de Abreu and João Tadeu Damian Souto Filho

Chapter 36   **Vest Chest Physiotherapy Airway Clearance is Associated with Nitric Oxide
Metabolism**   **234**
Joseph H. Sisson, Todd A. Wyatt, Jacqueline A. Pavlik, Pawanjit S. Sarna and
Peter J. Murphy

Chapter 37   **Is Mean Platelet Volume Really a Severity Marker for Obstructive Sleep Apnea
Syndrome without Comorbidities?**   **240**
Sinem Nedime Sökücü, Cengiz Özdemir, Levent Dalar, Levent Karasulu,
Fenay Aydın and Sedat Altın

Permissions

List of Contributors

Preface

Pulmonology is the field of medical science that deals with diseases related to lungs. The professionals or doctors working in this field are generally trained in dealing with diseases related to chest such as tuberculosis, asthma, emphysema, pneumonia and other complications. This also involves ventilator support in case of critical breathing problems. In this book, using case studies and examples, constant effort has been made to make the understanding of the difficult concepts of pulmonology practiced by clinicians as easy and informative as possible, for the readers. This book consists of contributions made by international experts which unravel the recent progress of this field. It is an essential guide for pulmonologists, academicians and those who wish to pursue this discipline further.

This book is the end result of constructive efforts and intensive research done by experts in this field. The aim of this book is to enlighten the readers with recent information in this area of research. The information provided in this profound book would serve as a valuable reference to students and researchers in this field.

At the end, I would like to thank all the authors for devoting their precious time and providing their valuable contributions to this book. I would also like to express my gratitude to my fellow colleagues who encouraged me throughout the process.

Editor

Trends in Pulmonary Hypertension Mortality and Morbidity

Alem Mehari, Orlando Valle, and Richard F. Gillum

Department of Medicine, Howard University, 2041 Georgia Avenue NW, Washington, DC 20060, USA

Correspondence should be addressed to Alem Mehari; alem.mehari@howard.edu
and Richard F. Gillum; rfg2.howard.edu@gmail.com

Academic Editor: Luisetti Maurizio

Context. Few reports have been published regarding surveillance data for pulmonary hypertension, a debilitating and often fatal condition. *Aims*. We report trends in pulmonary hypertension. *Settings and Design*. United States of America; vital statistics, hospital data. *Methods and Material*. We used mortality data from the National Vital Statistics System (NVSS) for 1999–2008 and hospital discharge data from the National Hospital Discharge Survey (NHDS) for 1999–2009. *Statistical Analysis Used*. We present age-standardized rates. *Results*. Since 1999, the numbers of deaths and hospitalizations as well as death rates and hospitalization rates for pulmonary hypertension have increased. In 1999 death rates were higher for men than for women; however, by 2002, no differences by gender remained because of the increasing death rates among women and the declining death rates among men; after 2003 death rates for women were higher than for men. Death rates throughout the reporting period 1999–2008 were higher for blacks than for whites. Hospitalization rates in women were 1.3–1.6 times higher than in men. *Conclusions*. Pulmonary hypertension mortality and hospitalization numbers and rates increased from 1999 to 2008.

1. Introduction

Pulmonary hypertension (PH) is a disorder of the pulmonary vasculature that results in increased pulmonary arterial pressure and is defined as a mean pulmonary arterial pressure (mPAP) ≥ 25 mm Hg at rest, the pressure being measured invasively with a pulmonary artery catheter [1–4]. Despite improvements in the diagnosis and management of PH over the past 2 decades with the introduction of targeted medical therapies leading to improved survival, the disease continues to have a poor long-term prognosis [5]. US death rates for PH as the underlying cause of death increased between 1979 and 1999 [6–8]. To assess more recent trends, this report describes national trends for all PH-related deaths and hospitalizations during 1999–2008.

2. Subjects and Methods

To examine trends in PH mortality, we analyzed data from the Centers for Disease Control (CDC) National Vital Statistics System (NVSS). The NVSS classified diseases and conditions reported on death certificates during 1999–2010 according to the *International Classification of Diseases, Tenth Revision* (ICD-10) codes for deaths [9–19]. For this analysis, we considered PH-associated deaths, those with ICD-10 codes I27.0, I27.8, or I27.9 during 1999–2002 and ICD-10 codes I27.0, I27.2, I27.8, or I27.9 during 2003–2008, as any contributing cause of death (i.e., any of the possible 20 conditions, including underlying cause) on their death certificate. We used resident populations from the U.S. Census Bureau to calculate death rates per 100,000 population. We age-standardized death rates to 2000 U.S. standard population [16, 17]. Because the numbers of deaths with PH were relatively small each year, we aggregated years according to the availability of drugs for PH, that is, when only epoprostenol was available (1999–2001), after availability of bosentan (2002–2005), and after sildenafil entered the market (2006–2009) to produce stable statistics and shed light on the possible role of these new drugs on mortality and hospitalization.

To examine trends in PH hospitalization, we analyzed data from the Centers for Disease Control (CDC) National Hospital Discharge Survey (NHDS) for 1999–2009 [20–22].

We report estimates of all-listed diagnoses of PH (ICD-9-CM codes 416.0, 416.8, or 416.9) based on counting up to seven medical diagnoses recorded in NHDS and using sampling weights (i.e., inflation factors) that allow estimation of US statistics from the sample.

We used the U.S. civilian population for the period 1999–2009 from the U.S. Census Bureau to calculate age- and sex-specific diagnosis rates per 100,000 population. To examine trends in diagnoses during 1999–2009, we aggregated data into one 3-year and two 4-year periods (1999–2001, 2002–2005) and (2006–2009) as for mortality (see above).

Supplementary Material provides detailed tables not included in this report. (See Supplementary Tables in the Supplementary Material available online at http://dx.doi.org/10.1155/2014/105864).

3. Results

3.1. Mortality. During 1999–2008, the total number of deaths with PH listed as any contributing cause of death increased from 15,046 in 1999 to 19,373 in 2008. For the reporting periods 1999–2002 and 2003–2008, 57.7% and 61%, respectively, of decedents with PH-related mortality were female. In 1999–2002, 11.2% of males and 9.7% of females were <45 years; in 2003–2008, 8.4% of males and 6.9% of females were aged <45 years. The proportion of decedents aged ≥85 years increased from 17.6% to 22.4%. At all ages in 1999–2008, the most common underlying cause of death was pulmonary hypertension (29.4–30.8%), followed by chronic lower respiratory disease (20.2–27.0%). Among decedents aged <45 years, the most common underlying causes of death were PH; congenital malformations; complications of pregnancy, childbirth, and the puerperium; or conditions originating in the perinatal period. Supplementary Material provides further detailed mortality data in supplementary Tables 1–9.

In 1999–2008, age-standardized death rates for the total U.S. population remained relatively stable from 1999 through 2008 (Table 1). However, age-standardized death rates increased among women; among men rates decreased during 1999–2006 then increased during 2007-2008 (Figure 1). Rates increased with age. Blacks had higher rates than whites for each year in the reporting period. Non-Hispanics had higher age-standardized death rates than Hispanics. There was an upward trend in age-specific death rates for people aged ≥85 years, most markedly during 2006–2008. In 1999–2001, men had slightly higher age-specific death rates than women, but in 2002–2008 women had higher age-specific death rates than men in the older age groups. At ages <75 years, blacks had higher age-specific death rates than whites during 1999–2001, but whites had higher death rates than blacks at ages ≥85 years. States with the 10 highest age-standardized death rates were Vermont (11.4), Wyoming (10), Colorado (8.9), Idaho (7.9), DC (7.7), Montana (7.5), North Carolina (7.5), Ohio (7.5), West Virginia (7.3), and New Mexico (7.4). Supplementary Material provides further detailed hospitalization data in supplementary Tables 10–13.

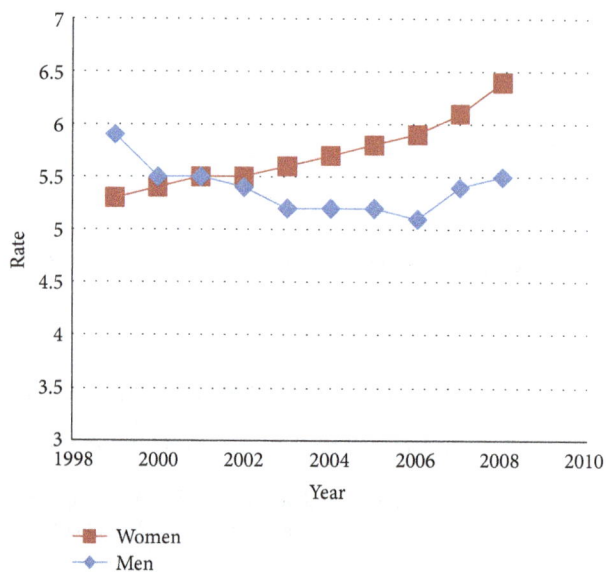

FIGURE 1: Age-standardized death rate per 100,000 population for decedents with pulmonary hypertension listed as any contributing cause of death by sex and year—United States 1999–2008. Age is standardized using the 2000 U.S. standard population.

TABLE 1: Age-standardized and age-specific death rates* for pulmonary hypertension† as any contributing cause of death for groups defined by selected characteristics and by period: United States, 1999–2008.

Characteristic	1999–2001	2002–2005	2006–2008
Age-standardized†† death rate			
All	5.5	5.5	5.8
Men	5.6	5.3	5.3
Women	5.4	5.7	6.1
Race			
Black	7.4	7.6	8.1
White	5.3	5.3	5.6
Asian/Pacific Islander	2.6	2.5	2.8
American Indian	4.0	3.9	3.9
Hispanic origin			
Hispanic	3.2	3.1	3.1
Non-Hispanic	5.6	5.7	5.9
Age-specific death rate			
0–44 yrs	0.9	0.8	0.7
45–54 yrs	2.8	2.7	2.8
55–64 yrs	7.2	7.0	7.0
65–74 yrs	19.4	19.0	18.3
75–84 yrs	37.1	39.0	43.0
>85 yrs	60.8	67.4	80.0

*Per 100,000 population; †International Classification of Diseases, Tenth Revision Codes I27.0, I27.2, I27.8, and I27.9; ††to the 2000 U.S. standard population.

3.2. Hospitalizations. From 1999 to 2009, the estimated number of all-listed diagnoses of PH increased by 1.5 times from 257 thousand to 386 thousand. Women accounted for

59.3–60.3% and patients aged ≥65 years accounted for 62.6–66.7% of all-listed diagnoses of PH. All-listed diagnosis rates in 2006–2009 were 1.2–1.4 times higher in men and 1.5 times higher in women than earlier (Table 2). The rate of all-listed diagnoses increased for all age groups; the greatest increase was among adults aged ≥65 years. Rates of diagnoses for PH among women were higher than those for men throughout the study period (Figure 2). Rates increased with age. Rates were highest in the northeast region.

4. Discussion

During 1999–2008, rates for PH as any contributing cause of death and as all-listed hospital diagnoses increased. The number of PH-related deaths and number of hospitalizations increased, particularly among women, blacks, and older adults. In addition, PH was the most common reported underlying cause of death among all decedents with PH as any contributing cause of death during 2000–2008. PH might have been diagnosed more often as diagnostic and therapeutic options improve. Increased survival of patients with PH receiving more effective therapy over the last two decades could also play a role.

The observed increases in reporting of PH as any-listed diagnosis on hospital records might indicate an actual increase in the number of patients or, more likely, a greater awareness among physicians. Increased awareness of PH as a fatal condition could lead to increased reporting of PH as a contributing cause of death [23, 24]. Even though patients with PH die due to right heart failure, heart failure is rarely reported on PH death certificates as the underlying cause because specific instructions on the death certificate state that "cardiac failure" should not be listed as the underlying cause of death.

Although the question cannot be directly addressed with these data, one may wish to consider the possible effect on PH mortality and hospitalizations of the introduction of new drugs for PH, namely, epoprostenol sodium, followed by bosentan and sildenafil to the US market. Epoprostenol (for injection) was approved for PH by the United States Food and Drug Administration (FDA) in 1995. Bosentan (oral) was approved for PH by the United States Food and Drug Administration (FDA) in 2001. Sildenafil (for injection and oral) is marketed for PH and was approved for PH by the United States Food and Drug Administration (FDA) in 2005 (Source Pulmonary Hypertension Association, http://www.phassociation.org/Treatments, last accessed 5/13/2014). These data are consistent with increased availability of approved drugs for the treatment of PH, some given by infusion, contributing to increased rates of hospitalization and listing of PH discharge diagnoses in the most recent period shown in Table 2 (2006–2009). Increasing frequency of premortem diagnoses also could have led to increased listing of PH as a contributing cause of death on death certificates leading to apparent increases in rates over the period shown in Table 1.

Our findings are similar to those of Davis et al., who suggested that annual age-adjusted mortality for idiopathic

TABLE 2: Estimated rate[*] of pulmonary hypertension[†] all-listed diagnoses during hospital stay, by selected characteristics and period: National Hospital Discharge Survey, United States, 1999–2009.

Characteristic	1999–2001 rate[*]	2002–2005 rate[*]	2006–2009 rate[*]
Total	96.3	90.8	115.1
Male	79.7	74.1	93.4
Female	112.2	106.9	135.4
15–44 years	14.1	18.3	20.2
45–64 years	103.4	104.5	100.0
65 and over	527.2	453.0	598.7
Northeast	120.8	103.4	132.6
Midwest	99.0	92.0	112.6
South	90.6	91.3	122.1
West	79.3	78.1	92.6

[*]Per 100,000 population; [†]International Classification of Diseases, Ninth Revision, Clinical Modification codes 416.0, 416.8, and 416.9.

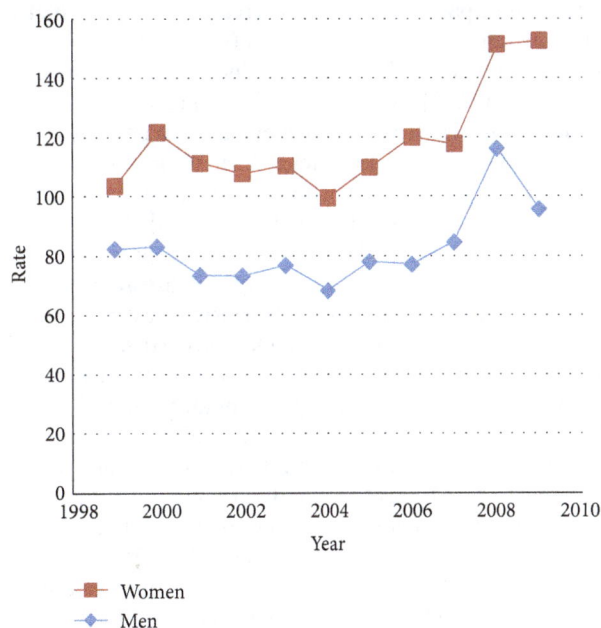

FIGURE 2: Estimated annual rate per 100,000 population of all-listed diagnoses of pulmonary hypertension by year and sex: National Hospital Discharge Survey, United States, 1999–2009.

pulmonary arterial hypertension increased between 1979–1996 and 1994–1998, the greatest increase was among black women and that the disease may not be uncommon in the elderly [6, 8]. Similarly, Hyduk et al. observed increasing rates of hospitalizations for PH and mortality with PH over the period 1980–2002, particularly among women, blacks, and older adults. In their report, 30% of the patients dying with PH were 75 years of age or older [7]. In addition, age-specific death rates for PH increased among men 65 years of age or older, whites 75 years of age or older, and blacks 65 years of age or older. Similar to our report, during 1990–2002 death rates were higher for blacks than whites. The proportion of patients dying with PH who were 75 years of age or older increased from 1980 to 2002; 30.6% of all patients dying with PH from 2000 to 2002 were 75 to 84 years of age, and 18.1% were 85 years of age or older, compared with 23.7% and 6.5%, respectively, from 1980 to 1984 [7]. Hence, these results combined with our results indicate long-term trends that may be expected to continue during the remainder of this decade. It will be important to learn what portion of the trends is due to increased physician awareness and changes in diagnosis and reporting.

Estimates for prevalence of idiopathic pulmonary arterial hypertension cannot be ascertained from our report. However, registry data suggest that the average age and percent female have increased in the last two decades [25–27]. In the Registry to Evaluate Early and Long-term Pulmonary Arterial Hypertension Disease Management, mean age at diagnosis was 47 years and 78% were female. Possible explanations for the increased female predominance include increased representation in the US population of ethnic groups (e.g., blacks, Hispanics) with a higher female:male ratio in patients with PH, increased environmental or iatrogenic and hormonal influences (particularly estrogens) in the pathogenesis of PH, and the increasing prevalence of severe obesity [28]. Another possible explanation is gender difference in health seeking behavior for reporting health problems and seeking treatment. A survivor bias may also exist with a greater proportion of female patients living longer or responding better to therapy [29]. Explanations for the older age include a change in the population age distribution, in the natural history of the disease itself (e.g., a change in some unrecognized intrinsic or extrinsic factor that delays disease manifestations), improved survival with therapy, or an increased prevalence of chronic lung disease in women due to secular trends in smoking among women. Our findings of excess PH mortality in blacks are generally consistent with the association between race and excess mortality from disease of the circulatory system in the United States [30]. Mechanisms for gender and racial differences in PH occurrence have been reviewed elsewhere [30, 31].

The highest hospital diagnosis rate was observed in the Northeast United States and highest death rates for PH were observed in Vermont and in the Rocky Mountain Western United States (Colorado, Idaho, Montana, New Mexico, and Wyoming). Possible explanations for this geographic pattern include the following: first, these cases might be more likely to be detected by physicians affiliated with PH centers that are located in Denver (CO) and Philadelphia (PA). Second, altitude might also play an important role in the development of PH in states such as Colorado, Montana, and Wyoming [6–8]. Identification of these patterns warrants further investigations.

Our study has several limitations. First, mortality data are subject to diagnosis and reporting errors by physicians, medical examiners, and coroners. Second, the current ICD classifications do not allow data users to differentiate specific diseases that are associated with PH. For example, the current ICD codes do not allow differentiation of the five major categories of PH [2, 3]. Thus, population estimates for WHO group I pulmonary arterial hypertension cannot be ascertained, a category of interest to researchers. Finally, hospital discharge data cannot be used to estimate prevalence or incidence of the disease because distinguishing between first hospitalizations or readmissions during the year is not possible and some patients may not be hospitalized. However, the NVSS and NHDS databases are useful for surveillance and monitoring trends.

Conflict of Interests

The authors declare that there is no conflict of interests regarding the publication of this paper.

Acknowledgments

The authors acknowledge the helpful comments by Rosanna Setse, M.D., Ph.D., Thomas O. Obisesan, M.D., M.P.H., Alicia N. Thomas, M.D., Alvin Thomas Jr., M.D., Octavius Polk, M.D., Wayne P. Davis, M.D., and Patricia O'Neal, M.D.

References

[1] D. B. Badesch, H. C. Champion, M. A. Gomez Sanchez et al., "Diagnosis and assessment of pulmonary arterial hypertension," *Journal of the American College of Cardiology*, vol. 54, no. 1, supplement, pp. S55–S66, 2009.

[2] G. Simonneau, N. Galiè, L. J. Rubin et al., "Clinical classification of pulmonary hypertension," *Journal of the American College of Cardiology*, vol. 43, no. 12, supplement, pp. 5S–12S, 2004.

[3] G. Simonneau, I. M. Robbins, M. Beghetti et al., "Updated Clinical Classification of Pulmonary Hypertension," *Journal of the American College of Cardiology*, vol. 54, no. 1, supplement 1, pp. S43–S54, 2009.

[4] N. F. Voelkel, R. A. Quaife, L. A. Leinwand et al., "Right ventricular function and failure: report of a National Heart, Lung, and Blood Institute working group on cellular and molecular mechanisms of right heart failure," *Circulation*, vol. 114, no. 17, pp. 1883–1891, 2006.

[5] V. V. McLaughlin, "Looking to the future: a new decade of pulmonary arterial hypertension therapy," *European Respiratory Review*, vol. 20, no. 122, pp. 262–269, 2011.

[6] K. K. Davis, D. E. Lilienfeld, and R. L. Doyle, "Increased mortality in African Americans with idiopathic pulmonary arterial hypertension," *Journal of the National Medical Association*, vol. 100, no. 1, pp. 69–72, 2008.

[7] A. Hyduk, J. B. Croft, C. Ayala, K. Zheng, Z.-J. Zheng, and G. A. Mensah, "Pulmonary hypertension surveillance–United States, 1980–2002," *MMWR Surveillance Summaries*, vol. 54, no. 5, pp. 1–28, 2005.

[8] D. E. Lilienfeld and L. J. Rubin, "Mortality from primary pulmonary hypertension in the United States, 1979–1996," *Chest*, vol. 117, no. 3, pp. 796–800, 2000.

[9] J. Link, C. Glazer, F. Torres, and K. Chin, "International classification of diseases coding changes lead to profound declines in reported idiopathic pulmonary arterial hypertension mortality and hospitalizations: implications for database studies," *Chest*, vol. 139, no. 3, pp. 497–504, 2011.

[10] S. Rich, E. Chomka, L. Hasara et al., "The prevalence of pulmonary hypertension in the United States. Adult population estimates obtained from measurements of chest roentgenograms from the NHANES II Survey," *Chest*, vol. 96, no. 2, pp. 236–241, 1989.

[11] R. N. Anderson, A. M. Miniño, D. L. Hoyert, and H. M. Rosenberg, "Comparability of cause of death between ICD-9 and ICD-10: preliminary estimates," *National Vital Statistics Reports*, vol. 49, no. 2, pp. 1–32, 2001.

[12] G. R. Bramer, "International statistical classification of diseases and related health problems. Tenth revision," *World Health Statistics Quarterly*, vol. 41, no. 1, pp. 32–36, 1988.

[13] E. Weitzenblum, "Chronic cor pulmonale," *Circulation*, vol. 27, no. 4, pp. 594–615, 1963.

[14] "MANUAL of the international statistical classification of diseases, injuries, and causes of death. Addendum 1. Supplementary interpretations and instructions for coding causes of death," *Bulletin of the World Health Organization. Supplement*, vol. 7, supplement 6, pp. 1–55, 1953.

[15] "The international conference for the tenth revision of the International Classification of Diseases. Strengthening of Epidemiological and Statistical Services Unit. World Health Organization, Geneva," *World Health Statistics Quarterly*, vol. 43, no. 4, pp. 204–245, 1990.

[16] R. N. Anderson and H. M. Rosenberg, "Age standardization of death rates: implementation of the year 2000 standard," *National Vital Statistics Reports*, vol. 47, no. 3, pp. 1–16, 20, 1998.

[17] R. J. Klein and C. A. Schoenborn, "Age adjustment using the 2000 projected U.S. population," *Healthy People 2000 Statistical Notes*, no. 20, pp. 1–9, 2001.

[18] Centers for Disease Control and Prevention, National Center for Health Statistics, *Underlying Cause of Death 1999–2009 on CDC WONDER Online Database*, 2012, http://wonder.cdc.gov/ucd-icd10.html.

[19] National Center for Health Statistics, *National Vital Statistics System*, US Department of Health and Human Services, CDC, National Center for Health Statistics, Hyattsville, Md, USA, 2009, http://www.cdc.gov/nchs/nvss.htm.

[20] W. R. Simmons and G. A. Schnack, *Development of the Design of the NCHS Hospital Discharge Survey. Vital Health Statistics*, series 2, no. 39, DHEW publication no. (HRA) 77-1199, Human Resources Administration, Rockville, Md, USA, 1977, http://www.cdc.gov/nchs/data/series/sr_02/sr02_039.pdf.

[21] L. J. Kozak, *Underreporting of Race in the National Hospital Discharge Survey*, Advance data no. 265, US Department of Health and Human Services, CDC, National Center for Health Statistics, Hyattsville, Md, USA, 1995, http://www.cdc.gov/nchs/data/ad/ad265.pdf.

[22] US Department of Health and Human Services. The International Classification of Diseases, *Ninth Revision, Clinical Modification*, DHHS publication no. (PHS) 91-1260, US Department of Health and Human Services, CDC, National Center for Health Statistics, Health Care Financing Administration, Hyattsville, Md, USA, 4th edition, 1991.

[23] D. Mukerjee, D. St George, B. Coleiro et al., "Prevalence and outcome in systemic sclerosis associated pulmonary arterial hypertension: application of a registry approach," *Annals of the Rheumatic Diseases*, vol. 62, no. 11, pp. 1088–1093, 2003.

[24] R. A. Israel, H. M. Rosenberg, and L. R. Curtin, "Analytical potential for multiple cause-of-death data," *The American Journal of Epidemiology*, vol. 124, no. 2, pp. 161–179, 1986.

[25] D. B. Badesch, G. E. Raskob, C. G. Elliott et al., "Pulmonary arterial hypertension: baseline characteristics from the REVEAL registry," *Chest*, vol. 137, no. 2, pp. 376–387, 2010.

[26] A. E. Frost, D. B. Badesch, R. J. Barst et al., "The changing picture of patients with pulmonary arterial hypertension in the United States: how REVEAL differs from historic and non-US contemporary registries," *Chest*, vol. 139, no. 1, pp. 128–137, 2011.

[27] G. E. D'Alonzo, R. J. Barst, S. M. Ayres et al., "Survival in patients with primary pulmonary hypertension: results from a national prospective registry," *Annals of Internal Medicine*, vol. 115, no. 5, pp. 343–349, 1991.

[28] K. M. Flegal, D. Carroll, B. K. Kit, and C. L. Ogden, "Prevalence of obesity and trends in the distribution of body mass index among US adults, 1999–2010," *Journal of the American Medical Association*, vol. 307, no. 5, pp. 491–497, 2012.

[29] M. Humbert, O. Sitbon, A. Chaouat et al., "Survival in patients with idiopathic, familial, and anorexigen-associated pulmonary arterial hypertension in the modern management era," *Circulation*, vol. 122, no. 2, pp. 156–163, 2010.

[30] A. T. Geronimus, J. Bound, T. A. Waidmann, M. M. Hillemeier, and P. B. Burns, "Excess mortality among blacks and whites in the United States," *The New England Journal of Medicine*, vol. 335, no. 21, pp. 1552–1558, 1996.

[31] E. D. Austin, T. Lahm, J. West et al., "Gender, sex hormones and pulmonary hypertension," *Pulmonary Circulation*, vol. 3, no. 2, pp. 294–314, 2013.

Fungal Exposure and Low Levels of IL-10 in Patients with Sarcoidosis

Marjeta Terčelj,[1] Sanja Stopinšek,[2] Alojz Ihan,[2] Barbara Salobir,[1] Saša Simčič,[2] and Ragnar Rylander[3]

[1] *Department of Respiratory and Allergic Diseases, The University Medical Centre, Ljubljana, Slovenia*
[2] *Institute of Microbiology and Immunology, Faculty of Medicine, University of Ljubljana, 1000 Ljubljana, Slovenia*
[3] *Biofact Environmental Health Research Center, Björkåsvägen 21, 44391 Lerum, Sweden*

Correspondence should be addressed to Ragnar Rylander; envhealth@biofact.se

Academic Editor: Leif Bjermer

Background and Objectives. Sarcoidosis is an inflammatory disease with increased levels of inflammatory cytokines. Previous studies have shown a relation between the degree of granuloma infiltration and serum cytokine levels, except for interleukin- (IL-) 10. The aim of the study was to further investigate the serum levels of IL-10 in patients with sarcoidosis and relate them to fungal exposure in terms of the amount of fungi in the air of their homes and β-glucan in bronchoalveolar lavage (BAL) fluid. *Methods*. Patients with sarcoidosis ($n = 71$) and healthy controls ($n = 27$) were enrolled. IL-10 was determined in serum. BAL was performed and the amount of β-glucan was measured. Domestic exposure to fungi was determined by measuring airborne β-N-acetylhexosaminidase (NAHA) in the bedrooms. *Results*. At high levels of fungal exposure (domestic fungal exposure and β-glucan in BAL), serum IL-10 values were lower than at low and intermediate exposure levels. *Conclusion*. The low serum IL-10 values at high fungal exposure suggest that fungal cell wall agents play a role in granuloma formation in sarcoidosis by inhibiting the secretion of the anti-inflammatory cytokine IL-10.

1. Introduction

Sarcoidosis is an inflammatory disease, often leading to granuloma formation [1, 2]. Several studies demonstrate that the amounts of inflammatory cytokines, particularly interleukin- (IL-) 10 and IL-12, are elevated in serum and in bronchoalveolar lavage fluid [3–6]. Previous studies have demonstrated that exposure to fungi is a risk factor for sarcoidosis [7–9]. One fungal cell wall agent (FCWA)—β-glucan—can induce different changes in the immune system and granulomas, depending on dose and means of administration (review in [10]). The formation of granuloma can be suppressed by IL-10 [11]. Chitin is another FCWA that can induce immune changes, depending on the size of the particles [12].

In *in vitro* studies on the reactivity of peripheral blood mononuclear cells (PBMC), particulate β-glucan was found to induce the secretion of TNFα, IL-6, IL-10, and IL-12 from PBMC [13] with a higher secretion from PBMC taken from patients with sarcoidosis [14].

A clinical study evaluated the relation between the extent of granuloma infiltration using an x-ray score and the amount of serum TNFα, IL-6, IL-10, IL-12, angiotensin converting enzyme (ACE), and chitotriosidase (CTO) [15]. There was a linear relationship for all inflammatory mediators and markers except for IL-10. For this cytokine, there was an initial increase with an increased X-ray score but the values were lower at the highest X-ray scores. This suggests that a blocking of the normal secretion of IL-10, due to inflammation, might be a mechanism related to the risk of granuloma formation in sarcoidosis. This observation prompted the present study which comprises an evaluation of serum levels of IL-10 in patients with sarcoidosis in relation to fungal exposure in terms of exposure to fungi at their home and the amount of β-glucan in BAL.

2. Material and Methods

2.1. Subjects.

The subjects were recruited from the Department for Respiratory and Allergic Diseases at the University Medical Centre, Ljubljana, Slovenia, from July 2007 to October 2013. The department is one of the national centres for patients with sarcoidosis. For the diagnosis the ERS/ATS criteria [16] are used. The routine at the clinic is to make bronchoscopy with 5 to 10 transbronchial biopsies of lung parenchyma and needle aspiration of mediastinal lymph nodes. Bronchoalveolar lavage (BAL) is made and the CD4+/CD8+ ratio is determined. The presence of non-caseating granulomas is verified histologically. If a biopsy is not considered representative, the patient undergoes surgical pulmonary or lymph node biopsy. Aspiration is performed from the right, upper lobe for culturing pathogenic fungi and bacteria including tuberculosis. Most biopsies are stained (silver staining, Gomori) to identify the presence of fungal infection. IgA, IgM, and IgG antibodies against *Candida* spp. and *Aspergillus* spp. are determined as well as mannan antigen in blood. Diagnostic BAL and sputum on subjects with sarcoidosis demonstrated an absence of pathogenic fungi and TB.

This study comprises newly diagnosed cases of pulmonary sarcoidosis ($n = 71$) and healthy subjects ($n = 26$) were examined. All subjects were nonsmokers. The study was approved by the Ethical Committee at the University Medical Centre, Ljubljana (198/05/04), and written, informed consent was obtained.

2.2. Clinical Assessments.

IL-10 was determined in serum using a commercial ELISA kit (Milenia Biotec, Germany, and Thermo Scientific, USA) and expressed as mmol/mL. Chitotriosidase (CTO) activity in serum was determined using $22 \mu M$ 4-methylumbelliferyl-β-D-N,N$'$,N$''$-triacetyl-chitotriosiose (Sigma) in citrate phosphate buffer (pH 5.2) and expressed as nmol/h/mL [17, 18].

2.3. Analysis of β-Glucan.

Samples of the BAL fluid were mixed with 20 mL of a solution containing 0.15 mol/L KOH, 0.3 mol/L KCl, and 0.1% polybrene and incubated at 37°C for 10 minutes. For the analysis of β-glucan, a commercially available method based on the reactivity of a Limulus extract was used. The BAL preparation was diluted in a protein blocking buffer (Biodispersing agent, Charles River, Charleston, SC, USA), kept in boiling water for two minutes, and further diluted in endotoxin free water (LAL, Charles River). Thereafter, 25 μL was added to each of the four wells in a plate preprepared with a Limulus reagent specific for β-glucan and read in an automatic analyser (Endosafe PTS, Charles River). The lower limit for detection is 1 pg/mL. Samples yielding a readout value of <100 pg/mL were given the uniform value of 90 to save on reagents. For ethical reasons BAL was only performed in nine control subjects.

2.4. Fungal Exposure at Home.

The exposure to fungi in the homes was determined by analysing the amount of airborne β-N-acetylhexosaminidase (NAHA) as a marker of fungal

TABLE 1: Basic characteristics of subjects with sarcoidosis. Mean and (SEM).

Parameter	Controls	Sarcoidosis	
n	26	71	
Age years	57.6 (5.2)	47.4 (1.4)	
Females %	63	49	
NAHA U/m^3	19.0 (5.0)	34.1 (3.9)	$P < 0.001$
B-glucan pg/mL	122.5 (16.1)	474.5 (38.6)	$P < 0.001$
CD4/CD8 ratio		7.5 (0.7)	
CTO nmol/h/mL		775 (68)	
sACE μKat/L		0.49 (0.03)	

TABLE 2: IL-10 values (pg/mL) in serum of subjects with sarcoidosis and controls. Mean, SEM and range.

Subjects	n	Mean	SEM	Minimum	Maximum	P
Controls	26	10.3	2.8	1	63	
Sarcoidosis	71	16.6	3.7	1	270	NS

cell biomass [19, 20]. Air samples (around 2000 L) were taken in the subject's bedroom using a filter and a fluorogenic enzyme substrate (4-methylumbelliferyl N-acetyl-β-D-glucosaminide, Mycometer A/S, Copenhagen, Denmark) was added to the filter. After an incubation period of around 30 minutes, set by room temperature, a developer was added, and the fluorescence of the liquid was read in a fluorometer (Picofluor, Turner Designs, Sunnyvale, CA, USA). The units read were divided by 10 to diminish methodological scatter and expressed as NAHA Units/m^3.

2.5. Statistical Analysis.

Values in the different groups were calculated using SPSS W7 and were expressed as mean and standard error of the mean (SEM). Differences between groups were evaluated using the t-test or Fisher's exact test. A P value of ≤0.05 was considered statistically significant.

3. Results

3.1. Characteristics of Test Subjects.

Basic characteristics of the subjects are shown in Table 1.

The clinical values are typical for newly diagnosed sarcoidosis. There were four cases of skin sarcoidosis.

Serum IL-10 values are reported in Table 2.

There were no significant differences in mean values between controls and sarcoidosis. The maximum value was higher among subjects with sarcoidosis. In controls all β-glucan values were less than 90 pg/mL and NAHA values were less than 30 U/m^3 except for one outlier (76).

Figure 1 illustrates serum levels of IL-10 among subjects with sarcoidosis in relation to β-glucan in BAL.

At higher amounts of β-glucan in BAL and NAHA in the homes, reflecting a higher exposure to fungi, there were no high levels of IL-10. At a break-off point of 750 pg/mL β-glucan, the mean IL-10 value in the lower β-glucan value group was 23.5/5.7 as compared to 3.8/0.5 for the higher value group ($P = 0.026$, Mann-Whitney's test). At a break-off point

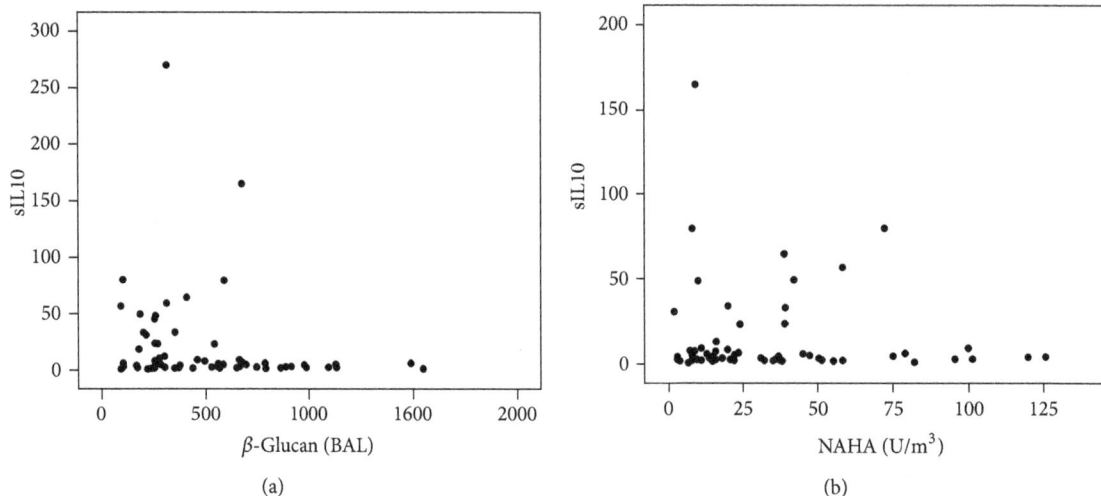

FIGURE 1: (a) Serum IL-10 in relation to the amount of β-glucan (BAL) pg/mL ($n = 70$) and (b) NAHA in homes ($n = 60$) of subjects with sarcoidosis.

of NAHA of 75, the corresponding IL-10 values were 20.6/8.9, $n = 65$, and 5.6/1.5, $n = 7$ ($P = 0.0001$, Fisher's exact test).

4. Discussion

The major findings from the study are that the serum values of IL-10 were low at higher exposure to fungi, as illustrated by the domestic exposure and the amount β-glucan in BAL.

There are some limitations to the study. The number of subjects is fairly small, particularly in the high fungal exposure group. Measurements of NAHA were made in the homes but significant exposures could also have been present at the workplace. BAL for β-glucan determination could not be performed in all subjects because of ethical reasons.

A previous study has shown that values of IL-10 were lower at higher levels of CTO, a marker of disease severity [15]. In this study a similar decrease was present in relation to the fungal exposure at home. This suggests that there is a depression of IL-10 secretory capacity at higher exposure levels. Almost all cells of both the innate and adaptive arms of the immune system can express IL-10 including dendritic cells, macrophages, mast cells, natural killer cells, eosinophils, neutrophils, and T regulatory cells [21, 22]. This cytokine is one of the most important anti-inflammatory and immune suppressive cytokines. It affects the vascular system through inhibition of leukocyte-endothelial cell interaction and inhibition of proinflammatory cytokine and chemokine production by macrophages and lymphocytes [23]. In an animal model low levels of IL-10 were a predisposing factor for chronic fibrosis [24]. Of particular interest in sarcoidosis is that IL-10 can inhibit an experimental granulomatous inflammation [11] and that corticosteroids, which are usually used to treat the disease, have the capacity to enhance IL-10 production [25].

This opens up a new possible mechanism to explain the relation between fungal exposure and sarcoidosis [9]. It

is tempting to speculate that the development of granulomas in sarcoidosis is initiated by an inflammation induced by inhaled β-glucan and that this inflammation at higher exposure levels depresses an important defence mechanism in terms of IL-10. Further work is required to assess this hypothesis. Although the focus in this context has been on fungi, it cannot be excluded that other microbial agents may induce similar reactions in terms of depression of the cellular capacity to secrete IL-10. To assess the importance of such agents, for example, Mycobacteria, studies on exposure levels as well as the effect on cellular mechanisms are required.

5. Conclusions

At a high environmental exposure to fungi, the level of serum IL-10 among subjects with sarcoidosis was low. This suggests that β-glucan could play a role in the granuloma formation in sarcoidosis by blocking a defence system in terms of IL-10 secretion. At high levels of fungal exposure patients with sarcoidosis have a depressed secretion of the anti-inflammatory cytokine IL-10. This suggests a new mechanism for the development of granulomas in sarcoidosis.

Conflict of Interests

The authors declare that there is no conflict of interests regarding the publication of this paper.

Authors' Contribution

M. Terčelj and Barbara Salobir were responsible for the clinical work, S. Stopinšek, A. Ihan, and S. Simčič were responsible for the PBMC work, and R. Rylander was responsible for the environmental and glucan measures and the analyses of the data. All authors agree on the content of the paper.

Acknowledgment

This paper received internal hospital funding only.

References

[1] M. C. Iannuzi, B. A. Rybicki, and A. S. Tierstein, "Sarcoidosis," *The New England Journal of Medicine*, vol. 357, pp. 2153–2165, 2007.

[2] R. P. Baughman, D. A. Culver, and M. A. Judson, "A concise review of pulmonary sarcoidosis," *The American Journal of Respiratory and Critical Care Medicine*, vol. 183, no. 5, pp. 573–581, 2011.

[3] S. Nureki, E. Miyazaki, M. Ando et al., "Circulating levels of both Th1 and Th2 chemokines are elevated in patients with sarcoidosis," *Respiratory Medicine*, vol. 102, no. 2, pp. 239–247, 2008.

[4] R. M. Mroz, M. Korniluk, A. Stasiak-Barmuta, and E. Chyczewska, "Increased levels of interleukin-12 and interleukin-18 in bronchoalveolar lavage fluid of patients with pulmonary sarcoidosis," *Journal of Physiology and Pharmacology*, vol. 59, supplement 6, pp. 507–513, 2008.

[5] M. Hata, K. Sugisaki, E. Miyazaki, T. Kumamoto, and T. Tsuda, "Circulating IL-12 p40 is increased in the patients with sarcoidosis, correlation with clinical markers," *Internal Medicine*, vol. 46, no. 17, pp. 1387–1394, 2007.

[6] U. Oltmanns, B. Schmidt, S. Hoernig, C. Witt, and M. John, "Increased spontaneous interleukin-10 release from alveolar macrophages in active pulmonary sarcoidosis," *Experimental Lung Research*, vol. 29, no. 5, pp. 315–328, 2003.

[7] L. S. Newman, C. S. Rose, E. A. Bresnitz et al., "A case-control etiological study of sarcoidosis—environmental and occupational risk factors," *American Journal of Respiratory and Critical Care Medicine*, vol. 170, no. 12, pp. 1324–1330, 2004.

[8] A. S. Laney, L. A. Cragin, L. Z. Blevins et al., "Sarcoidosis, asthma, and asthma-like symptoms among occupants of a historically water-damaged office building," *Indoor Air*, vol. 19, no. 1, pp. 83–90, 2009.

[9] M. Terčelj, B. Salobir, and R. Rylander, "Airborne enzyme in homes of patients with sarcoidosis," *Environmental Health*, vol. 10, pp. 8–13, 2011.

[10] R. Rylander, "Organic dust induced pulmonary disease - The role of mould derived B-Glucan," *Annals of Agricultural and Environmental Medicine*, vol. 17, no. 1, pp. 9–13, 2010.

[11] H. H. Herfarth, S. P. Mohanty, H. C. Rath, S. Tonkonogy, and R. B. Sartor, "Interleukin 10 suppresses experimental chronic, granulomatous inflammation induced by bacterial cell wall polymers," *Gut*, vol. 39, no. 6, pp. 836–845, 1996.

[12] R. A. A. Muzzarelli, "Chitins and chitosans as immunoadjuvants and non-allergenic drug carriers," *Marine Drugs*, vol. 8, no. 2, pp. 292–312, 2010.

[13] S. Stopinšek, A. Ihan, B. Wraber et al., "Fungal cell wall agents suppress the innate inflammatory cytokine responses of human peripheral blood mononuclear cells challenged with lipopolysaccharide in vitro," *International Immunopharmacology*, vol. 11, no. 8, pp. 939–947, 2011.

[14] M. Terčelj, S. Stopinšek, A. Ihan et al., "In vitro and in vivo reactivity to fungal cell wall agents in sarcoidosis," *Clinical and Experimental Immunology*, vol. 166, no. 1, pp. 87–93, 2011.

[15] M. Terčelj, B. Salobir, M. Zupancic, B. Wraber, and R. Rylander, "Inflammatory markers and pulmonary granuloma infiltration in sarcoidosis," *Respirology*, vol. 19, pp. 225–230, 2014.

[16] "Association of sarcoidosis and other granulomatous disorders (WASOG) adopted by the ATS board of directors and by the ERS executive committee," *The American Journal of Respiratory and Critical Care Medicin*, vol. 160, pp. 736–755, 1999.

[17] E. Bargagli, D. Bennett, C. Maggiorelli et al., "Human chitotriosidase: a sensitive biomarker of sarcoidosis," *Journal of Clinical Immunology*, vol. 33, no. 1, pp. 264–270, 2013.

[18] M. Terčelj, B. Salobir, S. Simcic, B. Wraber, M. Zupancic, and R. Rylander, "Chitotriosidase activity in sarcoidosis and some other pulmonary diseases," *Scandinavian Journal of Clinical and Laboratory Investigation*, vol. 69, no. 5, pp. 575–578, 2009.

[19] A. M. Madsen, "NAGase activity in airborne biomass dust and relationship between NAGase concentrations and fungal spores," *Aerobiologia*, vol. 19, no. 2, pp. 97–105, 2003.

[20] R. Rylander, M. Reeslev, and T. Hulander, "Airborne enzyme measurements to detect indoor mould exposure," *Journal of Environmental Monitoring*, vol. 12, no. 11, pp. 2161–2164, 2010.

[21] R. Sabat, "IL-10 family of cytokines," *Cytokine and Growth Factor Reviews*, vol. 21, no. 5, pp. 315–324, 2010.

[22] T. H. S. Ng, G. J. Britton, E. V. Hill, J. Verhagen, B. R. Burton, and D. C. Wraith, "Regulation of adaptive immunity; the role of interleukin-10," *Frontiers in Immunology*, vol. 4, pp. 1–13, 2013.

[23] D. A. Smith, S. D. Irving, J. Sheldon, D. Cole, and J. C. Kaski, "Serum levels of the antiinflammatory cytokine interleukin-10 are decreased in patients with unstable angina," *Circulation*, vol. 104, no. 7, pp. 746–749, 2001.

[24] L. J. Zhang, W. D. Zheng, Y. X. Chen et al., "Antifibrotic effects of interleukin-10 on experimental hepatic fibrosis," *Hepato-Gastroenterology*, vol. 54, no. 79, pp. 2092–2098, 2007.

[25] D. F. Richards, M. Fernandez, J. Caulfield, and C. M. Hawrylowicz, "Glucocorticoids drive human CD8$^+$ T cell differentiation towards a phenotype with high IL-10 and reduced IL-4, IL-5, and IL-13 production," *European Journal of Immunology*, vol. 30, no. 8, pp. 2344–2354, 2000.

3

Association of Serum Magnesium Levels with Frequency of Acute Exacerbations in Chronic Obstructive Pulmonary Disease: A Prospective Study

Aziz Gumus,[1] **Muge Haziroglu,**[1] **and Yilmaz Gunes**[2]

[1] *Department of Pulmonary Medicine, Recep Tayyip Erdogan University, 53000 Rize, Turkey*
[2] *Cardiology Department, Hisar Intercontinental Hospital, 34375 Istanbul, Turkey*

Correspondence should be addressed to Aziz Gumus; azizgumus@gmail.com

Academic Editor: Charlie Strange

Background. The course of chronic obstructive pulmonary disease (COPD) is accompanied by acute exacerbations. The purpose of this study is to determine the association of serum magnesium level with acute exacerbations in COPD (COPD-AE). *Materials and Methods.* Eighty-nine patients hospitalized with COPD-AE were included. Hemogram, biochemical tests, and arterial blood gases were analyzed. Pulmonary function tests were performed in the stable period after discharge. Patients were followed up at 3 monthly periods for one year. *Results.* Mean age of the patients was 70.4 ± 7.8 (range 47–90) years. Mean number of COPD-AE during follow-up was 4.0 ± 3.6 (range 0–15). On Spearman correlation analysis there were significant negative correlations between number of COPD-AE and predicted FEV1% ($P = 0.001$), total protein ($P = 0.024$), globulin ($P = 0.001$), creatinine ($P = 0.001$), and uric acid levels ($P = 0.036$). There were also significant positive correlations between number of COPD-AE and serum magnesium level ($P < 0.001$) and platelet count ($P = 0.043$). According to linear regression analysis predicted FEV1% ($P = 0.011$), serum magnesium ($P < 0.001$), and globulin ($P = 0.006$) levels were independent predictors of number of COPD-AE. *Conclusions.* In this small prospective observational study we found that serum magnesium level during exacerbation period was the most significant predictor of frequency of COPD-AE.

1. Introduction

Chronic obstructive pulmonary disease (COPD) is a preventable and treatable disease, generally progressive in nature, characterized by chronic inflammatory response of the airways and lungs to harmful gasses and particles, particularly tobacco and biomass fuel smoke (GOLD 2014) [1]. Acute exacerbations that compromise quality of life, accelerate a decline in respiratory functions, and increase economic costs may occur during the course of stable COPD [2, 3]. COPD exacerbation was defined as an acute worsening of respiratory symptoms (increased dyspnea, increased cough or change in amount, and purulence of sputum) that was beyond normal day-to-day variations of symptoms [1]. COPD acute exacerbation (COPD-AE) frequently appears with respiratory tract infections. It is a significant cause of mortality and morbidity [4].

Few studies have investigated the factors leading to exacerbations. Advanced age, low FEV1%, advanced stage of disease, poor performance status, accompanying anxiety and/or depression, poor quality of life, history of frequent exacerbation, hypercapnia, and prolonged duration of disease have all been identified as factors causing frequent exacerbation [5–8].

Magnesium is involved in such important functions as bronchodilation and contraction in respiratory tract smooth muscles, mast cell stabilization, neurohumoral mediator release, and mucociliary clearance [9]. Magnesium is thought to have a protective effect against chronic respiratory tract diseases. It has been suggested that insufficient magnesium intake through diet may lead to development of asthma and COPD [10]. However, insufficient information is available concerning the effect of magnesium on frequency of COPD-AE. The purpose of this study was to determine the factors associated with COPD-AE and to investigate the effect of magnesium levels on incidence of exacerbations.

2. Materials and Methods

The study was performed at the Recep Tayyip Erdogan University Faculty of Medicine Chest Diseases Clinic. Local ethical committee approval and written informed consent of patients were obtained. Ninety-four consecutive patients aged 40 or above, hospitalized with diagnosis of COPD-AE meeting the unit admission criteria [11] between May 2012 and March 2013, were included in the study. Five patients died during 1-year follow-up and were excluded from study. Arterial blood gasses, C-reactive protein (C-RP), hemogram, sedimentation rate, and serum electrolyte concentrations including magnesium, creatinine, uric acid, liver function tests, troponin-I, D-dimer, blood glucose, cholesterol, and triglyceride levels were measured within 24 hours of admission. Pulmonary function tests were performed in the stable period after discharge. Patients were followed up at 3 monthly intervals for one year. Patients experiencing acute exacerbations were treated on either an in- or outpatient basis. Patients requiring intensive care due to acute exacerbations, patients with active cancer, cirrhosis, and acute or chronic kidney or heart failure, and who died during monitoring were excluded from the study.

2.1. Statistical Analysis. Statistical analyses were performed on IBM-SPSS (SPSS version 21; SPSS Inc., Chicago, IL, USA) software. Constant variables were expressed as mean ± standard deviation and categorical variables as %. The independent samples t-test was used for continuous variables. Chi square test was used to compare categorical variables. Correlations between variables were investigated using Pearson correlation analysis for parametric variables and Spearman correlation analysis for nonparametric variables. Linear regression analysis was performed in order to identify independent factors affecting the number of exacerbations in 1 year. ROC curve analysis was performed in order to reveal the effect of serum magnesium level on exacerbation in 1 year. $P < 0.05$ value was considered statistically significant.

3. Results

Mean age of patients with COPD-AE was 70.4 ±7.8 (range 47–90). Almost all were male (88 male, 1 female). Nineteen (21%) patients were current smokers, 69 (78%) were ex-smoker, and 1 (1%) had never smoked. Pulmonary function tests were predicted FVC%: 54 ± 16, predicted FEV1%: 39 ± 14, and predicted FEV1/FVC%: 56±11. COPD staging was performed on the basis of these results. Very severe COPD was determined in 22 (%25) patients (stage 4), severe in 49 (55%) (Stage 3), and moderate COPD in 18 (20%) (Stage 2). None of the patients in the study group had mild COPD. Demographic characteristics of the patients are given in Table 1.

On Spearman correlation analysis the number of exacerbations during one year follow-up was negatively correlated with predicted FEV1% ($P = 0.001$), total protein ($P = 0.024$),

TABLE 1: The demographic characteristics of patients.

Parameters	$n = 89$ (100%)
Age (year, mean ± sd) (range)	70.4 ± 7.8 (47–90)
Sex	
Female (%)	1 (1%)
Male (%)	88 (99%)
BMI (kg/m^2)	25.5 ± 5.1
Smoking status	
Smoker	19 (21%)
Ex-smoker	69 (78%)
Nonsmoker	1 (1%)
Comorbidities	
HT	22 (25%)
Type 2 DM	13 (15%)
CAD	10 (11%)
BPH	6 (7%)
Bronchiectasis	4 (5%)
COPD stage	
Stage I	0 (0%)
Stage II	18 (20%)
Stage III	49 (55%)
Stage IV	22 (25%)

n: the number of patients; BMI: body mass index; mean ± sd: mean ± standard deviation; HT: hypertension; Type 2 DM: type 2 diabetes mellitus; CAD: coronary artery disease; BPH: benign prostatic hypertrophy.

TABLE 2: Linear regression analysis showing factors affecting frequency of COPD-AE.

	Standardized coefficients (Beta)	t	P value
Predicted FEV1%	−0.227	−2.590	**0.011**[*]
Serum creatinine	0.050	0.499	0.619
Serum uric acid	−0.040	−0.392	0.696
Serum protein	0.005	0.032	0.975
Serum globulin	−0.250	−2.839	**0.006**[*]
Serum magnesium	0.431	4.929	**<0.001**[*]
Platelet count	0.119	1.329	0.188

[*]Statistically significant.

globulin ($P = 0.001$), creatinine ($P = 0.001$), and uric acid levels ($P = 0.036$) and positively correlated with serum magnesium level ($P < 0.001$) (Figure 1) and platelet count ($P = 0.043$). According to linear regression analysis predicted FEV1% (beta = −0,227, $P = 0.011$), serum magnesium (beta = 0.431, $P < 0.001$), and globulin (beta = −0.250, $P = 0.006$) levels were independent predictors of number of exacerbations (Table 2).

The mean number of exacerbations in 1 year was 4.0 ± 3.6 (range 0–15). The distribution of exacerbations is shown in Figure 2. Patients were divided into two groups, those with a COPD-AE less than 3 and those with COPD-AE ≥ 3 per year. Predicted FEV% ($P = 0.001$), blood glucose ($P < 0.001$), creatinine ($P < 0.001$), uric acid ($P = 0.021$), and total

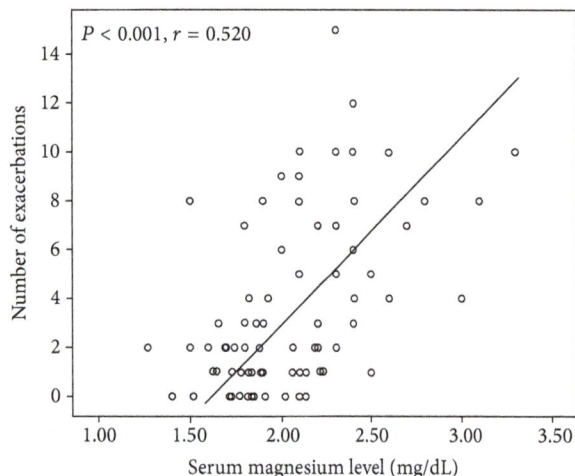

FIGURE 1: Scatterplot showing the positive correlation between number of exacerbations and serum magnesium level.

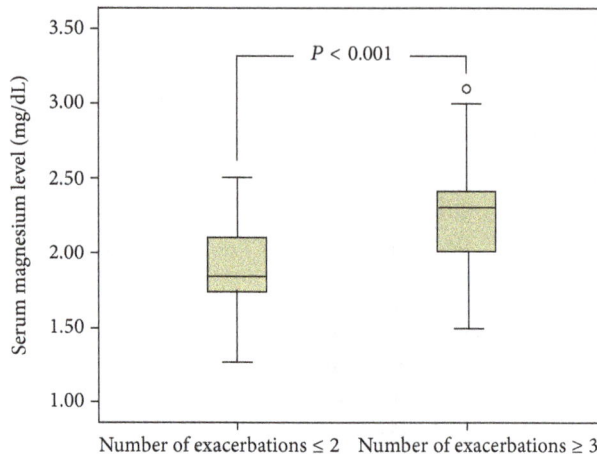

FIGURE 3: Box-plot showing the variation in magnesium levels between frequent and rare exacerbation groups.

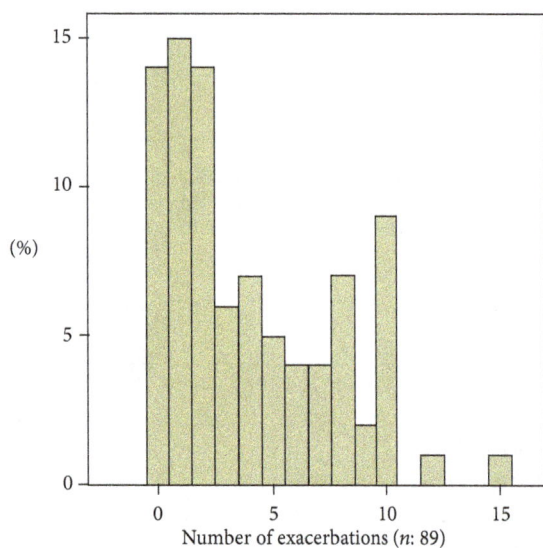

FIGURE 2: Histogram showing distribution of exacerbations.

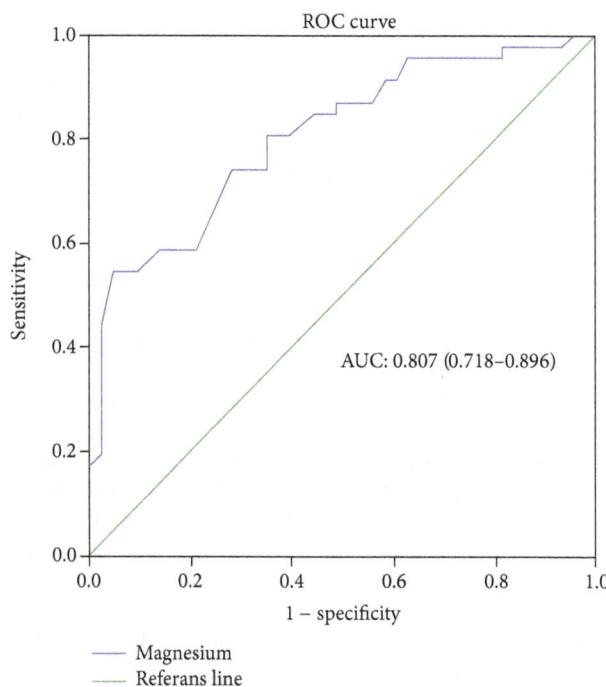

FIGURE 4: ROC curve analysis of serum magnesium level on frequency of COPD-AE.

protein ($P = 0.006$) levels were lower in the group with ≥3 exacerbations compared to those with ≤2, while platelet count ($P = 0.028$) and serum magnesium levels ($P < 0.001$) were higher (Table 3, Figure 3).

As seen in ROC curve analysis serum magnesium level is a valuable predictor of frequent exacerbations in COPD (Figure 4). Area under curve (AUC) was determined at =0.807 (0.718–0.896), at a cut-off value of 2.26 mg/dL, and serum magnesium predicted the occurrence of 3 attacks or more per year with a sensitivity of 54.3% and specificity of 95.3%.

4. Discussion

Few studies have investigated the factors giving rise to acute exacerbations in patients with COPD. In this study, predicted FEV1%, serum globulin, and serum magnesium levels were

identified as independent predictors of acute exacerbations of COPD and serum magnesium level was the most significant of these predictors.

A negative correlation was determined between predicted FEV1% and number of exacerbations. That is an expected outcome. Frequent exacerbations occur as the disease progresses. A low FEV1% has been associated with frequent exacerbations [12–14]. Coa et al. [6] determined a correlation between FEV1% <50% and frequent hospitalization due to acute exacerbations. Our study results also show that number of attacks rises as predicted FEV1% decreases. Another independent predictor of acute exacerbations in our study

TABLE 3: Comparison of variables between groups established on the basis of number of exacerbations.

	COPD-AE ≤ 2/year (n: 43)	COPD-AE ≥ 3/year (n: 46)	P value
Age, years (mean ± sd)	72 ± 8	69 ± 7	0.181
Sex, (M/F)	43/0	45/1	1.000
BMI, body mass index	25.6 ± 3.7	24.2 ± 4.5	0.301
Smoking, pack-year	65 ± 34	63 ± 35	0.815
FEV1, % of predicted	45 ± 16	34 ± 10	**0.001***
FVC, % of predicted	58 ± 19	51 ± 12	**<0.001***
pH	7.39 ± 0.06	7.40 ± 0.05	0.262
PaO2, mmHg	58 ± 10	57 ± 10	0.740
PaCO2, mmHg	42 ± 8	42 ± 11	0.711
Hb, gr/dL	14.2 ± 2.3	14.3 ± 1.7	0.961
Glucose, mg/dL	133 ± 47	106 ± 53	**<0.001***
Platelet, ×10³	243 ± 65	280 ± 88	**0.028***
Urea, mg/dL	44 ± 17	46 ± 19	0.582
Creatinine, mg/dL	1.03 ± 0.31	0.86 ± 0.23	**<0.001***
Uric acid, mg/dL	6.5 ± 1.6	5.7 ± 1.7	0.021
Magnesium, mg/dL	1.88 ± 0.26	2.27 ± 0.37	**<0.001***
Protein, g/dL	7.3 ± 0.7	6.9 ± 0.8	**0.006***
Albumin, g/dL	3.8 ± 0.5	3.7 ± 0.4	0.659
Globülin, g/dL	3.6 ± 0.6	3.1 ± 0.7	**0.004***
TSH, IU/mL	0.75 ± 1.28	0.69 ± 0.73	0.078

n: the number of patients; M: male; F: female; FEV1: expiratory volume percent at the first second of forced vital capacity over expected value; PaO2: arterial partial oxygen pressure; PaCO2: arterial partial carbon dioxide pressure.
* Statistically significant.

was serum globulin level. Total protein consists of albumin and globulin. No correlation between albumin level and exacerbation frequency was observed in this study. However, a negative correlation was determined between globulin level and COPD-AE. Globulin proteins consist of four groups, alpha 1, alpha 2, beta, and gamma. Subgroups were not investigated in this study. It is therefore not possible to state whether or not subgroup globulin levels may have an association frequency of COPD-AE. Alpha 1-antitrypsin deficiency is known to be a significant genetic risk factor for COPD [15].

The most important finding of this study is the positive correlation between serum magnesium level during acute exacerbation and annual number of COPD-AE. Number of attacks increased in association with serum magnesium levels. This is a significant finding. To the best of our knowledge, this is the first time that this correlation has been identified. Although it has not been proved, it is generally believed that due to its bronchodilating effect, a decreased level of magnesium increases COPD exacerbations. Unfortunately, we have not measured serum magnesium levels during stable period. Limited numbers of studies have investigated the relationship between magnesium and COPD-AE. Corradi et al. [16] determined higher serum magnesium levels in periods of COPD-AE compared to stable periods. A negative correlation was shown between magnesium and predicted FEV1%. However, they did not search the correlation between frequency of COPD-AE and magnesium levels. In a retrospective study, Aziz et al. [17] compared a group of COPD patients in the

stable period with a different group of COPD patients during acute exacerbation. Serum magnesium levels were higher in the stable period group compared to the COPD-AE group. Fiaccadori et al. [18] could not find a significant difference in serum magnesium levels of COPD-AE in the ICU and a control healthy group. Contrary to our finding Bhatt et al. [19] found a reverse correlation between serum magnesium level and frequency of COPD-AE. However, there are important problems requiring criticism in that study; contrary to expectation, it is noteworthy that FEV1% and the frequencies of influenza and pneumococcal vaccination were higher in the group with frequent COPD-AE compared to the rare COPD-AE group.

Our study has certain limitations. First, the study population consisted almost entirely of males. Our study results may not therefore reflect all individuals with COPD-AE. However, this was not planned beforehand; the patients were included consecutively. We attribute this to COPD being more common in males than females in Turkish society. Second, there were no patients with mild (Stage 1) COPD in our study group. Third, serum magnesium levels were measured in the acute exacerbation period on admission to hospital. Magnesium levels in the stable period were not examined. Magnesium levels could not, therefore, be compared between the stable and COPD-AE patients. We speculate that the increased Mg levels in frequent exacerbation phenotypes of COPD may be from the body's attempt to optimize bronchodilation. Whether magnesium levels define a new phenotype of COPD or explain existing high exacerbation frequency phenotypes of COPD will require additional studies.

In conclusion, serum magnesium level during acute exacerbation period might be correlated with frequency of COPD-AE. The mechanism involved is as yet unclear. Larger and further studies are needed to search this association.

Conflict of Interests

The authors declare that there is no conflict of interests regarding the publication of this paper.

References

[1] Global Initiative for Chronic Obstructive Lung Disease (GOLD), *Global Strategy for the Diagnosis, Management, and Prevention of Chronic Obstructive Pulmonary Disease*, Global Initiative for Chronic Obstructive Lung Disease (GOLD), 2014.

[2] J. R. Hurst and J. A. Wedzicha, "Management and prevention of chronic obstructive pulmonary disease exacerbations: a state of the art review," *BMC Medicine*, vol. 7, article 40, 2009.

[3] J. Vestbo, S. S. Hurd, A. G. Agustí et al., "Global strategy for the diagnosis, management, and prevention of chronic obstructive pulmonary disease: GOLD executive summary," *American Journal of Respiratory and Critical Care Medicine*, vol. 187, no. 4, pp. 347–365, 2013.

[4] J. A. Wedzicha, T. A. R. Seemungal, P. K. MacCallum et al., "Acute exacerbations of chronic obstructive pulmonary disease are accompanied by elevations of plasma fibrinogen and serum IL-6 levels," *Thrombosis and Haemostasis*, vol. 84, no. 2, pp. 210–215, 2000.

[5] G. Gudmundsson, T. Gislason, C. Janson et al., "Risk factors for rehospitalisation in COPD: role of health status, anxiety and depression," *European Respiratory Journal*, vol. 26, no. 3, pp. 414–419, 2005.

[6] Z. Cao, K. C. Ong, P. Eng, W. C. Tan, and T. P. Ng, "Frequent hospital readmissions for acute exacerbation of COPD and their associated factors," *Respirology*, vol. 11, no. 2, pp. 188–195, 2006.

[7] S. Vidal Serrano, N. González, I. Barrio et al., "Predictors of hospital admission in exacerbations of chronic obstructive pulmonary disease," *International Journal of Tuberculosis and Lung Disease*, vol. 17, no. 12, pp. 1632–1637, 2013.

[8] R. Carneiro, C. Sousa, A. Pinto, F. Almeida, J. R. Oliveira, and N. Rocha, "Risk factors for readmission after hospital discharge in chronic obstructive pulmonary disease. The role of quality of life indicators," *Revista Portuguesa de Pneumologia*, vol. 16, no. 5, pp. 759–777, 2010.

[9] K. I. Gourgoulianis, G. Chatziparasidis, A. Chatziefthimiou, and P.-A. Molyvdas, "Magnesium as a relaxing factor of airway smooth muscles," *Journal of Aerosol Medicine*, vol. 14, no. 3, pp. 301–307, 2001.

[10] J. Britton, I. Pavord, K. Richards et al., "Dietary magnesium, lung function, wheezing, and airway hyper-reactivity in a random adult population sample," *The Lancet*, vol. 344, no. 8919, pp. 357–362, 1994.

[11] G. Karadeniz, G. Polat, G. Senol, and M. Buyuksirin, "C-reactive protein measurements as a marker of the severity of chronic obstructive pulmonary disease exacerbations," *Inflammation*, vol. 36, no. 4, pp. 948–953, 2013.

[12] J. Farkas, M. Kosnik, M. Flezar, S. Suskovic, and M. Lainscak, "Self-rated health predicts acute exacerbations and hospitalizations in patients with COPD," *Chest*, vol. 138, no. 2, pp. 323–330, 2010.

[13] D. M. G. Halpin, M. Decramer, B. Celli, S. Kesten, D. Liu, and D. P. Tashkin, "Exacerbation frequency and course of COPD," *International Journal of Chronic Obstructive Pulmonary Disease*, vol. 7, no. 7, pp. 653–661, 2012.

[14] H. Yang, P. Xiang, E. Zhang et al., "Predictors of exacerbation frequency in chronic obstructive pulmonary disease," *European Journal of Medical Research*, vol. 19, no. 1, article 18, 2014.

[15] American Thoracic Society and European Respiratory Society, "American thoracic society/European respiratory society statement: standards for the diagnosis and management of individuals with alpha-1 antitrypsin deficiency," *The American Journal of Respiratory and Critical Care Medicine*, vol. 168, no. 7, pp. 818–900, 2003.

[16] M. Corradi, O. Acampa, M. Goldoni et al., "Metallic elements in exhaled breath condensate and serum of patients with exacerbation of chronic obstructive pulmonary disease," *Metallomics*, vol. 1, no. 4, pp. 339–345, 2009.

[17] H. S. Aziz, A. I. Blamoun, M. K. Shubair, M. M. F. Ismail, V. A. DeBari, and M. A. Khan, "Serum magnesium levels and acute exacerbation of chronic obstructive pulmonary disease: a retrospective study," *Annals of Clinical and Laboratory Science*, vol. 35, no. 4, pp. 423–427, 2005.

[18] E. Fiaccadori, S. Del Canale, E. Coffrini et al., "Muscle and serum magnesium in pulmonary intensive care unit patients," *Critical Care Medicine*, vol. 16, no. 8, pp. 751–760, 1988.

[19] S. P. Bhatt, P. Khandelwal, S. Nanda, J. C. Stoltzfus, and G. T. Fioravanti, "Serum magnesium is an independent predictor of frequent readmissions due to acute exacerbation of chronic obstructive pulmonary disease," *Respiratory Medicine*, vol. 102, no. 7, pp. 999–1003, 2008.

4

Pleural Fluid Cholesterol in Differentiating Exudative and Transudative Pleural Effusion

A. B. Hamal, K. N. Yogi, N. Bam, S. K. Das, and R. Karn

Department of Internal Medicine, Tribhuvan University Teaching Hospital (TUTH), Maharajgunj, Kathmandu, Nepal

Correspondence should be addressed to A. B. Hamal; abhamal@gmail.com

Academic Editor: Marc A. Judson

Objectives. To study the diagnostic value of pleural fluid cholesterol in differentiating transudative and exudative pleural effusion. To compare pleural fluid cholesterol level for exudates with Light's criteria. *Design.* Cross sectional descriptive study. *Settings.* Medical wards of Tribhuvan University Teaching Hospital. *Methods.* Sixty two cases of pleural effusion with definite clinical diagnosis admitted in TUTH were taken and classified as transudates (19) and exudates (43). The parameters pleural fluid protein/serum protein ratio (pfP/sP), pleural fluid LDH/ serum LDH ratio, pleural fluid LDH (pfLDH) and pleural fluid cholesterol (pCHOL) were compared with clinical diagnosis with regard to their usefulness for distinguishing between pleural exudates and transudates. *Results.* The pCHOL values determined were 1.92 ± 0.75 for exudates, 0.53 ± 0.28 for transudates, the differences between the transudates and others are statistically significant ($P < 0.0001$). It is seen that pfP/sP ratio has a sensitivity of 81.4% and specificity of 82.6%; pfLDH/sLDH ratio has a sensitivity of 86% and specificity of 94.7% and pCHOL with sensitivity of 97.7% and specificity of 100% for differentiating exudative and transudative PE. *Conclusion.* The determination of pCHOL is of great value for distinguishing between pleural exudates and transudates and should be included in routine laboratory analysis of pleural effusion.

1. Introduction

Light et al. in 1972 found criteria to have sensitivity and specificity of 99% and 98%, respectively, for differentiating transudative and exudative PEs (ratio of protein in pleural fluid and serum >0.5; ratio of LDH in pleural fluid and serum >0.6; pleural fluid LDH >2/3rd of upper limit of serum LDH) [1].

But the other investigators could only reproduce specificities of 70–86% using Light's criteria. Also it is found that 25% of patients with transudates pleural effusion are mistakenly identified as having exudative effusion by Light's criteria. In cases of heart failure on diuretic therapy, the transudative PE has high protein [2].

Pleural fluid cholesterol can be used to classify exudates and transudates as it misclassifies fewer cases than any other Light's parameters [3]. From meta-analysis, Heffner et al. 2002 have identified pleural effusion of exudative type with at least one of the following conditions [4].

(i) Pleural fluid protein >2.9 gm/dL.

(ii) Pleural fluid cholesterol >45 mg/dL (1.16 mmol/L).

(iii) Pleural fluid LDH >2/3rd of upper limit of serum.

Pleural cholesterol is thought to be derived from degenerating cells and vascular leakage from increased permeability. Though the cause of the rise in cholesterol levels in pleural exudates is unknown, two possible explanations have been put forward.

According to the first, the cholesterol is synthesized by pleural cells themselves for their own needs [5] (extrahepatic synthesis of cholesterol is now known to be much greater than was once thought, depends on the metabolic needs of cells, and is in dynamic equilibrium with cholesterol supply by LDL and cholesterol removal by HDL) [6], and the concentration of cholesterol in pleural cavity is increased by the degeneration of leukocytes and erythrocytes, which contain large quantities.

The second possible explanation is that pleural cholesterol derives from plasma; some 70 percent of plasma cholesterol is bound to low density, high molecular weight lipoproteins (LDL), and the rest to HDL or very low density lipoproteins

(VLDL), and the increased permeability of pleural capillaries in pleural exudate patients would allow plasma cholesterol to enter the pleural cavity.

The reason to select the cutoff value of pleural fluid cholesterol as 45 (1.16 mmol/L) is that this cutoff value eliminates the possibility of being equivocal to transudates and exudates, and measurement of pleural cholesterol >45 mg/dL (1.16 mmol/L) has been used to improve the accuracy of differentiating transudative and exudative effusions [7].

2. Methods

Sample size of 62 consecutive pleural effusion cases that fulfilled the inclusion criteria and were admitted in the Department of Internal Medicine, TUTH were taken. The study period was conducted for one year from July 2010 to August 2011.

2.1. Inclusion Criteria

(1) Age ≥ 16 yrs,

(2) patients giving consent,

(3) patients with definite clinical diagnosis and pleural effusion evidenced by radiological imaging.

2.2. Exclusion Criteria

(1) Patients not willing to participate in the study,

(2) age < 16 years,

(3) patients without definite clinical diagnosis,

(4) patients with pulmonary embolism or renal insufficiency with pleural effusion,

(5) patients previously diagnosed and already on treatment.

2.3. Study Procedure. After a detailed history and clinical examination, chest X-ray was done to localize pleural effusion. Diagnostic tapping of the pleural fluid was done in every case, and the help of ultrasonography of chest to localize the fluid was taken in some cases. All pleural fluid samples were tested for cell count, protein, glucose, LDH, pCHOL, Gram stain, bacterial culture, acid fast stain, and cytology. A concomitant blood sample was taken and tested for counts and biochemical parameters such as protein and LDH. Further investigations, such as computed tomography scan of chest, bronchoscopy, and fine needle aspiration cytology (FNAC), were also done to determine etiology of pleural effusion when needed.

The first sample of pleural fluid obtained in each patient was considered for analysis. Protein was measured by the biuret method, LDH by UV spectrophotometry at 37°C and 340 nm [8], and cholesterol with the Boehringer-Mannheim enzymatic method CHOD PAP (cholesterol oxidase peroxidise) [9].

Clinical diagnosis (i.e., etiological diagnosis) was made, and the pleural fluid parameters were analyzed with it. The

following evidences were used to include or exclude the cases [10].

(1) Congestive heart failure: presence of clinical features (increased jugular venous pulse, tachycardia, and ventricular gallop) with cardiomegaly or echocardiac evidence of cardiac dysfunction.

(2) Renal diseases: elevated urea (>20 mmol/L) or creatinine > 167 micomol/L with or without signs or symptoms of fluid overload.

(3) Malignancy: confirmed by cytology or histological proof of malignant tumor and in absence of all other conditions associated with pleural effusion.

(4) Liver cirrhosis: positive ultrasonography or CT findings with clinical, and lab evidence of hepatic derangements and portal hypertension.

(5) Infective effusion: clear evidence of infection (positive microbiologic culture), elevated CRP or leukocytosis, or positive sputum stain.

(6) Hypoalbuminemia: serum albumin < 20 gm/L.

Pleural effusions associated with congestive cardiac failure, hypoalbuminemia, and liver cirrhosis were classified as transudates and all others as exudates. Cases of renal diseases and pulmonary embolism were excluded.

Thus, pleural fluid was categorized as transudative and exudative pleural effusion on the basis of etiology which was contributed by clinical, imaging, and pathological evaluations. The pleural effusions were classified as exudative and transudative on the basis of etiological diagnosis, Light's criteria, and pCHOL (taken a cutoff value of 1.16 mmol/L or 45 mg/dL, given by Heffner et al. 2002) [4].

Quiroga et al. [11], using 45 mg/dL of cholesterol as the cutoff in 80 patients, also reported a sensitivity of 83% and a specificity of 100%. The statistical significance of the parameters for etiological diagnosis was measured to find their usefulness.

3. Observations and Results

A total of 62 patients with definite clinical diagnosis, eligible for the study, were included in which 30.6% (19) cases were transudates, and 69.4% (43) cases were exudates (Figure 1).

It is seen that tubercular effusion was the most common PE in the study. It counted 21 out of 62 cases (33.9%). Carcinoma lung was the second most common cause accounting for 14.5% (9), followed by parapneumonic effusion 11.3% (7), empyema thoracis 8.1% (5), hepatic hydrothorax 4.8% (3), hypoalbuminemia (2 cases), and 1 case each for atelectasis and splenic abscess. Transudates counted for 21% (13 cases) (see Figure 2).

In this study, it is found that mean pCHOL level (mmol/L) was 1.92 ± 0.75 for exudates, 0.53 ± 0.28 for transudates, 1.81 ± 0.59 for parapneumonic effusion, 2.08 ± 0.58 for tubercular, and 1.58 ± 0.65 for malignancy as shown in Figures 3 and 4, respectively.

It is seen that out of 62 cases (exudates 43 and transudates 19), protein ratio, as Light's parameter, identified 39 cases as

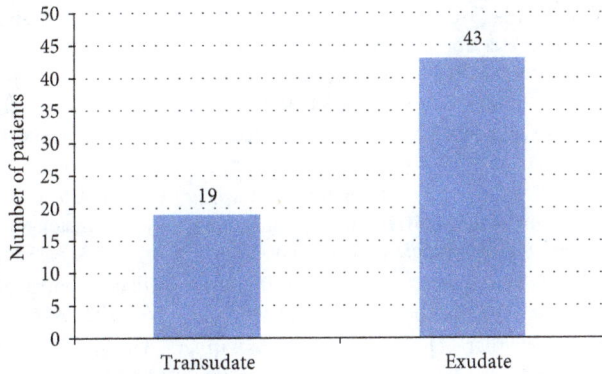

FIGURE 1: Distribution of type of pleural effusion.

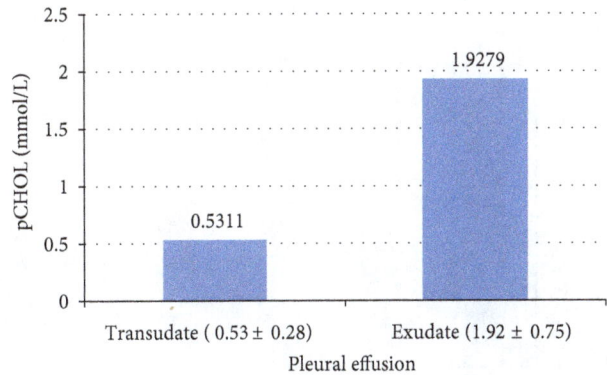

FIGURE 2: Distribution of causes (clinical diagnosis) of pleural effusion.

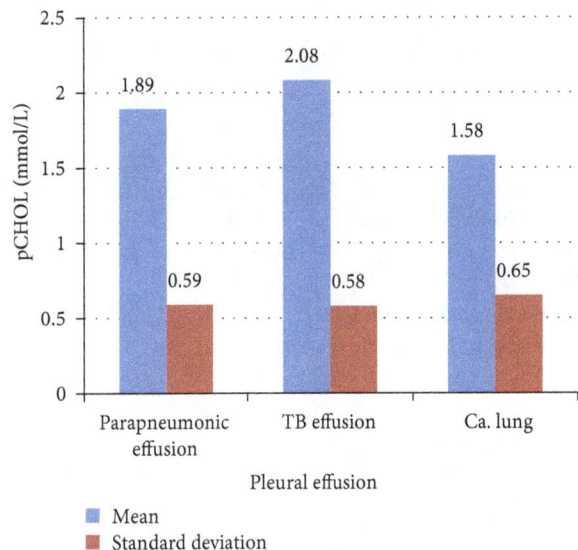

FIGURE 3: Mean values (±SD) of pCHOL (mmol/L) in type of pleural effusion.

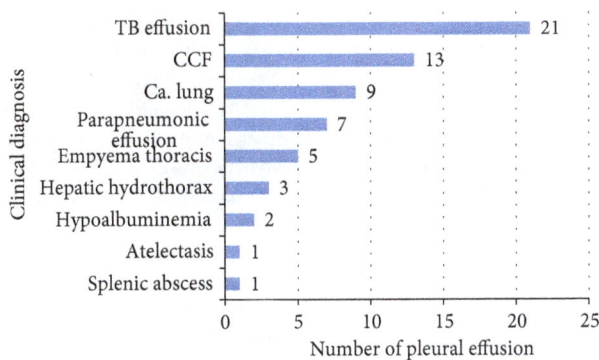

FIGURE 4: Mean values (±SD) of pCHOL (mmol/L) in different pleural effusion.

TABLE 1: Diagnostic comparison of PF parameters with clinical diagnosis.

Parameters	Sensitivity	Specificity	PPV	NPV	P value
Protein ratio	81.4%	82.6%	89.7%	70.4%	<0.0001
LDH ratio	86%	94.7%	97.4%	75%	<0.0001
pfLDH	100%	57.8%	84.3%	100%	<0.0001
pCHOL	97.7%	100%	100%	95%	<0.0001

exudates and 23 cases as transudates; LDH ratio identified 38 cases as exudates and 24 cases as transudates, while pCHOL identified 42 cases as exudate, and 20 cases as transudates (see Figure 5).

It is seen that pfP/sP ratio has a sensitivity of 81.4% and specificity of 82.6%; pfLDH/sLDH ratio has a sensitivity of 86% and specificity of 94.7%, and pCHOL with sensitivity of 97.7% and specificity of 100% for differentiating exudative and transudative PEs. All these parameters have a significant P value that is, <0.0001 (see Table 1).

Also on Pearson correlation test, pCHOL correlation is 0.963 and protein ratio (pfP/sP) is 0.591 which suggests that pCHOL is highly correlated than protein ratio with clinical diagnosis for exudate which is significant at the 0.01 level.

4. Discussion

In this study, a total of 62 patients, 19 with transudates and 43 with exudates, were considered according to the clinical diagnosis. The most frequent cause of pleural exudates is tuberculosis followed by lung cancer which is similar to the result of a study done in Malaysia where there is high incidence of tuberculosis [12]. Protein ratio identified exudates with a sensitivity of 81.4% and specificity of 82.6%. The pleural fluid to serum LDH ratio has a sensitivity and specificity of 86% and 94.7%, respectively. Also on Pearson correlation test, pCHOL correlation, and protein ratio (pfP/sP) are 0.963 and 0.591, respectively. It suggests that pCHOL is highly correlated than protein ratio with clinical diagnosis for exudate which is significant at the 0.01 level.

It is found that in transudates, parapneumonic, tubercular, and neoplastic pleural effusions, pCHOL levels were 0.53 ± 0.28 mmol/L, 1.81 ± 0.59 mmol/L, 2.08 ± 0.58 mmol/L,

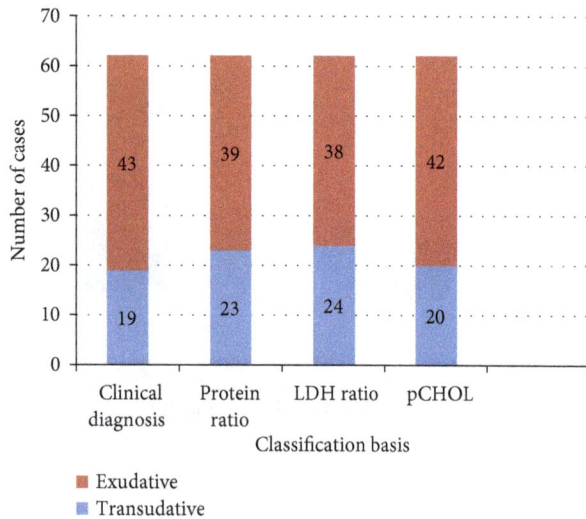

FIGURE 5: Cases classified by Light's criteria and pCHOL with clinical diagnosis.

and 1.58 ± 0.65 mmol/L, respectively. With a classifying threshold of 1.16 mmol/L, pCHOL has a sensitivity of 97.7 percent and specificity of 100 percent for diagnosis of exudates with a PPV of 100 percent in this study.

It was found that pCHOL criterion misclassified only one case of malignant effusion as transudate and that happened with the protein ratio of Light's criteria too. Similar findings have been reported by others, who suggested that the misclassified exudates had low cell component concentrations because the pleura had only recently been affected by the tumor [3, 13].

Other authors [14, 15] believe that a more likely explanation is that the pathogenesis of neoplastic exudates involves more than one mechanism more frequently than that of other kinds.

5. Conclusion

It is concluded that pCHOL has a better sensitivity, specificity, and PPV in differentiating transudates and exudates than the parameters of Light's criteria. This also avoids the plasma protein, sLDH and pleural fluid protein, and LDH. Therefore, it is, a more efficient, easier, and a more cost effective method to differentiate exudates from transudates. This study also suggests that determination of pCHOL should be in routine practice in cases of pleural effusion.

References

[1] R. W. Light, M. I. Macgregor, P. C. Luchsinger, and W. C. Ball Jr., "Pleural effusions: the diagnostic separation of transudates and exudates," *Annals of Internal Medicine*, vol. 77, no. 4, pp. 507–513, 1972.

[2] S. C. Chakko, S. H. Caldwell, and P. P. Sforza, "Treatment of congestive heart failure. Its effect on pleural fluid chemistry," *Chest*, vol. 95, no. 4, pp. 798–802, 1989.

[3] L. Valdes, A. Pose, J. Suarez et al., "Cholesterol: a useful parameter for distinguishing between pleural exudates and transudates," *Chest*, vol. 99, no. 5, pp. 1097–1102, 1991.

[4] J. E. Heffner, S. A. Sahn, and L. K. Brown, "Multilevel likelihood ratios for identifying exudative pleural effusions," *Chest*, vol. 121, no. 6, pp. 1916–1920, 2002.

[5] D. K. Spady and J. M. Dietschy, "Sterol synthesis in vivo in 18 tissues of the squirrel monkey, guinea pig, rabbit, hamster, and rat," *Journal of Lipid Research*, vol. 24, no. 3, pp. 303–315, 1983.

[6] M. S. Brown and J. L. Goldstein, "Receptor mediated control of cholesterol metabolism," *Science*, vol. 63, pp. 695–702, 1976.

[7] J. E. Heffner, L. K. Brown, and C. A. Barbieri, "Diagnostic value of tests that discriminate between exudative and transudative pleural effusions," *Chest*, vol. 111, no. 4, pp. 970–980, 1997.

[8] F. Wroblewski and J. S. La Due, "Lactate dehydrogenase activity in blood," *Proceedings of the Society for Experimental Biology and Medicine*, vol. 90, pp. 210–213, 1955.

[9] R. Deeg and J. Ziegenhorn, "Kinetic enzymic method for automated determination of total cholesterol in serum," *Clinical Chemistry*, vol. 29, no. 10, pp. 1798–1802, 1983.

[10] M. P. G. Leers, H. A. Kleinveld, and V. Scharnhorst, "Differentiating transudative from exudative pleural effusion: should we measure effusion cholesterol dehydrogenase?" *Clinical Chemistry and Laboratory Medicine*, vol. 45, no. 10, pp. 1332–1338, 2007.

[11] T. Quiroga, M. Costa, F. J. Sapunar et al., "Uulidad de la concentration de cholesterol en derrames pleurales para diferenciar entre transudados y exudados," *Enfermedades Respiratorias y Cirugía Torácica*, vol. 5, pp. 128–130, 1989.

[12] C. K. Liam, L. I. M. Kim-Hatt, and C. M. M. Wong, "Causes of pleural exudates in a region with a high incidence of tuberculosis," *Respirology*, vol. 5, no. 1, pp. 33–38, 2000.

[13] A. Martinez- Berganaza Asenio and P. CiaGomez, "Epidemiologia de las enfermedades de la pleura: a proposito de 562 casos," *Medicina Clínica*, vol. 90, pp. 311–315, 1988.

[14] S. A. Sahn, "The pleura," *American Review of Respiratory Disease*, vol. 138, no. 1, pp. 184–234, 1988.

[15] B. Chernow and S. A. Sahn, "Carcinomatous involvement of the pleura: an analysis of 96 patients," *American Journal of Medicine*, vol. 63, no. 5, pp. 695–702, 1977.

5

Comparison Study of Airway Reactivity Outcomes due to a Pharmacologic Challenge Test: Impulse Oscillometry versus Least Mean Squared Analysis Techniques

Elena Rodriguez,[1,2,3] **Charrell M. Bullard,**[4] **Milena H. Armani,**[1]
Thomas L. Miller,[5] **and Thomas H. Shaffer**[1,2,5]

[1] *Nemours Research Lung Center, Nemours/Alfred I. duPont Hospital for Children, Wilmington, DE 19803, USA*
[2] *Nemours Biomedical Research, Nemours/Alfred I. duPont Hospital for Children, Wilmington, DE 19803, USA*
[3] *Division of Clinical Pharmacology, Thomas Jefferson University, Philadelphia, PA 19107, USA*
[4] *Division of Neonatology, Thomas Jefferson University Hospital, Philadelphia, PA 19107, USA*
[5] *Department of Pediatrics, Thomas Jefferson University, Philadelphia, PA 19107, USA*

Correspondence should be addressed to Elena Rodriguez; merodrig@nemours.org

Academic Editor: S. L. Johnston

The technique of measuring transpulmonary pressure and respiratory airflow with manometry and pneumotachography using the least mean squared analysis (LMS) has been used broadly in both preclinical and clinical settings for the evaluation of neonatal respiratory function during tidal volume breathing for lung tissue and airway frictional mechanical properties measurements. Whereas the technique of measuring respiratory function using the impulse oscillation technique (IOS) involves the assessment of the relationship between pressure and flow using an impulse signal with a range of frequencies, requires less cooperation and provides more information on total respiratory system resistance (chest wall, lung tissue, and airways). The present study represents a preclinical animal study to determine whether these respiratory function techniques (LMS and IOS) are comparable in detecting changes in respiratory resistance derived from a direct pharmacological challenge.

1. Introduction

The use of animal models for studying respiratory mechanics under airway challenge tests has led to a sudden increase of information regarding the behavior of the different areas of the respiratory system. Despite the large amount of research in the adult and pediatric groups, we still lack significant knowledge in the neonatal subgroup. The present study represents a preclinical animal study to determine whether two respiratory function techniques are comparable in detecting changes in respiratory resistance derived from a direct pharmacological challenge.

The technique of measuring transpulmonary pressure and respiratory airflow with esophageal manometry, airway manometry, and pneumotachography has been previously described [1]. Transpulmonary pressure derived from proximal airway pressures and intrapulmonary esophageal pressure detected from a water-filled catheter [2, 3] are measured by differential pressure transducers. The airflow is measured with a low dead-space volume pneumotachometer and a differential pressure transducer. The least mean squared analysis (LMS) has been used broadly in both preclinical and clinical settings for the evaluation of neonatal lung function during tidal volume breathing [1, 4, 5].

The technique of measuring respiratory function using forced oscillation technique (FOT), or impulse oscillometry, involves the assessment of the relationship between pressure and flow using a forced/impulse signal composed with a range of frequencies. The response to this signal is called the respiratory impedance, which is the frequency-dependent relationship between transrespiratory pressure and flow. The impedance of the respiratory system includes the respiratory resistance (R_{rs}) and the respiratory reactance. The R_{rs} is the component of the pressure-flow relationship of the pressure oscillation that is in phase with the airflow; it is measured by the forward sound impulse and includes the total resistance of the respiratory system (chest wall, lung tissue, and airways). The technique was introduced in the initial study conducted by Dubois et al. in the 1950s [6].

Since then, many advances have been made in refining and using this technique for clinical research. Further modification of the technique has included the introduction of a computer friendly device that applies a respiratory pressure impulse, the impulse oscillometry system (IOS), which differs from the initial FOT in its setup. It uses signals lasting 5 ms and containing 5 Hz harmonics up to 50 Hz [7].

Multiple authors have published data using these oscillatory techniques for studies that evaluated airway and respiratory tissue mechanic responses after airway challenges in adolescents and children [8–16]. The techniques differentiated between proximal and distal airway obstruction and are a sensitive approach to determine bronchial hyperreactivity. In this regard, it has been demonstrated that oscillation does not modify the airway smooth muscle tone [17].

Despite the variable use of reference values, the techniques hold promise because the patients do not need to complete respiratory maneuvers, measurements are taken during quiet respiration, and invasive procedures (e.g., placement of an esophageal balloon) are not required to measure the resistance of the respiratory tract. Despite the amount of past research to establish these techniques as valid methods for assessment of respiratory function in both children and infants [18–25], additional validation is required for the neonatal population.

Significant remodeling of the respiratory system occurs even after birth in humans [26] and animals [27]; however, when compared with adults, neonates/infants have an increased upper airway resistance, increased lower airway resistance, decreased lung volume, decreased efficiency of respiratory muscles, and increased chest wall compliance. Extrapolation of outcomes regarding respiratory physiology-function and pharmacological challenge is not feasible.

The neonatal subgroup has been the focus of recent work, and published data supports the investigation of the oscillometry assessment in the youngest patients, with some technical modifications, which included the stimulation of a minimum of 2-second breathing pause at the end of inspiration using the Hering-Breuer inflation reflex (reflex triggered to prevent overinflation of the lungs by creating an apneic pause) in unsedated neonates by means of a shutter valve and a face mask [28, 29]. The IOS approach in neonates has not been validated against an accepted "gold standard" technique of respiratory function measurement (i.e., the use of an esophageal balloon to determine transpulmonary pressures to separate the chest wall and lung components of the resistance spectrum).

Appropriately, the development and validation of oscillometry techniques for clinical use in neonates will allow assessment of respiratory function in this group of patients to accurately measure lung development, respiratory disease, and the response to drug or therapeutic challenges. The

clinical applicability of the neonatal piglet model has been extensively studied for developmental respiratory biological processes and pre-clinical endpoints by our group [30] as well as numerous other investigators [31–37]. However, to validate this methodology for broad clinical use, we believe that accurate in vivo testing (a neonatal animal model) of an airway challenge is warranted.

Therefore, the main aims of this study were to detect significant pharmacological increases in resistance (% of change) with both respiratory function techniques and to assess the level of agreement between them in detecting this airway reactivity outcome. The overall study aim is to validate the IOS technique as a noninvasive means of evaluating respiratory mechanics in the neonatal setting through a range of resistance values representing the airway and tissue mechanical proprieties; this validation is to be compared with an older technique that is still currently accepted as a standard for respiratory mechanics evaluation but requires patient cooperation and placement of an esophageal pressure catheter [2].

To explore this gap in research, we conducted this pilot study to investigate the hypothesis that the IOS (new technique) could be interchangeably used to measure the effects of airway reactivity in neonatal settings.

2. Methods and Materials

2.1. Animal Preparation and Instrumentation Protocol. Neonatal piglets ($n = 8$, 6.6 ± 0.8 kg, and 20 ± 1 days of age) were anesthetized, intubated by tracheotomy, and allowed to breathe spontaneously. Piglets were anesthetized initially with two 1 mL/kg intramuscular injections, separated by 10 min, of an anesthesia cocktail (ketamine: 23 mg/kg; acepromazine: 0.58 mg/kg; xylazine: 0.8 mg/kg [KAX]) adapted from previously described piglet protocols [30, 38]. Local anesthesia was delivered to the skin and soft tissues around the surgical sites with 0.5% lidocaine HCl (4 mg/kg). For venous access and arterial blood sampling, respectively, 5- or 8-French umbilical catheters were inserted into the external jugular vein and carotid artery. A tracheotomy was performed to allow for continued spontaneous breathing through a 3.0- to 5.0-mm-ID endotracheal tube (ETT) (Hi-Lo™ Jet tube; Mallinckrodt, Saint Louis, MO, USA). The size of the trachea in this model facilitated the use of a standard neonatal/pediatric ETT. The tracheotomy procedure was necessary to ensure a tight seal for more accurate measures of respiratory mechanics and to eliminate upper airway shunting and flow contribution.

Subsequent anesthesia was maintained with intravenous infusion of KAX at 0.4 mL/kg/hr. Maintenance fluid was provided by a continuous venous infusion of 5% dextrose solution at a rate of 6 mL/kg/hr. Arterial blood pressure was monitored by attaching the arterial catheter to a standard pressure transducer via bedside patient monitor (model M1175A, Hewlett Packard, Palo Alto, CA, USA). ECG electrodes were also placed for monitoring the heart rate and cardiac rhythm and to detect any significant bradycardia. Throughout the protocol, the animal's rectal temperature was monitored and maintained at 37-38°C on a radiant warmer bed (Resuscitaire; Hill-Rom Air-Shields, Hatboro, PA, USA). Once the physiologic stability of the animal was confirmed by the analysis of the arterial blood chemistry (Stat profile; Nova Biomedical, Waltham, MA, USA), ECG, and blood pressure monitoring; the animal's respiratory measurements were recorded as described below. Intravenous midazolam was used as an anxiolytic to ease the work of breathing. Following the completion of the protocol, animals were euthanized with pentobarbital (50 mg/kg) and saturated potassium chloride (2 mEq). All procedures for the animal preparation were approved by the Institutional Animal Care and Use Committee. Functional respiratory parameters of interest were recorded after the animal was stabilized. The piglet then was connected to the PEDS circuit for baseline measurements. Immediately following LMS baseline assessment (average of 5 min), the piglet was connected to the IOS system for baseline oscillatory measurements, and testing was performed as soon as the transrespiratory pressure returned to 10 cmH$_2$O as described below. Also, Figure 1 illustrates the test paradigm that was followed in order to compare respiratory function assessment between the LMS and IOS methods both before and after pharmacologically induced airway constriction.

2.2. Respiratory Function Assessment-Least Mean Squared Analysis.

For the conventional tidal breathing resistance measurements, the ETT was connected to the pneumotachometer port. A three-valve stopcock was used to block the pressure port. The negative flow port was manually occluded to prevent flow artifact since there was no additional flow via ventilator tubing. A water-filled balloon was placed via the mouth into the esophagus to measure the intrathoracic pressure during respiration. Optimum placement of the balloon was confirmed by real-time monitoring of pressure tracings, using criteria of maximum negative deflection during inspiration with minimum cardiac artifacts. Only spontaneous breaths (at least 10 breaths) were analyzed, and breaths with distortion of the signal were excluded from the average data.

Piglets were observed for 30 seconds on the circuit. Respiratory volumes were determined by electronic integration of flow signals, and the following parameters were calculated: dynamic pulmonary resistance (R) in cmH$_2$O/L/s, respiratory rate, tidal volume, and minute ventilation. Resistance values were recorded while positive pressure was applied to induce opposition to flow and calculated by least mean squared (LMS) algorithms incorporated into the computer system.

2.3. Respiratory Function Assessment-Impulse Oscillometry Analysis.

The impedance of the total respiratory system was measured using a commercially available IOS that has been described previously. During tidal breathing through an ETT, an impulse generator delivered brief pulses at intervals of 0.2 sec, superimposed on the spontaneous breathing pattern. The digitalized pressure and flow signals were fed into the fast Fourier transformation, where 32 samples were considered. For experimental proposes, no system correction was used.

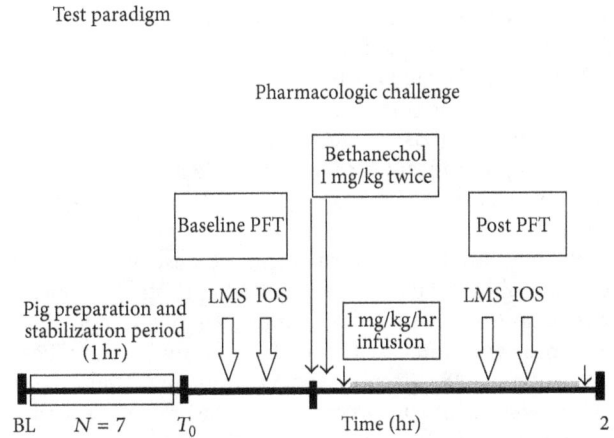

Test paradigm

FIGURE 1: A schematic diagram illustrating the current test paradigm. LMS, least mean squares; IOS, impulse oscillatory system; PFT, pulmonary function testing; N, number of animals; BL, baseline; Post, after bethanechol administration. Time between the first and second bethanechol doses was 10 min.

Daily calibration using a calibration pump (3.0 ± 0.01 L SD, Jaeger; Höechberg, Germany) and a reference impedance of 10 cmH$_2$O/L/s were performed, and a maximum error of 10% was permitted. Piglets were connected via ETT adapter to the pneumotach of the IOS, were tested for 30 seconds on the circuit with a transrespiratory pressure of 10 cmH$_2$O, and were saved for later evaluation; epoch of measurements was discarded if the time flow and pressure pattern in the primary data time and time results trends showed interruption of the oscillatory signal, which occurred occasionally (approximately 10–15%) in the current study. In the evaluation phase, the minimum time period for reporting these measurements was 2 seconds. The impedance of the respiratory system (Z_{rs}) and R_{rs} in cmH$_2$O/L/s were calculated at 3, 5, 10, 15, 20, 25, and 35 Hz. Replicate oscillatory values were performed by JLAB 4.65.1.0 software (Erich Jaeger GmbH, Würzburg, Germany) and analyzed by JLAB 5.20.0.52 software (VIASYS Healthcare GmbH, Höechberg, Germany). Since parameters were assessed within the same piglet over time/delta changes, a correction for the impedance of the ETT was not needed.

Each piglet provided a matched set of data from the MasterScreen PFT IOS (Jaeger, Höechberg, Germany) and the PEDS pulmonary function unit (MAS, Hatfield, PA) for the oscillometry and LMS analyses, respectively. Each piglet was measured with each device under two conditions: baseline (pre) and after intervention (post).

Following baseline measures, bethanechol was used as the intervention to pharmacologically induce bronchoconstriction and subsequent elevated airway resistance. Bethanechol powder (carbamyl-β-methylcholine, Sigma-Aldrich) was mixed with saline (5 mg of bethanechol : 1 mL of saline) and administered as two intravenous injections at a dose of 1 mg/kg of bethanechol chloride in 0.2 mL/kg of saline set 10 min apart to achieve an increase in the respiratory resistance. Decay in the elevated resistance was compensated with an infusion of 1 mg/kg/hr of bethanechol chloride started through the venous line following the initial bolus. This dosing regimen was adapted from a previously described piglet protocol [30]. To compare the two methodologies described herein, we were interested in establishing a large range of pulmonary changes (baseline to maximum dose response without evoking significant cardiovascular changes) instead of a standard dose response assessment with small pulmonary changes.

Bethanechol bolus and maintenance dose were given as described above. Piglets were observed until stable bronchoconstriction was assumed (3–5 min after the second dose) when resistance increased at least 40% from baseline. Postintervention LMS measurements were obtained, followed by IOS measurements, to prevent any unfavorable effect from the impulses on LMS parameters. Parameters of interest were documented for each technique, each time in the same sequence.

2.4. Statistics. Continuous variables were summarized overall by mean and standard error of the mean (SEM), unless indicated otherwise. All assumptions were tested for normality; in the case of violation of any assumption, nonparametric tests were performed. The delta changes were compared using paired t-test for the dependent continuous normal variables or Wilcoxon signed rank test for the nonnormal dependent variables, testing for positive mean or median differences, respectively. Significance was set at alpha level of 0.05 (1-sided). A comparative analysis of agreement between the two methods was detailed for the pharmacological challenge using the Bland-Altman plot analysis; the bias, or the average of the differences, and the 95% limits of agreement (LOA) were reported for all frequencies along with their linear regression analysis (r^2, slope, and P values). Statistical analysis was done using a combination of statistical software packages (GraphPad Prism version 5.02 for Windows; GraphPad Software, San Diego, CA, USA, and SPSS version 19; IBM, Chicago, IL, USA).

3. Results

In this animal model, measurements of respiratory mechanics were possible, and detection of an increase in resistance was achieved with both systems after bethanechol administration in seven of the piglets. One animal died during the postbethanechol measurements (post) secondary to cardiac arrest. Following intravenous (IV) administration of bethanechol, a small but statistically significant decrease was seen in heart rate (mean ± SD, 151 ± 12 versus 133 ± 6, –12%, $P = 0.03$) and arterial pressure (mean ± SD, 79 ± 5 versus 67 ± 5, –15%, $P = 0.002$) for the remaining 7 piglets; although these changes were not physiologically relevant for hemodynamic instability, there were no significant changes in respiratory rate, tidal volume, and minute ventilation following bethanechol administration.

Respiratory mechanics measurements showed a significant increase in dynamic pulmonary resistance measured by the LMS (+53%, $P = 0.003$) following bethanechol administration (Figure 2). Pressure-volume loops also verified that,

when compared with baseline, bethanechol administration resulted in increased pressure requirements as well as a widening and decrease in the slope of the pressure-volume loops.

Following bethanechol administration, a significant overall increase in the respiratory resistance measured by IOS was demonstrated by positive changes in R_{rs} from 10 to 25 Hz (+96%, $P = 0.018$; Figure 3). Significant increases in specific respiratory resistances were demonstrated by positive changes in the intermediate frequency spectrum (frequencies: $R_{rs\,10\,Hz}$ [+106%, $P = 0.031$], $R_{rs\,15\,Hz}$ [+96%, $P = 0.013$], $R_{rs\,20\,Hz}$ [+95%, $P = 0.026$], and $R_{rs\,25\,Hz}$ [+85%, $P = 0.037$]). No statistically significant differences between the prebethanechol (pre) and postbethanechol (post) outcomes for any remaining frequencies were observed: $R_{rs\,3\,Hz}$ (+67%, $P = 0.131$), $R_{rs\,5\,Hz}$ (+67%, $P = 0.09$), and $R_{rs\,35\,Hz}$ (+95%, $P = 0.084$), and the resistance spectrum of R_{rs} demonstrated increased positive frequency dependence (Figure 4).

The Bland-Altman analysis demonstrated that 95% of the differences between methods (IOS and LMS) lay within ±1.96 SD from the mean difference indicated by the LOA. Overall, there was a consistent linear sloped trend with a systematic bias (negative bias presented at lower values and positive bias presented at higher values of the measurement range) across the Bland-Altman plots, but within the LOA (Figure 5); this effect becomes less biased towards lower frequencies (Figures 5(a) and 5(b)) as do the slopes of the linear regression analysis.

4. Discussion

In the present study, we demonstrated that both respiratory function techniques assessed the effects of intravenous bethanechol on the respiratory system. Our results showed that delta changes of oscillometric resistances in the middle frequency range ($R_{rs\,10}$, 106%; $R_{rs\,15}$, 96%; $R_{rs\,20}$, 95%; $R_{rs\,25}$, 85%) were higher than LMS dynamic pulmonary resistance (R, 53%).

The smooth muscle of the respiratory tract has both parasympathetic and sympathetic innervations; carbamyl-β-methylcholine (bethanechol) is a choline ester and an agonist of muscarinic receptors that stimulates these receptors on the smooth muscle of the respiratory tract, causing airway narrowing and perhaps tissue constriction. Bethanechol belongs to the same group of drugs as acetylcholine, carbachol, and methacholine [39]. The piglet model used in this study was chosen based on its comparable size to the neonate/pediatric human and its common use for the investigation of ventilatory therapies [31–37].

In addition, bethanechol-induced airway challenges have been previously reported as an appropriate experimental intervention in the laboratory [40–44], and similar analogs (i.e., methacholine) have been used for clinical research purposes [45–47]. In humans, bethanechol is approved only for oral administration use; in veterinary medicine, it is available as an injection for subcutaneous (SC), intramuscular, or IV administration. Cardiac arrest is a severe, rare adverse reaction documented in humans, and in animals, it is a likely

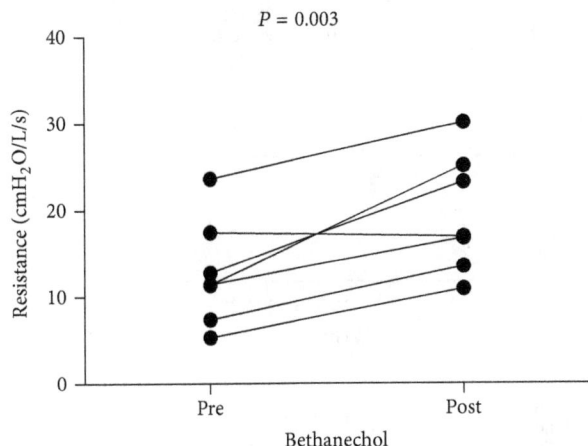

FIGURE 2: Plots of mean values for dynamic pulmonary resistance (resistance) before (pre) and after (post) bethanechol for each piglet. $P = 0.003$, paired t-test one tailed.

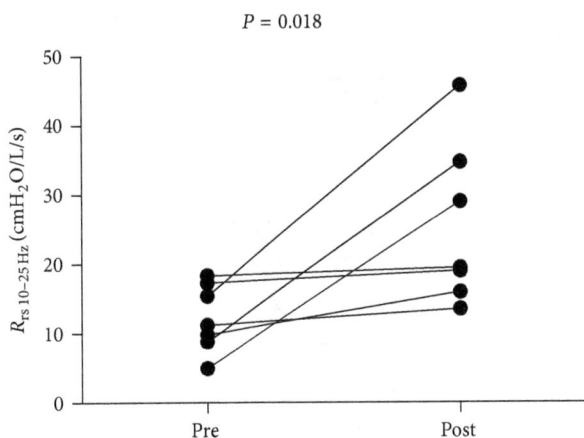

FIGURE 3: Plots of mean values for respiratory resistance (R_{rs}) from 10 Hz to 25 Hz before (pre) and after (post) bethanechol for each piglet. $P = 0.018$, paired t-test one tailed for the average.

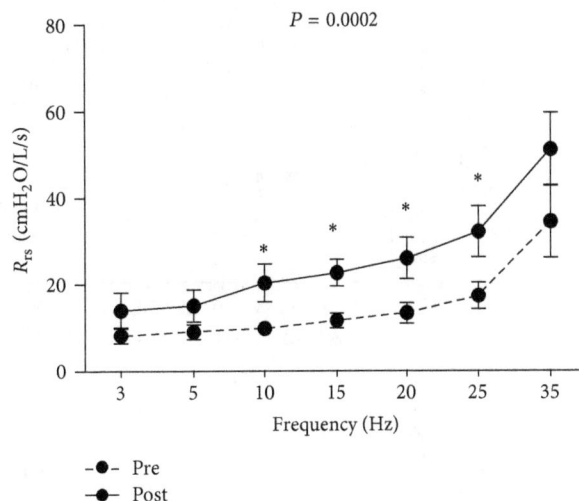

FIGURE 4: Plots of mean ($\pm$SEM) values for respiratory resistance (R_{rs}), as a function of oscillatory frequency, before (pre) and after (post) bethanechol ($n = 7$). As shown, significant differences in the middle oscillatory frequencies range are displayed ($^*P < 0.05$); paired t-test one tailed at each frequency and overall ($P = 0.0002$).

severe cholinergic reaction if given IV or in overdosage. It is recommended that atropine be immediately available when given IV or SC [48–51].

After bethanechol administration, a greater percentage of change was seen in airway resistance mainly represented by $R_{rs\,10}$–$R_{rs\,25}$ (+106–85%) when compared with the lung resistance mostly represented by $R_{rs\,3}$–$R_{rs\,5}$ (+69–63%), indicating a greater nonperipheral airway constriction response than peripheral airway/lung tissue response. Regarding the lung tissue contribution versus airway contributions to the total respiratory resistance, differences in the degree of tissue versus airway contribution exist between species [52, 53], including humans [54], and within induced-physiological and pharmacological conditions [44]; thus, caution should be taken in translating these findings between species.

It is widely recognized that the use of an esophageal balloon for resistance measurements separates the lung and chest wall component, therefore, excluding the chest wall resistance [4], while R_{rs} includes the resistance of the chest wall (i.e., lung resistance) and airway resistance. The lower the specific oscillatory frequency is, the more sensitive the measurement is to the periphery of the respiratory system. Measurement of the resistance using methods that require placement of an esophageal balloon for respiratory function testing procedures to assess the respiratory system in neonates is not easy. Noninvasive respiratory function techniques (i.e., impulse oscillometry) require less patient cooperation and provide more information about the total respiratory system resistance [19].

We also demonstrated that no pause in breathing was necessary for recording reliable data at low frequencies for R_{rs} using the impulse oscillation technique in neonatal piglets spontaneously breathing through an ETT. In this regard, the Hering-Breuer inflation reflex and face mask were not used in our study in comparison to previously cited studies in unsedated neonates/infants [28, 29].

The Bland-Altman analysis showed good agreement between the two techniques (IOS and LMS) for measuring resistance properties, and the agreement between these techniques depended on the oscillation frequency. From a mechanistic view point, R measured by the LMS in the study represents resistance of the lung tissue and airway frictional mechanical properties, whereas R_{rs} measured by IOS represents total respiratory resistance, so the two techniques are not directly interchangeable at lower frequencies. However, as mentioned in Section 3, the bias and slope decrease towards lower frequencies. In this regard, respiratory resistance at 5 Hz ($R_{rs\,5}$) and respiratory resistance at 3 Hz ($R_{rs\,3}$) may be closely interchangeable in the appropriate settings. However, the difference of ± 1.96 SD from the mean difference for $R_{rs\,35}$ (Figure 5(g)) was demonstrated to be unacceptable for interchangeability.

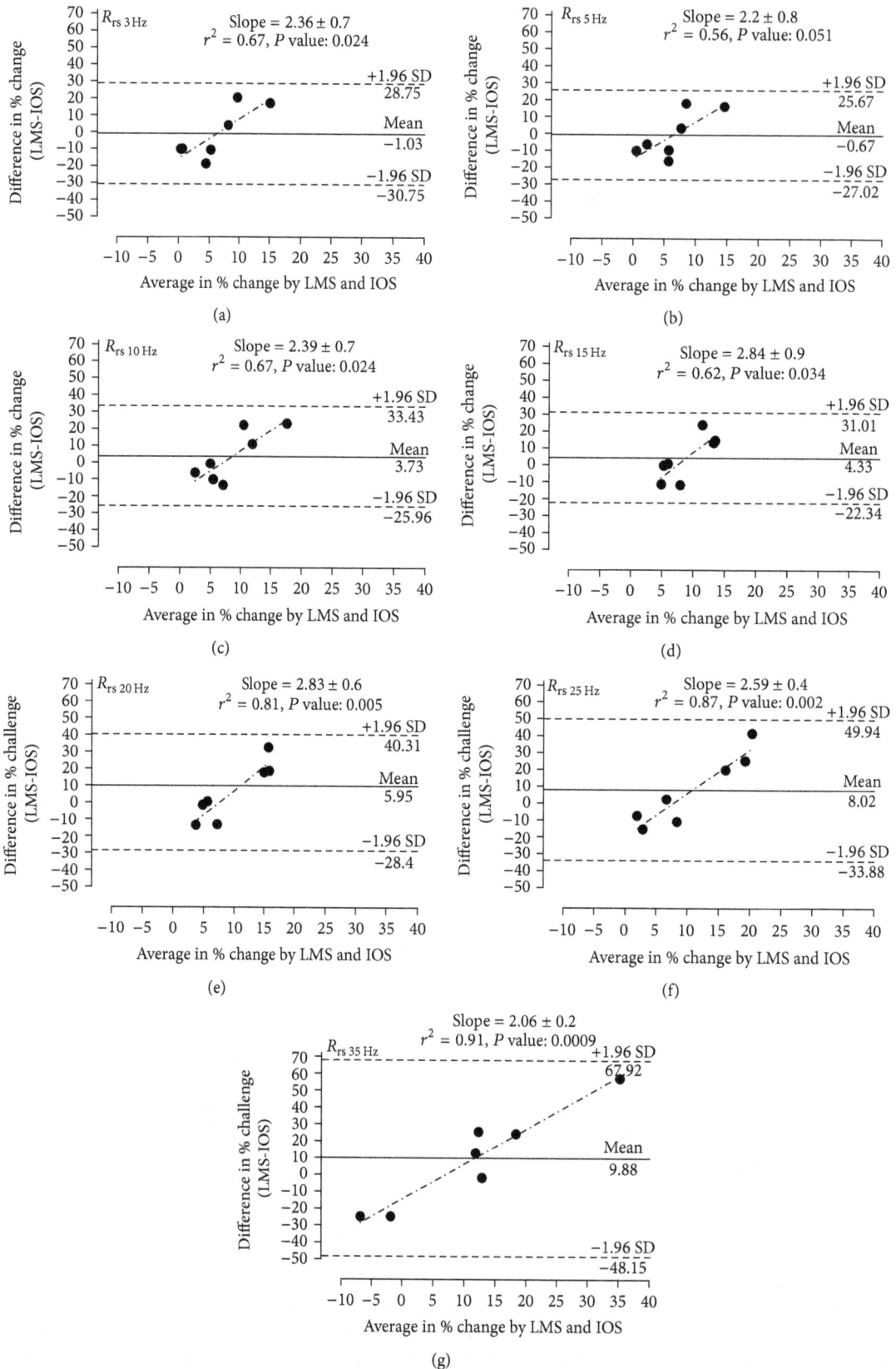

FIGURE 5: Bland-Altman plots constructed from the least mean square (LMS) and impulse oscillometry (IOS) data at each specific frequency (percentage of change) with mean (bias), ±LOA, and best-fit values of linear regression (slope, r^2, P value) after administration of intravenous bethanechol. LOA, limit of agreement; Upper LOA, mean difference (bias) + 1.96 SD; Lower LOA, mean difference (bias) −1.96 SD; r^2, R squares. The P value is testing the null hypothesis that the overall slope is zero.

Like many preliminary studies, the present study has some experimental limitations. Along these lines, the current study is an experimental preclinical model comparing the IOS and the LMS approach as an indicator of airway reactivity behavior to a pharmacologic intervention in a small number of animals. Additional work is required in the performance, reproducibility, and safety of the oscillation technique, including validation and qualification as a biomarker, before it can be proposed for standard clinical practice in the neonatal population.

5. Conclusions

In conclusion, we documented significant airway reactivity using both respiratory function techniques and demonstrated the magnitude of the change in airway resistance component at baseline and after administration of intravenous bethanechol. In a similar scenario, the measurements of respiratory resistance from the impulse oscillation technique (from 3 Hz to 25 Hz) may be used in lieu of the dynamic pulmonary resistance measurements from the LMS technique to determine resistance changes secondary to induced airway reactivity during spontaneous breaths.

The IOS technique as a noninvasive means of evaluating the different components of the respiratory system and pulmonary mechanics in the neonatal setting is very appealing; it gives further information through a range of resistance values representing the airway, tissue, and chest mechanical proprieties. However, further modification in the technique setup, incorporation of the appropriate references values for the neonatal population, and collaboration with experienced physicians and scientists in respiratory physiology/respiratory function techniques are required before broader clinical use is pursued in the neonatal population.

Funding

This study was funded through Nemours Research Programs/Nemours Foundation, NIH COBRE Grant no. 8 P20 GM103464 (T. H. Shaffer), and NIH Grant no. 5T32 GM008562-17 (E. Rodriguez) pediatric pharmacology fellow funded by NICHD under the Best Pharmaceuticals for Children Act. This work was performed at the Nemours/Alfred I. duPont Hospital for Children.

Acknowledgment

The authors thank Ms. Anne Hesek for her assistance with the animal surgical preparation.

References

[1] V. K. Bhutani, E. M. Sivieri, S. Abbasi, and T. H. Shaffer, "Evaluation of neonatal pulmonary mechanics and energetics: a two factor least mean square analysis," *Pediatric Pulmonology*, vol. 4, no. 3, pp. 150–158, 1988.

[2] C. S. Beardsmore, P. Helms, J. Stocks, D. J. Hatch, and M. Silverman, "Improved esophageal balloon technique for use in infants," *Journal of Applied Physiology Respiratory Environmental and Exercise Physiology*, vol. 49, no. 4, pp. 735–742, 1980.

[3] A. Baydur, P. K. Behrakis, and W. A. Zin, "A simple method for assessing the validity of the esophageal balloon technique," *American Review of Respiratory Disease*, vol. 126, no. 5, pp. 788–791, 1982.

[4] V. K. Bhutani, T. H. Shaffer, and D. Vidyasagar, Eds., *Neonatal Pulmonary Function Testing: Physiological, Technical and Clinical Considerations*, Perinatology Press, Ithaca, NY, USA, 1988.

[5] L. S. Goldsmith, J. S. Greenspan, S. D. Rubenstein, M. R. Wolfson, and T. H. Shaffer, "Immediate improvement in lung volume after exogenous surfactant: alveolar recruitment versus increased distention," *Journal of Pediatrics*, vol. 119, no. 3, pp. 424–428, 1991.

[6] A. B. Dubois, A. W. Brody, D. H. Lewis, and B. F. Burgess Jr., "Oscillation mechanics of lungs and chest in man," *Journal of Applied Physiology*, vol. 8, no. 6, pp. 587–594, 1956.

[7] H. J. Smith, P. Reinhold, and M. D. Goldman, "Forced oscillation technique and impulse oscillometry," *European Respiratory Monograph*, vol. 31, pp. 72–105, 2005.

[8] H. Bisgaard and B. Klug, "Lung function measurement in awake young children," *European Respiratory Journal*, vol. 8, no. 12, pp. 2067–2075, 1995.

[9] C. Delacourt, H. Lorino, M. Herve-Guillot, P. Reinert, A. Harf, and B. Housset, "Use of the forced oscillation technique to assess airway obstruction and reversibility in children," *American Journal of Respiratory and Critical Care Medicine*, vol. 161, no. 3, part 1, pp. 730–736, 2000.

[10] F. M. Ducharme and G. M. Davis, "Respiratory resistance in the emergency department: a reproducible and responsive measure of asthma severity," *Chest*, vol. 113, no. 6, pp. 1566–1572, 1998.

[11] B. Klug and H. Bisgaard, "Measurement of lung function in awake 2–4-year-old asthmatic children during methacholine challenge and acute asthma: a comparison of the impulse oscillation technique, the interrupter technique, and transcutaneous measurement of oxygen versus whole-body plethysmography," *Pediatric Pulmonology*, vol. 21, no. 5, pp. 290–300, 1996.

[12] B. Klug and H. Bisgaard, "Repeatability of methacholine challenges in 2- to 4-year-old children with asthma, using a new technique for quantitative delivery of aerosol," *Pediatric Pulmonology*, vol. 23, no. 4, pp. 278–286, 1997.

[13] B. Klug and H. Bisgaard, "Specific airway resistance, interrupter resistance, and respiratory impedance in healthy children aged 2–7 years," *Pediatric Pulmonology*, vol. 25, no. 5, pp. 322–331, 1998.

[14] B. Klug and H. Bisgaard, "Lung function and short-term outcome in young asthmatic children," *European Respiratory Journal*, vol. 14, no. 5, pp. 1185–1189, 1999.

[15] B. Klug, K. G. Nielsen, and H. Bisgaard, "Observer variability of lung function measurements in 2–6-yr-old children," *European Respiratory Journal*, vol. 16, no. 3, pp. 472–475, 2000.

[16] D. Stănescu, N. E. Moavero, C. Veriter, and L. Brasseur, "Frequency dependence of respiratory resistance in healthy children," *Journal of Applied Physiology Respiratory Environmental and Exercise Physiology*, vol. 47, no. 2, pp. 268–272, 1979.

[17] E. Oostveen, D. MacLeod, H. Lorino et al., "The forced oscillation technique in clinical practice: methodology, recommendations and future developments," *European Respiratory Journal*, vol. 22, no. 6, pp. 1026–1041, 2003.

[18] J. J. Pillow, P. D. Sly, and Z. Hantos, "Monitoring of lung volume recruitment and derecruitment using oscillatory mechanics

during high-frequency oscillatory ventilation in the preterm lamb," *Pediatric Critical Care Medicine*, vol. 5, no. 2, pp. 172–180, 2004.

[19] E. Rodriguez, M. B. Bober, L. Davey et al., "Respiratory mechanics in an infant with perinatal lethal hypophosphatasia treated with human recombinant enzyme replacement therapy," *Pediatric Pulmonology*, vol. 47, pp. 917–922, 2012.

[20] U. Frey, M. Silverman, R. Kraemer, and A. C. Jackson, "High-frequency respiratory impedance measured by forced-oscillation technique in infants," *American Journal of Respiratory and Critical Care Medicine*, vol. 158, no. 2, pp. 363–370, 1998.

[21] K. N. Desager, W. Buhr, M. Willemen et al., "Measurement of total respiratory impedance in infants by the forced oscillation technique," *Journal of Applied Physiology*, vol. 71, no. 2, pp. 770–776, 1991.

[22] K. N. Desager, M. Cauberghs, J. Naudts, and K. P. van de Woestijne, "Influence of upper airway shunt on total respiratory impedance in infants," *Journal of Applied Physiology*, vol. 87, no. 3, pp. 902–909, 1999.

[23] K. N. Desager, M. Willemen, H. P. Van Bever, W. De Backer, and P. A. Vermeire, "Evaluation of nasal impedance using the forced oscillation technique in infants," *Pediatric Pulmonology*, vol. 11, no. 1, pp. 1–7, 1991.

[24] U. Frey, "Forced oscillation technique in infants and young children," *Paediatric Respiratory Reviews*, vol. 6, no. 4, pp. 246–254, 2005.

[25] G. L. Hall, Z. Hantos, J. H. Wildhaber, F. Peták, and P. D. Sly, "Methacholine responsiveness in infants assessed with low frequency forced oscillation and forced expiration techniques," *Thorax*, vol. 56, no. 1, pp. 42–47, 2001.

[26] C. J. Lanteri and P. D. Sly, "Changes in respiratory mechanics with age," *Journal of Applied Physiology*, vol. 74, no. 1, pp. 369–378, 1993.

[27] T. H. Shaffer, V. K. Bhutani, M. R. Wolfson, R. B. Penn, and N. N. Tran, "In vivo mechanical properties of the developing airway," *Pediatric Research*, vol. 25, no. 2, pp. 143–146, 1989.

[28] G. L. Hall, Z. Hantos, F. Petak et al., "Airway and respiratory tissue mechanics in normal infants," *American Journal of Respiratory and Critical Care Medicine*, vol. 162, no. 4, part 1, pp. 1397–1402, 2000.

[29] J. J. Pillow, J. Stocks, P. D. Sly, and Z. Hantos, "Partitioning of airway and parenchymal mechanics in unsedated newborn infants," *Pediatric Research*, vol. 58, no. 6, pp. 1210–1215, 2005.

[30] T. L. Miller, C. J. Singhaus, T. I. Sherman, J. S. Greenspan, and T. H. Shaffer, "Physiologic implications of helium as a carrier gas for inhaled nitric oxide in a neonatal model of Bethanecol-induced bronchoconstriction," *Pediatric Critical Care Medicine*, vol. 7, no. 2, pp. 159–164, 2006.

[31] E. A. Mates, J. Hildebrandt, J. C. Jackson, P. Tarczy-Hornoch, and M. P. Hlastala, "Shunt and ventilation-perfusion distribution during partial liquid ventilation in healthy piglets," *Journal of Applied Physiology*, vol. 82, no. 3, pp. 933–942, 1997.

[32] M. A. Enrione, M. C. Papo, C. L. Leach et al., "Regional pulmonary blood flow during partial liquid ventilation in normal and acute oleic acid-induced lung-injured piglets," *Critical Care Medicine*, vol. 27, no. 12, pp. 2716–2723, 1999.

[33] D. M. Steinhorn, M. C. Papo, A. T. Rotta, A. Aljada, B. P. Fuhrman, and P. Dandona, "Liquid ventilation attenuates pulmonary oxidative damage," *Journal of Critical Care*, vol. 14, no. 1, pp. 20–28, 1999.

[34] S. Wolf, H. Lohbrunner, T. Busch et al., ""Ideal PEEP" is superior to high dose partial liquid ventilation with low PEEP in experimental acute lung injury," *Intensive Care Medicine*, vol. 27, no. 12, pp. 1937–1948, 2001.

[35] R. K. M. Krishnan, P. A. Meyers, C. Worwa, R. Goertz, G. Schauer, and M. C. Mammel, "Standardized lung recruitment during high frequency and conventional ventilation: similar pathophysiologic and inflammatory responses in an animal model of respiratory distress syndrome," *Intensive Care Medicine*, vol. 30, no. 6, pp. 1195–1203, 2004.

[36] J. L. Nold, P. A. Meyers, C. T. Worwa et al., "Decreased lung injury after surfactant in piglets treated with continuous positive airway pressure or synchronized intermittent mandatory ventilation," *Neonatology*, vol. 92, no. 1, pp. 19–25, 2007.

[37] A. L. Lampland, P. A. Meyers, C. T. Worwa, E. C. Swanson, and M. C. Mammel, "Gas exchange and lung inflammation using nasal intermittent positive-pressure ventilation versus synchronized intermittent mandatory ventilation in piglets with saline lavage-induced lung injury: an observational study," *Critical Care Medicine*, vol. 36, no. 1, pp. 183–187, 2008.

[38] T. L. Miller, T. J. Blackson, T. H. Shaffer, and S. M. Touch, "Tracheal gas insufflation-augmented continuous positive airway pressure in a spontaneously breathing model of neonatal respiratory distress," *Pediatric Pulmonology*, vol. 38, no. 5, pp. 386–395, 2004.

[39] J. L. Schlatter and J. L. Saulnier, "Bethanechol chloride oral solutions: stability and use in infants," *Annals of Pharmacotherapy*, vol. 31, no. 3, pp. 294–296, 1997.

[40] E. N. Keklikian, M. R. Wolfson, and T. H. Shaffer, "Caffeine potentiates airway responsiveness in the neonatal lamb," *Pediatric Pulmonology*, vol. 12, no. 1, pp. 17–22, 1992.

[41] V. K. Bhutani, R. J. Koslo, and T. H. Shaffer, "The effect of tracheal, smooth muscle tone on neonatal airway collapsibility," *Pediatric Research*, vol. 20, no. 6, pp. 492–495, 1986.

[42] R. B. Penn, M. R. Wolfson, and T. H. Shaffer, "Effect of tracheal smooth muscle tone on collapsibility of immature airways," *Journal of Applied Physiology*, vol. 65, no. 2, pp. 863–869, 1988.

[43] R. B. Penn, M. R. Wolfson, and T. H. Shaffer, "Influence of smooth muscle tone and longitudinal tension on the collapsibility of immature airways," *Pediatric Pulmonology*, vol. 5, no. 3, pp. 132–138, 1988.

[44] H. B. Panitch, I. Talmaciu, J. Heckman, M. R. Wolfson, and T. H. Shaffer, "Quantitative bronchoscopic assessment of airway collapsibility in newborn lamb tracheae," *Pediatric Research*, vol. 43, no. 6, pp. 832–839, 1998.

[45] H. B. Panitch, E. N. Keklikian, R. A. Motley, M. R. Wolfson, and D. V. Schidlow, "Effect of altering smooth muscle tone on maximal expiratory flows in patients with tracheomalacia," *Pediatric Pulmonology*, vol. 9, no. 3, pp. 170–176, 1990.

[46] S. M. Stick, D. J. Turner, and P. N. LeSouëf, "Lung function and bronchial challenges in infants: repeatability of histamine and comparison with methacholine challenges," *Pediatric Pulmonology*, vol. 16, no. 3, pp. 177–183, 1993.

[47] C. Delacourt, M. R. Benoist, S. Waernessyckle et al., "Repeatability of lung function tests during methacholine challenge in wheezy infants," *Thorax*, vol. 53, no. 11, pp. 933–938, 1998.

[48] J. L. Schlatter and J. L. Saulnier, "Bethanechol chloride oral solutions: stability and use in infants," *Annals of Pharmacotherapy*, vol. 31, no. 3, pp. 294–296, 1997.

[49] L. V. Allen Jr. and M. A. Erickson, "Stability of bethanechol chloride, pyrazinamide, quinidine sulfate, rifampin, and tetracycline

hydrochloride in extemporaneously compounded oral liquids," *American Journal of Health-System Pharmacy*, vol. 55, no. 17, pp. 1804–1809, 1998.

[50] M. C. Nahata, V. B. Pai, and T. F. Hipple, Eds., *Pediatric Drug Formulations*, Harvey Whitney Books, Cincinnati, Ohio, USA, 5th edition, 2004.

[51] D. C. Plumb, *Veterinary Drug Handbook*, Iowa State Press, St. Paul, Minn, USA, 4th edition, 2002.

[52] Z. Hantos, B. Daroczy, B. Suki, and S. Nagy, "Low-frequency respiratory mechanical impedance in the rat," *Journal of Applied Physiology*, vol. 63, no. 1, pp. 36–43, 1987.

[53] Z. Hantos, B. Daroczy, B. Suki, S. Nagy, and J. J. Fredberg, "Input impedance and peripheral inhomogeneity of dog lungs," *Journal of Applied Physiology*, vol. 72, no. 1, pp. 168–178, 1992.

[54] B. G. Ferris Jr., J. Mead, and L. H. Opie, "Partitioning of respiratory flow resistance in man," *Journal of Applied Physiology*, vol. 19, pp. 653–658, 1964.

Effects of Inactivated *Bordetella pertussis* on Phosphodiesterase in the Lung of Ovalbumin Sensitized and Challenged Rats

Ya-Juan Wang,[1,2] Shun-De Song,[1] Jun-Chun Chen,[3] Xue-Feng Wang,[4] Ya-Li Jiang,[1] Qiang-Min Xie,[1] Ji-Qiang Chen,[1] Zi-Gang Li,[5] and Hui-Fang Tang[1]

[1] *Zhejiang Respiratory Drugs Research Laboratory of SFDA of China, School of Medicine, Zhejiang University, Hangzhou 310058, China*
[2] *Clinical College of Integrated Traditional and Western Medicine, Anhui University of Chinese Medicine, Hefei 230038, China*
[3] *First Affiliated Hospital, Zhejiang University, School of Medicine, Hangzhou 310000, China*
[4] *Second Affiliated Hospital, Zhejiang Chinese Medical University, Hangzhou 310005, China*
[5] *Women's Hospital, School of Medicine, Zhejiang University, Hangzhou 310006, China*

Correspondence should be addressed to Hui-Fang Tang; tanghuifang@zju.edu.cn

Academic Editor: Andrew Sandford

This paper indicated that inactivated *Bordetella pertussis* (iBp) can enhance the lung airway hyperreactivity of the rats sensitized and challenged with OVA. The mechanisms were involved in the upregulation of cAMP-PDE activity and PDE4A, PDE4D, and PDE3 gene expression in the lungs. But only PDE4 activity was different between the OVA and OVA+iBp groups, and PDE4D expression was significantly increased in iBp rats alone. So, our data suggested that cosensitization with OVA and iBp affects lung airway reactivity by modulating the lung cAMP-PDE activity and PDE4D gene expression.

1. Introduction

Inactivated *Bordetella pertussis* (iBp) has been used as a strong Th2 adjuvant to boost allergic responses to antigen such as house dust mite antigen (HDM), ovalbumin (OVA), and ragweed pollen in animal models of asthmatic hypersensitivity from 1968 [1–4]. Systemic administration of iBp enhances these sensitization processes and enhances the pulmonary and systemic immune responses to locally administered HDM [5]. Our experiments have also suggested that simultaneous exposure to OVA and intramuscularly iBp can enhance the bronchial hyperresponsiveness [6]. But how this occurs at the molecular level has not been elucidated.

The phosphodiesterase (PDE) superfamily participates in the only cellular pathways for degradation of the ubiquitous intracellular second messengers. It comprises eleven biochemically and pharmacologically distinct enzyme families (PDEs 1-11) that hydrolyze cAMP and/or cGMP [7]. PDE4 is specific for cAMP and comprises four subtypes (A, B, C, and D). It is predominantly expressed and plays an important role in the regulation of cellular functions in inflammatory and immune cells. There has been significant interest in PDE4 inhibitors as a potential therapy for inflammatory diseases such as allergy and asthma [8]. Cyclic adenosine monophosphate (cAMP) relaxes airway smooth muscles in the lung. Our previous study using iBp adjuvants suggested that PDE4 is upregulated in the lung of allergic rats [6]. But whether the adjuvants had effects on PDE activity and expression was unclear.

Growing evidence suggests that the D subtype of PDE4-PDE4D plays a key role in balancing relaxation and contraction in airway smooth muscle [9]. The airway smooth muscle contractility of PDE4D-deficient mice is disrupted and no longer responsive to cholinergic stimulation [10]. Interestingly, animals exposed prenatally but not postnatally to cigarette smoke show increased airway hyperresponsiveness after a single intratracheal injection of *Aspergillus fumigatus* extract. This increased airway hyperresponsiveness is causally related to decreased lung cAMP levels, increased PDE4 enzymatic activity, and PDE4D isoform-specific mRNA expression in the lung [11].

Therefore, we set out to investigate the effects of OVA and iBp in airway responsiveness and the possible role of phosphodiesterase. Our study suggested that the response of the airways was different between OVA model with iBp (OVA+iBp) and OVA model without iBp (OVA). Interestingly, PDE4D expression was also increased in the lung of allergic rats using iBp adjuvants, while this result was not observed in the allergic rats without using iBp adjuvants. So, our study first suggested that PDE4D upregulation was induced by iBp and was involved in airway hyperresponsiveness.

2. Materials and Methods

2.1. Animal Model Preparation [12]. Male Sprague-Dawley rats (140–160 g, Laboratory Animal Center of Zhejiang University School of Medicine, Hangzhou, China) were maintained under a 24 h light/dark cycle with food and water *ad libitum.* Animals were treated in accordance with the National Institutes of Health Guide for the Care and Use of Laboratory Animals. Animal experiments were approved by the Zhejiang Medical Laboratory Animal Administration Committee.

Rats were sensitized by subcutaneous injection (1 mL) of a saline suspension containing 0.2% OVA (Sigma, St. Louis, MO) and 10% aluminum hydroxide into two footpads, neck, back, groin (0.1 mL each), and abdomen (0.5 mL) on day 0, with or without intramuscular injection of 2×10^{10} heat-killed *B. Pertussis* (iBp; 1 mL) into the hindlimbs. Other rats were sensitized with OVA as above but without iBpinjection. From day 14 after sensitization, those rats were challenged once daily for 7 days by 20 min of exposure to aerosolized 1% OVA in saline generated by a jet nebulizer (PARI MASTER, Pari GmbH, Starnberg, Germany; droplet diameter: 1–5 μm). *B. pertussis* control (iBp) rats received intramuscular injection of 2×10^{10} iBp (1 mL) only. Blank control rats were "sensitized" and "challenged" with a saline aerosol.

2.2. Measurement of Airway Hyperresponsiveness (AHR) [13]. The rat was tracheal cannulated after anesthetized with urethane (40 mg/kg), then placed in a whole-body plethysmograph for the measurement of lung resistance (R_L) and lung dynamic compliance (Cdyn) with a real-time data analysis system (MedLab Biological Signal Collection System V 5.0, Medease Scientific Technic Co. Ltd, Nanjing, China). After 5 min for stabilization, AHR was induced by exposure to methacholine aerosols (MCh, Sigma Chemical Co., St. Louis, MO) of increasing doses (0.2, 0.4, 0.8, 1.2, 1.6, 2.0, 4.0, 8.0, 12, and 16 g/L) through the tracheal cannula for 10 s with the jet nebulizer. The signals from all pressure transducers were continuously processed by fitting flow, volume, and pressure to an equation of motion. R_L and Cdyn were monitored for 5 min and maximal changes from baseline for each parameter were recorded. Ten- to fifteen-minute intervals were allowed between concentrations.

2.3. Preparation of Bronchoalveolar Lavage Fluids (BALF). After the last OVA challenge, rats were anaesthetized with urethane (2 g/kg, i.p.). Bronchoalveolar lavage was performed by gently instilling D-Hanks' solution into the lung *via* a tracheal catheter followed by withdrawal. This process was repeated three times with a total volume of 5 mL D-Hanks. Total BALF cells counts were determined with a hemocytometer. Cell pellets' slides were stained with Wright's stain; the number of neutrophils, eosinophils, lymphocytes, and monocytes on each slide was recorded. The total number of cells in each sample was then determined according to the volume of BALF recovered.

2.4. Histological Examination. The lungs were infused via the trachea with 1 mL of 10% neutral formalin and immersed in the same fixative for seven days. Tissues were paraffined, and 5 μm sections were cut and stained with H&E for examining cell infiltration under a light microscope. Inflammatory cell infiltration and peribronchial inflammatory cell counts were used to evaluate the severity.

2.5. Assays for cAMP-PDE and cGMP-PDE Activities [14]. On day 21, animals were sacrificed, and the lungs were immediately removed, frozen in liquid nitrogen, and then stored at −80°C until analysis. The frozen lungs were thawed and cut into small cubes. Twenty-five milligrams of the lung was homogenized in 100 μL of ice-cold 30 mM HEPES (pH 7.4) containing 0.1% Triton X-100. The PDE assay mixture (200 μL) in PBS (pH 7.4) contained 137 mM NaCl, 2.7 mM KCl, 8.8 mM Na_2HPO_4, 1.5 mM KH_2PO_4, 1 mM $CaCl_2$, 1 mM $MgCl_2$, 1 μM cAMP or 1 μM cGMP (Sigma), and lung homogenate. The PDE reaction was started by the addition of 10 μL lung homogenate and was performed at 37°C for 10 min. The reaction was stopped by boiling the mixture for 3 min. The assay mixture was cooled on ice, followed by centrifugation at 12,850 ×g for 30 μmin at 4°C. The amount of cAMP or cGMP present in the supernatant was determined by HPLC (Hypersil ODS 4.0 × 250 mm; Hewlett-Packard, Palo Alto, CA) using a standard curve for cAMP. The PDE inhibitors, theophylline (nonselective), rolipram (PDE4-selective), SKF94836 (PDE3-selective), and zaprinast (PDE5-selective), were used to inhibit the PDE activity and to analyze the components of PDE activity in the lung. In brief, 100 μM PDE inhibitor was added to the PDE assay mixture as above and then mixed with lung homogenate. The rest of the process was as above. The total amounts of protein were determined by the Bradford method using BSA as standard [15]. The results were expressed as nanomoles of PDE activity per milligram of protein.

2.6. Analysis of PDE Subtype mRNAs. Total RNA was isolated from each tissue frozen in liquid nitrogen using TRIzol reagent (Invitrogen, Carlsbad, CA). Preparation of first-strand cDNA from rat and total RNA was performed using First-Strand cDNA Synthesis kit (Shanghai Sangon Biological Engineering Technology and Service, Shanghai, China) and Advantage RT-for-PCR kit (Clontech, Palo Alto, CA), respectively. The PCR primer sets of PDE were listed in Table 1. Each of the PCR primer sets was able to detect all known

TABLE 1: Primer sequences of rats PDEs.

Gene	Primer sequences (5'-3')	Length (bp)	T_m (°C)
β-Actin	Sense: AACCCTAAGGCCAACCGTGAAAAG Antisense: GCTCGAAGTCTAGGGCAACATA	343	57
PDE1	Sense: TGGAAGCTGCACTACAGGTG Antisense: CTTCAGGTCCACAGCTGACA	375	59
PDE2	Sense: GAGGACATCGAGATCTTTGC Antisense: TCTTTGTAGATCAGCTCCGC	442	57
PDE3	Sense: TCTTTGCCACTCCTACGACT Antisense: CTGTGCCTGATAAACACTGC	265	57
PDE4A	Sense: TCAACACCAATTCGGAGCTGG Antisense: GTCTTCAGGTCAGCCAGGAGG	216	61
PDE4B	Sense: AGGATTCTGAAGGACCGG Antisense: AGATTATGTGTCGATCAG	154	56
PDE4C	Sense: ACTGAGTCTGCGCAGGATGG Antisense: CACTCCTCTTCCTCTGCTCTCCTC	539	62
PDE4D	Sense: GGCTTCATAGACTACATTG Antisense: TTACACTGTTACGTGTCAGG	418	56
PDE5	Sense: CTGTCTGATCTGGAAACAGC Antisense: GCAATCAGCAATGCAAGCGT	250	57
PDE7	Sense: TCGTATGCTAGGAGATGTCCG Antisense: GCTTACTAGACTATTTCCATTTG	334	55
PDE8	Sense: GGAGAACCAACTCCTTCCTGTG Antisense: AGGCATCCCATGCATCAAAC	592	58
PDE9	Sense: ATGGACCGAGACAAAGTGAC Antisense: AGGCGAACGGTCTTCATTGT	275	57
PDE10	Sense: CTGAGGGGGATGAGATGAAG Antisense: TCAGTTGCTAGGCAGACATCA	322	58
PDE11	Sense: TTCAGCTCGGACAGTCCTAAA Antisense: TCCACTAGCAAAGGAGACGAA	374	58

variants derived from the appropriate PDE gene. PCR amplification was performed in a PCR buffer (10 mM Tris-HCl, pH 9.0, 100 mM KCl, 80 mM $(NH_4)_2SO_4$, and 0.1% NP-40) containing 0.2 mM of each dNTP, 1.5 mM of $MgCl_2$, 500 nM of each primer, and 1 U of Taq DNA polymerase (Sangon) in a total volume of 25 μL for 30 cycles, with the following cycle parameters: denaturing, 94°C for 45 sec; annealing, 58°C for 70 sec; and extension, 72°C for 2 min. After PCR amplification, 8 μl of each reaction mixture was resolved by electrophoresis on a 1.5% agarose gel containing ethidium bromide, and the PCR product bands were quantified using the UVP Gel Documentation system (UVP, Upland, CA). The levels of PDE mRNAs were calculated relative to β-actin. It was confirmed that under these conditions the PCR product accumulation did not reach plateau levels (data not shown).

2.7. Statistical Analysis. Data are expressed as mean ± SEM. Statistical analysis was performed with one-way ANOVA (SPSS11.0, USA) to evaluate PDE activity, PDE mRNA expression and lung resistance, and dynamic compliance. Differences with $P < 0.05$ were considered statistically significant.

3. Results

3.1. Intramuscular iBp Enhanced the AHR. The baseline values before aerosol challenge with MCh were similar in control rats, OVA sensitized and challenged rats with iBp as an adjuvant (OVA+iBp), iBp alone (iBp), and OVA sensitized and challenged rats without iBp (OVA). There were no significant differences in basal R_L and Cdyn among groups. Inhaled MCh caused a dose-dependent bronchoconstriction that peaked within 60 s. In our rat model of allergic asthma, OVA sensitization and challenge caused a significant decrease in Cdyn and increase in R_L compared to control rats (Figure 1). Simultaneous exposure to OVA and intramuscular iBp enhanced the decrease in Cdyn and increase in R_L at lower concentrations of MCh, but at high MCh concentrations, the responses of the OVA and OVA+iBP groups were equivalent. Interestingly, a single iBp injection had an effect similar to OVA sensitization and challenge.

3.2. Intramuscular iBp Increased the Eosinophils in BALF. To investigate the molecular mechanisms underlying the differences between our rat models, we used another series of

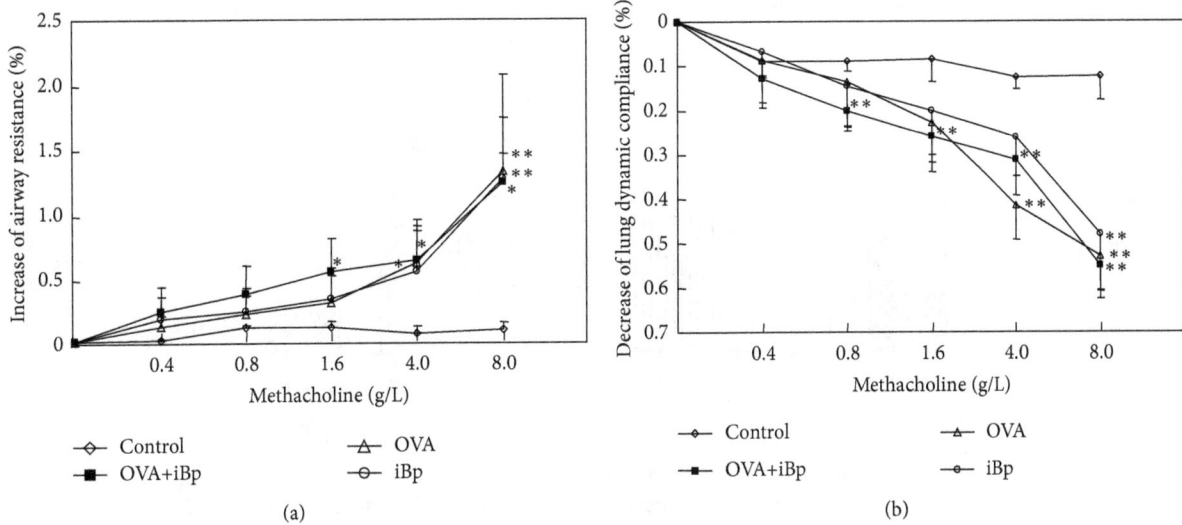

FIGURE 1: (a) R_L as a marker of AHR induced by MCh in normal ($n = 6$), OVA+iBp ($n = 8$), iBp ($n = 6$), and OVA rats ($n = 6$); (b) Cdyn as a marker of AHR induced by MCh (mean ± SEM; $^*P < 0.05$; $^{**}P < 0.01$ versus normal rats).

TABLE 2: Antigen-induced lung inflammatory cells in bronchoalveolar fluid.

Group	n	Total number	Eosinophils	Lymphocytes ($\times 10^4$ cells/L)	Neutrophils	Monocytes
Control	6	35.0 ± 12.6	0.12 ± 0.11	31.34 ± 12.31	1.90 ± 0.54	1.64 ± 0.39
OVA+iBp	6	$169.6 \pm 48.4^{**}$	$31.73 \pm 7.46^{**}$	$86.13 \pm 23.42^{**}$	$23.45 \pm 0.99^{**}$	$13.20 \pm 10.75^{*}$
OVA	6	$94.0 \pm 11.27^{**}$	$16.54 \pm 5.35^{**}$	$61.90 \pm 7.56^{**}$	$8.93 \pm 1.12^{**}$	$7.38 \pm 2.94^{**}$
iBp	6	31.0 ± 14.41	$1.23 \pm 0.73^{**}$	22.31 ± 9.21	$6.48 \pm 3.72^{*}$	2.77 ± 1.95

$^*P < 0.05$, $^{**}P < 0.01$, versus control group.

rats to study the BALF and the lung. The total number of cells (Table 2) and eosinophils in BALF increased in the OVA+iBp and OVA groups, as compared to controls ($P < 0.01$). At the same time, the numbers of total leukocytes, eosinophils, and neutrophils in BALF from OVA+iBp group were significantly higher than the OVA group. While iBp groupshowed a total number similar to the blank control group, the eosinophils and neutrophils were significantly higher than those in the blank control.

3.3. Simultaneous Exposure to Ovalbumin and Intramuscularly iBp Enhanced cAMP-PDE Activity.
With regard to PDE regulation in the lung, OVA sensitization and challenge with or without iBp significantly elevated the cAMP-PDE activity, resulting in 2.5-fold or 2-fold higher activity than that of normal animals, although the difference between OVA and OVA+iBp groups was not statistically significant (Figure 2(a)). But iBp did not affect the cAMP-PDE activity; the level was equivalent to the normal control. The total cGMP-PDE activity in the normal control and the OVA groups was high, while in OVA+iBp and iBp groups the activity was decreased (Figure 2(b)).

To further determine which PDE subtype plays a key role in the total PDE activity, we used the theophylline (nonselective PDE inhibitor), rolipram (PDE4 inhibitor), SKF94836 (PDE3 inhibitor), and zaprinast (PDE5 inhibitor)

to determine the overall PDE activity of each subtype. Rolipram (100 μM) sensitive cAMP-PDE activity (i.e., PDE4 activity) was 1.4-fold or 1.6-fold higher in the OVA or OVA+iBp rats than in normal rats (Figure 3(d)). These results suggest that the increase in total cAMP-PDE activity by OVA sensitization and challenge is primarily due to upregulation of PDE4. Zaprinast (100 μM) sensitive cGMP-PDE activity (i.e., PDE5 activity) was the major resource of cGMP-PDE activity, but the OVA or the OVA+iBp rats were similar to normal rats (Figure 4(c)).

3.4. Intramuscular iBp Enhanced mRNA Expression of PDE4D.
To investigate whether the elevation of PDE activity was due to enhanced PDE subtype gene expression, we measured the lung mRNA levels of subtypes PDE1 to PDE11 in control, OVA, OVA+iBp, and iBp rats. There were no significant changes in the expression of PDEs 1, 2, 9, 10, and 11 (data not shown). The expression of PDEs 3, 4A, 4D, 5, 7, and 8 was upregulated in OVA+iBp rats. Although PDE4A and PDE4D were significantly increased in the OVA+iBp rats, PDE4A did not increase in the OVA or iBprats, while simultaneous exposure to OVA and intramuscular iBpenhanced the PDE4A expression. Interestingly, the expression of PDE4D was significantly increased in iBprats, while in the OVA group it did not increase. This suggested that iBpspecially upregulated PDE4D (Figure 5). At the same time, this result

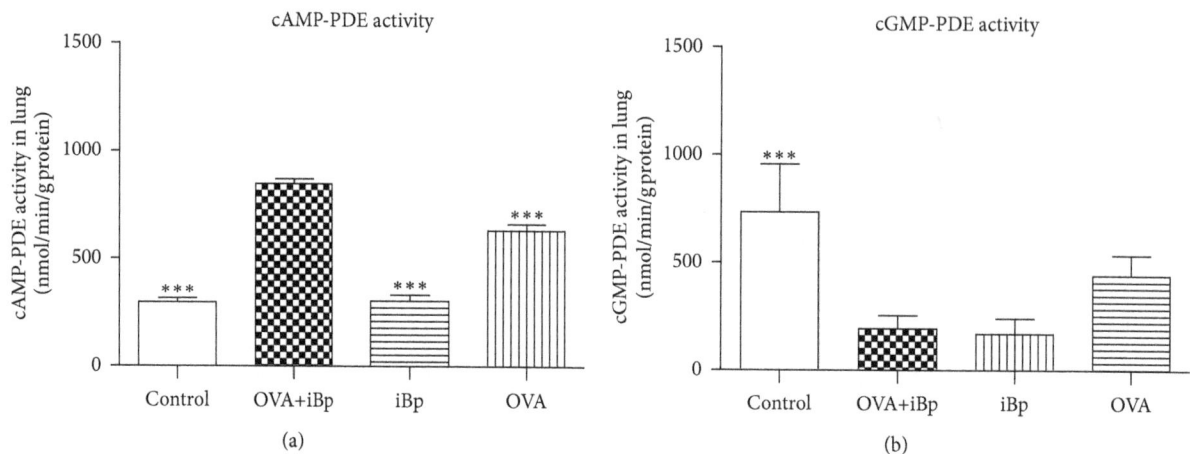

FIGURE 2: (a) Lung cAMP-PDE activity in normal ($n = 8$), OVA+iBp, iBp ($n = 6$), and OVA rats ($n = 8$); (b) lung cGMP-PDE activity in normal ($n = 8$), OVA+iBp, iBp ($n = 6$), and OVA rats ($n = 8$) (mean ± SEM; $^{*}P < 0.05$; $^{**}P < 0.01$ versus OVA+iBp; $^{#}P < 0.05$; $^{##}P < 0.01$ versus normal).

also suggested that the increased cAMP-PDE activity might be due to enhanced PDE7 and PDE8 gene expression by simultaneous exposure to OVA and iBp, at least in part.

The expression of PDE3 and PDE5 was complex. In OVA group, PDE5 was downregulated. Interestingly, in iBp rats, PDE5 was significantly increased, while in OVA+iBp group, the level of PDE5 expression was located in the middle of the OVA group and OVA+iBp group. PDE3 was upregulated in OVA or iBp groups, while in OVA+iBp group PDE3 was lower than OVA or iBp groups. This suggested that iBp specially upregulated PDE5, there was not siginificant difference.

3.5. Simultaneous Exposure to OVA and Intramuscular iBp Enhanced the Infiltration of Eosinophils. In the lung histology, increased numbers of infiltrated eosinophils were observed in peribronchial and perivascular tissues in the OVA and OVA+iBp groups, with more eosinophils in the latter. In iBp group, the lung histology was similar to normal controls (Figure 6).

4. Discussion

Inactivated *B. pertussis* has long been used as an effective adjuvant for eliciting IgE responses to a variety of antigens in experimental animals, while being also an antigen [16–19]. Because of this specific property, iBp has also been used in animal models of hypersensitivity to boost allergic responses to HDM, OVA, and ragweed pollen. As early as 1980, Bartell and Busse revealed that administration of *B. pertussis* vaccine to mice is associated with the development of impaired β-adrenoceptor responsiveness and in many respects resembles human asthma. The relaxant effects of isoprenaline are impaired in tracheal smooth muscle isolated from *B. pertussis*-vaccinated mice [20]. Further, Giembycz suggested that β2-adrenoceptor desensitization is based on the accelerated degradation of cAMP by phosphodiesterase [21]. Recently, Xiang et al. not only suggested that PDE4D

is an integral component of the β2-adrenoceptor signaling complex but also underscored the critical role of subcellular cAMP regulation in the complex control of receptor signaling [22]. So, we assumed that administration of iBp would be associated with the upregulation of PDE4D activity and expression.

Our allergic model described here provided an experimental system that could be used to further investigate the potential role of iBp on the development of allergy and asthma. This study also confirmed the capabilities of iBp. After subsequent pulmonary antigen challenge, presensitized animals displayed many features of allergic asthma including increased bronchial hyperresponsiveness, eosinophilic inflammation, and mucus production. These data suggested that iBp enhances this sensitization process. The AHR induced by iBp has long been known [23, 24], but the mechanism of this effect was unclear. The effects of iBp may be attributed to lipopolysaccharide (LPS) or pertussis toxin. Importantly, both are agonists of Toll-like receptor 4 but have different downstream effects.

In the present study, we investigated PDE regulation in the lung of OVA+iBp, OVA, and iBp rats. OVA sensitization and challenge increased the cAMP-PDE activity which might be primarily due to upregulation of PDE4 and PDE3, but the decreased cGMP-PDE activity might be primarily due to the downregulation of PDE5. There was no significant contribution of iBp to cAMP-PDE activity and cGMP-PDE activity; this result was consistent with the fewer changes in histology and BALF. The main contribution of iBp was to AHR, rather than to inflammation. Our data suggested that *B. pertussis* specifically enhances AHR and specifically enhances the PDE4 activity and PDE4D expression.

Regulation of PDE4 in allergy and asthma has been investigated by many groups but only in human blood leukocytes, and the data are inconsistent. Some groups reported a significant increase in PDE4 activity in asthmatic or allergic patients [25–29], whereas others found no significant difference in the enzyme activity in such patients

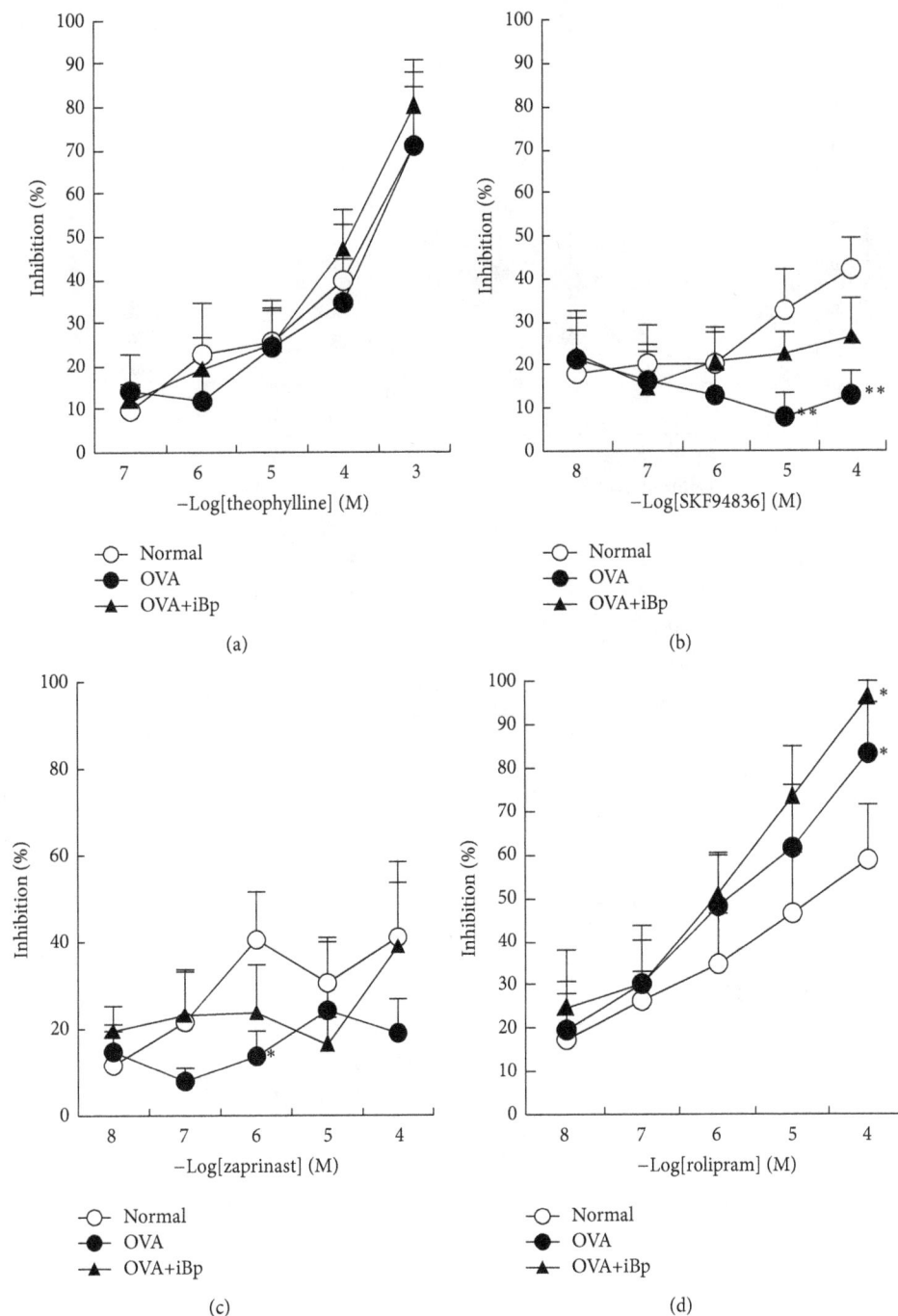

FIGURE 3: Inhibitory effects (%) of theophylline (a), SKF94836 (b), zaprinast (c), and rolipram (d) on the cAMP-PDE activity in the lung homogenates harvested from OVA+iBp and OVA rats (mean ± SEM; $^{*}P < 0.05$; $^{**}P < 0.01$ versus normal).

as compared with healthy individuals [30–33]. PDE4B is involved in the inflammatory process in airways [34]. The only other significant PDE4 gene inducer known thus far is lipopolysaccharide (LPS), which specifically activates the PDE4B gene in monocytes/macrophages [35, 36]. However, in the lungs of allergic rats, expression of the PDE4A and PDE4D genes, but not the PDE4B gene, was upregulated, suggesting that the expression of these genes might be induced by a mechanism(s) distinct from those cAMP or LPS

mechanisms. Our result showing upregulation of PDE4 in the lungs of allergic rats supports the use of PDE4 inhibitors in asthma. Thus, if PDE4 does play a role in the pathogenesis of asthma, lung PDE4 may be as important as, if not more important than, leukocyte PDE4. Various PDE4 subtypes are known to be expressed in different tissues and play distinct biological roles. PDE4B is the predominant subtype in blood neutrophils and monocytes [37] but not in lung, which may explain the unchanged PDE4B mRNA expression.

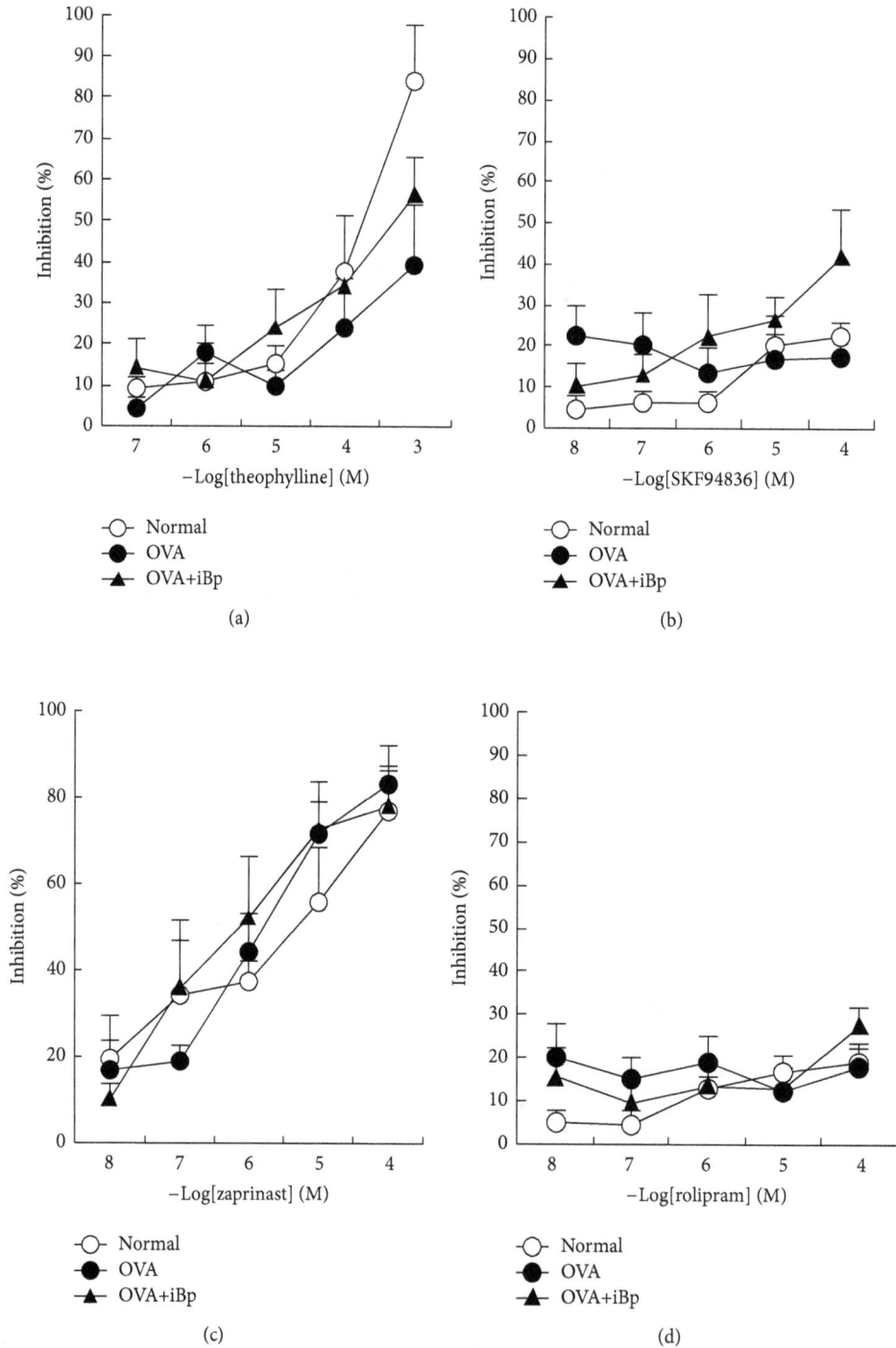

FIGURE 4: Inhibitory effects (%) of theophylline (a), SKF94836 (b), zaprinast (c), and rolipram (d) on the cGMP-PDE activity in the lung homogenates harvested from OVA+iBp and OVA rats (mean ± SEM).

Interestingly, PDE4D gene expression was specially increased in iBp rats. So we assumed there is a relationship between PDE4D and iBp. PDE4A is involved in the inflammatory process in airways [34]. PDE4D gene is involved in emesis [38], which limits the therapeutic use of PDE4 inhibitors. At the same time, PDE4D is also involved in AHR PDE4D-null mice which no longer respond to cholinergic stimulation, and AHR on exposure to antigen is abolished [11]. In addition, animals exposed prenatally but not postnatally to cigarette smoke exhibited increased AHR causally associated with PDE4D mRNA expression in the lung [12]. Recently, PDE4D has been shown to play an important role in vascular diseases, including stroke [39]. These findings demonstrate that the PDE4D gene plays an

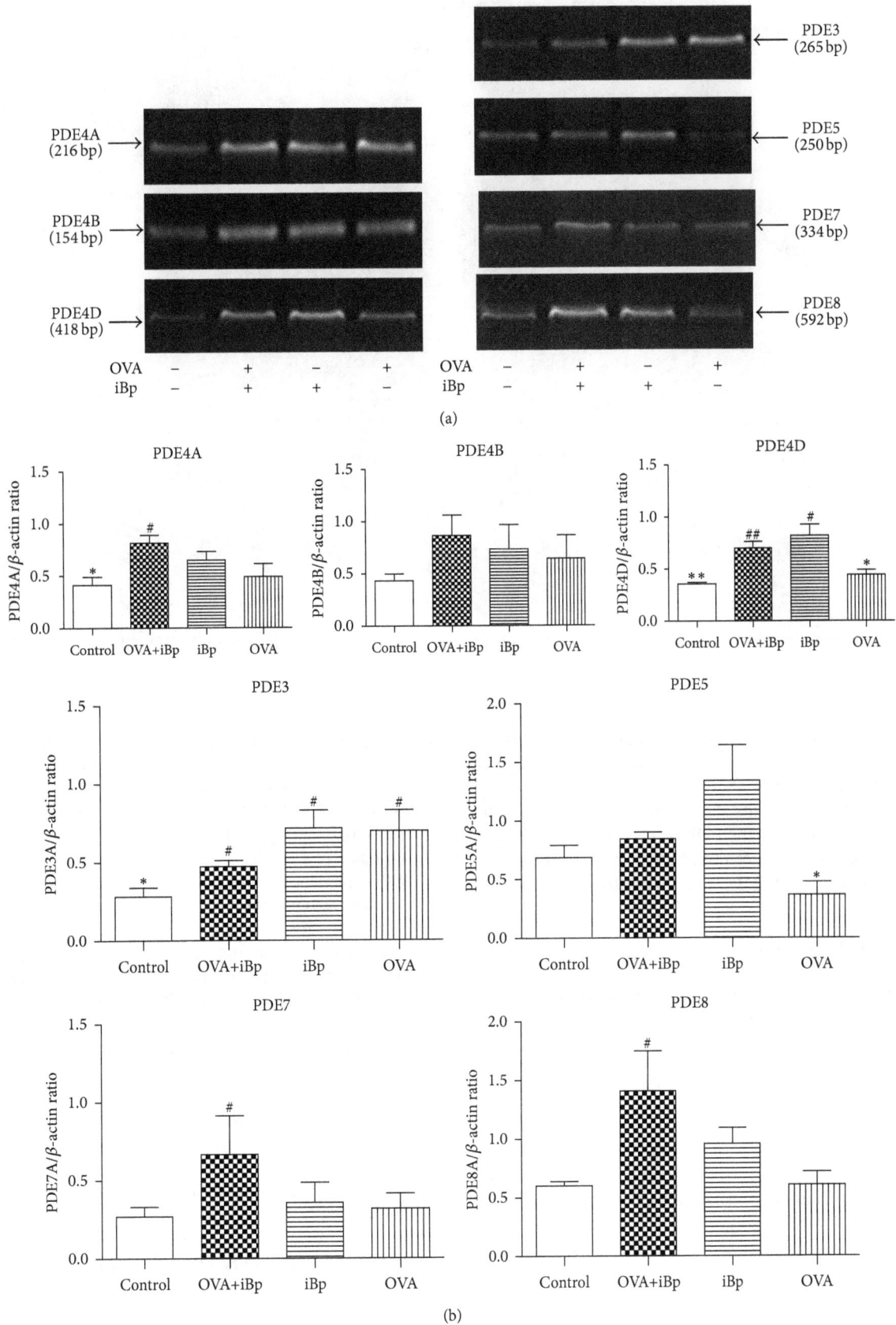

FIGURE 5: (a) Representative image of PDE subtype mRNA expression. (b) Levels of mRNA expression of lung PDE subtypes in normal ($n = 8$), OVA+iBp, iBp ($n = 6$), and OVA rats ($n = 8$). Data are expressed relative to β-actin ($^{*}P < 0.05$; $^{**}P < 0.01$ versus OVA+iBp; $^{#}P < 0.05$; $^{##}P < 0.01$ versus normal).

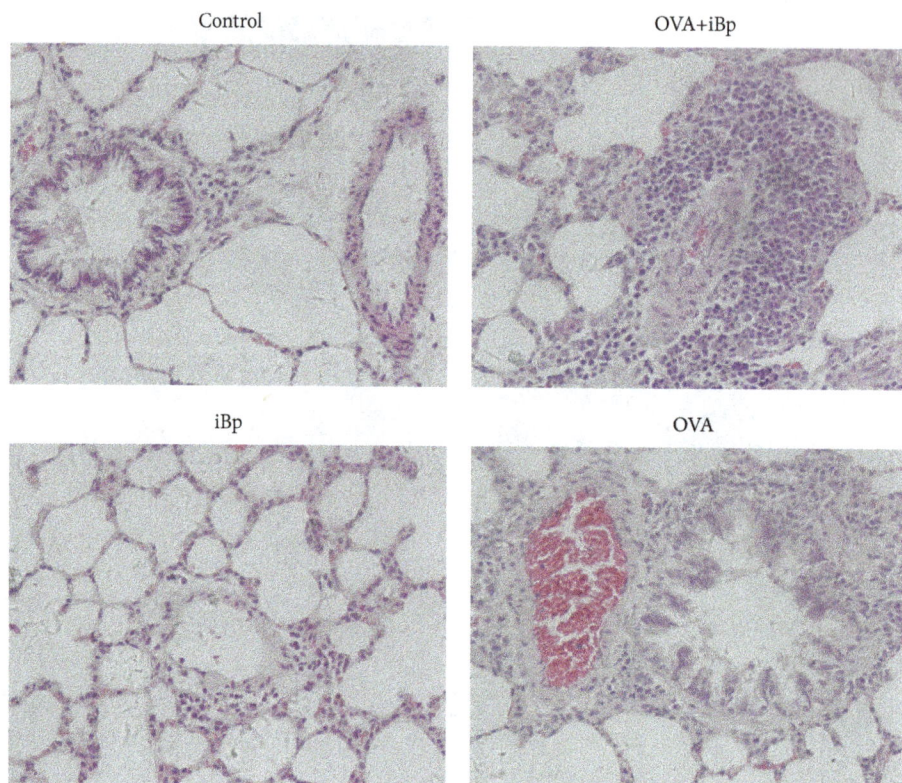

FIGURE 6: Representative histological alterations of the small airways and small blood vessels in control, OVA+iBp, iBp, and OVA rats.

essential role in the development of some disease. How to benefit from PDE4D and avoid the adverse emesis effect is still an important question.

In summary, our results showed that inactivated *B. pertussis* specifically induces the PDE4D expression and airway hyperresponsiveness, rather than inducing inflammation in the lung and upregulating the total PDE activity.

Conflict of Interests

The authors declare that there is no conflict of interests regarding the publication of this paper.

Acknowledgments

The authors thank Professor IC Bruce (Zhejiang University School of Medicine, Zhejiang, China) for modification of the paper. This work is supported by the Zhejiang Provincial Natural Science Foundation (Z204198), the National Natural Science Foundation of China (81170536, 30800497), and Annual Scientific Project of Anhui Province (1301043040).

References

[1] C. E. Reed, "Pertussis sensitization as an animal model for the abnormal bronchial sensitivity of asthma," *Yale Journal of Biology and Medicine*, vol. 40, no. 5, pp. 507–521, 1968.

[2] S. Waserman, R. Olivenstein, P. Renzi, L. J. Xu, and J. G. Martin, "The relationship between late asthmatic responses and antigen-specific immunoglobulin," *Journal of Allergy and Clinical Immunology*, vol. 90, no. 4 I, pp. 661–669, 1992.

[3] H. O. Heuer, B. Wenz, H. Jennewein, and K. Urich, "Characterisation of a novel airway late phase model in the sensitized guinea pig which uses silica and Bordetella pertussis as adjuvant for sensitization," *European Journal of Pharmacology*, vol. 317, no. 2-3, pp. 361–368, 1996.

[4] I. C. Chang and R. Y. Gottshall, "Sensitization to ragweed pollen in Bordetella pertussis infected or vaccine injected mice," *Journal of Allergy and Clinical Immunology*, vol. 54, no. 1, pp. 20–24, 1974.

[5] W. Dong, M. J. K. Selgrade, and M. I. Gilmour, "Systemic administration of Bordetella pertussis enhances pulmonary sensitization to house dust mite in juvenile rats," *Toxicological Sciences*, vol. 72, no. 1, pp. 113–121, 2003.

[6] H. Tang, Y. Song, J. Chen, and P. Wang, "Upregulation of phosphodiesterase-4 in the lung of allergic rats," *American Journal of Respiratory and Critical Care Medicine*, vol. 171, no. 8, pp. 823–828, 2005.

[7] M. Conti, W. Richter, C. Mehats, G. Livera, J. Park, and C. Jin, "Cyclic AMP-specific PDE4 phosphodiesterases as critical components of cyclic AMP signaling," *Journal of Biological Chemistry*, vol. 278, no. 8, pp. 5493–5496, 2003.

[8] M. A. Giembycz, "Development status of second generation PDE4 inhibitors for asthma and COPD: the story so far," *Monaldi Archives for Chest Disease*, vol. 57, no. 1, pp. 48–64, 2002.

[9] C. Méhats, S.-C. Jin, J. Wahlstrom, E. Law, D. T. Umetsu, and M. Conti, "PDE4D plays a critical role in the control of airway smooth muscle contraction," *The FASEB Journal*, vol. 17, no. 13, pp. 1831–1841, 2003.

[10] G. Hansen, S.-. C. Jin, D. T. Umetsu, and M. Conti, "Absence of muscarinic cholinergic airway responses in mice deficient in the cyclic nucleotide phosphodiesterase PDE4D," *Proceedings of the National Academy of Sciences of the United States of America*, vol. 97, no. 12, pp. 6751–6756, 2000.

[11] S. P. Singh, E. G. Barrett, R. Kalra et al., "Prenatal cigarette smoke decreases lung cAMP and increases airway hyperresponsiveness," *American Journal of Respiratory and Critical Care Medicine*, vol. 168, no. 3, pp. 342–347, 2003.

[12] Q. M. Xie, J. Q. Chen, W. H. Shen, and R. L. Bian, "Correlative changes of interferon-γ and interleukin-4 between cortical layer and pulmonary airway of sensitized rats," *Acta Pharmacologica Sinica*, vol. 23, no. 3, pp. 248–252, 2002.

[13] Q. Xie, J. Chen, W. Shen, Q. Yang, and R. Bian, "Effects of cyclosporin A by aerosol on airway hyperresponsiveness and inflammation in guinea pigs," *Acta Pharmacologica Sinica*, vol. 23, no. 3, pp. 243–247, 2002.

[14] Y. H. Song, J. Q. Chen, and H. L. Zhou, "Cyclic nucleotides phosphodiesterase activity in a rat lung model of asthma," *Zhejiang Da Xue Xue Bao Yi Xue Ban*, vol. 31, pp. 127–130, 2002 (Chinese).

[15] M. M. Bradford, "A rapid and sensitive method for the quantitation of microgram quantities of protein utilizing the principle of protein dye binding," *Analytical Biochemistry*, vol. 72, no. 1-2, pp. 248–254, 1976.

[16] C. Clausen, J. Munoz, and R. K. Bergman, "Lymphocytosis and histamine sensitization of mice by fractions from Bordetella pertussis," *Journal of Bacteriology*, vol. 96, no. 5, pp. 1484–1487, 1968.

[17] C. R. Clausen, J. Munoz, and R. K. Bergman, "A reaginic type of antibody stimulated by extracts of Bordetella pertussis in inbred strains of mice," *Journal of Immunology*, vol. 104, no. 2, pp. 312–319, 1970.

[18] D. S. J. Lindsay, R. Parton, and A. C. Wardlaw, "Adjuvant effect of pertussis toxin on the production of anti-ovalbumin IgE in mice and lack of direct correlation between PCA and ELISA," *International Archives of Allergy and Immunology*, vol. 105, no. 3, pp. 281–288, 1994.

[19] S. B. Lehrer, "Role of mouse IgG and IgE homocytotropic antibodies in passive cutaneous anaphylaxis," *Immunology*, vol. 32, no. 4, pp. 507–511, 1977.

[20] T. E. Bartell and W. W. Busse, "Effect of Bordetella pertussis vaccination in mice and the isolated tracheal response to isoprenaline," *Allergy*, vol. 35, no. 4, pp. 291–296, 1980.

[21] M. A. Giembycz, "Phosphodiesterase 4 and tolerance to β_2-adrenoceptor agonists in asthma," *Trends in Pharmacological Sciences*, vol. 17, no. 9, pp. 331–336, 1996.

[22] Y. Xiang, F. Naro, M. Zoudilova, S.-L. C. Jin, M. Conti, and B. Kobilka, "Phosphodiesterase 4D is required for $\beta2$ adrenoceptor subtype-specific signaling in cardiac myocytes," *Proceedings of the National Academy of Sciences of the United States of America*, vol. 102, no. 3, pp. 909–914, 2005.

[23] A. J. M. Schreurs and F. P. Nijkamp, "Contribution of bacterial cell wall compounds to airway hyperreactivity," *European Journal of Respiratory Diseases*, vol. 65, no. 135, pp. 164–167, 1984.

[24] A. Imaizumi, J. Lefort, D. Leduc, A. Lellouch-Tubiana, and B. B. Vargaftig, "Pertussis toxin induces bronchopulmonary

hyperresponsiveness in guinea-pigs while antagonizing the effects of formyl-L-methionyl-L-leucyl-L-phenylalanine," *European Journal of Pharmacology*, vol. 212, no. 2-3, pp. 177–186, 1992.

[25] J. G. Castillo, P. M. Gamboa, B. E. Garcia, and A. Oehling, "Effect of ketotifen on phosphodiesterase activity from asthmatic individuals," *Allergologia et Immunopathologia*, vol. 18, no. 4, pp. 197–201, 1990.

[26] I. C. Crocker, M. K. Church, S. E. Ohia, and R. G. Townley, "Beclomethasone decreases elevations in phosphodiesterase activity in human T lymphocytes," *International Archives of Allergy and Immunology*, vol. 121, no. 2, pp. 151–160, 2000.

[27] J. M. Hanifin and S. C. Chan, "Monocyte phosphodiesterase abnormalities and dysregulation of lymphocyte function in atopic dermatitis," *Journal of Investigative Dermatology*, vol. 105, S84, no. 1, p. S88, 1995.

[28] S. Mue, T. Ise, S. Shibahara, M. Takahashi, and Y. Ono, "Leukocyte cyclic 3′,5′ nucleotide phosphodiesterase activity in human bronchial asthma," *Annals of Allergy*, vol. 37, no. 3, pp. 201–207, 1976.

[29] T. Sawai, K. Ikai, and M. Uehara, "Cyclic adenosine monophosphate phosphodiesterase activity in peripheral blood mononuclear leucocytes from patients with atopic dermatitis: correlation with respiratory atopy," *British Journal of Dermatology*, vol. 138, no. 5, pp. 846–848, 1998.

[30] I. H. Coulson, S. N. Duncan, and C. A. Holden, "Peripheral blood mononuclear leukocyte cyclic adenosine monophosphate specific phosphodiesterase activity in childhood atopic dermatitis," *British Journal of Dermatology*, vol. 120, no. 5, pp. 607–612, 1989.

[31] F. Gantner, H. Tenor, V. Gekeler, C. Schudt, A. Wendel, and A. Hatzelmann, "Phosphodiesterase profiles of highly purified human peripheral blood leukocyte populations from normal and atopic individuals: a comparative study," *Journal of Allergy and Clinical Immunology*, vol. 100, no. 4, pp. 527–535, 1997.

[32] L. J. Landells, D. Spina, J. E. Souness, B. J. O'Connor, and C. P. Page, "A biochemical and functional assessment of monocyte phosphodiesterase activity in healthy and asthmatic subjects," *Pulmonary Pharmacology and Therapeutics*, vol. 13, no. 5, pp. 231–239, 2000.

[33] L. J. Landells, C. M. Szilagy, N. A. Jones et al., "Identification and quantification of phosphodiesterase 4 subtypes in CD4 and CD8 lymphocytes from healthy and asthmatic subjects," *British Journal of Pharmacology*, vol. 133, no. 5, pp. 722–729, 2001.

[34] C. D. Manning, M. Burman, S. B. Christensen et al., "Suppression of human inflammatory cell function by subtype-selective PDE4 inhibitors correlates with inhibition of PDE4A and PDE4B," *The British Journal of Pharmacology*, vol. 128, no. 7, pp. 1393–1398, 1999.

[35] D. Ma, P. Wu, R. W. Egan, M. M. Billah, and P. Wang, "Phosphodiesterase 4B gene transcription is activated by lipopolysaccharide and inhibited by interleukin-10 in human monocytes," *Molecular Pharmacology*, vol. 55, no. 1, pp. 50–57, 1999.

[36] S.-. C. Jin and M. Conti, "Induction of the cyclic nucleotide phosphodiesterase PDE4B is essential for LPS-activated TNF-α responses," *Proceedings of the National Academy of Sciences of the United States of America*, vol. 99, no. 11, pp. 7628–7633, 2002.

[37] P. Wang, P. Wu, K. M. Ohleth, R. W. Egan, and M. M. Billah, "Phosphodiesterase 4B2 is the predominant phosphodiesterase species and undergoes differential regulation of gene expression in human monocytes and neutrophils," *Molecular Pharmacology*, vol. 56, no. 1, pp. 170–174, 1999.

[38] A. Robichaud, P. B. Stamatiou, S.-L. C. Jin et al., "Deletion of phosphodiesterase 4D in mice shortens $\alpha 2$-adrenoceptor-mediated anesthesia, a behavioral correlate of emesis," *The Journal of Clinical Investigation*, vol. 110, no. 7, pp. 1045–1052, 2002.

[39] H. Hakonarson, "Role of FLAP and PDE4D in myocardial infarction and stroke: target discovery and future treatment options," *Current Treatment Options in Cardiovascular Medicine*, vol. 8, no. 3, pp. 183–192, 2006.

Clinical Investigation of Benign Asbestos Pleural Effusion

**Nobukazu Fujimoto,[1] Kenichi Gemba,[2,3] Keisuke Aoe,[4]
Katsuya Kato,[5,6] Takako Yokoyama,[7] Ikuji Usami,[7] Kazuo Onishi,[8]
Keiichi Mizuhashi,[9] Toshikazu Yusa,[10] and Takumi Kishimoto[11]**

[1] Department of Medical Oncology, Okayama Rosai Hospital, 1-10-25 Chikkomidorimachi, Okayama 7028055, Japan

[2] Department of Respiratory Medicine, Okayama Rosai Hospital, 1-10-25 Chikkomidorimachi, Okayama 7028055, Japan

[3] Department of Respiratory Medicine, Chugoku Chuo Hospital, Fukuyama 7200001, Japan

[4] Department of Medical Oncology, Yamaguchi-Ube Medical Center, 685 Higashikiwa, Ube 7550241, Japan

[5] Department of Radiology, Okayama University Hospital, 2-5-1 Shikatacho, Okayama 7008558, Japan

[6] Department of Diagnostic Radiology 2, Kawasaki Medical School, Okayama 7008505, Japan

[7] Department of Respiratory Medicine, Asahi Rosai Hospital, 61 Hirakochokita, Owariasahi 4880875, Japan

[8] Department of Respiratory Medicine, Kobe Rosai Hospital, 4-1-23 Kagoikedori, Chuoku, Kobe 6510053, Japan

[9] Department of Respiratory Medicine, Toyama Rosai Hospital, 992 Rokuromaru, Uozu 9370042, Japan

[10] Department of Thoracic Surgery, Chiba Rosai Hospital, 2-16 Tatsumidaihigashi, Ichihara 2900003, Japan

[11] Department of Internal Medicine, Okayama Rosai Hospital, 1-10-25 Chikkomidorimachi, Okayama 7028055, Japan

Correspondence should be addressed to Nobukazu Fujimoto; nfuji@okayamah.rofuku.go.jp

Academic Editor: Denis Caillaud

There is no detailed information about benign asbestos pleural effusion (BAPE). The aim of the study was to clarify the clinical features of BAPE. The criteria of enrolled patients were as follows: (1) history of asbestos exposure; (2) presence of pleural effusion determined by chest X-ray, CT, and thoracentesis; and (3) the absence of other causes of effusion. Clinical information was retrospectively analysed and the radiological images were reviewed. There were 110 BAPE patients between 1991 and 2012. All were males and the median age at diagnosis was 74 years. The median duration of asbestos exposure and period of latency for disease onset of BAPE were 31 and 48 years, respectively. Mean values of hyaluronic acid, adenosine deaminase, and carcinoembryonic antigen in the pleural fluid were 39,840 ng/mL, 23.9 IU/L, and 1.8 ng/mL, respectively. Pleural plaques were detected in 98 cases (89.1%). Asbestosis was present in 6 (5.5%) cases, rounded atelectasis was detected in 41 (37.3%) cases, and diffuse pleural thickening (DPT) was detected in 30 (27.3%) cases. One case developed lung cancer (LC) before and after BAPE. None of the cases developed malignant pleural mesothelioma (MPM) during the follow-up.

1. Introduction

Asbestos-related pathological changes of the pleura include pleural plaques, malignant pleural mesothelioma (MPM), diffuse pleural thickening (DPT), and benign asbestos pleural effusion (BAPE). BAPE is a nonmalignant pleural disease initially described in 1964 [1]. It is also termed asbestos pleuritis. Once a patient is diagnosed with BAPE, he or she is compensated by workers' compensation in Japan. Epler et al. [2] advocated diagnostic criteria for BAPE, which include (1) previous asbestos exposure, (2) determination of pleural effusion by chest X-ray or thoracentesis, and (3) the absence of other causes of effusion. They also stated that follow-up assessments for at least 3 years were essential to confirm the diagnosis and to exclude the development of malignant diseases such as MPM or lung carcinomatous pleuritis. Later, Hillerdal and Ozesmi [3] described that a 1-year follow-up would be sufficient based on a detailed exploration including computed tomographic (CT) scanning. Most of the previous studies included small numbers of patients and were undertaken in the 1980s, so no detailed information is available about the disease.

In the current study, we retrospectively analysed the clinical features of BAPE in patients in Japan. The aim of the study was to clarify the clinical features of BAPE and to suggest more practical diagnostic standard for the disease.

2. Patients and Methods

2.1. Subjects. Enrolled patients were referred to Rosai Hospital and affiliated hospitals in Japan for an examination for pleural effusion and were finally diagnosed with BAPE. The criteria of enrolled patients were as follows: (1) previous history of asbestos exposure obtained by an in-person questionnaire or interview; (2) presence of pleural effusion determined by chest X-ray, CT, and thoracentesis; and (3) the absence of other causes of effusion. The pleural fluid was collected by thoracentesis or thoracoscopy, and information on cell classification, cytological analysis, and the biochemical examination was extracted from the medical records. Hyaluronic acid (HA), adenosine deaminase (ADA), and carcinoembryonic antigen (CEA) were included among the clinical laboratory tests. The HA concentration was determined using a latex agglutination turbidimetric immunoassay. ADA was measured using an enzymatic technique. CEA was measured using a chemiluminescent immunoassay.

2.2. Data Collection and Analysis. Clinical and demographic information was obtained from the medical records at each facility. The information included age, gender, smoking status, initial symptoms, and results of laboratory testing of the pleural effusion. The work histories, those of the family members, and residential histories were investigated to assess the patient's history of asbestos exposure.

The radiological images were sent to Okayama Rosai Hospital for review. Characteristic radiological findings associated with asbestos exposure were assessed as the presence of pleural effusion, asbestosis, rounded atelectasis, pleural plaques, and DPT. Asbestosis was classified on chest X-rays according to perfusion rate (PR) based on the International Labour Organization (ILO) criteria [4]. DPT was defined as pleural thickening of more than 5 mm on chest X-rays, extending for more than half of the lateral thoracic wall (LTW) in cases of unilateral DPT or more than quarter of the LTW in cases of bilateral DPT [5]. The presence of pleural effusion, rounded atelectasis, and pleural plaques was assessed on chest CT.

Survival data were determined from the day pleural effusion was detected to the day of death or last follow-up and analysed using the Kaplan-Meier method with SPSS 11.0 software (SPSS, Inc., Chicago, IL, USA).

This study was done according to the Ethical Guidelines for Epidemiological Research by the Japanese Ministry of Education, Culture, Sports, Science, and Technology and the Ministry of Health, Labour, and Welfare. This study was approved by Japan Labour Health and Welfare Organization and the institutional review boards of each institution. Patient confidentiality was strictly maintained. This study was carried

TABLE 1: Patient characteristics.

Age (n = 110)	
Median (range)	74 (36–90)
Gender (n = 110)	
Male/female	110/0
Smoking history (n = 63)	
Ever/current	56
Never	7
Symptoms (n = 65, multiple answers)	
Dyspnea	34
Cough	15
Chest pain	13
Fever	3
Palpitation	2
Sputum	1
Wheezing	1
Back pain	1
Weight loss	1
Fatigue	1

out according to the principles set out in the Declaration of Helsinki.

3. Results

3.1. Patient Characteristics. One hundred ten patients from 9 institutions fulfilled the enrolled criteria based on the descriptions in their medical records and review of the radiographs between 1991 and 2012. Characteristics of the patients are shown in Table 1. Smoking history was obtained in 63 cases including 56 ever/current smokers and 7 never smokers, with the median (range) pack-years of 34.5 (0–112). Pleural effusion was found in 56 cases in the right, 25 in the left, and 27 in both thoracis. Sixty-five patients visited the clinic for subjective symptoms, and pleural effusion was detected at the regular medical check-up in 35 cases without any symptoms. Pleural effusion was detected during the treatment of other diseases in another 15 cases. Thoracentesis was performed in all patients to collect pleural fluid. Thoracoscopic exploration was done in 78 patients to exclude carcinomatous pleuritis or MPM and to confirm the diagnosis of BAPE.

3.2. Asbestos Exposure History. A history of asbestos exposure was reported by 109 patients, with one patient whose detailed information of asbestos exposure was not obtained. Among the 109 patients, 108 patients had a history of occupational asbestos exposure and one patient had a history of environmental asbestos exposure. The occupational categories associated with asbestos exposure are shown in Table 2. The median (range) age of the first exposure to asbestos was 21.5 (14–58) years. The median (range) duration of asbestos exposure was 31 (0.75–50) years and the median (range) period of latency for disease onset of BAPE was 48 (17–76) years.

TABLE 2: Occupational category related to asbestos exposure.

Shipbuilding	25
Construction	20
Chemical facility	10
Asbestos products manufacturing	8
Electrical work	8
Plumbing	7
Asbestos transportation	5
Moisturizing work	4
Asbestos spraying	3
Steel production	3
Demolition work	2
Automobile manufacturing	2
Heat insulation	2
Firebrick manufacturing	2
Glasswork	1
Metallic product manufacture	1
Furnace installation	1
Coating industry	1
Shipman	1
Others	2
Total	108

TABLE 3: Concomitant asbestos-related radiological findings.

Findings		n	%
Pleural plaques		98	89.1
Calcified		76	
Asbestosis		6	5.7
	1	3	
PR[†]	2	2	
	3	1	
Rounded atelectasis		41	37.3
DPT[‡]		30	27.3

[†]Perfusion rate, [‡]diffuse pleural thickening.

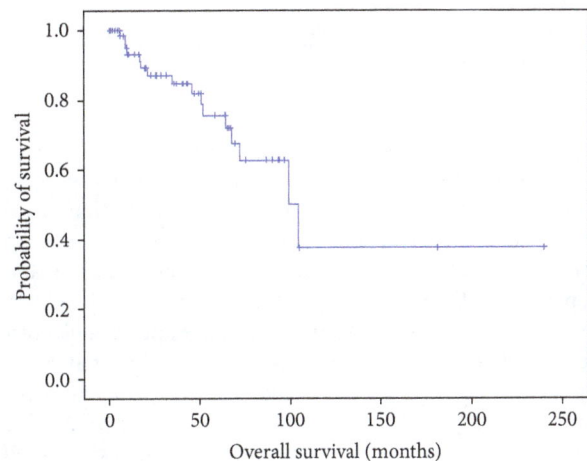

FIGURE 1: Overall survival of patients with benign asbestos-related pleural effusions at Okayama Rosai Hospital.

3.3. Characteristics of the Pleural Effusion.

Information regarding the pleural effusion was obtained in 104 cases. The gross impression of the pleural fluid was bloody in 75 cases, light yellow in 27, and light brown and dark red in 1 case each. The effusions were exudative in all cases. A cellular classification of the fluid was obtained in 57 cases and the median proportions of lymphocytes, macrophages, neutrophils, and eosinophils were 77.7%, 9.7%, 8.0%, and 8.0%, respectively. The HA concentration was determined in 106 cases and the mean (standard deviation) concentration was 39,840 (40,228) ng/mL. Mean (standard deviation) values of ADA and CEA were 23.9 (24.9) IU/L and 1.8 (1.3) ng/mL, respectively.

3.4. Concomitant Asbestos-Related Findings.

As shown in Table 3, pleural plaques were detected in 98 cases (89.1%), among which 76 cases were calcified. Asbestosis was present in 6 cases, rounded atelectasis was detected in 41 cases (37.3%), and DPT was detected in 30 cases (27.3%). One of the cases developed lung cancer (LC) before and after diagnosis of BAPE. The patient had undergone right upper lobectomy for LC two years before his BAPE diagnosis and left partial lobectomy for another LC two years after his BAPE diagnosis.

3.5. Clinical Course.

In most of the cases, thoracentesis and/or thoracotomy were done to collect the fluid and drain the pleural effusion. Oral steroids were prescribed in 5 cases and one of them demonstrated temporal decrease of the effusion. Survival data was obtained in 70 cases from Okayama Rosai Hospital. As shown in Figure 1, median overall survival was 104.2 months (95% confidence interval (CI), 67.3–141.0 months) after a median observation period of

73.0 months (95% CI, 16.2–268.2 months). There were 17 dead cases out of 70 cases at the analysis. The causes of death were determined in 11 cases including 7 respiratory failure cases and each 1 of renal failure, suicide, septic shock due to urinary tract infection, and death of old age. There were 9 cases that developed DPT out of the 17 cases, including the 7 dead cases of respiratory failure. At the time of the analysis, none of the cases had developed MPM.

4. Discussion

In the current study, we examined the clinical features of BAPE and demonstrated that BAPE developed after long-term asbestos exposure. In a previous report, BAPE occurred 15–20 years after exposure and was more common in younger patients aged 21–40 years [6]. In another report, the interval between asbestos exposure and presentation of BAPE varied between 5 and more than 30 years, and early onset was correlated with higher asbestos exposure [7]. Wagner reported that BAPEs were usually unilateral, and the most common manifestation of asbestos-related pleural disease occurred 10 to 20 years after exposure [8]. A limitation of these earlier studies is that the diagnosis criteria of BAPE were ambiguous in the studies. The median latency period between asbestos exposure and BAPE development in the current study was

TABLE 4: Proposed diagnostic criteria of benign asbestos pleural effusion.

Diagnostic criteria
(1) Asbestos exposure history.
(2) Exudative effusion.
(3) Exclusion of other pleuritides such as lung cancer, MPM[†], and tuberculous pleuritis by radiological examination and pleural biopsy via thoracoscopy.
Additional diagnostic information
(1) In cases thoracoscopy could not be undergone, the diagnosis should be discussed based on the bacteriological examination and biochemical markers below.
(a) Elevated carcinoembryonic antigen (>5 ng/mL) suggests carcinomatous pleuritis.
(b) Elevated adenosine deaminase (>35 IU/L) suggests tuberculous pleuritis.
(c) Elevated hyaluronic acid (>100,000 ng/dL) suggests MPM.
(2) In cases with some concomitant medical problem such as autoimmune diseases, the activity of the disease should be carefully evaluated.

[†]Malignant pleural mesothelioma.

48 years, which was similar to that observed for MPM (41 years), LC (47 years), and asbestos-induced DPT (46 years) in our previous reports [4, 9, 10]. We consider that BAPE develops after a long latency period in those with a history of asbestos exposure. There is one point, however, that most of the patients of BAPE in the current study have associated with other asbestos-related lesions such as rounded atelectasis and/or diffuse pleural thickening. It is possible that BAPE might have been developed earlier in these cases, and this could be an explanation of the longer latency of BAPE than previously published. The current study suggests that BAPE can develop after moderate-to-high levels of exposure to asbestos, because the occupational category of the subjects in the current study included those of relatively high levels of asbestos exposure such as asbestos product manufacturing, construction, and shipbuilding, although the correlation between the exposure amount and development of BAPE is unclear. The subjects in the current study included substantial portion of those with smoking history. To our knowledge, the correlation between BAPE and smoking history has not been reported.

The diagnosis of BAPE should be based on a history of asbestos exposure and an exclusion of other causes of effusion such as tuberculous pleuritis, bacterial pleuritis, collagen diseases, heart failure, and malignant conditions such as MPM and LC. In our analysis, the gross impression of the pleural fluid was bloody in 72% of the cases, and cellular classification of the fluid demonstrated lymphocyte dominancy. These results are similar to those of a previous report showing that the effusion was exudative and could be hemorrhagic, as well as predominantly eosinophilic [11].

In cases of LC, tumor cells are detected in the fluid in more than 60% of cases [12]. In cases with MPM, tumor cells can be detected in the pleural fluid, but the detection rate has been reported as less than 30% [13]. Tuberculosis pleuritis or bacterial pleuritis could be diagnosed by staining for acid-fast bacteria, polymerase chain reaction detection, or bacterial culture, although the detection rate is usually low. These analyses may not always determine the diagnosis but should be undergone to exclude MPM, LC, and tuberculosis or bacterial pleuritis and to make the diagnosis of BAPE.

In addition, we analysed some markers such as HA concentration, ADA, and CEA. Recently, we reported the clinical usefulness of HA for the differential diagnosis of MPM and BAPE [14]. In cases with tuberculosis pleuritis, elevated values of ADA could help in the diagnosis [15]. However, elevated ADA may not be limited to tuberculous pleuritis, as it is also present in LC or MPM [16]. In cases with elevated CEA values, carcinomatous pleuritis is strongly suggested [17]. These markers should be determined to exclude these conditions and to confirm a diagnosis of BAPE. However, the differential diagnosis of MPM and BAPE is especially difficult, even when based on these markers. Especially in cases with exudative pleural effusions, thoracoscopic exploration and pleural biopsy should be performed to exclude MPM and confirm the diagnosis of BAPE [18].

Based on the findings in the current study and previous reports, we propose more practical diagnostic standard for the diagnosis of BAPE including (1) asbestos exposure history, (2) exudative effusion, and (3) exclusion of other pleuritides such as LC, MPM, and tuberculous pleuritis by radiological examination and pleural biopsy via thoracoscopy. Additional diagnostic information is as follows: (1) in cases thoracoscopy could not be undergone, the diagnosis should be discussed based on the bacteriological examination and biochemical markers such as CEA, ADA, and HA; in cases with elevated CEA (>5 ng/mL), ADA (>35 IU/L), or HA (>100,000 ng/dL), carcinomatous pleuritis, tuberculous pleuritis, or MPM is more likely, respectively; and (2) in cases with some concomitant medical problem such as autoimmune diseases, the activity of the disease should be carefully evaluated, because autoimmune diseases such as systemic lupus erythematosus or rheumatoid arthritis could involve the pleura and cause pleural effusion (Table 4).

"Benign" is meant to refer to a nonmalignant process, but these effusions can be associated with significant morbidity [19]. The effusion generally takes a long time to resolve. It may resolve spontaneously or be followed by DPT, which causes extrapulmonary restriction and may thereby ultimately become disabling. Previous studies reported that a considerable number of patients with BAPE subsequently developed DPT [2, 3]. Actually, in our previous study, half the patients with asbestos-induced DPT had a history of BAPE [4]. Furthermore, in the current study one patient developed LC before and after being diagnosed with BAPE. The risks of developing MPM or LC in patients with BAPE are increased compared with those of the general population because of their past history of asbestos exposure. Particular attention should be paid to the management of patients with BAPE.

There are a few limitations to the current study. First, this was a retrospective study. Second, pathological analyses including immunohistochemistry were not reviewed. In addition, there are recent reports that increased uptake of fluorodeoxyglucose (FDG) by positron emission tomography (PET) may be a useful marker to distinguish MPM from benign pleural disease [20, 21]. In addition, recent reports revealed that biomarkers such as soluble mesothelin-related peptides (SMRP) are selectively elevated in patients with MPM [22, 23]. A clinical study to evaluate the utility of PET and/or SMRP for the differentiation between MPM and BAPE is warranted.

5. Conclusions

BAPE develops after a long latency period after past asbestos exposure. The diagnosis of BAPE should be based on the exclusion of other pleural diseases. A thorough evaluation, including diagnostic thoracentesis and cytological and bacterial analysis, must be performed. Clinical markers such as HA, ADA, and CEA might help with the differential diagnosis. However, thoracoscopic exploration and pleural biopsy should be performed to confirm a diagnosis of BAPE.

Disclosure

This study is a part of "the research and development and the dissemination projects related to the 9 fields of occupational injuries and illnesses" of Japan Labour Health and Welfare Organization. This organization had no involvement in the study design, collection, analysis, and interpretation of the data, writing of the paper, or decision to submit the paper for publication.

Conflict of Interests

The authors declare that there is no conflict of interests in their submitted paper.

References

[1] H. B. Eisenstadt, "Asbestos pleurisy," *Diseases of the Chest*, vol. 46, pp. 78–81, 1964.

[2] G. R. Epler, T. C. McLoud, and E. A. Gaensler, "Prevalence and incidence of benign asbestos pleural effusion in a working population," *The Journal of the American Medical Association*, vol. 247, no. 5, pp. 617–622, 1982.

[3] G. Hillerdal and M. Ozesmi, "Benign asbestos pleural effusion: 73 exudates in 60 patients," *European Journal of Respiratory Diseases*, vol. 71, no. 2, pp. 113–121, 1987.

[4] N. Fujimoto, K. Kato, I. Usami et al., "Asbestos-related diffuse pleural thickening," *Respiration*, vol. 88, no. 4, pp. 277–284, 2014.

[5] American Thoracic Society, "Medical Section of the American Lung Association: the diagnosis of nonmalignant diseases related to asbestos," *American Review of Respiratory Disease*, vol. 134, pp. 363–368, 1986.

[6] P. Ernst and J. Zejda, "Pleural and airway diseases associated with mineral fibers," in *Mineral Fibers and Health*, D. Lidderll and K. Miller, Eds., pp. 121–134, CRC, Boca Raton, Fla, USA, 1991.

[7] B. W. S. Robinson and A. W. Musk, "Benign asbestos pleural effusion: diagnosis and course," *Thorax*, vol. 36, no. 12, pp. 896–900, 1981.

[8] G. R. Wagner, "Asbestosis and silicosis," *The Lancet*, vol. 349, no. 9061, pp. 1311–1315, 1997.

[9] T. Kishimoto, K. Gemba, N. Fujimoto et al., "Clinical study on mesothelioma in Japan: relevance to occupational asbestos exposure," *American Journal of Industrial Medicine*, vol. 53, no. 11, pp. 1081–1087, 2010.

[10] T. Kishimoto, K. Gemba, N. Fujimoto et al., "Clinical study of asbestos-related lung cancer in Japan with special reference to occupational history," *Cancer Science*, vol. 101, no. 5, pp. 1194–1198, 2010.

[11] A. J. Ghio and V. L. Roggli, "Diagnosis and initial management of nonmalignant diseases related to asbestos," *American Journal of Respiratory and Critical Care Medicine*, vol. 170, no. 6, pp. 691–715, 2004.

[12] K. B. Sriram, V. Relan, B. E. Clarke et al., "Diagnostic molecular biomarkers for malignant pleural effusions," *Future Oncology*, vol. 7, no. 6, pp. 737–752, 2011.

[13] A. Medford and N. Maskell, "Pleural effusion," *Postgraduate Medical Journal*, vol. 81, no. 961, pp. 702–710, 2005.

[14] N. Fujimoto, K. Gemba, M. Asano et al., "Hyaluronic acid in the pleural fluid of patients with malignant pleural mesothelioma," *Respiratory Investigation*, vol. 51, no. 2, pp. 92–97, 2013.

[15] A. Gopi, S. M. Madhavan, S. K. Sharma, and S. A. Sahn, "Diagnosis and treatment of tuberculous pleural effusion in 2006," *Chest*, vol. 131, no. 3, pp. 880–889, 2007.

[16] Y. Ogata, K. Aoe, A. Hiraki et al., "Is adenosine deaminase in pleural fluid a useful marker for differentiating tuberculosis from lung cancer or mesothelioma in Japan, a country with intermediate incidence of tuberculosis?" *Acta Medica Okayama*, vol. 65, no. 4, pp. 259–263, 2011.

[17] H.-Z. Shi, Q.-L. Liang, J. Jiang, X.-J. Qin, and H.-B. Yang, "Diagnostic value of carcinoembryonic antigen in malignant pleural effusion: a meta-analysis," *Respirology*, vol. 13, no. 4, pp. 518–527, 2008.

[18] A. Scherpereel, P. Astoul, P. Baas et al., "Guidelines of the European Respiratory Society and the European Society of Thoracic Surgeons for the management of malignant pleural mesothelioma," *European Respiratory Journal*, vol. 35, no. 3, pp. 479–495, 2010.

[19] R. Myers, "Asbestos-related pleural disease," *Current Opinion in Pulmonary Medicine*, vol. 18, no. 4, pp. 377–381, 2012.

[20] F. Bénard, D. Sterman, R. J. Smith, L. R. Kaiser, S. M. Albelda, and A. Alavi, "Metabolic imaging of malignant pleural mesothelioma with fluorodeoxyglucose positron emission tomography," *Chest*, vol. 114, no. 3, pp. 713–722, 1998.

[21] H. Yildirim, M. Metintas, E. Entok et al., "Clinical value of fluorodeoxyglucose-positron emission tomography/computed tomography in differentiation of malignant mesothelioma from

asbestos-related benign pleural disease: an observational pilot study," *Journal of Thoracic Oncology*, vol. 4, no. 12, pp. 1480–1484, 2009.

[22] A. Scherpereel, B. Grigoriu, M. Conti et al., "Soluble mesothe-lin-related peptides in the diagnosis of malignant pleural mesothelioma," *American Journal of Respiratory and Critical Care Medicine*, vol. 173, no. 10, pp. 1155–1160, 2006.

[23] N. Fujimoto, K. Gemba, M. Asano et al., "Soluble mesothelin-related protein in pleural effusion from patients with malignant pleural mesothelioma," *Experimental and Therapeutic Medicine*, vol. 1, no. 2, pp. 313–317, 2010.

Retrospective Observations on the Ability to Diagnose and Manage Patients with Asthma through the Use of Impulse Oscillometry: Comparison with Spirometry and Overview of the Literature

Constantine Saadeh,[1,2,3] **Blake Cross,**[1,2] **Charles Saadeh,**[1,2,3] **and Michael Gaylor**[1,2,4]

[1] *Amarillo Center for Clinical Research (ACCR), TX, USA*
[2] *Allergy, Asthma, Rheumatology Treatment Specialist (Allergy ARTS), 6842 Plum Creek Dr, Amarillo, TX 79124, USA*
[3] *Texas Tech University Health Sciences Center, USA*
[4] *University of North Texas School for Osteopathic Medicine, USA*

Correspondence should be addressed to Constantine Saadeh; aarts@allergyarts.com

Academic Editor: Hisako Matsumoto

Objective. Impulse oscillometry (IOS) is an evolving technology for the diagnosis and followup of patients with asthma. Our objective is to review the findings on patients who underwent both spirometry and IOS during clinical evaluations of their asthma. The goal was to retrospectively evaluate IOS during the initial diagnosis and followup of patients with asthma in comparison with spirometry. *Methods.* We routinely perform IOS and spirometry evaluation in patients with suspected asthma during baseline visits and at followup. We reviewed the data on 39 patients over the age of 13 with asthma at baseline and following treatment with inhaled corticosteroids. IOS and spirometry were both done at baseline, following short acting bronchodilator administration, and at followup after at least three months of inhaled corticosteroid treatment. *Results.* IOS showed improvement in airway function both initially, following short acting bronchodilator introduction, and later after initiation of long term inhaled corticosteroid treatment, even when the spirometry did not reveal improvement. We noted the IOS improvement in the reactance or AX as well as the resistance in smaller airways or R5. *Conclusion.* IOS may provide a useful measure towards identifying an asthma diagnosis and followup without inducing the extra respiratory effort spirometry requires.

1. Introduction and Background

Impulse oscillometry measures both small and large airways resistance and resonance capacitance of the lung [1]. Its main advantage is its ability to perform these measurements in a noninvasive, relatively effort independent, and minimally intrusive manner during spontaneous normal tidal breathing [1–3].

In contrast to traditional spirometry, impulse oscillometry or IOS traces its findings independent of age, height, weight or gender on adolescents and adults aged 13 years or older [1, 4]. The most relevant outcome of IOS measures include R5 (resistance in small airways), R15 or higher (resistance in larger airways), and AX (low frequency integrated impedance reactance at R5).

These values can be compared to baseline following short acting bronchodilator use or longitudinally while patients are under treatment for chronic asthma via inhaled corticosteroids [5, 6].

IOS has been applied in few studies in asthma diagnosis and management. In these studies [4, 5, 7–13] asthma had already been diagnosed, and patients were included based upon symptoms and baseline abnormal spirometry. In this report, we reviewed the data on patients with initial symptoms of allergic asthma and allergic rhinitis in our clinic who had spirometry and IOS at baseline, following bronchodilator administration, and later, after treatment with inhaled corticosteroids. In this report the role of IOS utilization in routine clinical practice is examined retrospectively at both baseline and followup.

2. Methods

(a) 39 patients aged 13 years and older with a history of asthma or unexplained shortness of breath with allergic rhinitis were routinely evaluated at baseline with spirometry and IOS. The diagnosis of asthma was made by history of wheezing, cough, or shortness of breath. Some of the patients also reported history of asthma prior to coming to this office for evaluation. However, they have not been treated for asthma before. Family history of asthma was also confirmed in at least 30 of these patients. Patients with smoking history have been excluded. Also, by reviewing the charts as well patients with history of secondhand smoke were also excluded. The patients were routinely given a nebulized bronchodilator and the same measurements were obtained following its administration. Patients were then followed up at a minimum of three months of treatment regimens with various inhaled corticosteroids. The same measurements were obtained and recorded. IRB approval was granted for this study.

(b) Spirometry and IOS diagnostics were conducted utilizing a Jaeger (c) instrument. The technique of IOS measurement was as described in [1, 14]. Briefly patients were seated comfortably in a nonswivel chair. Nose clips were applied, and a special mouthpiece was used. Patients were allowed to breathe normally while a loudspeaker component of the instrument delivered intermittent multifrequency impulses over a minimum of 30 second duration. A trained technician guided, comforted, and assisted the patient in following the tracing as at least 3 sinusoidal readings were obtained. We chose the recording with the best coherence at frequencies from 5 to 30 Hz. The ideal coherence was 0.9, 1, 1, and 1 at 5, 10, 15, and 20 Hz, respectively. The technician was also trained to capture subclinical leaks through the mouthpiece and leak recordings were discarded. The values we obtained were recorded as R5, R15, and AX (the integrated impedance reactance at R5 and above). We then recorded spirometry after IOS in the same setting. Forced expiratory volume of the first second, or FEV1, was recorded and the results were obtained according to the guidelines of the American Thoracic Society.

(c) We tabulated results as outlined below. Interference from cough, swallowing, or breath holding was identified and discarded during spirometry. Patients were treated with various inhaled corticosteroids (ICS) or ICS/LABA (inhaled corticosteroid and long acting beta agonist combination). We noted posttreatment results for at least three months later. We gathered histories and conducted exams also.

All patients had reported symptoms and a history of asthma with or without allergic rhinitis.

(d) Statistics. Data were analyzed via the (Welch's) t-test utilizing the t-test comparison. A statistically significant difference was considered at P value of less than or equal to 0.05.

3. Results

Table 1 summarizes the demographic and background information of the patients as well as the results of pre- and post-ronchodilator and Table 2 summarizes the follow-up treatment of at least three months. In both situations the IOS, and particularly the AX, provided a reliable indicator of improvement. FEV1 did show improvement in some patients, but AX consistently showed improvement in almost every patient followed after consistent inhaled corticosteroid use. Figure 1 illustrates a typical patient with asthma and the IOS measurement before and after administration of a short acting Beta agonist (levalbuterol) at baseline evaluation. Also in Figure 1, we included in the third column the type of inhaled corticosteroids, alone or in combination, that the patients were placed on at presentation. Figure 2 shows the same patient following treatment with inhaled corticosteroids and improvement in AX. The retrospective clinical data we utilized and present appear to support the hypothesis that IOS may play an important role in evaluating and following patients with asthma—even when the baseline FEV1 is normal or does not change with treatment.

FEF 25–75% was also measured in the same patients. Improvement from a low abnormal (<80% level of predicted) was noted in only five patients. Improvement from a normal baseline of ≥80% of predicted was noted in nine patients. The improvement was defined as a change of 15% of predicted over baseline after nebulizer from baseline or after inhaled corticosteroid treatment.

Based on our data, even though the FEF 25–75% was helpful in few patients, the majority of patients did not show a response pattern for FEF 25–75% (data not shown).

4. Discussion

In adults aged 13 years and older, the R5 value in cm of H_2O is the summation of large and small airways [1, 15, 16]. Typically R5 is approximately 3 cm H_2O or less. R15 is a direct measure of larger airways and R15 is about 2 cm H_2O or less. Therefore, absolute measurement of small airways is R5–R15 [1, 15, 16]. R5 in general is the larger number than R15 or R20. Therefore, R5 is a reflection of small airways while R15 is directly correlated with larger airways. It is possible that R5 can be equal to R15 or R20 and the difference, therefore, will be 0. In this situation, it only reflects that the airways are completely normal [1].

AX by definition is the area under X curve and is reflective of the reactance of the lung in response to the instrument's loudspeaker stimuli. This value reflects the integral reactance of small airways, and may by itself be an index of small airway response to the external application of multiple frequency

TABLE 1: Patient Spirometry and IOS Baseline.

Asthma patient	Age	Inhaled steroid	Before FEV1	Post bronchodilator FEV1	% Chg	Before AX	Post bronchodilator AX	% Chg	Before R5	Post bronchodilator R5	% Chg	Before R15	After R15	% Chg
1	41	Mometasone furoate	4.03	3.27	-19.00%	11.98	6.94	-42.10%	4.12	3.41	-17.30%	3.2	2.62	-18.30%
2	41	Fluticasone/salmeterol	4.16	4.12	-1.00%	10.37	6.36	-38.70%	4.03	3.86	-4.10%	2.83	2.77	-1.90%
3	45	Ciclesonide	3.6	2.94	-18.30%	4.44	5.24	17.90%	2.78	2.47	-10.90%	1.99	1.64	-17.50%
4	78	Mometasone furoate	2.26	2.74	21.60%	7.05	3.13	-55.50%	2.79	72.2	-15.90%	1.87	1.74	-7.20%
5	65	Budesonide/formoterol	1.5	1.79	19.10%	6.22	3.81	-38.70%	3.02	2.36	-21.80%	2.07	1.69	-18.20%
6	71	Beclomethasone dipropionate	1.37	1.28	-6.40%	32.15	24.39	-24.20%	6.18	5.25	-15.00%	3.74	3.71	-1.10%
7	44	Budesonide/formoterol	3.54	3.87	9.20%	11.82	2.49	-78.90%	4.55	3.21	-29.40%	3.85	2.91	-24.40%
8	47	Mometasone furoate	2.18	2.65	21.40%	7.74	5.59	-27.80%	3.62	3.48	-3.90%	2.53	2.62	3.70%
9	59	Ciclesonide	2.26	2.26	0.20%	8.71	6.75	-22.50%	3.71	3.24	-12.60%	2.49	2.21	-11.00%
10	35	Mometasone furoate	3.81	4.01	5.10%	7.4	6.5	-12.20%	3.01	3.56	18.20%	2.32	2.46	5.80%
11	60	Mometasone furoate	1.91	1.95	2.40%	23.86	19.05	-20.20%	6.47	5.29	-18.20%	3.98	3.31	-16.80%
12	31	Ciclesonide	4.13	4.13	-0.10%	2.28	1.04	-54.60%	2.72	2.43	-10.60%	2.29	2.29	-0.30%
13	51	Budesonide/formoterol	1.97	1.85	-6.00%	14.32	11.78	-17.70%	4.64	4.14	-11.00%	2.72	2.64	-2.80%
14	29	Mometasone furoate	3.93	4.18	5.30%	4.08	2.99	-26.70%	2.39	2.45	2.60%	1.92	1.8	-6.20%
15*	36	Mometasone furoate	3.61	3.89	7.80%	6.32	4.59	-27.30%	3.14	3.37	7.20%	2.76	2.94	6.70%
16	51	Budesonide	2.32	2.36	1.90%	7.43	5.63	-24.30%	2.79	3.11	11.50%	2.29	2.39	4.20%
17	50	Budesonide	3.11	3.25	4.70%	3.05	1.88	-38.20%	3.63	3.05	-15.90%	3.19	2.67	-16.30%
18	83	Fluticasone/salmeterol	2.49	2.21	-11.30%	6.36	9.18	44.30%	2.25	2.66	18.20%	1.84	1.8	-2.20%
19	57	Fluticasone/salmeterol	1.91	1.94	1.50%	22.44	20.31	-9.50%	4.3	4.18	-2.80%	2.75	2.67	-3.20%
20	37	Mometasone furoate	3.78	3.51	-7.10%	7.41	5.34	-28.00%	3.69	3.37	-8.60%	2.85	2.66	-6.90%
21	51	Ciclesonide	2.64	2.73	3.50%	9.4	7.54	-19.80%	4.01	3.31	-17.40%	2.88	2.48	-14.00%
22	24	Mometasone furoate	3.95	3.72	-5.70%	5.55	2.95	-46.80%	2.92	2.41	-17.40%	2.17	1.91	-12.00%
23	35	Budesonide/formoterol	2.38	2.86	20.50%	6.23	2.35	-62.20%	3.56	2.18	-38.70%	3.15	1.95	-38.20%
24	61	Budesonide/formoterol	2.48	2.56	3.20%	10.87	9.11	-16.20%	3.86	3.58	-7.30%	2.62	2.43	-7.30%
25	33	Mometasone furoate	2.74	2.73	-0.30%	9.86	9.56	-3.00%	3.66	4.09	11.80%	2.41	2.49	3.30%
26	49	Mometasone furoate	2.96	2.99	1.20%	7.66	6.06	-20.80%	3.97	3.86	-2.90%	3.06	3.05	-0.10%
27	65	Fluticasone/salmeterol	1.73	1.87	7.90%	4.78	5.55	16.10%	2.97	3.99	34.20%	2.4	3.66	52.50%
28	31	Mometasone furoate	2.56	2.19	-14.40%	5.37	2.96	-44.90%	3.73	3.38	-9.40%	2.64	2.8	6.00%
29	74	Mometasone furoate	1.6	1.67	4.90%	14.06	11.15	-20.70%	3.65	3.23	-11.50%	2.54	2.38	-6.30%
30	54	Ciclesonide	2.36	2.7	14.10%	5.23	2.08	-60.20%	2.6	2.18	-15.90%	2.05	1.87	-8.80%
31	54	Ciclesonide	2.53	2.54	0.40%	9.46	7.24	-23.50%	2.85	2.76	-3.10%	1.94	1.87	-3.60%
32	53	Ciclesonide	3.01	3.1	3.10%	20.7	18.9	-8.70%	4.83	4.97	2.80%	3.28	3.17	-3.30%
33	60	Budesonide/formoterol	1.63	1.7	4.40%	15.32	4.46	-70.90%	4.91	3.83	-22.20%	3.9	3.34	-14.20%
34	80	Mometasone furoate	2.3	2.54	10.10%	19.97	5.98	-70.00%	4.2	2.97	-29.40%	2.85	2.29	-19.80%
35	65	Fluticasone/salmeterol	1.69	1.8	6.70%	16.32	7.38	-54.80%	4.45	3.41	-23.20%	2.95	2.47	-16.30%
36	71	Mometasone furoate	1.56	1.67	6.70%	5.68	7.31	28.80%	2.11	3.08	46.20%	1.7	2.42	42.20%
37	23	Fluticasone/salmeterol	3.36	3.74	11.30%	21.19	5.63	-73.40%	4.39	2.85	-35.00%	2.86	2.38	-16.90%
38	63	Beclomethasone dipropionate	2.73	2.77	1.60%	6.05	4.69	-22.40%	3.07	2.83	-8.00%	2.33	2.22	-4.90%
39	52	Budesonide	1.81	1.97	8.60%	15.74	6.46	-58.90%	3.8	2.66	-30.00%	2.4	1.72	28.20%

*denotes patient that is referenced in Figure 1.

TABLE 2: Patient followup.

Asthma patient	Followup FEV1	Followup AX	Followup R5	Followup R15	FEV1 % chg	AX % chg	R5 % chg	R15 % chg
1	4.01	9.69	3.51	2.67	−0.50%	−19.12%	−14.81%	−16.56%
2	4.33	6.9	3.86	2.72	4.09%	−33.46%	−4.22%	−3.89%
3	3.25	7.87	2.88	1.85	−9.72%	77.25%	3.60%	−7.04%
4	2.57	4.03	2.5	1.84	13.72%	−42.84%	−10.39%	−1.60%
5	1.78	7.46	2.32	1.59	18.67%	19.94%	−23.18%	−23.19%
6	1.24	26.32	5.59	3.81	−9.49%	−18.13%	−9.55%	1.87%
7	3.42	7.82	3.74	2.97	−3.39%	−33.84%	−17.80%	−22.86%
8	3.44	7.77	3.14	2.12	57.80%	0.39%	−13.26%	−16.21%
9	—	6.81	3.05	2.14	—	−21.81%	−17.79%	−14.06%
10	4.08	4.94	2.62	2.06	7.09%	−33.24%	−12.96%	−11.21%
11	2.29	17.6	5.49	3.82	19.90%	−26.24%	−15.15%	−4.02%
12	3.68	1.3	2.19	1.89	−10.90%	−42.98%	−19.49%	−17.47%
13	2.01	8.58	3.61	2.28	2.03%	−40.08%	−22.20%	−16.18%
14	3.94	1.97	2.36	2.08	0.25%	−51.72%	−1.26%	8.33%
15[*]	3.99	1.26	2.71	2.8	10.53%	−80.06%	−13.69%	1.45%
16	2.45	5.07	2.9	2.31	5.60%	−31.76%	3.94%	0.87%
17	3.21	1.64	2.7	2.43	3.22%	−46.23%	−25.62%	−23.82%
18	2.44	7.3	2.66	1.75	−2.01%	14.78%	18.22%	−4.89%
19	1.92	31.8	5.04	2.83	0.52%	41.71%	17.21%	2.91%
20	3.6	7.59	3.55	2.63	−4.76%	2.43%	−3.79%	−7.72%
21	2.64	9.65	3.32	2.27	0.00%	2.66%	−17.21%	−21.18%
22	3.58	3.04	2.53	1.96	−9.37%	−45.23%	−13.36%	−9.68%
23	2.53	5.35	3.01	2.5	6.30%	−14.13%	−15.45%	−20.63%
24	2.46	10.18	4.1	2.82	−0.81%	−6.35%	6.22%	7.63%
25	2.69	8.68	3.7	2.36	−1.82%	−11.97%	1.09%	−2.07%
26	2.88	6.06	3.76	2.95	−2.70%	−20.89%	−5.29%	−3.59%
27	—	4.15	3.02	2.51	—	−13.18%	1.68%	4.58%
28	—	4.97	3.27	2.68	—	−7.45%	−12.33%	1.52%
29	1.74	13.77	3.52	2.3	8.75%	−2.06%	−3.56%	−9.45%
30	2.96	3.23	2.7	2.04	25.42%	−38.24%	3.85%	−0.49%
31	2.43	9.41	3.33	2.05	−3.95%	−0.53%	16.84%	5.67%
32	2.95	9.42	4.11	2.81	−1.99%	−54.49%	−14.91%	−14.33%
33	—	6.29	4.17	3.86	—	−58.94%	−15.07%	−1.03%
34	—	10.36	2.97	2.25	—	−48.12%	−29.29%	−21.05%
35	—	11.2	4.02	2.55	—	−31.37%	−9.66%	−13.56%
36	—	6.8	2.32	1.69	—	19.72%	9.95%	−0.59%
37	—	12.02	3.39	2.4	—	−43.28%	−22.78%	−16.08%
38	2.81	3.15	2.51	1.96	2.93%	−47.93%	−18.24%	−15.88%
39	1.69	10.27	2.94	1.86	−6.63%	−34.75%	−22.63%	−22.50%
				Mean	0.04	−0.21	−0.09	−0.08
				Number	31	39	39	39
				Test statistic	1.6	−4.41	−4.49	−5.41
				Critical value of $t.05, n-1$				
				1 tailed	2.04	2.02	2.02	2.02
				2 tailed	1.7	1.68	1.66	1.64
				P value	$0.10 > x > 0.05$	$x < 0.005$	$x < 0.005$	$x < 0.005$

[*] denotes patient referenced in Figure 1.

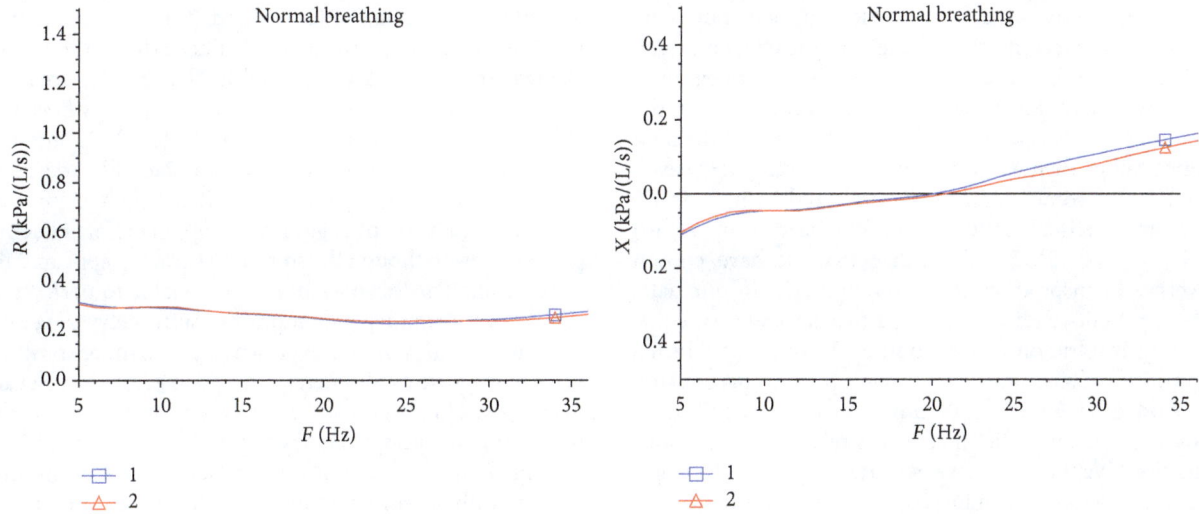

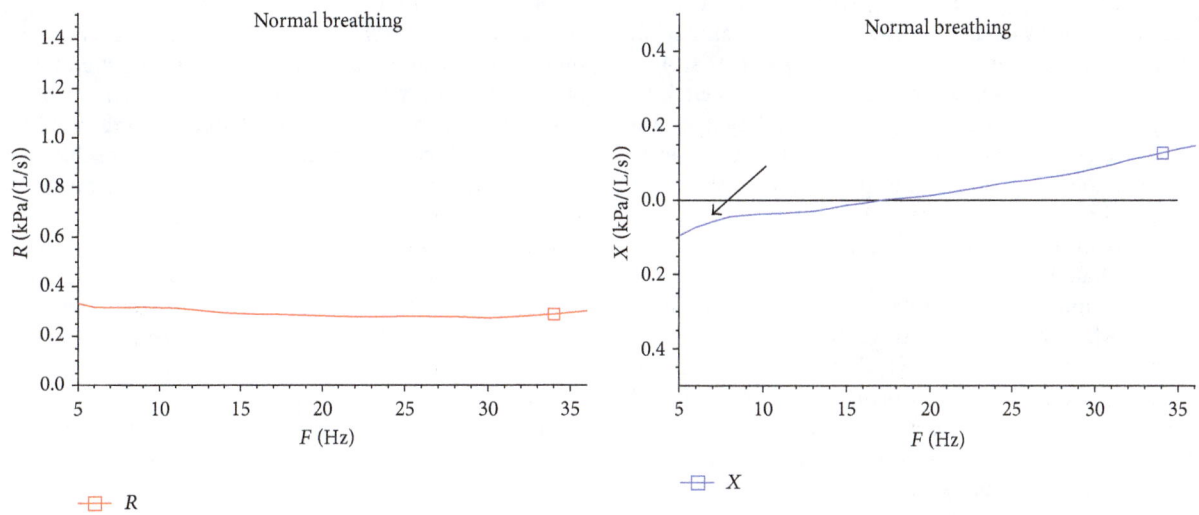

FIGURE 1: (a) Patient 15 before bronchodilator. (b) Patient 15 after bronchdilator.

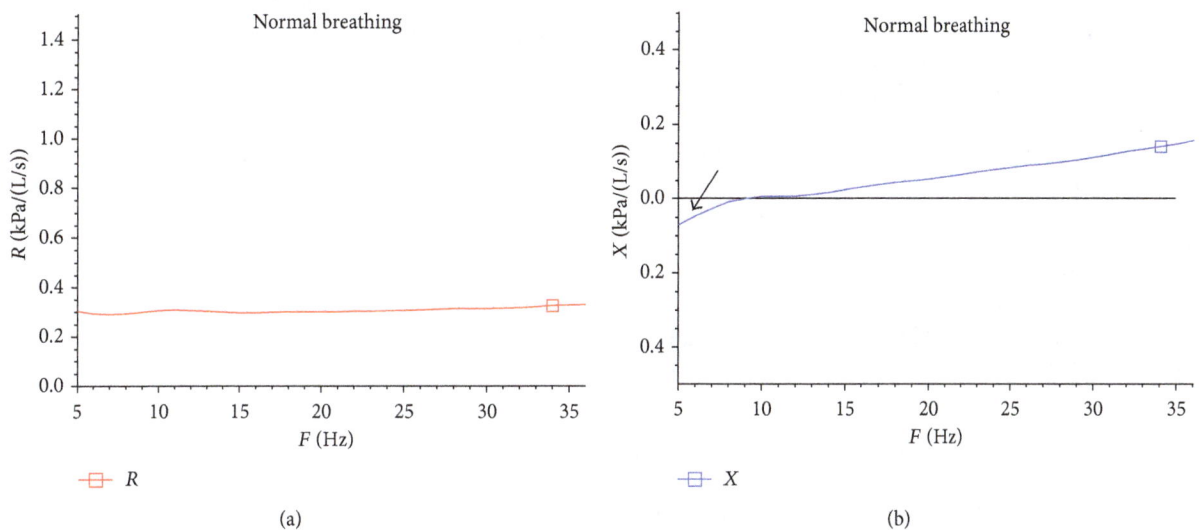

FIGURE 2: Patient 15 followup (post) (shadowed area AX).

signals through a transducer. X5 or resonant frequency is the point on the curve reflective of the same reactance as AX or at 5 Hz. Since AX is reflective of physiologic integration of small frequency signals rather than a specific point in the respiratory cycle, we elected to choose AX to reflect the lung reactance rather than X5. This was our reasoning. However, we realize that some studies have preferred to include X5 rather than AX. The literature is still not clear in this regard at this point [1, 15]. We do realize that we have chosen the average of inspiration and expiration AX. In our data, we chose patients with clear asthma that have almost equal AX during inspiration and expiration. In our unpublished observations, we have noted that in some patients particularly with COPD, the AX on expiration is at least twice that of inspiration. It is our belief that this is related to vocal cord dysfunction. We therefore have excluded patients with major differences between AX on inspiration and expiration.

The concept of forced oscillation technique or FOT was initiated in 1956 by Dubois [1]. Later, Lancer in 1976 introduced it as a resonant frequency between 6 and 11 Hz [1]. However, measurements of resistive frequencies at 4 to 32 Hz were noted to comprise small airway resistance [1]. In 2003 we presented data on IOS responses including decrease in R5 and AX, even in patients who had normal spirometry, including patients who had normal spirometry via the FEV1 or those who have decreased initial FEV1 [2].

These patients had an FEV1 with minimal to no improvement with inhaled corticosteroids [17]. Yet, their impulse oscillometry improved significantly. The IOS is a modification of FOT whereby the IOS delivers a regular square wave of pressure five times per second [1]. This has the advantage of generating a larger sample during measurements and omitting a continuous spectrum of frequencies (5–35 Hz) that provide a more detailed characterization of respiratory function [1, 6]. IOS therefore measures the properties of the lung to an externally applied stimulus. This is achieved through applying pressure variations at the mouth of the subject via a loudspeaker component of the instrument. Respiratory impedance is then obtained as resistance (R5 and above) and reactance (AX).

In our clinic, we utilize IOS routinely to determine the status. In this study, we chose our patients at random and as part of their asthma evaluation and management. These patients presented with allergic rhinitis and history of shortness of breath. Some of them were told that they had asthma by the referring provider. These patients were only treated by the referring provider with as needed short acting beta agonist inhaler only.

We realize the limitations of this study. First, this is retrospective evaluation. Ideally, prospective evaluation is more appropriate to study the effects of IOS in the diagnosis of asthma. However, since we perform IOS routinely and have well trained technicians, we thought that the retrospective data presentation may give awareness of the technical use of this modality in studying the pulmonary status of patients suspected to have asthma.

Second, there were three patients in our cohort that showed decrease or no reversibility in the FEV1 following bronchodilator treatment as shown in Table 1. These were patients 1, 2, and 18. Patients 1 and 18 had decrease in the FEV1 by 19 and 11%, respectively. Patient 2 did not show much change in FEV1 following hand-held nebulizer treatment. This is not unusual in clinical practice perhaps because of either poor cooperation or fatigue factor. It is important to note, however, that, even though the FEV1 decreased, in all of these three patients the IOS values significantly improved. This might suggest that support effort effect may play a role even though the spirometry tracing appeared to be appropriate. For this reason, it is reasonable to perform IOS since it is effort independent prior to spirometry to get more accurate readings. In our experience, performing spirometry prior to impulse oscillometry can lead to erroneous elevation in the AX. This is perhaps due to the provoking of the lung mechanics during spirometry (unpublished observations).

Third, the followup of these patients was a minimum of three months to a maximum of 18 months. In this case, the FEV1 may decrease with age but only slightly within a period of 18 months. The IOS values, however, should not change. In patients with severe obesity, there might be a minor effect on impulse oscillometry in terms of elevating the value of X5 or AX [18]. In reviewing the status of our patients based on what has been reported in the literature, there should not a significant effect on the values of the impulse oscillometry.

Fourth, our patients represent a heterogeneous group since they were placed on different types of inhaled corticosteroids. However, they were all evaluated by the same short acting beta agonist nebulizer which was levalbuterol hydrochloride. We could have chosen albuterol but based on the literature the effects are similar. However, irrespective of which kind of corticosteroid was used, the improvement in IOS appeared to be uniform.

Despite these limitations, we may have been able to demonstrate that IOS is useful in the diagnosis and followup of patients with adult asthma. Previously, IOS has been regarded as equivalent but not as an alternative to spirometry [4, 6]. Marotta et al. showed that, for children at risk for asthma, IOS is a better predictor than spirometry [16]. In a study by Al-Mutairi et al. [19] patients with COPD and asthma diagnoses were tested via IOS and spirometry. The authors concluded that IOS may be an alternative method to evaluate lung function at baseline when compared to spirometry.

Our observations, however, were directed towards evaluating patients at baseline following bronchodilator administration and at followup with ICS or ICS/LABA. These observations were retrospective and involved a relatively small number of adult asthma patients. It is noteworthy, however, that longitudinal studies in adult asthma with IOS evaluation should be considered in a larger cohort of patients.

In children, IOS has been more evaluated, even prospectively. Ortiz and Menendez showed that salmeterol alone showed IOS improvement in children between the ages of 2 and 5 when spirometry could not be performed in this age group [20]. In another larger cohort study, Komarow et al. demonstrated the efficacy of IOS in 117 children even as an alternative to FEV1 in asthmatic children [21].

In a study by Schermer et al. [22], IOS was studied in metropolitan firefighters. Similar to our findings, R5 and

X5 (equivalent to AX; see earlier) were better predictors of airway dysfunction, even when the spirometry was normal in most of these subjects. In airway dynamics IOS offers an advantage in measuring bronchomotor tone in adolescents who have asthma with daily variation, even when spirometry was unchanged (Goldman and Carter) [23]. In another study by Meraz et al. [13], IOS indices were sensitive indicators of small and large airway resistance in patients with asthma and cystic fibrosis independent of the upper airway shunt capacitance.

Other investigators have shown that X5 can be useful parameter of bronchial hyperresponsiveness in children [24]. X5 was suggested to be a useful correlate and adjunct to nitric oxide measurement in COPD and asthma [25]. In reality X5 referred to as resonant frequency is a direct reflection of AX [1, 6]. FEF 25–75% is obtained during routine pulmonary function testing. It measures the air flow during the mid-expiration cycle. It is supposed to be reflective of small airway resistance. In reality, however, it is a variable parameter and is also dependent on comparative parameters such as age, height, weight, and gender [26]. In our data the FEF 25–75% was helpful in a minority of patients (total of fourteen patients). In a study by Drewek et al., the FEF 25–75% was noted to be a valuable parameter to measure small airway decline in methacholine responsiveness in children [27]. Alberts et al. demonstrated that FEF 25/75 is useful in the diagnosis of asthma when the cut-off value at baseline is less than 60% [28]. Rao et al. showed that FEF 25/75 can be a predictor of childhood asthma and severity when the FEV1 is normal [29]. These studies did not utilize IOS in their evaluation of small airway disease. In a recent study by Anderson et al., baseline values of FEV1 in patients with persistent asthma according to the British Thoracic Society asthma treatment steps did not differ after inhaled corticosteroids while the R5 did show improvement [30]. AX as utilized in our study was not noted in this study. In another study, Yamaguchi et al. examined IOS and specifically AX in patients with asthma and noted improvement in AX from baseline when using HFA-BDP (Hydrofluoroalkane-beclomethasone dipropionate) compared to chlorofluorocarbon-beclomethasone dipropionate (or CFC-BDP). In their study, there was no comparison to spirometry, but they did affirm the role of IOS in the evaluation of small airway disease [31]. In our study and with our limited observations, the role of IOS and especially AX has been noted to be clinically significant. It did not correlate with FEV1 or FEF 25/75. This observation is important and warrants further investigation in a prospective large scale trial analysis.

Additional applications of IOS which we applied in our clinic and others as well include response to exercise in patients with symptoms suggestive of asthma who have normal spirometry and AX [32]. Also, it has been utilized in methacholine challenge testing [11] and in pregnancy when patients could not perform spirometry [33].

As previously stated, AX is easier to observe since it is reflective of the integral of reactance at various frequencies, particularly the small airways. We relied on R5 and AX in our study to evaluate these patients. In order to account for reliability and accuracy of IOS testing, the concept of coherence was used. Coherence is the estimate of the quality of impedance measurements. This approach provides an index of discrepancy between input and measure signals. The appropriate coherence established at each frequency of resistance is as follows: Co5 is 0.9, Co10 is 1.0, Co15 is 1.0, and Co20 is 1.0 (R15 is considered a measurement of larger airway resistance) [1, 6]. Based on the above, interpretation of the IOS requires more training and experience on the part of both the technician and interpreting physician. The technician should be alert to the patient's breathing, mouthpiece position, tidal breathing, and selection of the best normal breathing wave in relationship to coherence and absence of leak through the mouthpiece. The physician interpreter should have the basic knowledge of the pathophysiology of IOS and the ability to detect aberrancies in AX or R5 [1, 6].

Some of the pitfalls of IOS include airway leak and poor holding of the cheeks (which is particularly important in children and COPD patients). Tongue effect, cough, swallowing, shallow breaths, and vocalization are other pitfalls [1]. An experienced technician is able to identify these pitfalls and perform an appropriate test. Our technicians were well trained in identifying these pitfalls.

Other uses and future utilizations of IOS include respiratory impedance model measurements [34], heart failure models, and ventilatory changes following head-up tilt standing in healthy subjects [35–37].

Despite the above limitations, IOS has been shown to be useful in interpreting small airway dysfunction and, perhaps, superior to the FEF 25–75 [38]. FEF 25–75 measurement, because of its dependence on effort, can lead to false positive findings since its effect can diminish with time [30].

5. Conclusion

In our small observational study, we noted retrospectively that when IOS is performed appropriately it can potentially be an additional and perhaps be considered an alternative tool in the diagnosis and followup of adult asthma patients. The limitation of our study being retrospective and heterogeneous undermines a firmer conclusion. Future studies in a prospective group of of patients with adult asthma should help define a clearer role of IOS utility in asthma diagnosis and followup.

Conflict of Interests

The authors report no conflict of interests. Although they are using the IOS equipment manufactured by Jaeger, they purchased equipment like any other customer and do not have any financial interest in the company. This is a retrospective and clinical observation. Patients were treated based on FDA guidelines for asthma. Lung functions were evaluated via traditional spirometry and impulse oscillometry.

Acknowledgments

This work is dedicated to the memory of Michael D. Goldman, M.D., a colleague, a friend, and a mentor in the study of pulmonary physiology and forced oscillation. The authors have special appreciation for Dr. Andrew Liu. His willingness to review this paper, and provide suggestions was most helpful.

References

[1] M. D. Goldman, C. K. Saadeh, and D. Ross, "Clinical applications of forced oscillation to assess peripheral airway function," *Respiratory Physiology & Neurobiology*, vol. 148, no. 1-2, pp. 179–194, 2005.

[2] G. R. Vink, H. G. M. Arets, J. van der Laag, and C. K. van der Ent, "Impulse oscillometry: a measure for airway obstruction," *Pediatric Pulmonology*, vol. 35, no. 3, pp. 214–219, 2003.

[3] C. M. Houghton, N. Lawson, Z. L. Borrill et al., "Comparison of the effects of salmeterol/fluticasone propionate with fluticasone propionate on airway physiology in adults with mild persistent asthma," *Respiratory Research*, vol. 8, article 52, 2007.

[4] M. Hoshino, "Comparison of effectiveness in ciclesonide and fluticasone propionate on small airway function in mild asthma," *Allergology International*, vol. 59, no. 1, pp. 59–66, 2010.

[5] H. Ohbayashi, N. Shibata, T. Hirose, and M. Adachi, "Additional effects of pranlukast in salmeterol/fluticasone combination therapy for the asthmatic distal airway in a randomized crossover study," *Pulmonary Pharmacology & Therapeutics*, vol. 22, no. 6, pp. 574–579, 2009.

[6] C. M. Houghton, S. J. Langley, S. D. Singh et al., "Comparison of bronchoprotective and bronchodilator effects of a single dose of formoterol delivered by hydrofluoroalkane and chlorofluorocarbon aerosols and dry powder in a double blind, placebo-controlled, crossover study," *British Journal of Clinical Pharmacology*, vol. 58, no. 4, pp. 359–366, 2004.

[7] J. H. Lee, Y. W. Lee, Y. S. Shin, Y. H. Jung, C. S. Hong, and J. W. Park, "Exercise-induced airway obstruction in young asthmatics measured by impulse oscillometry," *Journal of Investigational Allergology and Clinical Immunology*, vol. 20, no. 7, pp. 575–581, 2010.

[8] A. Nieto, R. Pamies, F. Oliver, A. Medina, L. Caballero, and A. Mazon, "Montelukast improves pulmonary function measured by impulse oscillometry in children with asthma (Mio study)," *Respiratory Medicine*, vol. 100, no. 7, pp. 1180–1185, 2006.

[9] K. N. Sjöswärd, M. Hmani, A. Davidsson, P. Söderkvist, and B. Schmekel, "Single-isomer R-salbutamol is not superior to racemate regarding protection for bronchial hyperresponsiveness," *Respiratory Medicine*, vol. 98, no. 10, pp. 990–999, 2004.

[10] M. Hoshino, H. Handa, and T. Miyazawa, "Effects of salmeterol and fluticasone propionate combination versus fluticasone propionate on airway function and eosinophilic inflammation in mild asthma," *Allergology International*, vol. 58, no. 3, pp. 357–363, 2009.

[11] A. H. Mansur, S. Manney, and J. G. Ayres, "Methacholine-induced asthma symptoms correlate with impulse oscillometry but not spirometry," *Respiratory Medicine*, vol. 102, no. 1, pp. 42–49, 2008.

[12] J. W. Park, Y. W. Lee, Y. H. Jung, S. E. Park, and C. S. Hong, "Impulse oscillometry for estimation of airway obstruction and bronchodilation in adults with mild obstructive asthma," *Annals of Allergy, Asthma & Immunology*, vol. 98, no. 6, pp. 546–552, 2007.

[13] E. Meraz, H. Nazeran, M. Goldman, P. Nava, and B. Diong, "Impulse oscillometric features of lung function: towards computer-aided classification of respiratory diseases in children," in *Proceedings of the 30th Annual International Conference of the IEEE Engineering in Medicine and Biology Society (EMBS '08)*, pp. 2443–2446, August 2008.

[14] B. Klug, "The impulse oscillation technique applied for measurements of respiratory function in young children," *Pediatric Pulmonology*, vol. 16, pp. 240–241, 1997.

[15] J. Hellinckx, M. Cauberghs, K. de Boeck, and M. Demedts, "Evaluation of impulse oscillation system: comparison with forced oscillation technique and body plethysmography," *European Respiratory Journal*, vol. 18, no. 3, pp. 564–570, 2001.

[16] A. Marotta, M. D. Klinnert, M. R. Price, G. L. Larsen, and A. H. Liu, "Impulse oscillometry provides an effective measure of lung dysfunction in 4-year-old children at risk for persistent asthma," *Journal of Allergy and Clinical Immunology*, vol. 112, no. 2, pp. 317–322, 2003.

[17] C. K. Saadeh, M. Goldman, P. Gaylor et al., "Forced oscillation using impulse oscillometry (IOS) detects false negative spirometry in symptomatic patients with reactive airways," *Journal of Allergy and Clinical Immunology*, vol. 111, no. 1, p. 136, 2003.

[18] F. Zerah-Lancner, L. Boyer, S. Rezaiguia-Delclaux et al., "Airway responsiveness measured by forced oscillation technique in severely obese patients, before and after bariatric surgery," *Journal of Asthma*, vol. 48, no. 8, pp. 818–823, 2011.

[19] S. S. Al-Mutairi, P. N. Sharma, A. Al-Alawi, and J. S. Al-Deen, "Impulse oscillometry: an alternative modality to the conventional pulmonary function test to categorise obstructive pulmonary disorders," *Clinical and Experimental Medicine*, vol. 7, no. 2, pp. 56–64, 2007.

[20] G. Ortiz and R. Menendez, "The effects of inhaled albuterol and salmeterol in 2- to 5-year-old asthmatic children as measured by impulse oscillometry," *Journal of Asthma*, vol. 39, no. 6, pp. 531–536, 2002.

[21] H. D. Komarow, J. Skinner, M. Young et al., "A study of the use of impulse oscillometry in the evaluation of children with asthma: analysis of lung parameters, order effect, and utility compared with spirometry," *Pediatric Pulmonology*, vol. 47, pp. 18–26, 2012.

[22] T. Schermer, W. Malbon, W. Newbury et al., "Spirometry and impulse oscillometry (IOS) for detection of respiratory abnormalities in metropolitan firefighters," *Respirology*, vol. 15, no. 6, pp. 975–985, 2010.

[23] M. D. Goldman, R. Carter, R. Klein, G. Fritz, B. Carter, and P. Pachucki, "Within- and between-day variability of respiratory impedance, using impulse oscillometry in adolescent asthmatics," *Pediatric Pulmonology*, vol. 34, no. 4, pp. 312–319, 2002.

[24] H. M. Jee, J. H. Kwak, D. W. Jung, and M. Y. Han, "Useful parameters of bronchial hyperresponsiveness measured with an impulse oscillation technique in preschool children," *Journal of Asthma*, vol. 47, no. 3, pp. 227–232, 2010.

[25] P. A. Williamson, K. Clearie, D. Menzies, S. Vaidyanathan, and B. J. Lipworth, "Assessment of small-airways disease using alveolar nitric oxide and impulse oscillometry in asthma and COPD," *Lung*, vol. 189, no. 2, pp. 121–129, 2011.

[26] M. R. Simon, V. M. Chinchilli, B. R. Phillips et al., "Forced expiratory flow between 25% and 75% of vital capacity and FEV1/forced vital capacity ratio in relation to clinical and physiological parameters in asthmatic children with normal FEV1 values," *The Journal of Allergy and Clinical Immunology*, vol. 126, no. 3, pp. 527–534, 2010.

[27] R. Drewek, E. Garber, S. Stanclik, P. Simpson, M. Nugent, and W. Gershan, "The FEF25-75 and its decline as a predictor of

methacholine responsiveness in children," *Journal of Asthma*, vol. 46, no. 4, pp. 375–381, 2009.

[28] W. M. Alberts, M. C. Ferris, S. M. Brooks, and A. L. Goldman, "The FEF25-75% and the clinical diagnosis of asthma," *Annals of Allergy*, vol. 73, no. 3, pp. 221–225, 1994.

[29] D. R. Rao, J. M. Gaffin, S. N. Baxi, W. J. Sheehan, E. B. Hoffman, and W. Phipatanakul, "The utility of forced expiratory flow between 25% and 75% of vital capacity in predicting childhood asthma morbidity and severity," *Journal of Asthma*, vol. 49, no. 6, pp. 586–592, 2012.

[30] W. J. Anderson, E. Zajda, and B. J. Lipworth, "Are we overlooking persistent small airways dysfunction in community-managed asthma?" *Annals of Allergy, Asthma & Immunology*, vol. 109, no. 3, pp. 185–189, 2012.

[31] M. Yamaguchi, A. Niimi, T. Ueda et al., "Effect of inhaled corticosteroids on small airways in asthma: investigation using impulse oscillometry," *Pulmonary Pharmacology and Therapeutics*, vol. 22, no. 4, pp. 326–332, 2009.

[32] T. M. Evans, K. W. Rundell, K. C. Beck, A. M. Levine, and J. M. Baumann, "Airway narrowing measured by spirometry and impulse oscillometry following room temperature and cold temperature exercise," *Chest*, vol. 128, no. 4, pp. 2412–2419, 2005.

[33] K. Bidad, H. Heidarnazhad, A. Kazemnejad, and Z. Pourpak, "Impulse oscillometry in comparison to spirometry in pregnant asthmatic females," *European Respiratory Journal*, vol. 32, no. 6, pp. 1673–1675, 2008.

[34] T. U. Nguyen, B. Diong, and M. Goldman, "A study of IOS data using the aRIC+I(p) model of respiratory impedance," in *Proceedings of the Annual International Conference of the IEEE Engineering in Medicine and Biology Society (EMBS '09)*, pp. 2875–2878, 2009.

[35] D. G. Spyratos, G. P. Glattki, L. T. Sichletidis, and D. Patakas, "Assessment of respiratory mechanics by impulse oscillometry in orthopneic patients with acute left ventricular failure," *Heart & Lung*, vol. 40, no. 2, pp. 97–104, 2011.

[36] K. K. Witte, A. Morice, A. L. Clark, and J. G. Cleland, "Airway resistance in chronic heart failure measured by impulse oscillometry," *Journal of Cardiac Failure*, vol. 8, no. 4, pp. 225–231, 2002.

[37] A. T. Chang, R. J. Boots, M. G. Brown, J. D. Paratz, and P. W. Hodges, "Ventilatory changes following head-up tilt and standing in healthy subjects," *European Journal of Applied Physiology*, vol. 95, no. 5-6, pp. 409–417, 2005.

[38] T. W. Song, K. W. Kim, E. S. Kim, J. W. Park, M. H. Sohn, and K. E. Kim, "Utility of impulse oscillometry in young children with asthma," *Pediatric Allergy and Immunology*, vol. 19, no. 8, pp. 763–768, 2008.

9

Markers of Myocardial Ischemia in Patients with Obstructive Sleep Apnea and Coronary Artery Disease

Misa Valo, Annette Wons, Albert Moeller, and Claudius Teupe

Center of Sleep Medicine, Department of Medicine, Krankenhaus Sachsenhausen, 60594 Frankfurt, Germany

Correspondence should be addressed to Claudius Teupe; teupe@em.uni-frankfurt.de

Academic Editor: Akio Niimi

Obstructive sleep apnea (OSA) is characterized by intermittent hypoxia during sleep. We tested the hypothesis that nocturnal myocardial ischemia is detectable by ST segment depression and elevation of high sensitive troponin T (hsTrop T) and B-type natriuretic peptide (NT-proBNP) in patients with OSA and coexisting coronary artery disease (CAD). Twenty-one patients with OSA and CAD and 20 patients with OSA alone underwent in-hospital polysomnography. Blood samples for hsTrop T and NT-proBNP measurements were drawn before and after sleep. ST segment depression was measured at the time of maximum oxygen desaturation during sleep. The apnea-hypopnea-index (AHI), oxygen saturation nadir, and time in bed with oxygen saturation of ≤80% were similar in both groups. Levels of hsTrop T and NT-proBNP did not differ significantly before and after sleep but NT-proBNP levels were significantly higher in patients suffering from OSA and CAD compared to patients with OSA alone. No significant ST depression was found at the time of oxygen saturation nadir in either group. Despite the fact that patients with untreated OSA and coexisting CAD experienced severe nocturnal hypoxemia, we were unable to detect myocardial ischemia or myocyte necrosis based on significant ST segment depression or elevation of hsTrop T and NT-proBNP, respectively.

1. Introduction

Obstructive sleep apnea (OSA) is associated with an increased risk of cardiovascular morbidity and mortality [1]. OSA is characterized by intermittent hypoxia during sleep, which is associated with elevated sympathetic activity, cardiovascular variability, and intrathoracic pressure changes. OSA also provokes systemic inflammation, oxidative stress, endothelial dysfunction, insulin resistance, and thrombosis [2]. Atrial fibrillation, coronary artery disease, congestive heart failure, and arterial hypertension are clinical manifestations and are more common in patients with OSA [3, 4]. Stress imposed on the myocardium by repeated severe hypoxemia during sleep and an increased oxygen demand by sympathetic overstimulation in OSA may result in subclinical myocardial injury [5]. Cardiac troponin T is an important biomarker in myocardial injury and a predictor of clinical outcome [6]. Cardiac myocytes constitute the major source of N-terminal pro B-type natriuretic peptide (NT-proBNP). This is secreted by myocytes after myocardial hypoxemia and ventricular volume overload [7]. NT-proBNP production is strongly upregulated in cardiac failure and locally in the area surrounding a myocardial infarction [8].

We hypothesized that moderate to severe OSA may precipitate myocardial ischemia in patients with coexisting CAD, reflected by ST-segment depression. We also evaluate whether repetitive nocturnal hypoxia in these patients may cause low-grade myocardial injury, as demonstrated by increased levels of NT-proBNP and highly sensitive troponin T (hsTrop T).

2. Methods

The prospective study was approved by the ethics committee of the State Medical Council of Hessen, Germany (approval number FF 6/2912). Informed consent was obtained from each patient.

2.1. Study Population. Consecutive patients were screened by polygraphy for the presence of moderate to severe OSA with a minimum oxygen desaturation of ≤80% during apnea. The study ultimately enrolled a group of 21 patients with untreated

OSA and concomitant CAD proven by coronary angiography (group 1) who were referred for complete polysomnography (PSG). A group of 20 patients with untreated OSA but without a history of CAD and free from CAD symptoms served as a control (group 2).

Inclusion criteria were as follows: age >18 years, apnea-hypopnea-index (AHI) ≥15/h, oxygen desaturation ≤80% at PSG, proven history of CAD (group 1), and untreated OSA. Exclusion criteria were heart failure (left ventricular ejection fraction <40% measured by echocardiography) and renal insufficiency (glomerular filtration rate <50 mL/min estimated using the Cockcroft-Gault formula).

2.2. Polysomnography. The presence and severity of OSA were determined by overnight complete polysomnography using a computerized system (Alice 5, Philips Respironics, Herrsching, Germany). Standard techniques such as EEG, electrooculography, electromyography, electrocardiogram, thermistor measurements of air flow, thoracoabdominal motion, pulse oximetry of arterial oxyhemoglobin saturation (SPO_2), and body position were used to monitor sleep disordered breathing. Bedtime was 10 p.m. to 6 a.m. Sleep stages were scored according to the standard criteria of the American Academy of Sleep Medicine [9]. Apnea was defined as an absence of airflow for >10 s. Hypopnea was defined as a more than 30% reduction in airflow accompanied by a decrease in SPO_2 of >4%. AHI was calculated as the average number of apneas and hypopneas per hour of sleep. An AHI ≥15/h was defined as moderate to severe OSA.

2.3. Measurement of hsTrop T and NT-proBNP. Quantitative measurement of hsTrop T was achieved via an immunoassay for the in vitro quantitative determination of cardiac troponin T in human serum and plasma (Cobas e 411 Roche Troponin T hs STAT; Roche Diagnostics Inc.) with the upper limit of normal of 14 pg/mL representing the 99th percentile in a normal reference population and a coefficient of variation of <10%. HsTrop T values below the Limit of Blank are reported as <3 ng/L.

NT-proBNP levels were measured with an immunoassay for the in vitro quantitative determination of NT-proBNP in heparinized venous blood (Cobas Roche Cardiac proBNP+; Roche Diagnostics Inc.). Values below the Limit of Blank are reported as <60 ng/L.

Venous blood samples (5 mL) were collected at different time points: before (9 p.m.) and after (7 a.m.) polysomnography. The measurements were performed immediately after the second set of blood samples were drawn.

2.4. ST Segment Analysis in the Electrocardiogram. A continuous ECG recording was performed simultaneously during sleep in all patients to screen for ST segment depression episodes as an indicator of myocardial ischemia. Lead II was used to analyze the ST segment for myocardial ischemia. Additional leads I, III, aVL, aVR, and aVF were used as backup for further evaluation of features suggestive of cardiac ischemia observed in the main ECG lead. An ischemic episode was defined as a horizontal or downsloping ST segment depression of ≥1 mm (100 μV) from baseline, measured 80 ms after the J point. The time point of maximum oxygen desaturation during sleep was determined by continuous oximetry. The analysis of the ST segments was performed 10 cardiac cycles after the oxygen saturation nadir. The ST segments in the next 10 consecutive cardiac cycles were analyzed and averaged.

2.5. Statistics. The results are expressed as mean ± standard deviation (SD) for continuous variables. For the descriptive statistics, the arithmetic mean, SD, median, minimum and maximum, and 1st and 3rd quartiles were calculated. For comparison of the two groups, the Fisher exact test and the Wilcoxon-Mann-Whitney U test (U test) were used. The Wilcoxon Matched Pairs Test was applied for paired samples. Statistical analyses were performed using a statistical software package (BiAS for Windows, Version 10.05). P values <0.05 were considered statistically significant.

3. Results

The study population included a group of 21 patients with OSA and cooccurring CAD (group 1). Within this group, previous coronary artery bypass graft operation had been performed in 5 patients and percutaneous coronary interventions in 16 patients, and CAD proven by angiogram was treated medically in 2 patients. A group of 20 patients with OSA but with no history of CAD and free from CAD symptoms served as a control (group 2). Anthropometric characteristics and clinical data are presented in Table 1.

There were no statistically significant differences between the two groups other than the presence of hypercholesterolemia, history of myocardial infarction, and medication with ACE-inhibitors and β-blockers.

AHI and oxygen saturation nadir were similar in both groups (Figure 1). Additional polysomnographic variables are presented in Table 2. There were no significant differences between the two groups.

The levels and distribution of the cardiac markers hsTrop T and NT-proBNP did not differ significantly before and after sleep within the same group. However, NT-proBNP levels were higher before sleep as well as after sleep in patients with OSA and coexisting CAD compared to patients with OSA alone. HsTrop T was detectable (≥3 ng/L) in 18 (86%) patients before as well as after polysomnography in group 1 and in 16 (80%) patients before and after polysomnography in group 2. Mean hsTrop T levels before and after sleep were 10 ± 7 ng/L and 10 ± 9 ng/L in patients in group 1 and 6 ± 4 ng/L and 7 ± 4 ng/L in group 2, respectively. Mean NT-proBNP levels were 499 ± 758 pg/mL and 400 ± 592 pg/mL before and after sleep in patients in group 1 and 123 ± 93 pg/mL and 101 ± 68 pg/mL in group 2 (Figure 2).

ST segment analysis revealed no significant ST depression (≥100 μV) at the time of the deepest oxygen desaturation, neither in patients with OSA and coexisting CAD nor in the control group. However, ST segment depression was significantly more pronounced in group 1 patients than in group 2 patients (Figure 3).

TABLE 1: Clinical characteristics.

	OSAS + CAD ($n = 21$)	OSAS ($n = 20$)	P value
Demographics			
Gender (female/male)	5/16	3/17	n.s.
Age (yr)	61 ± 11	54 ± 12	n.s
Body mass index (kg/m^2)	35 ± 7	33 ± 6	n.s.
Medical history			
Hypertension	19 (90%)	13 (65%)	n.s.
Hypercholesterolemia	17 (81%)	5 (25%)	<0.001
Diabetes mellitus	10 (48%)	5 (25%)	n.s.
Arrhythmia	6 (29%)	1 (5%)	n.s.
Stroke	2 (10%)	0 (0%)	n.s.
Myocardial infarction	12 (57%)	0 (0%)	<0.001
COPD	4 (19%)	2 (10%)	n.s.
Medication			
Nitrates	3 (14%)	0 (0%)	n.s.
β-Blockers	19 (90%)	7 (35%)	<0.001
Renin inhibitor	0 (0%)	1 (5%)	n.s.
ACE inhibitors	14 (67%)	3 (15%)	<0.01
Angiotensin II receptor blockers	3 (14%)	5 (25%)	n.s.
Diuretics	11 (52%)	5 (25%)	n.s.
Calcium channel blockers	9 (43%)	5 (25%)	n.s.
α-Blockers	1 (5%)	2 (10%)	n.s.
Cardiac and renal function			
LVEF (%)	59 ± 9	65 ± 2	n.s.
GFR (mL/min)	121 ± 53	137 ± 43	n.s.
Polygraphy (screening)			
AHI (n/h)	39 ± 18	43 ± 18	n.s.
Oxygen saturation nadir (%)	70 ± 10	71 ± 8	n.s.

Data are presented as mean ± SD or No. ACE: angiotensin-converting enzyme; AHI: apnea-hypopnea-index; GFR: glomerular filtration rate; LVEF: left ventricular ejection fraction.

TABLE 2: Polysomnographic data.

	OSAS + CAD ($n = 21$)	OSAS ($n = 20$)	P value
Polysomnography			
AHI (n/h)	53 ± 21	49 ± 20	n.s.
Oxygen saturation nadir (%)	71 ± 12	71 ± 15	n.s.
Percentage of time with SaO$_2$ <90% (%)	18 ± 17	18 ± 18	n.s.
Percentage of time with SaO$_2$ <80% (%)	2 ± 4	4 ± 7	n.s.
Arousal index (n/h)	40 ± 17	40 ± 26	n.s.
Desaturation index (n/h)	53 ± 29	45 ± 26	n.s.
Maximal duration of SRBD (sec)	89 ± 56	82 ± 23	n.s.

Data are presented as mean ± SD. AHI: apnea-hypopnea-index; SaO$_2$: oxygen saturation; SRBD: sleep-related breathing disorder.

4. Discussion

It is well known that OSA is associated with adverse effects on cardiac structure and function. There is a linear relationship between the severity of OSA and patient morbidity and mortality [10]. Cardiac damage in OSA may be caused by activation of the sympathetic nervous system due to hypoxia and changes in negative intrathoracic pressure and increased oxidative stress [11].

Previous studies have suggested that the main risk factor for myocardial ischemia in patients with OSA is inadequate oxygen supply in the presence of CAD, while others assume an increase in oxygen demand due to tachycardia and sympathetic activation following the rebreathing phase after an apnea event [12–14]. The potential cellular mechanism in intermittent hypoxia-induced cardiac damage is an increase in apoptosis and cardiac fibrosis, a decreased arterial vessel and capillary density, and the loss of troponin I [15].

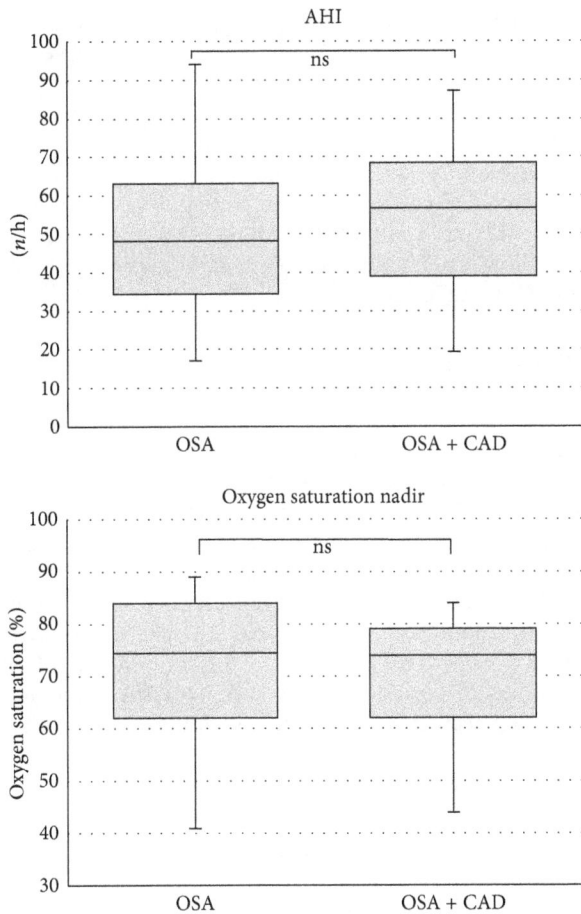

FIGURE 1: Comparison of polysomnography data (AHI: apnea-hypopnea-index; CAD: coronary artery disease; OSA: obstructive sleep apnea). Middle horizontal line inside box indicates median. Bottom and top of the box are 25th and 75th percentiles, and the error bars outside the box represent maximum and minimum values, respectively.

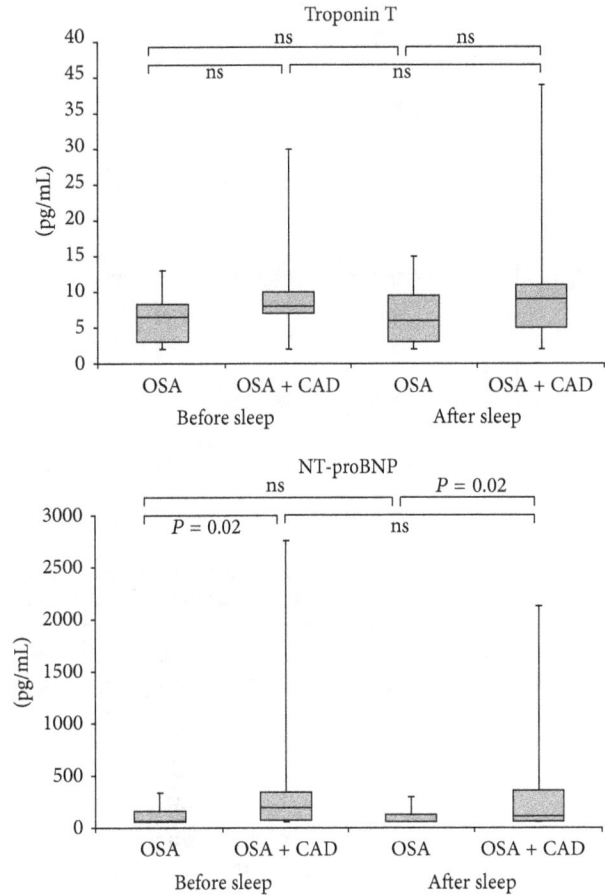

FIGURE 2: Distribution of troponin T and NT-proBNP levels before and after sleep (CAD: coronary artery disease; OSA: obstructive sleep apnea). Middle horizontal line inside box indicates median. Bottom and top of the box are 25th and 75th percentiles, and the error bars outside the box represent maximum and minimum values, respectively.

In the current study, we found no evidence of myocardial ischemia or myocyte necrosis in patients with moderate to severe OSA and coexisting CAD based on significant ST segment depression or elevation of hsTrop T. NT-proBNP levels were significantly higher in patients who suffered from OSA and CAD compared to controls but were unchanged after sleep.

The results of previously presented studies which investigated the relation between OSA and myocardial damage measured by different troponins are not univocal. Similar to our findings, a study by Gami et al. reported no myocardial injury detectable by troponin T assay despite the fact that patients with OSA and concomitant CAD experience nocturnal ischemia [16]. In this study, the AHI was comparable to our study but the mean nocturnal oxygen saturation nadir was less distinct (SPO$_2$ 83 ± 6%). Two other studies found higher levels of hsTrop T and hsTrop I, respectively, independently correlated with OSA severity, suggesting that frequent apneas or hypoxemia in OSA may cause low-grade myocardial injury and play a role in the association between

OSA and risk of heart failure [17, 18]. In a study including 505 subjects drawn from the general population, hsTrop T was detectable (≥3 ng/L) in 216 subjects. The proportion of subjects with detectable hsTrop T increased with increasing severity of OSA. But after adjustment for significant univariate predictors of detectable hsTrop T, the association between AHI and hsTrop T was no longer statistically significant [19].

The mechanism of ST segment depression during sleep in patients with OSA is not fully understood. Inspiration against occluded upper airways causing periodic negative changes in intrathoracic pressure and alterations in cardiac preload and afterload may result in myocardial ischemia in the absence of hypoxemia [20].

We found a more pronounced but not significant ST depression of ≥1 mm at the time of oxygen saturation nadir in patients suffering from OSA and CAD. Previous studies have noted ST segment depression in about one-third of OSA patients with CAD predominantly during apneas and reduced oxygen saturation [13, 14]. A study of 226 patients referred for coronary angiogram because of angina pectoris found nocturnal ST segment depression within 2 minutes

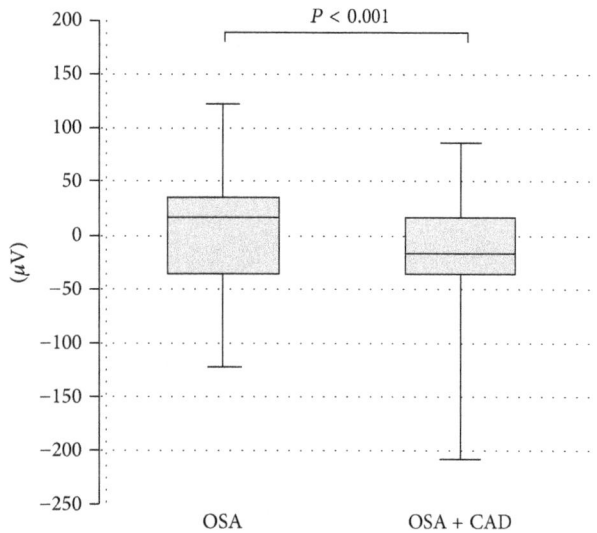

FIGURE 3: ST segment depression at the time of the deepest oxygen desaturation (CAD: coronary artery disease; OSA: obstructive sleep apnea). Middle horizontal line inside box indicates median. Bottom and top of the box are 25th and 75th percentiles, and the error bars outside the box represent maximum and minimum values, respectively.

after apnea-hypopnea or desaturation in only 12% of patients [21]. Apnea-associated ST segment depression was often preceded by a significant increase in heart rate, repetitive apneas, and severe oxygen desaturation. A temporal relationship between sleep-disordered breathing and myocardial ischemia was present only in a minority of patients. Hanly et al. also found asymptomatic ST depression during sleep in 30% of patients with OSA who did not have a history of CAD [22].

We found significantly higher NT-proBNP levels in patients with OSA and coexisting CAD compared to controls. Several studies found higher serum NT-proBNP values in patients with OSA, while other studies found no correlation between OSA severity and NT-proBNP levels [17, 23–26]. NT-proBNP is also an independent predictor for patients with CAD [27]. In patients with stable angina pectoris NT-proBNP serum concentrations showed a close relationship with the extent of CAD and inducible myocardial ischemia [28, 29]. A meta-analysis indicated strong associations between the circulating concentration of NT-proBNP and the long-term prognosis in patients with stable coronary artery disease [30]. NT-proBNP is also strongly associated with mortality in patients with suspected or confirmed unstable CAD [31].

The present study did have some limitations that deserve comment. First is the small number of the study group, which limits interpretation of the results, in particular the P values. Second, in patients with OSA alone, a concomitant CAD was excluded only by patient history, although there was a chance that some patients in this group suffered from unrecognized CAD. On the other hand, most patients with coexisting CAD had previous coronary interventions, which may also affect ischemic thresholds. Third, it is possible that the chosen time point for the analysis of ST segment depression after

oxygen saturation nadir might not represent the time of most severe myocardial ischemia. ST depression may have been more pronounced during postapnea tachycardia. We also did not take into account the duration of hypoxemia. Other mechanisms like sympathetic activation with increased heart rate and blood pressure were not considered in exploring the relationship between OSA and myocardial injury since most of the patients with OSA and coexisting CAD were on medications (β-blockers, ACE inhibitors) which may confound these findings.

5. Conclusion

In patients with moderate to severe OSA and coexisting CAD, repeated oxygen desaturation did not result in myocardial necrosis based on elevation of hsTrop T serum levels after sleep. At the time of maximum oxygen desaturation during sleep, we found no significant ST segment depression. Patients with OSA and concomitant CAD had higher NT-proBNP serum levels compared to patients with OSA alone, but NT-proBNP levels were not affected by severe nocturnal hypoxia. Cardiovascular injury in patients with significant OSA seems to be independent of direct ischemia-induced myocardial necrosis even in patients with manifest CAD.

Conflict of Interests

All authors have no conflict of interests to disclose.

Authors' Contribution

Misa Valo and Annette Wons contributed equally to this paper.

Acknowledgments

The authors would like to give special thanks to Simone Rack for her assistance in performing the polysomnography and the data acquisition.

References

[1] Y. Kaneko, J. S. Floras, K. Usui et al., "Cardiovascular effects of continuous positive airway pressure in patients with heart failure and obstructive sleep apnea," *The New England Journal of Medicine*, vol. 348, no. 13, pp. 1233–1241, 2003.

[2] T. D. Bradley and J. S. Floras, "Obstructive sleep apnoea and its cardiovascular consequences," *The Lancet*, vol. 373, no. 9657, pp. 82–93, 2009.

[3] A. S. Gami, G. Pressman, S. M. Caples et al., "Association of atrial fibrillation and obstructive sleep apnea," *Circulation*, vol. 110, no. 4, pp. 364–367, 2004.

[4] E. Shahar, C. W. Whitney, S. Redline et al., "Sleep-disordered breathing and cardiovascular disease: cross-sectional results of the Sleep Heart Health Study," *The American Journal of Respiratory and Critical Care Medicine*, vol. 163, no. 1, pp. 19–25, 2001.

[5] F. de Torres-Alba, D. Gemma, E. Armada-Romero, J. R. Rey-Blas, E. López-De-Sá, and J. L. López-Sendon, "Obstructive

sleep apnea and coronary artery disease: from pathophysiology to clinical implications," *Pulmonary Medicine*, vol. 2013, Article ID 768064, 9 pages, 2013.

[6] B. Lindahl, H. Toss, A. Siegbahn, P. Venge, and L. Wallentin, "Markers of myocardial damage and inflammation in relation to long-term mortality in unstable coronary artery disease," *The New England Journal of Medicine*, vol. 343, no. 16, pp. 1139–1147, 2000.

[7] J. P. Goetze, L. Friis-Hansen, J. F. Rehfeld, B. Nilsson, and J. H. Svendsen, "Atrial secretion of B-type natriuretic peptide," *European Heart Journal*, vol. 27, no. 14, pp. 1648–1650, 2006.

[8] C. Hall, "Essential biochemistry and physiology of (NT-pro)BNP," *European Journal of Heart Failure*, vol. 6, no. 3, pp. 257–260, 2004.

[9] C. Iber, S. Ancoli-Israel, A. Chesson, and S. F. Quan, *The AASM Manual for the Scoring of Sleep and Associated Events: Rules, Terminology and Technical Specification*, American Academy of Sleep Medicine, Westchester, Ill, USA, 1st edition, 2007.

[10] B. Shivalkar, C. van de Heyning, M. Kerremans et al., "Obstructive sleep apnea syndrome: more insights on structural and functional cardiac alterations, and the effects of treatment with continuous positive airway pressure," *Journal of the American College of Cardiology*, vol. 47, no. 7, pp. 1433–1439, 2006.

[11] W. T. McNicholas and M. R. Bonsignore, "Sleep apnoea as an independent risk factor for cardiovascular disease: current evidence, basic mechanisms and research priorities," *European Respiratory Journal*, vol. 29, no. 1, pp. 156–178, 2007.

[12] K. A. Franklin, J. B. Nilsson, C. Sahlin, and U. Naslund, "Sleep apnoea and nocturnal angina," *The Lancet*, vol. 345, no. 8957, pp. 1085–1087, 1995.

[13] H. Schäfer, U. Koehler, T. Ploch, and J. H. Peter, "Sleep-related myocardial ischemia and sleep structure in patients with obstructive sleep apnea and coronary heart disease," *Chest*, vol. 111, no. 2, pp. 387–393, 1997.

[14] N. Peled, E. G. Abinader, G. Pillar, D. Sharif, and P. Lavie, "Nocturnal ischemic events in patients with obstructive sleep apnea syndrome and ischemic heart disease: effects of continuous positive air pressure treatment," *Journal of the American College of Cardiology*, vol. 34, no. 6, pp. 1744–1749, 1999.

[15] Q. Han, S. C. Yeung, M. S. M. Ip, and J. C. W. Mak, "Cellular mechanisms in intermittent hypoxia-induced cardiac damage in vivo," *Journal of Physiology and Biochemistry*, vol. 70, no. 1, pp. 201–213, 2014.

[16] A. S. Gami, A. Svatikova, R. Wolk et al., "Cardiac troponin T in obstructive sleep apnea," *Chest*, vol. 125, no. 6, pp. 2097–2100, 2004.

[17] G. Q. Roca, S. Redline, N. Punjabi et al., "Sleep apnea is associated with subclinical myocardial injury in the community: the ARIC-SHHS study," *American Journal of Respiratory and Critical Care Medicine*, vol. 188, no. 12, pp. 1460–1465, 2013.

[18] G. Einvik, H. Rsøjø, A. Randby et al., "Severity of obstructive sleep apnea is associated with cardiac troponin I concentrations in a community-based sample: data from the Akershus Sleep Apnea Project," *Sleep*, vol. 37, no. 6, pp. 1111–1116, 2014.

[19] A. Randby, S. K. Namtvedt, G. Einvik et al., "Obstructive sleep apnea is associated with increased high-sensitivity cardiac troponin T levels," *Chest*, vol. 142, no. 3, pp. 639–646, 2012.

[20] J. M. Parish and J. W. Shepard Jr., "Cardiovascular effects of sleep disorders," *Chest*, vol. 97, no. 5, pp. 1220–1226, 1990.

[21] T. Mooe, K. A. Franklin, U. Wiklund, T. Rabben, and K. Holmström, "Sleep-disordered breathing and myocardial ischemia in patients with coronary artery disease," *Chest*, vol. 117, no. 6, pp. 1597–1602, 2000.

[22] P. Hanly, Z. Sasson, N. Zuberi, and K. Lunn, "ST-segment depression during sleep in obstructive sleep apnea," *American Journal of Cardiology*, vol. 71, no. 15, pp. 1341–1345, 1993.

[23] A. G. Kaditis, E. I. Alexopoulos, F. Hatzi et al., "Overnight change in brain natriuretic peptide levels in children with sleep-disordered breathing," *Chest*, vol. 130, no. 5, pp. 1377–1384, 2006.

[24] H. Kita, M. Ohi, K. Chin et al., "The nocturnal secretion of cardiac natriuretic peptides during obstructive sleep apnoea and its response to therapy with nasal continuous positive airway pressure," *Journal of Sleep Research*, vol. 7, no. 3, pp. 199–207, 1998.

[25] R.-H. Hübner, N. E. El Mokhtari, S. Freitag et al., "NT-proBNP is not elevated in patients with obstructive sleep apnoea," *Respiratory Medicine*, vol. 102, no. 1, pp. 134–142, 2008.

[26] N. Çifçi, M. Uyar, O. Elbek, H. Süyür, and E. Ekinci, "Impact of CPAP treatment on cardiac biomarkers and pro-BNP in obstructive sleep apnea syndrome," *Sleep and Breathing*, vol. 14, no. 3, pp. 241–244, 2010.

[27] N. Q. Wu, F. L. Ma, Y. L. Guo et al., "Association of N-terminal pro-brain natriuretic peptide with the severity of coronary artery disease in patients with normal left ventricular ejection fraction," *Chinese Medical Journal*, vol. 127, no. 4, pp. 627–632, 2014.

[28] M. Weber, T. Dill, R. Arnold et al., "N-terminal B-type natriuretic peptide predicts extent of coronary artery disease and ischemia in patients with stable angina pectoris," *American Heart Journal*, vol. 148, no. 4, pp. 612–620, 2004.

[29] K. Bibbins-Domingo, M. Ansari, N. B. Schiller, B. Massie, and M. A. Whooley, "B-type natriuretic peptide and ischemia in patients with stable coronary disease: data from the Heart and Soul study," *Circulation*, vol. 108, no. 24, pp. 2987–2992, 2003.

[30] G. Wei, R. Yaqi, W. Ningfu, and H. Xuwei, "N-terminal prohormone B-type natriuretic peptide and cardiovascular risk in stable coronary artery disease: a meta-analysis of nine prospective studies," *Reviews in Cardiovascular Medicine*, vol. 14, no. 2–4, pp. e92–e98, 2013.

[31] T. Jernberg, S. James, B. Lindahl, M. Stridsberg, P. Venge, and L. Wallentin, "NT-proBNP in unstable coronary artery disease—experiences from the FAST, GUSTO IV and FRISC II trials," *European Journal of Heart Failure*, vol. 6, no. 3, pp. 319–325, 2004.

10

The Pattern of Respiratory Disease Morbidity and Mortality in a Tertiary Hospital in Southern-Eastern Nigeria

Victor Aniedi Umoh,[1] **Akaninyene Otu,**[2] **Henry Okpa,**[3] **and Emmanuel Effa**[3]

[1] *Department of Internal Medicine, University of Uyo, Uyo, Akwa Ibom State, Nigeria*
[2] *University of Calabar, Nigeria*
[3] *Department of Internal Medicine, University of Calabar, Nigeria*

Correspondence should be addressed to Victor Aniedi Umoh; aaumoh@gmail.com

Academic Editor: Hisako Matsumoto

Background. Respiratory complaints are commonly encountered in medicine and respiratory diseases place a high burden on healthcare infrastructure. Healthcare planning should be based on adequate information: this study will help us to analyze the pattern of respiratory disease admissions in the medical wards in a developing country. *Methods.* The medical records of patients admitted into the medical wards over a 5-year period were retrieved and reviewed. Information obtained included demography, diagnosis, comorbid conditions, and risk factors for respiratory disease. *Results.* Three thousand four hundred and ninety patients were admitted into the medical wards with 325 (9.3%) of them diagnosed with a respiratory condition. There were 121 females and 204 males. The average age of the patients was 40.7 ± 14.7 years. Only 7% of the patients smoked cigarette. The commonest respiratory conditions were tuberculosis (66.8%) and pneumonia (24.9%). The commonest comorbidity was HIV infection (39.7%). Tuberculosis/HIV coinfection rate was 50.7%. HIV infection was the single most important predictor of an adverse outcome (OR 5.1, 95% CI 2.05–12.7, $P < 0.001$). *Conclusion.* Infective conditions make up a large percentage of respiratory diseases in low income countries with HIV infection constituting a significant risk factor for a poor disease outcome.

1. Introduction

Respiratory complaints such as cough and catarrh are some of the commonest symptoms encountered in medicine. This is due in part to the large surface area; nearly $70\,m^2$ of the lungs present to the atmosphere [1]. The atmosphere that we breathe is more than just "air." In reality, it is a complex mixture of ambient gases and environmental particulates to which pathogen containing droplets are added when respiratory secretions are coughed or sneezed out by others. Respiratory diseases constitute a major cause of morbidity and mortality worldwide. The top four respiratory diseases, lower respiratory tract infections, chronic obstructive pulmonary disease (COPD), tuberculosis, and lung cancer, are among the ten leading causes of death worldwide [2]. In Africa, lower respiratory tract infection and tuberculosis are ranked 2nd and 8th, respectively [3].

In developed countries, respiratory diseases feature prominently in the top ten causes of morbidity and mortality [4–7]. In Nigeria, lower respiratory tract infections constituted the second leading cause of death in all age brackets in 2002, a year in which TB was the seventh leading cause of death, accounting for 4% of all deaths [8]. In India another developing country, pneumonia and pulmonary tuberculosis ranked in the top five causes of death [9].

Health care demands are rapidly expanding and the trends are changing in developing countries. Upgrading of the health care system is a pressing need and the priorities are not always easy to define especially in a resource constrained system. The changes necessary to improve the health care systems should be evidence-based. There are few studies on the morbidity and mortality pattern of respiratory diseases in Africa and fewer still from Nigeria. This study was undertaken to address some of the issues concerning respiratory diseases in Nigeria.

2. Methods

This was a retrospective study conducted in the University of Calabar Teaching Hospital (UCTH), Calabar Cross River state in the South-Eastern part of Nigeria. This Hospital is a 400-bed hospital with 40 beds spaces for medical admissions. The hospital serves as a training centre for undergraduate medical students and postgraduate Resident Doctors. It is also a referral centre for other secondary health facilities in this part of Nigeria.

The medical records of all patients admitted into the medical wards of UCTH over a five-year period from April 2008 to March 2013 were retrieved and reviewed and the following information was extracted: demographic data, diagnosis of respiratory disease, comorbidities, complications, duration of hospitalisation, cigarette smoking habit, and treatment outcome. Treatment outcome was defined as favourable if the patient was successfully treated and discharged or unfavourable if the patient died while on admission or discharges against medical advice (DAMA). Data was analysed using the computer program Statistical Package for the Social Sciences, version 16.0 (SPSS Inc., Chicago, IL, USA). Descriptive and frequency statistics were obtained for the variables studied. The chi-square test was used to evaluate associations between the categorical variables, and values of $P < 0.05$ were considered statistically significant.

3. Results

3.1. General Characteristics of the Patients. Three thousand four hundred and ninety patients were admitted into the medical wards within the period of study. There were 2202 males and 1288 females with a male to female ratio of 1.7 : 1. Three hundred and twenty five patients were diagnosed with respiratory diseases constituting 9.3% of all the medical admissions. Two hundred and four were males (9.3% of all male patients) and one hundred and twenty one were females (9.4% of all female patients). The average age for the males was 41.4 ± 14.3 years with a range of 15–85 years, while for the females it was 39.3 ± 15.2 years with a range of 19–85 years. Sixty-four percent of the patients were less than 45 years old and 92% were less than 65 years old (Table 1). Most of the patients were farmers with <5% being unemployed. Smoking was not common among the patients with only 7% smoking rate and only the males indulged in smoking.

3.2. Respiratory Diagnosis. Figure 1 shows the frequency of respiratory diseases among the patients. 217 (66.8%) patients were diagnosed with pulmonary tuberculosis, 81 (24.9%) with pneumonia, 16 (4.9%) patients with asthma, 7 (2.2%) patients with COPD, and only 2 (0.6%) patients with lung cancer and interstitial lung disease. The distribution of the various conditions among the patients is shown in Table 2. There was no significant gender difference in frequency of chest disease. The age distribution of the chest diseases shows that tuberculosis and pneumonia were more common within the 30–44 years age bracket and least common within the 65+ age bracket. Asthma and COPD were more common within

TABLE 1: General characteristics of patients with respiratory diseases in UCTH.

	Female 121 (%)	Male 204 (%)	Total 325 (%)
Age			
15–29	41 (33.8)	42 (20.6)	83 (25.5)
30–44	38 (31.5)	87 (42.7)	125 (38.5)
45–64	33 (27.3)	58 (28.4)	91 (28)
65+	9 (7.4)	17 (8.3)	26 (8)
Occupation			
Farmer	42 (34.7)	78 (38.2)	120 (37.0)
Trader	15 (12.4)	35 (17.1)	50 (15.4)
Public servant	31 (25.6)	52 (25.5)	83 (25.5)
Semiskilled	23 (19.0)	34 (17.7)	57 (17.5)
Unemployed	10 (8.3)	5 (2.5)	15 (4.6)
Smoker	0 (0.0)	23 (11.3)	23 (7.1)

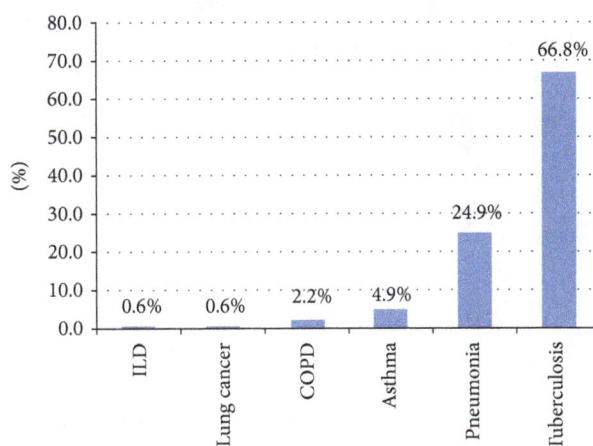

FIGURE 1: Frequency of respiratory conditions among patients in the medical wards.

the 45–64 years age bracket followed by the 15–29 and 30–44 years age bracket. There was also one case of interstitial lung disease (ILD) in the age brackets of 30–44 and 65+. There was one case of lung cancer among patients aged 34–44 years and 45–64 years. The differences were statistically significant ($P = 0.001$). Smoking was significantly associated with COPD, lung cancer, and chest infections ($P = 0.007$). HIV infection was significantly associated with tuberculosis and pneumonia ($P < 0.0001$).

3.3. Comorbid Conditions. Figure 2 shows the distribution of comorbidities among the patients with chest diseases. One hundred and fifty six (48%) of the patients had one comorbidity or the other. The commonest comorbidity was HIV infection (39.7%). Eleven (3.4%) of the patients had diabetes mellitus. Eight (2.5%) of the patients had congestive cardiac failure. There were three patients each with stroke, chronic liver disease, and septicaemia, while two patients had other malignancies other than lung cancer.

TABLE 2: Distribution of respiratory conditions among patients.

	Tuberculosis $N = 217$ (%)	Pneumonia $N = 81$ (%)	Asthma $N = 16$ (%)	COPD $N = 7$ (%)	Lung ca. $N = 2$ (%)	ILD $N = 2$ (%)	P
Gender							
Female	80 (36.9)	28 (34.6)	9 (56.2)	3 (42.9)	0 (0.0)	1 (50.0)	0.53
Male	137 (63.1)	53 (65.4)	7 (43.8)	4 (57.1)	2 (100)	1 (50.0)	
Age							
15–29	60 (27.6)	18 (22.2)	4 (25)	1 (14.3)	0 (0.0)	0 (0.0)	
30–44	90 (41.5)	29 (35.8)	4 (25)	0 (0.0)	1 (50.0)	1 (50)	0.001
45–64	58 (26.7)	20 (24.7)	7 (43.8)	5 (71.4)	1 (50.0)	0 (0.0)	
65+	9 (4.2)	14 (17.3)	1 (6.2)	1 (14.3)	0 (0.0)	1 (50)	
HIV+ve	110 (50.7)	18 (22.2)	1 (6.2)	0 (0.0)	0 (0.0)	0 (0.0)	<0.001
Smoking	17 (7.8)	5 (6.2)	0 (0.0)	2 (28.6)	2 (100)	0 (0.0)	0.007

Lung ca.: lung cancer
ILD: interstitial lung disease.

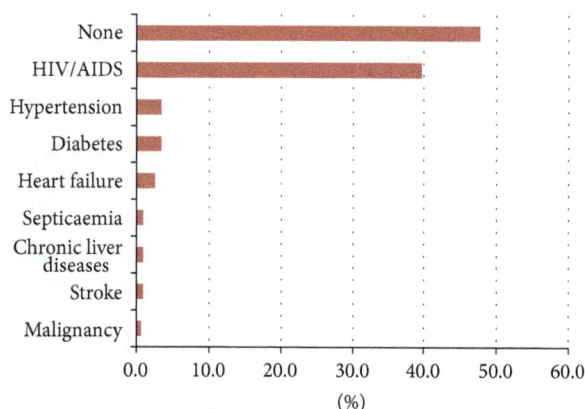

FIGURE 2: Frequency of comorbidities among respiratory diseases patients.

TABLE 3: Average duration of hospital stay based on the respiratory condition.

Diagnosis	Mean (SD)	95% CI	
		Lower	Upper
Asthma	8.25 (2.5)	6.91	9.59
Pneumonia	9.14 (5.0)	8.03	10.25
Tuberculosis	17.63 (5.2)	16.94	18.33
Lung cancer	17.0 (11.3)	−84.65	118.65
COPD	16.14 (5.7)	10.85	21.44
ILD	21.0 (9.89)	−67.94	109.94

ILD: interstitial lung disease.

3.4. *Duration of Hospitalisation.* The average duration of hospitalisation was 15.4 ± 6.4 days with a range between 3 and 35 days. Patients with interstitial lung disease spent the most days in hospital (21 ± 9.9) followed by patients with tuberculosis and lung cancer, 17.6 ± 5.2 days and 17 ± 11.3 days, respectively. Asthma patients spent the least number of days in hospital; 8.3 ± 2.5 days (Table 3). A one way analysis of variance test was conducted to explore the impact of the respiratory diagnosis on the duration of hospital stay. Patients were divided into six groups based on their diagnosis. There was a statistically significant difference in duration of hospital admission for the six groups $F(5,319) = 38.9$, $P < 0.0001$. The diagnosis had a large effect on the duration of hospitalisation (Eta squared 0.37). Post hoc analysis using Tukey-HSD indicated that the duration of stay for tuberculosis was significantly longer than that of asthma and pneumonia.

3.5. *Treatment Outcome.* Two hundred and ninety (89.2%) patients were treated successfully and discharged form hospital and 30 (9.2%) died while on admission, while five (1.6%)

patients DAMA; Figure 3. All 35 (10.8%) patients had an unfavourable outcome. There was no significant association between the diagnosis and the final outcome (Table 4).

Direct logistic regression analysis was performed to assess the impact of certain factors on an unfavourable outcome. The model contained seven variables: age, duration of hospital stay, gender, cigarette smoking, HIV infection, tuberculosis, and lung cancer. The full model was statistically significant $\chi^2 = 29.066$ and $P < 0.001$, indicating that the model could distinguish patients who had a favourable outcome from those with an unfavourable outcome. The model could explain up to 17.3% of the variance in outcome (Negelkerke R squared) and correctly classified 90% of the patients. Only HIV infection made a unique significant contribution to the model (OR 5.1, $P < 0.0001$) indicating that patients with HIV infection were over five times more likely to have an unfavourable outcome (Table 5).

4. Discussion

Respiratory diseases constituted 9.3% of medical admissions in this survey. Similar observations have been reported by other investigators. Desalu et al. [10] in Ilorin, North-Central Nigeria, reported that respiratory diseases make up 8.7% of all medical admissions. Respiratory diseases accounted for

TABLE 4: Diseases outcome according to respiratory condition.

	Asthma 16 (%)	Pneumonia 81 (%)	Tuberculosis 217 (%)	Lung ca. 2 (%)	COPD 7 (%)	ILD 2 (%)	P
Discharged	16 (100)	74 (91.4)	192 (88.5)	0 (0.0)	6 (85.7)	2 (100)	0.147
DAMA	0 (0.0)	1 (1.2)	4 (1.8)	0 (0.0)	0 (0.0)	0 (0.0)	
Died	0 (0.0)	6 (7.4)	21 (9.7)	2 (100)	1 (14.3)	0 (0.0)	

Lung ca.: lung cancer
ILD: interstitial lung disease.

TABLE 5: Predictors of unfavourable outcome among patients with respiratory conditions.

Parameter	OR	P	95% CI for OR	
			Lower	Upper
Age	0.99	0.96	0.97	1.03
Hospital stay	0.98	0.58	0.91	1.05
Gender	0.5	0.09	0.22	1.13
Smoking	2.74	0.17	0.65	11.5
HIV infection	5.1	<0.001	2.05	12.7
TB infection	1.03	0.94	0.36	2.97
Lung cancer	2.01×10^{10}	0.99	0.00	

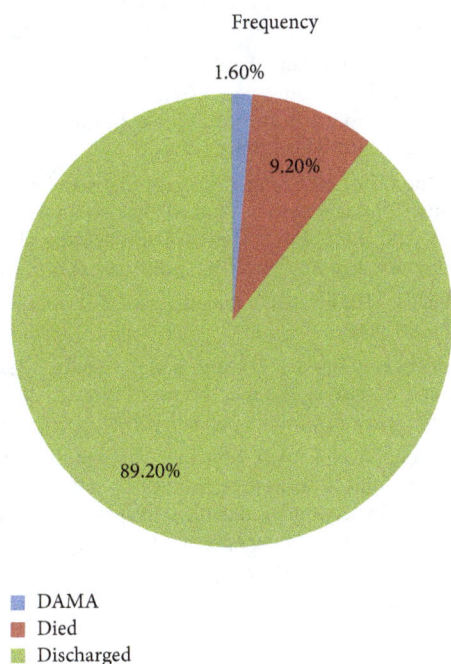

FIGURE 3: Outcome among patients with respiratory disease.

a higher percentage (14.5%) of medical admissions in Saudi Arabia [11] and 31.73% in Kathmandu, Nepal [12]. The much higher prevalence of respiratory diseases in the Saudi survey and Kathmandu may be due to the higher prevalence of a major risk factor for respiratory diseases in these desert areas with many pilgrims: cigarette smoking which may be as high as 53% in some of these areas [13, 14] among other factors. This stands in contrast to the observed smoking rate in this study (7%) as well as in a previous Nigerian report of 8.7% [15].

Tuberculosis was the commonest respiratory condition followed by pneumonia. Together they account for over 90% of respiratory admissions. In Ilorin Central Nigeria, chest infections were the most important causes of respiratory disease hospitalisation with tuberculosis and pneumonia occupying the first and third most frequent indications for hospitalisation [10]. This contrasts sharply with observations from other parts of the world where chronic noninfective respiratory diseases predominate [11, 12].

Young patients <45 years made up >60% of the admissions in this study. This picture is similar to what was observed in a previous study from Nigeria by Desalu et al. [10] in that study most of the patients were young adults <45 years. This can be explained by the demographic pattern of Nigeria where >80% of the population is <45 years [16]. This pattern contrasts with observations in the ward admissions of patients with respiratory diseases in other parts of the world where older patients make up the bulk of the respiratory diseases admissions [4–6, 11].

The most common comorbidity in this study was HIV infection with a prevalence of 39.7% and a tuberculosis coinfection rate of 50.7%. HIV has been shown to have a strong association with tuberculosis. Pennap et al. [17] in Keffi, North-Central Nigeria reported a prevalence of 44.2% for tuberculosis/HIV coinfection. Studies from regions with a low prevalence of HIV have reported a different pattern for the comorbidities; diabetes and hypertension being the most common comorbidities [11].

The average duration of hospitalisation was 15.4 ± 6.4 days. A previous local study reported the duration of hospitalisation for medical admissions of 15.6 ± 13.8 days [18]; this shows that on average respiratory disease patients did not spend more time on admission than medical conditions of other systems. Hospital stay in this study was significantly longer for ILD and tuberculosis patients compared with pneumonia and asthma ($P < 0.05$). This is similar to observations by Desalu et al. [10] where they reported the average duration of hospitalisation for respiratory diseases to be 14 days with pneumonia and asthma accounting for the shortest duration of hospitalisation. Alamoudi [11] in Saudi Arabia reported similar findings; a majority of asthma and pneumonia patients were hospitalised for less than a week, while ILD, tuberculosis, and bronchiectasis accounted for most of the patients that spent more than two weeks on admission.

Thirty (9.2%) patients died while five patients DAMA. Lung cancer recorded 100% mortality in this study. Mortality from lung cancer is high all over the world [19]. Smoking is a major risk factor for lung cancer [20]. In this study, all the patients with lung cancer had a significant smoking history. The smoking rate is on the increase in low income countries [3] as such we should expect an increase in the incidence and mortality from lung cancer in the coming years. In this study one death was attributed to COPD. With the increasing rate of smoking in low income countries we should also expect an increase in morbidity and mortality from this condition.

11.5% of patients with tuberculosis had an unfavourable outcome. Different investigators have reported varying mortality rates for tuberculosis. Our observations on mortality is similar to a report of mortality rate of 10.1% among 4000 tuberculosis patients in Ethiopia by Tessema et al. [21] and Busari et al. [22] in Ido-Ekiti South-West, Nigeria. A much higher mortality rate was observed by Salako and Sholeye in Sagamu, South-West, Nigeria. In their study 23.2% of the hospitalised patient had unfavourable outcome [23]. The different mortality rates may be a reflection of the difference in diseases severity in those centres.

HIV infection was the only condition with a unique significant contribution to an adverse outcome in this study after controlling for confounders (OR 5.1, 95% CI 2.05–12.7, and $P < 0.001$). The probability of dying or abandoning treatment among patients with respiratory disease was five times higher for patients with concomitant HIV infection than for patients without HIV infection. Several studies from Nigeria have described the critical role of HIV infection as a cause of morbidity and mortality in hospitalised patients [24, 25]. Studies have also revealed that HIV/AIDS patients in Nigeria tend to present late with advanced illnesses [26]. Thus compounding the outcome in this very serious disease condition.

There are several limitations of this study. First of all this was a retrospective study as such we encountered some poor and incomplete record keeping which affected our ability to quantify some variables. It is worthy to note that certain diseases, such as bronchiectasis, pulmonary vascular diseases, sleep apnoea, pneumocystis jirovecii pneumonia (PCP), sarcoidosis, collagen lung diseases, overlap syndromes of asthma and COPD, and pneumoconiosis were not reported. This may be due to a lack of awareness and a low index of suspicion from the attending physicians. In conclusion this study has highlighted the high burden of respiratory diseases in our hospital and the role of tuberculosis and HIV coinfections as a major cause of morbidity and mortality.

Disclosure

Dr. Victor Aniedi Umoh will act as the guarantor. This study in part or as a whole has not been published or presented in any journal or conference before. No other person or body has been given permission to reproduce any information or material in this paper.

Conflict of Interests

The authors have no conflict of interests whatsoever.

References

[1] M. Ochs and E. R. Weibel, "Functional design of the human lungs for gas exchange," in *Fishman's Pulmonary diseases and disorders*, vol. 10036, pp. 23–25, McGraw Hill, New York, NY, USA, 4th edition, 2008.

[2] R. Lozano, M. Naghavi, K. Foreman et al., "Global and regional mortality from 235 causes of death for 20 age groups in 1990 and 2010: a systematic analysis for the Global Burden of Disease Study 2010," *The Lancet*, vol. 380, pp. 2095–2128, 2012.

[3] WHO, "Global Burden of Disease: 2004 update," vol. 1211, World Health Organisation, Geneva, Switzerland, 2008 http://www.who.int/healthinfo/global_burden_disease/2004_report_update/en/index.html.

[4] BTS, "The burden of lung disease: a statistical report from the British Thoracic Society," 2nd ed., British Thoracic Society, London, UK, 2006, http://www.brit-thoracic.org.uk/delivery-of-respiratory-care/burden-of-lung-disease-reports.aspx.

[5] R. Hubbard, "The burden of lung disease," *Thorax*, vol. 61, no. 7, pp. 557–558, 2006.

[6] R. Loddenkemper, G. J. Gibson, and Y. Sibille, "Respiratory health and disease in Europe: the new European Lung White Book," *European Respiratory Journal*, vol. 42, pp. 559–563, 2013.

[7] D. E. Schraufnagel, F. Blasi, M. Kraft, M. Gaga, P. Finn, and K. F. Rabe, "An official American Thoracic Society and European Respiratory Society policy statement: disparities in respiratory health," *European Respiratory Journal*, vol. 42, pp. 906–915, 2013.

[8] WHO, "Country Health System Fact Sheet 2006: Nigeria," WHO, Geneva, Switzerland, 2006, http://www.afro.who.int/home/countries/fact_sheets/nigeria.pdf.

[9] A. Ramanakumar and C. Aparajita, "Respiratory disease burden in rural India: a review from multiple data sources," *The Internet Journal of Epidemiology*, vol. 2, no. 2, 2005.

[10] O. O. Desalu, J. A. Oluwafemi, and O. Ojo, "Respiratory diseases morbidity and mortality among adults attending a tertiary hospital in Nigeria," *Jornal Brasileiro de Pneumologia*, vol. 35, no. 8, pp. 745–752, 2009.

[11] O. S. Alamoudi, "Prevalence of respiratory diseases in hospitalized patients in Saudi Arabia: a 5 years study 1996–2000," *Annals of Thoracic Medicine*, vol. 1, no. 2, pp. 76–80, 2006.

[12] B. R. Pokharel, S. Humagain Pant P, R. Gurung, R. Koju, and T. R. Bedi, "Spectrum of diseases in a medical ward of a teaching hospital in a developing country," *Journal of College of Medical Sciences-Nepal*, vol. 8, no. 2, pp. 7–11, 2012.

[13] A. El-Menyar, M. Zubaid, A. Shehab et al., "Prevalence and impact of cardiovascular risk factors among patients presenting with acute coronary syndrome in the middle east," *Clinical Cardiology*, vol. 34, no. 1, pp. 51–58, 2011.

[14] C. T. Sreeramareddy, N. Ramakrishnareddy, H. N. Harsha Kumar, B. Sathian, and J. T. Arokiasamy, "Prevalence, distribution and correlates of tobacco smoking and chewing in Nepal: a secondary data analysis of Nepal Demographic and Health Survey-2006," *Substance Abuse*, vol. 6, no. 1, article 33, 2011.

[15] E. G. Adepoju, S. A. Olowookere, N. A. Adeleke, O. T. Afolabi, F. O. Olajide, and O. O. Aluko, "A population based study on the prevalence of cigarette smoking and smokers' characteristics at Osogbo, Nigeria," *Tobacco Use Insights*, vol. 6, pp. 1–5, 2013.

[16] National Population Commission (NPC) [Nigeria] and ICF Macro, "Nigeria Demographic and Health Survey 2008," National Populaton Commission and ICF Macro, Abuja, Nigeria, 2009, http://www.measuredhs.com/pubs/pdf/FR222/FR222.pdf.

[17] G. Pennap, S. Makpa, and S. Ogbu, "The prevalence of HIV/AIDS among tuberculosis patients in a tuberculosis/leprosy Referral Center in Alushi, Nasarawa State, Nigeria," *The Internet Journal of Epidemiology*, vol. 8, no. 1, 2010.

[18] E. O. Sanya, T. M. Akande, G. Opadijo, J. K. Olarinoye, and B. J. Bojuwoye, "Pattern and outcome of medical admission of elderly patients seen at University of Ilorin Teaching Hospital, Ilorin," *African Journal of Medicine and Medical Sciences*, vol. 37, no. 4, pp. 375–381, 2008.

[19] P. Paliogiannis, F. Attene, A. Cossu et al., "Lung cancer epidemiology in North Sardinia, Italy," *Multidisciplinary Respiratory Medicine*, vol. 8, no. 1, article 45, 2013.

[20] V. N. Davis, A. Lavender, R. Bayakly, K. Ray, and T. Moon, "Using current smoking prevalence to project lung cancer morbidity and mortality in Georgia by 2020," *Preventing Chronic Disease*, vol. 10, Article ID 120271, 2013.

[21] B. Tessema, A. Muche, A. Bekele, D. Reissig, F. Emmrich, and U. Sack, "Treatment outcome of tuberculosis patients at Gondar University Teaching Hospital, Northwest Ethiopia. A five - Year retrospective study," *BMC Public Health*, vol. 9, article 371, 2009.

[22] O. A. Busari, O. T. Olarewaju, and O. E. Busari, "Management and outcomes of suspected pulmonary tuberculosis in a resource-poor setting," *Internet Journal of Pulmonary Medicine*, vol. 11, no. 2, 2010.

[23] A. A. Salako and O. O. Sholeye, "Management outcomes of tuberculosis cases in a tertiary hospital in Southwestern Nigeria," *Journal of Community Medicine and Health Education*, vol. 2, no. 2, article 122, 2012.

[24] D. Ogoina, R. O. Obiako, H. M. Muktar, M. Adeiza, A. Babadoko, and A. Hassan, "Morbidity and mortality patterns of hospitalised adult HIV/AIDS patients in the era of highly active antiretroviral therapy: a 4-year retrospective review from Zaria, Northern Nigeria," *AIDS Research and Treatment*, vol. 2012, Article ID 940580, 10 pages, 2012.

[25] A. N. Gyuse, I. E. Bassey, N. E. Udonwa, I. B. Okokon, and E. E. Philip-Ephraim, "HIV/AIDS related mortality among adult medical patients in a tertiary health institution in South-South, Nigeria," *Asian Pacific Journal of Tropical Medicine*, vol. 3, no. 2, pp. 141–144, 2010.

[26] C. Akolo, C. O. Ukoli, G. N. Ladep, and J. A. Idoko, "The clinical features of HIV/AIDS at presentation at the Jos University Teaching Hospital," *Nigerian Journal of Medicine*, vol. 17, no. 1, pp. 83–87, 2008.

11

The Immediate Pulmonary Disease Pattern following Exposure to High Concentrations of Chlorine Gas

Pallavi P. Balte,[1] Kathleen A. Clark,[1] Lawrence C. Mohr,[2] Wilfried J. Karmaus,[3] David Van Sickle,[4] and Erik R. Svendsen[5]

[1] *Arnold School of Public Health, University of South Carolina, 800 Sumter Street, Room 210, Columbia, SC 29208, USA*

[2] *Medical University of South Carolina, 135 Cannon Street, Suite 405, P.O. Box 250838, Charleston, SC 29425, USA*

[3] *Division of Epidemiology, Biostatistics, and Environmental Health, School of Public Health, University of Memphis, 301 Robison Hall, 3825 De Soto Avenue, Memphis, TN 38152, USA*

[4] *Asthmapolis, 612 W. Main Street, Suite 201, Madison, WI 53703, USA*

[5] *Department of Global Environmental Health Sciences, Tulane University School of Public Health and Tropical Medicine, 1440 Canal Street, Suite 2100, New Orleans, LA 70112, USA*

Correspondence should be addressed to Pallavi P. Balte; balte.p@gmail.com

Academic Editor: Andrew Sandford

Background. Classification of pulmonary disease into obstructive, restrictive, and mixed patterns is based on 2005 ATS/ERS guidelines and modified GOLD criteria by Mannino et al. (2003), but these guidelines are of limited use for simple spirometry in situations involving mass casualties. *Aim.* The purpose of this study was to apply these guidelines to patients who underwent simple spirometry following high concentration of chlorine gas inhalation after a train derailment in Graniteville, South Carolina. *Methods.* We retrospectively investigated lung functions in ten patients. In order to classify pulmonary disease pattern, we used 2005 ATS/ERS guidelines and modified GOLD criteria along with our own criteria developed using available simple spirometry data. *Results.* We found predominant restrictive pattern in our patients with both modified GOLD and our criteria, which is in contrast to other chlorine exposure studies where obstructive pattern was more common. When compared to modified GOLD and our criteria, 2005 ATS/ERS guidelines underestimated the frequency of restrictive disease. *Conclusion.* Diagnosis of pulmonary disease patterns is of importance after irritant gas inhalation. Acceptable criteria need to be developed to evaluate pulmonary disease through simple spirometry in events leading to mass casualty and patient surge in hospitals.

1. Introduction

Chlorine gas is one of the most commonly used industrial chemicals and is a potential weapon of mass destruction [1–8]. The health effects of chlorine inhalation depend on chlorine concentration and duration of exposure. If inhaled in low concentration (<50 ppm) chlorine gas is known to cause mild irritation of mucus membranes, coughing, choking, and shortness of breath [9, 10]. Exposure to high concentrations (>50 ppm) may damage the lower respiratory tract and lung parenchyma causing complications such as rapid development of interstitial pneumonia, pulmonary edema, and death due to progressive respiratory failure [9–11]. Several studies have shown decrease in lung function

after acute inhalation of chlorine gas, but very few studies attempted to determine pulmonary disease pattern in these patients [11–14]. Although obstructive pulmonary disease was most commonly observed in all these studies, restrictive and mixed pulmonary disease were also seen in a few studies [12–14].

At present, 2005 ATS/ERS task force guidelines based on NHANES III data are considered the "gold standard" and are used universally to provide guidance to physicians and hospital based pulmonary function tests (PFTs) laboratories for interpreting PFTs [15]. These guidelines are based on availability of plethysmography to determine total lung capacity (TLC). On the other hand, Mannino et al. used a modification of the Global Initiative for Chronic Obstructive Lung Disease

(GOLD) criteria to determine pulmonary disease patterns in NHANES I cohort based on spirometry data alone [16].

The modified GOLD criteria [16] are a very useful tool for diagnosing and assessing the severity of COPD through simple spirometry without lung volume measurements in clinical settings [17]. However, there are no specific guidelines for diagnosing mixed pattern. The 2005 ATS/ERS guidelines [15] cannot be used with spirometry data alone due to lack of information on lung volumes.

Both ATS/ERS guidelines and modified GOLD criteria are extremely valuable to diagnose, characterize, and assess pulmonary disease in patients routinely admitted to hospitals [17–19]. These guidelines are also useful in diagnosing pulmonary disease in irritant gas exposure events with small number of people affected [20]. But in mass casualty events providing diagnostic PFTs is not possible within days of occurrence [21, 22]. In emergency situations like these where a large number of people are affected, healthcare services are more concentrated on making quick medical evaluation and providing appropriate emergent treatment. There are rarely major resources available to provide diagnostic testing like complete PFTs in such situations. Therefore, assessment of severity of pulmonary disease has to be based on available resources like spirometry. However, at present there are no known universally acceptable criteria or guidelines available that can be used to diagnose pulmonary disease during mass casualty or in situations where healthcare resources are limited due to patient surge in emergency departments. Irritant gas exposure is known to have long term sequelae, so it is also important to know different pulmonary disease patterns and the pathophysiology behind it for long term follow-up [23, 24].

The purpose of this study was to apply 2005 ATS/ERS and Mannino et al. (2003) guidelines along with our own criteria to determine pulmonary function patterns in ten patients who underwent simple spirometry following high concentration of chlorine gas inhalation after a train derailment in Graniteville, South Carolina.

2. Methods

2.1. Graniteville Train Accident. On January 6, 2005, a train derailment and tanker breach led to the largest chlorine spill in the United States history, releasing approximately 60 tons of chlorine gas in Graniteville, South Carolina. A report was published earlier describing exposure to the community, evacuation, and emergency medical response [21]. There were nine immediate fatalities and 525 emergency room visits with 71 hospitalizations initially reported. Twenty-three of these patients were intubated and placed on mechanical ventilation. The remaining 48 were admitted to acute care with various clinical manifestations attributed to high concentration of chlorine gas inhalation. All patients were admitted within the first 24 hours after exposure. The initial evaluation included physical examination, chest radiography, and arterial blood gas determinations. Spirometry was performed on ten patients. A detailed description of

sociodemographic characteristics, clinical signs and symptoms, hematological and biochemical findings, radiographic findings, and treatment in all 71 patients admitted to hospital was previously published [22].

2.2. Study Population and Protocol. We conducted a case series study of the ten patients who underwent simple spirometry testing while being admitted in the hospital. The data used for this report were part of a larger public health effort directed by South Carolina Department of Health and Environmental Control (SCDHEC) which focused on recovery and mitigation of disease in the exposed Graniteville community. A retrospective chart review was conducted under the public health authority within declared emergency situations. We accessed a de-identified SCDHEC database from that public health chart review. This study was approved by both SCDHEC and University of South Carolina (USC) institutional review boards (IRB).

2.3. Criteria for Classification of Pulmonary Disease Pattern. All spirometry tests were performed within one week of admission (on an average 5th day after admission). Spirometry tests were performed according to ATS/ERS guidelines [15]. The predicted and lower limits of normal (LLN) values were calculated using NHANES III prediction equations [25]. In order to classify pulmonary disease patterns in these patients we applied two widely used criteria: 2005 ATS/ERS task force guidelines [15] which are derived from NHANES III data and require lung volume parameters and criteria used by Mannino et al. which are based on simple spirometry [16]. In our study we had simple spirometry data without any lung volume parameters on ten patients. As 2005 ATS/ERS guidelines require lung volume parameters to diagnose pulmonary disease pattern and Mannino et al. (2003) did not have any specified criteria to diagnose mixed pattern, we were unable to use these two criteria to their full extent in our study. We therefore developed criteria that facilitate diagnosis of all three pulmonary disease patterns using available spirometry data. We do not consider these criteria as guidelines to be used in mass casualty events, as these are based on data from only ten patients. We use these criteria here as only a tool to get a complete picture of pulmonary disease pattern in the patients admitted to hospital and to compare them with existing guidelines (Table 1).

2.4. Statistical Analyses. This is a descriptive epidemiological study with a small sample size. We calculated the agreement between different criteria used to classify pulmonary disease patterns. The data analysis for this paper was generated using SAS 9.2. (SAS Institute Inc., Cary, NC, USA).

3. Results

Of the ten patients we evaluated, five were admitted to the intensive care unit (ICU), and two of these required intubation and mechanical ventilation due to acute lung injury. There were nine males and one female with a mean age of 44.7 ± 16.1 years. Among the ten patients four were

TABLE 1: Comparison of different criteria for classification of pulmonary disease patterns.

Pulmonary disease pattern	2003 Mannino et al. guidelines [16]	2005 ATS/ERS task force guidelines[#] [15]	Graniteville criteria
Obstructive	Mild: FEV_1/FVC ratio < 70%, $FEV_1 \geq 80\%$ of predicted Moderate: FEV_1/FVC ratio < 70%, $FEV_1 \geq 50\%$ but < 80% of predicted Severe: FEV_1/FVC ratio < 70%, $FEV_1 < 50\%$ of predicted	FEV_1/VC ratio below LLN[*]	FEV_1/FVC ratio ≤ 0.70 and normal, reduced, or increased FEV_1 and FVC percent predicted
Restrictive	FEV_1/FVC ratio ≥ 70 and FVC < 80% of predicted	TLC below LLN or FEV_1/VC ratio ≥ 85 and a reduced VC	FEV_1/FVC ratio ≥ 0.75, FEV_1 and FVC < 75% of predicted
Mixed	No criteria reported	FEV_1/VC ratio and TLC below LLN	FEV_1/FVC ratio > 0.70 and < 0.75 and both FEV_1 and FVC < 75% predicted

[#]Vital capacity (VC) measures were unavailable, so we used FEV_1/FVC ratio instead of FEV_1/VC ratio as suggested by 2005 ATS/ERS guidelines.
[*]Lower limit of normal.

TABLE 2: Sociodemographic characteristics of patients who underwent spirometry.

Characteristic	$N = 10$
Age (years), mean ± S.D.	44.7 ± 16.1
Gender, n	
Male	9
Female	1
Race, n	
Caucasian	6
African American	4
Smoker, n	
Current	4
Former	1
Nonsmoker	5

TABLE 3: Presenting symptoms and physical findings in patients who underwent spirometry.

Variable	N
Symptoms:	
Sore throat	35
Cough	9
Nose irritation	8
Shortness of breath	7
Choking	6
Chest pain	6
Productive cough	5
Dizziness	3
Headache	4
Eye irritation	4
Nausea/vomiting	2
Physical findings:	
Tachypnea	10
Tachycardia	9
Crackles	5
Wheeze	6
Decreased breath sounds	2

current smokers, five were nonsmokers, and one was a former smoker (Table 2). Presenting symptoms specific to chlorine exposure were shortness of breath, coughing, choking, chest pain, productive cough, eye irritation, nose irritation and sore throat (Table 3). Symptoms less specific to chlorine exposure were dizziness, headache, nausea, and vomiting. On physical examination tachypnea and tachycardia were the most common findings. Other notable findings on auscultation were wheeze, crackles, and decreased breath sounds.

Mean oxygen saturation upon admission to emergency department was 81.1 ± 18.1% (Table 4). Mean white blood cell (WBC) count in all patients was $13.91 \pm 3.25 \times 10^3$ cells/μL within the first 24 hours with an elevated neutrophil count in six patients, mean 79.7 ± 4.8%. The average blood pH and PCO_2 in nine patients were 7.32 ± 0.08 and 47.42 ± 9.02 mm of Hg, respectively. Chest radiography was performed on all patients. Seven patients showed evidence of pulmonary edema and one showed increased bronchovascular markings,

while two patients had a normal chest radiograph. Electrocardiography was performed on six patients and three showed nonspecific T-wave changes.

All patients received warm humidified oxygen on arrival at the emergency department along with inhaled short acting beta receptor agonists. Additionally, all patients were treated with either inhaled or oral steroids, six were treated with inhaled ipratropium bromide, and seven were treated with antibiotics. One patient also received intravenous sodium bicarbonate due to severe acid-base imbalance. The average stay in the hospital was 8.1 ± 5.4 days.

All spirometry tests were done within the first week (on an average 5th day after admission) of hospitalization after the

TABLE 4: Mean and standard deviation of pulmonary function parameters, hematological and biochemical findings, and oxygen saturation.

Variable	N	Mean ± S.D.
Pulmonary function tests (done within one week):		
Measured FVC	10	2.51 ± 0.39 mL
Measured FEV_1	10	1.84 ± 0.36 mL
FVC% predicted	10	57.2 ± 11.6%
FEV_1% predicted	10	53.4 ± 13.4%
FEV_1/FVC ratio	10	0.76 ± 0.09
LLN FVC	10	3.72 ± 0.68 mL
LLN FEV_1	10	2.97 ± 0.57 mL
LLN FEV_1/FVC ratio	10	0.70 ± 0.04
Hematological and biochemical findings (done within first 24 hours):		
Total WBC count	10	$13.9 ± 3.2 × 10^3$ cells/μL
Neutrophil count	6	79.7 ± 4.8%
Blood pH	9	7.32 ± 0.08
Blood CO_2	9	47.42 ± 9.02 mm Hg
Blood HCO_3	7	54 ± 79.86 mEq/L
Oxygen saturation (done in emergency department):		
Overall	10	81.1 ± 18.1%
With pulmonary edema	7	77.9 ± 21.2%
Without pulmonary edema	3	88.7 ± 3.8%

patient was stabilized. Mean FVC and FEV_1 were 2.51 ± 0.39 L and 1.84 ± 0.36 L, respectively (Table 4). Mean FEV_1 percent predicted was 53.4 ± 13.4%, mean FVC percent predicted was 57.2 ± 11.6%, and mean FEV_1/FVC ratio was 0.76 ± 0.09. Using 2005 ATS/ERS task force guidelines [13], we found an obstructive pattern in three and restrictive pattern in two patients. We were not able to determine the primary pulmonary disease pattern in the remaining five patients as information on TLC was not available (Table 5). Based on guidelines used by Mannino et al. (2003), we found a restrictive pattern in eight patients, and obstructive pattern in two patients. After applying our criteria based, we found a restrictive pattern in seven patients, obstructive pattern in two patients and mixed pattern in one patient (Table 5). The agreement between our criteria and guidelines provided by Mannino et al. (2003) was 75%. Agreement between our criteria and 2005 ATS/ERS task force guidelines resulted in only 16.7% agreement which is expected as we did not have lung volume parameters to use 2005 ATS/ERS guidelines to full extent. Among current smokers, three had restrictive and one had obstructive pattern, while among nonsmokers three had restrictive, one had mixed, and one had an obstructive pattern. One former smoker showed a restrictive pattern.

4. Discussion

Chlorine is one of the most commonly produced chemicals in the United States and the most common cause of household exposure to irritant gases resulting in lung injury [9]. Chlorine is also considered as a hazardous material with a constant threat of industrial accidental exposure and as a terrorist weapon [26]. Medical management decisions for acute chlorine inhalation are subjective and largely depend on presenting signs and symptoms and oxygen saturation [27]. Acute injury from chlorine gas exposure may induce chronic inflammation and fibrosis, which may then influence the rate of functional decline [24, 28] and lead to restrictive lung disease [29]. It is important to determine pulmonary disease pattern after acute inhalation of chlorine gas because the treatment modalities differ in obstructive and restrictive lung disease. Obstructive disease is primarily treated with bronchodilators and inhaled corticosteroids depending on the stage of disease whereas treatment of restrictive disease mainly focuses on immunosuppression using oral corticosteroids in early stages and drugs like cyclophosphamide in late stages [29].

In the present study, all ten patients exhibited symptoms consistent with high concentration of irritant gas exposure and moderate to severe hypoxemia, tachypnea, and tachycardia. Eight patients demonstrated adventitious breath sounds associated with adverse clinical symptoms such as dyspnea, wheezing, coughing, and chest pain. Pulmonary edema and increased bronchovascular markings were common on chest radiographs. After applying our criteria to determine pulmonary disease patterns we found that restrictive pattern ($n = 7$) was more common than the obstructive ($n = 2$) and mixed ($n = 1$) pattern. All patients received humidified oxygen and short acting beta agonists. Treatment should have improved pulmonary function after one-week period. However, we found that all patients who underwent pulmonary function testing had abnormal lung function. As mentioned earlier, obstructive lung disease is more common after exposure to high concentration of chlorine gas [12–14]. In contradiction to other studies we found that restrictive pulmonary disease was more common than obstructive pulmonary disease. We found no past medical history for preexisting underlying lung disease during chart review. Additionally, there were no specific differences in pulmonary disease patterns among smokers and nonsmokers.

There are several limitations to our study. Firstly, our sample size was very small, too small to draw any definite conclusions. Secondly, since the data came from a retrospective review of medical charts for public health reporting purposes, the information retrieved was very limited. Thirdly, TLC measurements were not available. Finally, we also did not have baseline pulmonary function measurements for comparison.

Several studies have examined the acute effects of high concentration of chlorine inhalation on pulmonary functions with differing results. Charan et al. studied 19 people exposed to chlorine gas in an accident in a pulp mill [14]. They found an obstructive disease pattern in ten out of 19 patients admitted within the first 24 hours. After a period of 10 days,

TABLE 5: Pulmonary function pattern and radiographic findings in patients who underwent spirometry.

Patient	Smoking status	Percent predicted		FEV$_1$/FVC ratio	LLN FEV$_1$/FVC ratio	Hematology		Chest radiographs		Pulmonary function pattern		
		FVC	FEV$_1$			Total WBC[#]	Neut[*]%	PE	IVM	ATS/ERS Task force[£]	Mannino et al.[¥] [16]	Graniteville criteria[$]
1	Current	59	43	0.55	0.63	9.3	73.8	Yes	Yes	O	Severe O	O
2	Current	40	37	0.75	0.71	14.2	Miss.	Yes	No	U	R	R
3	Current	50	58	0.79	0.67	15.2	Miss.	Yes	No	U	R	R
4	Current	45	45	0.85	0.74	19.7	Miss.	Yes	No	R	R	R
5	Nonsmoker	56	46	0.73	0.76	16	80	Yes	No	O	R	M
6	Nonsmoker	68	63	0.69	0.68	11	75	No	No	U	Moderate O	O
7	Nonsmoker	71	66	0.81	0.71	12.1	86	No	No	U	R	R
8	Nonsmoker	71	75	0.87	0.70	14.4	79.3	No	Yes	R	R	R
9	Nonsmoker	66	64	0.78	0.71	16.9	Miss.	Yes	No	U	R	R
10	Former	46	37	0.81	0.71	10.3	84	Yes	No	U	R	R

[#]×10^3 cells/μL, [*]neutrophils.

PE: pulmonary edema; IVM: increased vascular markings; Miss.: missing.

O: obstructive pattern; R: restrictive pattern; M: mixed pattern; U: undetermined pattern.

[£]Obstructive pattern: FEV1/VC ratio below LLN; Restrictive pattern: TLC below LLN or FEV$_1$/VC ratio ≥ 85% and a reduced VC; mixed: FEV$_1$/VC ratio and TLC below LLN.

[¥]Obstructive pattern: mild: FEV$_1$/FVC ratio < 70%, FEV$_1$ ≥ 80% of predicted, moderate: FEV$_1$/FVC ratio < 70%, FEV$_1$ ≥ 50%–< 80% of predicted, severe: FEV$_1$/FVC ratio < 70%, FEV$_1$ < 50% of predicted; restrictive pattern: FEV$_1$/FVC ratio ≥ 70% and FVC < 80% of predicted.

[$]Obstructive pattern: FEV$_1$/FVC ratio ≤ 0.70 and normal, reduced, or increased FEV$_1$ and FVC percent predicted; restrictive pattern FEV$_1$/FVC ratio ≥ 0.75, FEV$_1$ and FVC < 75% of predicted; mixed: FEV$_1$/FVC ratio > 0.70 and < 0.75 FEV$_1$ and FVC < 75% predicted.

only seven out of ten patients showed airflow obstruction. In another study Moulick et al. studied 82 patients exposed to chlorine leaked from a storage tank at a factory in Mumbai, India [12]. The investigators found an obstructive pattern in 22 (26.8%), restrictive patter in three (3.7%), and mixed pattern in 44 (53.4%) cases within the first 48 hours. Similarly, Barret and Faure after studying 129 patients admitted in Grenoble, France, who underwent spirometry in the acute period after exposure to chlorine found an obstructive pattern in 63%, restrictive pattern in 30%, and mixed pattern in 7% [13]. However, we were unable to obtain information on specific guidelines used for classifying pulmonary disease pattern in the above-mentioned studies. So, we applied three different criteria to classify pulmonary disease patterns using simple spirometry: (1) 2005 ATS/ERS guidelines; (2) modified GOLD criteria used by Mannino et al. (2003); and (3) Graniteville criteria. We found predominant restrictive pattern in our patients by using both modified GOLD and Graniteville criteria, in contrast with above-mentioned studies. The obstructive pattern after chlorine inhalation can be attributed to the irritating action of hypochlorous and hydrochloric acid along with bronchospasm [30, 31]. The restrictive patterns seen in our review could be due to neutrophil sequestration in the respiratory system (as evidenced by elevated neutrophil counts) leading to acute, early onset of inflammation and pulmonary edema [30]. Accumulation of fluid in the alveoli would produce restrictive pattern [30]. In this study, we found radiographic evidence of pulmonary edema in six out of seven patients with a restrictive spirometry pattern and four of them had elevated neutrophil counts. While comparing our criteria to Mannino et al. (2003), we saw strong agreement on obstructive and restrictive disease patterns but no agreement on mixed pattern. With 2005 ATS/ERS guidelines, we agreed on two restrictive patterns and one obstructive pattern mainly due to unavailability of TLC measurements and also due to small sample size. However, our findings are consistent with Aggarwal and Agarwal [32], who studied simple spirometry (without any lung volume measurements) in 2,527 patients prospectively over a period of six months at the Postgraduate Institute of Medical Education and Research, Chandigarh, India. They compared 2005 ATS/ERS task force guidelines with 1991 ATS guidelines and reported that the 2005 ATS/ERS guidelines underestimated the frequency and severity of the restrictive disease pattern [32].

Any mass casualty disaster can overtax and paralyze the local health care system as it demands emergency medical responses on a large scale. Irritant or chemical gas exposure events are known to occur all around the world. The most notable examples are Bhopal Gas Tragedy [33, 34] and Chernobyl accident [35]. Not all healthcare institutions have infrastructure to routinely perform PFTs and if they do only few have facilities to perform a complete diagnostic work-up with lung volume measurements. Most of the energy focuses on providing symptomatic relief to patients with minor symptoms and stabilization of more critical patients, thus limiting resources for providing diagnostic testing [36–38]. However, after the initial spirometry patients should be followed up with full diagnostic PFTs. Several studies have suggested that the exposure to high concentration of irritant gas exposure may lead to long term pulmonary complications [14, 23, 39]. We are aware of the hesitancy to perform diagnostic testing immediately after an event. But serial complete PFTs can alert the physician as to the inflammatory processes that occur along with remodeling after the obstructive pattern subsides [23, 24]. Additionally, acceptable criteria should be developed to diagnose restrictive pattern through simple spirometry to aid in therapeutic recommendations.

5. Conclusions

We found reduction in lung function and predominant restrictive pulmonary pattern in our patients on simple spirometry done within the first week of admission to hospital after exposure to high concentrations of chlorine gas. This finding was in contrast to other studies done in patients exposed to chlorine gas where obstructive disease was more prominent. There is a need to develop acceptable criteria to evaluate pulmonary disease using parameters available through simple spirometry in events such as irritant gas exposure leading to mass casualty and patient surge in hospitals.

Abbreviations

ATS/ERS: American Thoracic Society/European Respiratory Society
GOLD: Global Initiative for Chronic Obstructive Lung Disease
ppm: Parts per million
NHANES: National Health and Nutrition Examination Survey
PFT: Pulmonary function testing
TLC: Total lung capacity
SCDHEC: South Carolina Department of Health and Environmental Control
USC: University of South Carolina
IRB: Institutional review board
ICU: Intensive care unit
LLN: Lower limit of normal
FEV_1:   Forced expiratory volume in one second
FVC: Forced vital capacity
FEV_1/FVC: Forced expiratory volume in one second/forced vital capacity
VC: Vital capacity
SAS: Statistical Analysis Software
WBC: White blood count.

Conflict of Interests

All authors declare that they have no conflict of interests.

Acknowledgment

The authors would like to thank South Carolina Department of Health and Environmental Control for their support and help with the study.

References

[1] D. K. Horton, Z. Berkowitz, and W. E. Kaye, "The public health consequences from acute chlorine releases, 1993–2000," *Journal of Occupational and Environmental Medicine*, vol. 44, no. 10, pp. 906–913, 2002.

[2] P. Z. Ruckart, W. A. Wattigney, and W. E. Kaye, "Risk factors for acute chemical releases with public health consequences: Hazardous Substances Emergency Events Surveillance in the U.S., 1996–2001," *Environmental Health: A Global Access Science Source*, vol. 3, article 10, 2004.

[3] J. S. Parrish and D. A. Bradshaw, "Toxic inhalational injury: gas, vapor and vesicant exposure," *Respiratory Care Clinics of North America*, vol. 10, no. 1, pp. 43–58, 2004.

[4] R. A. Greenfield, B. R. Brown, J. B. Hutchins et al., "Microbiological, biological, and chemical weapons of warfare and terrorism," *American Journal of the Medical Sciences*, vol. 323, no. 6, pp. 326–340, 2002.

[5] K. P. Ernst, W. A. Wattigney, and W. E. Kaye, "Releases from improper chemical mixing, hazardous substances emergency events surveillance system, 1996–2001," *Journal of Occupational and Environmental Medicine*, vol. 47, no. 3, pp. 287–293, 2005.

[6] P. C. Muskat, "Mass casualty chemical exposure and implications for respiratory failure," *Respiratory Care*, vol. 53, no. 1, pp. 58–63, 2008.

[7] A. D. Laita, S. N. Xarau, and F. P. Roa, "Chemical terrorist attacks: basis for health care," *Medicina Clinica*, vol. 117, no. 14, pp. 541–554, 2001.

[8] D. G. Bell, "Management of acute respiratory distress syndrome (ARDS) following chlorine exposure," *American Journal of Respiratory and Critical Care Medicine*, vol. 176, p. A314, 2008.

[9] C. Winder, "The toxicology of chlorine," *Environmental Research*, vol. 85, no. 2, pp. 105–114, 2001.

[10] V. Nodelman and J. S. Ultman, "Longitudinal distribution of chlorine absorption in human airways: comparison of nasal and oral quiet breathing," *Journal of Applied Physiology*, vol. 86, no. 6, pp. 1984–1993, 1999.

[11] C. Gülolu, I. H. Kara, and P. G. Erten, "Acute accidental exposure to chlorine gas in the southeast of Turkey: a study of 106 cases," *Environmental Research*, vol. 88, no. 2, pp. 89–93, 2002.

[12] N. D. Moulick, S. Banavali, A. D. Abhyankar et al., "Acute accidental exposure to chlorine fumes–a study of 82 cases," *The Indian Journal of Chest Diseases & Allied Sciences*, vol. 34, no. 2, pp. 85–89, 1992.

[13] L. Barret and J. Faure, "Chlorine poisoning," *The Lancet*, vol. 1, no. 8376, pp. 561–562, 1984.

[14] N. B. Charan, S. Lakshminarayan, G. C. Myers, and D. D. Smith, "Effects of accidental chlorine inhalation on pulmonary function," *The Western Journal of Medicine*, vol. 143, no. 3, pp. 333–336, 1985.

[15] R. Pellegrino, G. Viegi, V. Brusasco et al., "Interpretative strategies for lung function tests," *European Respiratory Journal*, vol. 26, no. 5, pp. 948–968, 2005.

[16] D. M. Mannino, A. S. Buist, T. L. Petty, P. L. Enright, and S. C. Redd, "Lung function and mortality in the United States: data from the First National Health and Nutrition Examination Survey follow up study," *Thorax*, vol. 58, no. 5, pp. 388–393, 2003.

[17] R. Rodriguez-Roisin, J. Vestbo, S. S. Hurd et al., "Global strategy for the diagnosis, management and prevention of chronic obstructive pulmonary disease," Global Initiative for Chronic Obstructive Lung Disease, 2011, http://www.goldcopd.org/.

[18] W. M. Vollmer, P. Gíslason, P. Burney et al., "Comparison of spirometry criteria for the diagnosis of COPD: results from the BOLD study," *European Respiratory Journal*, vol. 34, no. 3, pp. 588–597, 2009.

[19] L. Jarenbäck, J. Ankerst, L. Bjermer, and E. Tufvesson, "Flow-volume parameters in COPD related to extended measurements of lung volume, diffusion, and resistance," *Pulmonary Medicine*, vol. 2013, Article ID 782052, 10 pages, 2013.

[20] G. Bonetto, M. Corradi, S. Carraro et al., "Longitudinal monitoring of lung injury in children after acute chlorine exposure in a swimming pool," *American Journal of Respiratory and Critical Care Medicine*, vol. 174, no. 5, pp. 545–549, 2006.

[21] M. A. Wenck, D. Van Sickle, D. Drociuk et al., "Rapid assessment of exposure to chlorine released from a train derailment and resulting health impact," *Public Health Reports*, vol. 122, no. 6, pp. 784–792, 2007.

[22] D. Van Sickle, M. A. Wenck, A. Belflower et al., "Acute health effects after exposure to chlorine gas released after a train derailment," *American Journal of Emergency Medicine*, vol. 27, no. 1, pp. 1–7, 2009.

[23] T. A. Kowitz, R. C. Reba, R. T. Parker, and W. S. Spicer Jr., "Effects of chlorine gas upon respiratory function," *Archives of Environmental Health*, vol. 14, no. 4, pp. 545–558, 1967.

[24] S. M. Brooks, M. A. Weiss, and I. L. Bernstein, "Reactive airways dysfunction syndrome (RADS). Persistent asthma syndrome after high level irritant exposures," *Chest*, vol. 88, no. 3, pp. 376–384, 1985.

[25] G. L. Ruppel, *Manual of Pulmonary Function Testing*, Mosby, St. Louis, Mo, USA, 8th edition, 2003.

[26] R. Jones, B. Willis, and C. Kang, "Chlorine gas: an evolving hazardous material treat and unconventional weapon," *Western Journal of Emergency Medicine*, vol. 11, no. 2, pp. 151–156, 2010.

[27] C. W. White and J. G. Martin, "Chlorine gas inhalation: human clinical evidence of toxicity and experience in animal models," *Proceedings of the American Thoracic Society*, vol. 7, no. 4, pp. 257–263, 2010.

[28] D. Gautrin, L.-P. Boulet, M. Boutet et al., "Is reactive airways dysfunction syndrome a variant of occupational asthma?" *Journal of Allergy and Clinical Immunology*, vol. 93, no. 1, pp. 12–22, 1994.

[29] D. L. Kasper, E. Braunwald, A. S. Fauci et al., *Harrison's Principles of Internal Medicine*, vol. II, McGraw Hill, New York, NY, USA, 16th edition, 2005.

[30] R. P. Gie, C. M. Doerschuk, D. English, H. O. Coxson, and J. C. Hogg, "Neutrophil-associated lung injury after the infusion of activated plasma," *Journal of Applied Physiology*, vol. 70, no. 6, pp. 2471–2478, 1991.

[31] A. K. Yadav, A. Bracher, S. F. Doran et al., "Mechanisms and modification of chlorine-induced lung injury in animals," *Proceedings of the American Thoracic Society*, vol. 7, no. 4, pp. 278–283, 2010.

[32] A. N. Aggarwal and R. Agarwal, "The new ATS/ERS guidelines for assessing the spirometric severity of restrictive lung disease differ from previous standards," *Respirology*, vol. 12, no. 5, pp. 759–762, 2007.

[33] P. K. Mishra, R. M. Samarth, N. Pathak, S. K. Jain, S. Banerjee, and K. K. Maudar, "Bhopal gas tragedy: review of clinical and experimental findings after 25 years," *International Journal of Occupational Medicine and Environmental Health*, vol. 22, no. 3, pp. 193–202, 2009.

[34] S. Sriramachari, "The Bhopal gas tragedy: an environmental disaster," *Current Science*, vol. 86, no. 7, pp. 905–920, 2004.

[35] J. Havenaar, G. Rumyantzeva, A. Kasyanenko et al., "Health effects of the Chernobyl disaster: illness or illness behavior? A comparative general health survey in two former Soviet regions," *Environmental Health Perspectives*, vol. 105, no. 6, pp. 1533–1537, 1997.

[36] A. C. Ramesh and S. Kumar, "Triage, monitoring, and treatment of mass casualty events involving chemical, biological, radiological, or nuclear agents," *Journal of Pharmacy and Bioallied Sciences*, vol. 2, no. 3, pp. 239–247, 2010.

[37] E. R. Frykberg, "Principles of Mass Casualty Management Following Terrorist Disasters," *Annals of Surgery*, vol. 239, no. 3, pp. 319–321, 2004.

[38] R. J. Brennan, J. F. Waeckerle, T. W. Sharp, and S. R. Lillibridge, "Chemical warfare agents: emergency medical and emergency public health issues," *Annals of Emergency Medicine*, vol. 34, no. 2, pp. 191–204, 1999.

[39] D. A. Schwartz, D. D. Smith, and S. Lakshminarayan, "The pulmonary sequelae associated with accidental inhalation of chlorine gas," *Chest*, vol. 97, no. 4, pp. 820–825, 1990.

12

Sarcoidosis Treatment with Antifungal Medication: A Follow-Up

Marjeta Terčelj,[1] Barbara Salobir,[1] Mirjana Zupancic,[2] and Ragnar Rylander[3]

[1]Clinic of Pulmonary Diseases and Allergy, University Medical Centre, Zaloska 7, 1000 Ljubljana, Slovenia
[2]Laboratory Department, Children's Hospital, University Medical Center, 1000 Ljubljana, Slovenia
[3]BioFact Environmental Health Research Center, 44391 Lerum, Sweden

Correspondence should be addressed to Marjeta Terčelj; marjeta.tercelj@kclj.si

Academic Editor: Sebastian L. Johnston

Introduction. The aim of the study was to compare treatment of sarcoidosis with antifungal or corticosteroid medication. *Methods.* In patients with sarcoidosis antifungal medication ($n = 29$), corticosteroids ($n = 21$) or a combination ($n = 27$) was given. Nine patients allotted to antifungal medication were later given corticosteroids because of the lack of regression of the disease. X-ray scores for the severity of granuloma infiltration were determined. Chitotriosidase and angiotensin converting enzyme were determined. The time in months till remission was observed as well as the number of recurrences.

1. Introduction

Sarcoidosis is an inflammatory, granulomatous disease present in populations worldwide and with a higher incidence in some ethnic groups [1, 2]. The conventional treatment is with corticosteroids. During recent years there have been an increasing number of studies reporting a connection between sarcoidosis and environmental exposure to fungi [3–5]. Fungal exposure at home was higher among patients with sarcoidosis as compared to controls and highest among those with recurrence of the disease. β-Glucan, a major constituent of the fungal cell wall, has been determined in bronchoalveolar lavage (BAL) fluid in patients with sarcoidosis and controls [6]. The amounts were significantly higher among patients with sarcoidosis and were related to the fungal exposure at home as well as to serum levels of IL-2R and IL-12.

These studies showing a relation between exposure to fungi and different experimental and clinical effects have prompted studies where antifungal medication has been given, together with or without simultaneous corticosteroid treatment. In a first study, 18 patients with chronic sarcoidosis were given antifungal medication in addition to the usual corticosteroid treatment. 15 of these patients improved after 6 months [7]. In a subsequent study 39 newly diagnosed patients received corticosteroids for 6 months and 18 received antifungal medication [8]. Pulmonary granuloma infiltration

was significantly less severe in the antifungal group as were the values of angiotensin converting enzyme (ACE) and chitotriosidase (CTO). In a case study on osseous sarcoidosis, treatment with antifungal medication improved the condition [9].

These treatment studies covered a relatively short time period and the time till remission or the risk of recurrence was not studied. Before a final conclusion regarding the efficiency of antifungal treatment can be drawn, further studies are required with a larger number of subjects, followed over a longer time period.

The present study was undertaken to compare the effects of corticosteroid and antifungal treatment with regard to remission and recurrence of the disease after termination of treatment.

2. Material and Methods

Patients with sarcoidosis attend the Clinic of Respiratory Diseases and Allergy at the University Medical Centre, Ljubljana, Slovenia. The diagnosis of sarcoidosis at the clinic adheres to the ATS criteria [10] and comprises the following steps. Bronchoscopy is made and 5 to 10 transbronchial biopsies of lung parenchyma and lymph nodes are taken. BAL is performed with 200 mL saline to determine CD8+ cells and the CD4+/CD8+ ratio. The presence of noncaseating granulomas is verified histologically. If a biopsy is not considered representative, the patient undergoes surgical pulmonary or lymph node biopsy. Aspiration is performed from one lobe for culturing fungi and bacteria including tuberculosis. Most biopsies are stained (silver staining, Gomori) to verify the absence of pathogenic fungi.

The subjects in the present study were 77 Caucasian patients with sarcoidosis who had undergone treatment during the years 2006–2011. After a three-month expectation period to avoid including patients with a spontaneous regression, treatment was initiated. Criteria for treatment were symptoms such as fatigue, joint pains, and dyspnoea, X-ray changes indicating granuloma formation, and involvement of organs other than the lung, such as spleen, liver, and eyes at the time for treatment decision.

The patients were given the choice of antifungal (posaconazole 300 mg/day or ketoconazole 200 mg/day) or corticosteroid (methylprednisolone initially 0.4 mg/kg body weight/day for the first month and then 20 mg every second day) medication. The dose of antifungal was low for precautionary reasons and because there was no sign of fungal infection.

A double-blind, placebo design was not possible as all patients needed treatment at the time when medication was chosen. A randomized study was also not possible as the subjects had to be informed about the side effects, and some subjects insisted on antifungal medication, aware of the results from previous studies. The side effects were explained and some patients chose the antifungal and others the corticosteroid treatment. Those who let the physician choose were given antifungal treatment. In summary 21 subjects were given corticosteroid medication (C group) and 56 antifungal medication. Among those with antifungal treatment, corticosteroid was added later in 27 subjects because of increased symptoms of fatigue, joint pains, and shortness of breath (AF + C group). Nine subjects in the antifungal group showed no clinical improvement or had worsening of symptoms or X-rays at 6 months after initiation of treatment. They received an additional treatment with corticosteroids. These patients are reported separately. In summary 20 subjects were thus given antifungal only (AF group).

X-rays were taken and a grading scheme for the presence of granuloma was used as described previously [7, 8]. The X-rays were read by two experienced radiologists, unaware of the status of the patient, grading granuloma infiltration according to a numerical score (0–4) and judging the size and extension of the infiltrates (0 normal, 1 about 25% of lung field involved, 2 up to 50%, 3 up to 75%, and 4 virtually the whole lung field involved). Repeat evaluations on two successive occasions showed only minor deviations in the score classification. Pulmonary function (VC, DLco) was determined and expressed as a percentage of the expected.

Serum samples were taken and ACE was determined using a colorimetric method and expressed as μKat/L [11]. CTO was determined using 22 μM 4-methylumbelliferyl-β-D-N,N$'$,N$''$-triacetylchitotriosiose (Sigma) in citrate phosphate buffer (pH 5.2) and expressed as nmol/h/mL [12].

TABLE 1: Characteristics of subjects in different groups at initiation of treatment. Number (n) or arithmetic mean/SEM.

Treatment	Corticosteroid	Antifungal	AF + C
n	21	20	27
Age years	44.0/3.4	42.4/2.3	41.1/2.0
Smokers n	3	1	4
Females n	10	9	12
Stage 2 n	19	20	21
Stage 3 n	2	0	6
Extrapulmonary n	12	8	9
CD4/CD8	6.9/0.9	6.4/0.9	6.5/0.8
VC %	89.3/2.9	97.3/1.0	93.7/1.9
FEV$_1$ %	89.1/3.0	94.3/2.3	92.5/2.3
DLco %	80.5/3.6	92.3/3.3	89.6/3.5

The disease was monitored using X-ray, and inflammatory cytokines in serum were determined at the time of diagnosis, after about 6 months, and at the end of treatment (remission). Remission comprised absence of symptoms, signs of active disease and ACE, and CTO lower than the initial values. Time till remission in months was determined for all subjects. In addition the number of patients with a recurrence of the disease was determined.

2.1. Statistics. Group data were reported as mean and SEM. Differences between groups were evaluated using the Mann-Whitney test and Fisher's exact test. Correlations were evaluated using Spearman's test. A P value of ≤ 0.05 was considered the level of significance.

3. Results

Table 1 reports the characteristics of the study subjects at initiation of treatment.

The demographic characteristics were very similar in the different groups except that there were more cases with extrapulmonary involvement in the C group and that DLco was lower in the C group ($P = 0.008$).

The average duration of treatment till remission was 12.1/0.7 months in the AF group, 13.7/0.8 months in the C group (NS), and 17.6/2.2 in the AF + C group which was significant from AF group ($P = 0.023$).

Table 2 reports the clinical parameters at initiation of treatment, after 6 months of treatment, and at remission.

Before treatment the X-ray score was slightly higher, although not statistically significant, in the AF + C group as compared to the AT group and the C group. CTO was significantly lower in the AF group as compared to the C group ($P = 0.001$) and the AF + C group (NS). DLco was lower in the C group as compared to the AF and AF + C groups ($P = 0.07$ and 0.039, resp.).

Over time there was an improvement in X-ray scores in all groups but a larger recovery in the AF group as compared to the C group at remission ($P = 0.003$ and NS, resp.).

TABLE 2: Clinical parameters at initiation of treatment, after 6 months of treatment, and at remission. Mean/SEM.

Treatment	Corticosteroid	Antifungal	AF + C
n	21	20	27
X-ray score			
Before	1.7/0.1	1.9/0.2	2.2/0.2
6 months	1.1/0.1	0.6/0.2	0.8/0.1
Remission	0.6/0.2	0.1/0.1	0.3/0.1
CTO nmol/h/mL			
Before	843/86	454/70	632/108
6 months	260/44	372/149	184/52
Remission	342/57	271/66	178/37
ACE μKat/L			
Before	0.44/0.05	0.44/0.04	0.41/0.03
6 months	0.20/0.02	0.38/0.04	0.26/0.03
Remission	0.24/0.03	0.34/0.03	0.24/0.02
DLco % pred.			
Before	80.5/3.6	92.3/3.3	89.6/3.5
6 months	79.0/5.5	92.9/3.7	91.1/4.7
Remission	90.8/3.6	95.7/3.5	93.4/3.6

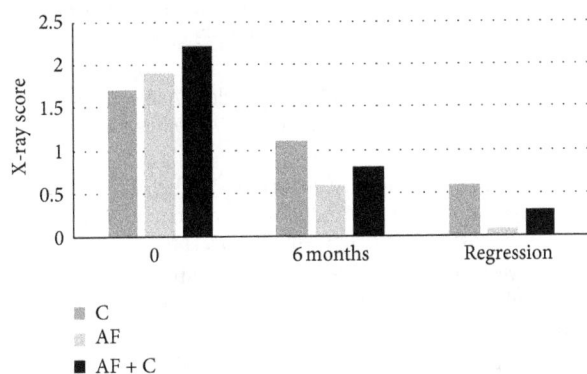

■ C
■ AF
■ AF + C

FIGURE 1: X-ray scores at different times after initiation of treatment with corticosteroid (C, n = 21), with antifungal medication (AF, n = 20), and with antifungal + corticosteroid (AF + C, n = 27).

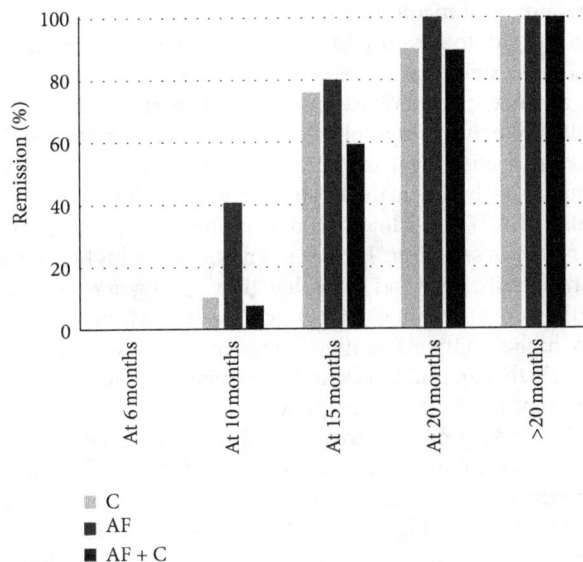

■ C
■ AF
■ AF + C

FIGURE 2: Proportion of patients with remission at different times after initiation of treatment for those treated with corticosteroid (C, n = 21), with antifungal medication (AF, n = 20), and with antifungal + corticosteroid (AF + C, n = 27).

A similar trend was found for CTO, but here the decrease was most marked in the AF + C group. Also ACE and DLco values improved in all groups with no significant differences between the groups.

At remission the X-ray scores were lower in the AF and AF + C groups as compared to the C group (P = 0.015 and NS, resp.). Also the CTO values were lower in the AF group and the AF + C group as compared to the C group (NS and P = 0.017, resp.).

Figure 1 illustrates the X-ray scores at different times from initiation of treatment.

Figure 2 reports the proportion of patients with remission at different times after initiation of treatment in the C, AF, and AF + C groups.

At 10 months a larger proportion of subjects in the AF group had remission as compared to the C and AF + C groups

(P = 0.033 and NS). At 20 months the proportion with remission in the AF + C group was lower than in the other groups (NS). Among those who took longer than 20 months to remission, there was one subject in the C group (25 months till remission) and five in the AF + C group (24, 26, 28, 50, and 56 months till remission).

Regarding recurrence of sarcoidosis after treatment, there were seven cases in the C group, one in the AF group, and two in the AF + C group (different from C group, P = 0.021 and 0.026, resp.).

The disease characteristics were analysed for the nine subjects initially given antifungal treatment, but corticosteroid treatment was added. One subject had developed involvement of the central nervous system, two had sarcoidosis in the eyes, and one subject developed side effects from the antifungal medication. The initial X-ray score in this group was higher than in the C group (2.33/2.2 versus 1.71/0.1, P = 0.035). ACE was also higher (0.55/0.7 versus 0.24/0.03, NS). The duration of therapy till remission was 15.3/3.8 months. There were no differences for the other parameters.

4. Discussion

The main result from this study was a larger proportion of patients with remission after 6–10 months of treatment, a lower X-ray score at remission, and fewer cases of recurrence among subjects treated with antifungal medication.

The study has some limitations. The number of subjects is small and the study is thus of an exploratory nature. There were, however, marked differences between the treated groups, which were statistically significant. Medication with corticosteroids and antifungal was not distributed randomly or in a double blind fashion. The absence of a randomized distribution of medication could induce a selection of cases with regard to severity at the initiation of treatment. It is also possible that a precaution regarding treatment and the absence of experience in the initial parts of the study could make the responsible physician choose corticosteroids instead of antifungal medication in more severe cases. A comparison between the C and AF groups showed higher values of CTO and lower values of DLco in the C group, suggesting a selection. The AF + C group had a higher X-ray score initially, but it was lower than the C groups at remission. Furthermore the values of CTO were lower and those of DLco were higher in the AF group at remission. In view of this it is unlikely that an initial selection had a major influence on the treatment results in the AF group.

In the AF group corticosteroids had to be added for nine patients due to the clinical development of the disease. These patients could have had a more severe form of the disease (as suggested by the higher X-ray score at start of treatment), resisting the antifungal treatment or a form of sarcoidosis not related to fungal exposure. Another possibility is that they might have had a lower than normal absorption of the antifungal medication. Furthermore the dose for antifungal medication used was below the recommended therapeutical dose because of safety reasons. This might also explain the need for additional treatment in these patients.

The antifungal treatment was efficient although analysis of BAL and lung tissue could not demonstrate the presence of pathogenic fungi. In the environment, however, the major fungal burden is nonpathogenic fungi such as *Penicillium*. Previous studies have reported that fungal exposure at home was higher among patients with sarcoidosis than controls [5]. There is also a relation between fungal exposure at home and the amount of β-glucan in BAL of subjects with sarcoidosis [6]. From an environmental exposure point of view the finding that antifungal medication is efficient in sarcoidosis is thus not surprising.

5. Conclusion

The results demonstrate that the effect of antifungal medication in newly diagnosed cases of sarcoidosis was similar to that after treatment with corticosteroids in 21 out of 30 patients. At six months after initiation of treatment and at remission, the X-ray changes were less severe among those treated with antifungal medication. The risk of recurrence was also significantly lower in this group. The results suggest that patients should be informed about the possibility to take antifungal medication and that attention should be given to their possible exposure to high levels of fungi. Further studies on patients with severe forms of sarcoidosis and using higher levels of antifungal medication are warranted.

Abbreviations

ACE: Angiotensin converting enzyme
CTO: Chitotriosidase
DLco: Pulmonary diffusion capacity
VC: Vital capacity.

Disclosure

This study was funded by University Hospital Funds. This research received no specific grant from any funding agency in the public, commercial, or not-for-profit sectors.

Conflict of Interests

The authors declare that there is no conflict of interests regarding the publication of this paper.

References

[1] M. C. Iannuzi, B. A. Rybicki, and A. S. Tierstein, "Sarcoidosis," *The New England Journal of Medicine*, vol. 357, pp. 2153–2165, 2007.

[2] R. P. Baughman, D. A. Culver, and M. A. Judson, "A concise review of pulmonary sarcoidosis," *American Journal of Respiratory and Critical Care Medicine*, vol. 183, no. 5, pp. 573–581, 2011.

[3] L. S. Newman, C. S. Rose, E. A. Bresnitz et al., "A case control etiologic study of sarcoidosis: environmental and occupational risk factors," *The American Journal of Respiratory and Critical Care Medicine*, vol. 170, no. 12, pp. 1324–1330, 2004.

[4] A. S. Laney, L. A. Cragin, L. Z. Blevins et al., "Sarcoidosis, asthma, and asthma-like symptoms among occupants of a historically water-damaged office building," *Indoor Air*, vol. 19, no. 1, pp. 83–90, 2009.

[5] M. Terčelj, B. Salobir, and R. Rylander, "Airborne enzyme in homes of patients with sarcoidosis," *Environmental Health*, vol. 10, pp. 8–13, 2011.

[6] M. Terčelj, B. Salobir, M. Zupancic, B. Wraber, and R. Rylander, "Inflammatory markers and pulmonary granuloma infiltration in sarcoidosis," *Respirology*, vol. 19, no. 2, pp. 225–230, 2014.

[7] M. Tercelj, T. Rott, and R. Rylander, "Antifungal treatment in sarcoidosis—a pilot intervention trial," *Respiratory Medicine*, vol. 101, no. 4, pp. 774–778, 2007.

[8] M. Terčelj, B. Salobir, M. Zupancic, and R. Rylander, "Antifungal medication is efficient in the treatment of sarcoidosis," *Therapeutic Advances in Respiratory Disease*, vol. 5, no. 3, pp. 157–162, 2011.

[9] K. Murakami, T. Tamada, K. Abe et al., "Rapid improvement of osseous sarcoidosis after the treatment of pulmonary aspergillosis by itraconazole," *Sarcoidosis, Vasculitis and Diffuse Lung Diseases*, vol. 28, no. 1, pp. 75–78, 2011.

[10] ATS/ERS Joint, "Statement on sarcoidosis," *The American Journal of Respiratory and Critical Care Medicine*, vol. 160, no. 2, pp. 736–755, 1999.

[11] Y. Kasahara and Y. Ashihara, "Colorimetry of angiotensin-I converting enzyme activity in serum," *Clinical Chemistry*, vol. 27, no. 11, pp. 1922–1925, 1981.

[12] M. Terčelj, B. Salobir, S. Simcic, B. Wraber, M. Zupancic, and R. Rylander, "Chitotriosidase activity in sarcoidosis and some other pulmonary diseases," *Scandinavian Journal of Clinical & Laboratory Investigation*, vol. 69, no. 5, pp. 575–578, 2009.

13

The Role of the High-Sensitivity C-Reactive Protein in Patients with Stable Non-Cystic Fibrosis Bronchiectasis

Meng-Heng Hsieh,[1] Yueh-Fu Fang,[1] Guan-Yuan Chen,[1] Fu-Tsai Chung,[1] Yuan-Chang Liu,[2] Cheng-Hsien Wu,[2] Yu-Chen Chang,[3] and Horng-Chyuan Lin[1]

[1] *Department of Thoracic Medicine, Chang Gung Medical Foundation, Department of Chest Medicine, Chang Gung University, College of Medicine, Taoyuan 33342, Taiwan*
[2] *Department of Radiology, Chang Gung Medical Foundation, Department of Chest Medicine, Chang Gung University, College of Medicine, Taoyuan 33342, Taiwan*
[3] *Department of Nuclear Medicine, Chang Gung Medical Foundation, Department of Chest Medicine, Chang Gung University, College of Medicine, Taoyuan 33342, Taiwan*

Correspondence should be addressed to Horng-Chyuan Lin; lin53424@msl3.hinet.net

Academic Editor: Akio Niimi

Study Objectives. The aim of this study is to investigate the correlation between serum high-sensitivity C-reactive protein (hs-CRP) and other clinical tools including high-resolution computed tomography (HRCT) in patients with stable non-CF bronchiectasis. *Design.* A within-subject correlational study of a group of patients with stable non-CF bronchiectasis, who were recruited from our outpatient clinic, was done over a two-year period. *Measurements.* Sixty-nine stable non-CF bronchiectasis patients were evaluated in terms of hs-CRP, 6-minute walk test, pulmonary function tests, and HRCT. *Results.* Circulating hs-CRP levels were significantly correlated with HRCT scores ($n = 69$, $r = 0.473$, $P < 0.001$) and resting oxygenation saturation ($r = -0.269$, $P = 0.025$). HRCT severity scores significantly increased in patients with hs-CRP level of 4.26 mg/L or higher (mean ± SD 28.1 ± 13.1) compared to those with hs-CRP level less than 4.26 mg/L (31.7 ± 9.8, $P = 0.004$). Oxygenation saturation at rest was lower in those with hs-CRP level of 4.26 mg/L or higher (93.5 ± 4.4%) compared to those with hs-CRP level less than 4.26 mg/L (96.4 ± 1.6%, $P = 0.001$). *Conclusion.* There was a good correlation between serum hs-CRP and HRCT scores in the patients with stable non-CF bronchiectasis.

1. Introduction

Despite improvements in childhood immunization and tuberculosis control, bronchiectasis remains a significant clinical issue worldwide [1, 2]. It is a chronic, debilitating lung disease characterized by irreversible dilatation of the bronchi from airway remodeling due to chronic airway inflammation and infection. Underlying etiologies include autoimmune diseases, severe infections, genetic abnormalities, and acquired disorders; however, its pathogenesis and progression remain poorly understood [1–5]. Exacerbations occur at rates of 1.5–6.5 per patient per year [6, 7] and are associated with an increased risk of admission and readmission to hospitals and high healthcare costs [8].

High-resolution computed tomography (HRCT) is a proven, reliable, and noninvasive method for assessing bronchiectasis [9]. It can accurately diagnose bronchiectasis and localize and describe areas of parenchymal abnormality. A link between morphological HRCT parameters and clinical functional correlation has been established [9–14]. However, concerns over radiation exposure and high cost limit its frequent use in stable bronchiectasis patients.

Inflammation in bronchiectasis is characterized by persistence and intensity. Airway inflammation is neutrophil-predominant, and inflammatory profiles show increased levels of proinflammatory cytokines such as IL-1, IL-6, and TNF-α and low levels of anti-inflammatory cytokines such as IL-10 [3, 15, 16]. Elevation of systemic inflammatory markers, such as C-reactive protein (CRP) and total white cell count, has been found to correlate with the extent of the disease and poor lung function [17]. CRP is a pentraxin structure composed of five 23 kDa subunits. It is highly stable and allows measurements to be made accurately in both fresh and frozen plasma, without requiring special collection procedures. Moreover, high-sensitivity assays for CRP have been standardized across many commercial platforms. The long plasma half-life of CRP (18 to 20 hours), stability over a long period of time, and almost no circadian variation make it an accurate and sensitive marker of low-grade systemic inflammation [18, 19]. While the use of hs-CRP in cardiovascular diseases has been documented [20–24], its role in stable bronchiectasis remains unknown. Thus, the aim of this study was to explore the relationship between hs-CRP and severity scores on HRCT and other clinical variables in stable non-CF bronchiectasis patients.

2. Methods

2.1. Study Population and Design. One hundred and twenty-five (125) patients with bronchiectasis were recruited from the Thoracic Outpatient Clinic of Chang Gung Memorial Hospital in Taiwan from January 2006 to December 2007. The inclusion criteria were as follows: bronchiectasis documented on chest HRCT, idiopathic etiology of bronchiectasis (none of the patients with background suggests cystic fibrosis such as chronic dysfunction of the pancreas or liver or intestine or an electrolyte imbalance, disease onset before adolescence, and family history), chronic sputum production (daily sputum ≥ 10 mL), absence of other major pulmonary diagnoses, and a steady state defined by the absence of changes in symptoms noted by the patient over the past 3 weeks. The exclusion criteria were as follows: bronchiectasis with defined etiology (i.e., primary ciliary dyskinesia and allergic bronchopulmonary aspergillosis), common variable immunodeficiency, and use of antibiotics within the last three weeks. Patients with hepatic failure, malignancy, or pregnancy were also excluded.

The study design was conducted with approval of the Institutional Review Board (IRB) of Chang Gung Medical Foundation (IRB no. 97-1105A3). All patients provided written informed consent to participate in this study. The methodology and patient confidentiality were also approved by our IRB.

2.2. Measurement of Serum High-Sensitivity C-Reactive Protein Levels. Blood was drawn for measurement of serum inflammatory markers. The blood samples were then centrifuged at 3000 rpm at 4°C for 15 minutes, and aliquots were stored at −70°C. A latex turbidimetric immunoassay with a sensitivity of 0.01 mg/L was used to measure circulating levels of hs-CRP (Biomedical Laboratory Inc.).

2.3. High-Resolution Computed Tomography (HRCT). The scoring system for HRCT described by Brody was used, and a score sheet was completed for each lobe of the lung [25]. Briefly, each lung lobe (considering the lingula and middle lobe as independent) was scored as 0 (no bronchiectasis),

1 (cylindrical bronchiectasis in a single lung segment), 2 (cylindrical bronchiectasis > 1 lung segment), or 3 (cystic bronchiectasis). The maximum score for each lobe was 12 points and a single radiologist with five years of experience in thoracic CT interpretation assessed the HRCT images in random order, without clinical functional information. This scoring system was used in a previous study, with the bronchiectasis score ranging from 0 to 72.

Two experienced radiologists, both pulmonary division consultants with more than 5 years of experience, scored the HRCT of these patients without any clinical data information. The interobserver agreement was 0.946 (data not shown).

2.4. Six-Minute Walk Test (6 MWT). The 6-minute walk tests using the standard protocol described in the 2002 American Thoracic Society (ATS) statement [26] were performed at the outpatient clinic visit by well-trained technicians with at least three years of experience in performing 6 MWTs. Pre- and posttest oxygenation saturation under room air, walking distance, and standard spirometry before the test were recorded.

2.5. Body Mass Index (BMI). Height was measured with a rigid stadiometer, and weight was measured by a calibrated digital scale. Body mass index (BMI) was calculated by dividing the weight (kilograms) by the height (meters squared), and then the quotient was converted into age- and sex-adjusted percentiles based on population data from NHANES 2000.

2.6. Statistical Analysis. Data were presented as mean ± SD, and all statistical analyses were performed using SPSS version 13.0 (SPSS Inc., Chicago, IL, USA). Independent Student t-tests or chi-square tests were performed to compare the clinical parameters, as appropriate. For bivariate analysis, we stratified the participants, using a cutoff point of serum hs-CRP of 4.26 mg/L, into two groups according to previous exacerbation-related hospitalizations (less than 2 times versus 2 times and above). To compare hs-CRP with other clinical variables, we used age (years), BMI (kg/m^2), FVC (L), FEV$_1$ (L), FEV$_1$/FVC, IgE (KU/L), ECP (mcg/L), rest O_2%, lowest O_2%, ΔO_2%, 6-minute walking distance (6 MWD, meters), and HRCT scores for correlation analysis. Correlations between data were analyzed using Pearson's correlation tests. A P value of less than 0.05 was considered significant.

3. Results

3.1. Patient Characteristics. During the study period, 125 patients with bronchiectasis were recruited in the chest outpatient department, and 78 patients were evaluated for this study. Sixty-nine patients who met the inclusion criteria were enrolled in the study (Figure 1), and their demographic data are shown in Table 1. Three patients with a serum hs-CRP level of more than 30 mg/L without overt clinical symptoms or signs of infection at enrolment were excluded from the final data analysis because of the exacerbations and oral

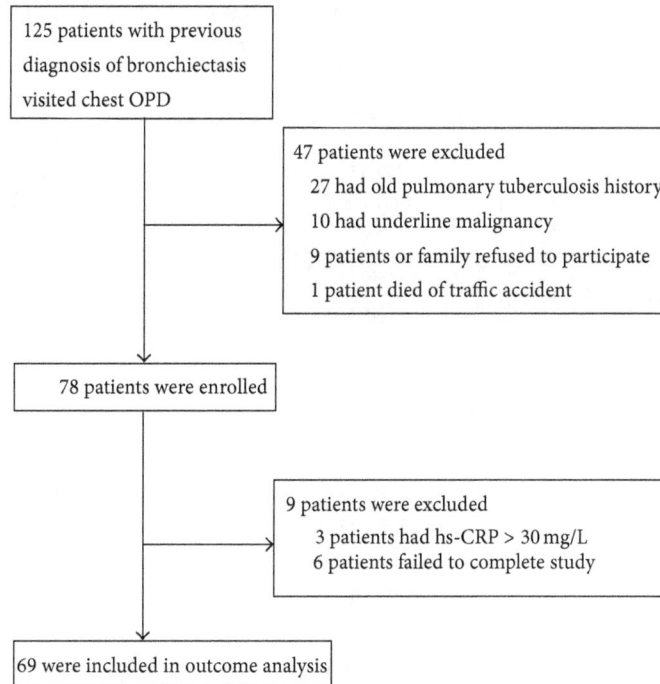

FIGURE 1: Flowchart of patients in the study cohort.

TABLE 1: Demographic data of the 69 stable bronchiectasis patients.

Demographic factor	Mean (SD)	95% CI
Age (years)	57.5	54.2–60.8
BMI (kg/m^2)	22.0	21.2–22.8
FVC (L)	2.1	1.9–2.3
FVC% predicted	67.4	62.7–72.0
FEV$_1$ (L)	1.5	1.4–1.7
FEV$_1$% predicted	62.6	57.1–68.1
6 MWD (m)	454.4	432.4–476.4
Rest O$_2$S%	95.1	94.3–95.9
HRCT score	26.2	23.1–29.3
hs-CRP (mg/L)	4.5	3.6–5.5

Abbreviations: BMI: body mass index, FVC: forced vital capacity, FEV$_1$: volume that has been exhaled at the end of the first second of forced expiration, 6 MWD: 6-minute walk test distance, HRCT: high-resolution computed tomography, and hs-CRP: high-sensitivity C-reactive protein.

antibiotics given in the following weeks. Their serum hs-CRP levels were 45.51, 55.47, and 78.41 mg/L, respectively.

Following the initial evaluation of hs-CRP, the patients were divided into two groups according to their previous exacerbation-related hospitalizations: those with an hs-CRP level less than 4.26 mg/L ($n = 38$) and those with an hs-CRP level of 4.26 mg/L or higher ($n = 31$) (Figure 2). We defined exacerbation-related hospitalizations as those with symptoms/signs of lower respiratory tract infection including cough, increased sputum production, changes in the sputum characteristics, hemoptysis, poor appetite accompanied by body weight loss, and need for further bronchodilator treatment, requiring treatment with systemic steroids or accompanied by respiratory failure. The characteristics and outcomes

of the two groups of patients with stable bronchiectasis are shown in Table 2.

3.2. Circulating hs-CRP and Clinical Assessments. There were no statistical differences in age, sex distribution, smoking status, BMI, pulmonary function test, and 6 MWT between the two groups. Bacteriology and regular treatment regimens (data not shown) were also similar. The HRCT scores were significantly increased in the higher hs-CRP group compared with the lower group (Table 3 and Figure 3). Resting oxygenation saturation was significantly decreased in the higher group than in the lower group, and there was a trend that patients with a lower hs-CRP had higher pulmonary functions (FVC and FEV$_1$). Circulating hs-CRP levels were also significantly correlated with HRCT scores ($n = 69$, $r = 0.318$, $P = 0.009$) (Figure 4) and inversely correlated with rest oxygenation saturation ($r = -0.349$, $P = 0.004$) (Figure 5). The correlation between resting oxygenation saturation and HRCT score severity showed a moderately negative linear relationship ($P < 0.001$, $r = -0.478$, figure not shown).

4. Discussion

The pathogenetic mechanism leading to bronchiectasis is complex and still not well understood [1–5]. The current point of view considers that idiopathic bronchiectasis, chronic bronchial infection, and inflammation interact with each other leading to progressive lung damage [3]. The associated airway inflammation in bronchiectasis has been studied more widely recently; however, little is known about the intensity of low-grade systemic inflammation. To the best of our knowledge, this is the first study to describe the relationship

TABLE 2: Characteristics and outcomes of the 69 stable bronchiectasis patients.

	hs-CPR < 4.26 \n $n = 38$	hs-CRP $\geq$ 4.26 \n $n = 31$	P value
Age (years)	56.2 ± 13.7	59.0 ± 13.9	0.406
Gender (M/F)	21/17	18/13	0.815
BMI (kg/m^2)	22.0 ± 3.4	22.0 ± 3.4	0.990
Smoking			
Never	30	25	0.862
Ex/current	8	6	
PFT			
FVC (L)	2.25 ± 0.81	1.85 ± 0.71	0.034
FVC (%)	72.5 ± 16.4	61.1 ± 21.0	0.014
FEV$_1$ (L)	1.69 ± 0.74	1.34 ± 0.59	0.038
FEV$_1$ (%)	67.6 ± 21.4	56.6 ± 23.5	0.046
FEV$_1$/FVC (%)	73.5 ± 11.0	71.3 ± 10.4	0.401
Total IgE (KU/L)	137.8 ± 320.3	170.9 ± 490.6	0.737
ECP (mcg/L)	17.5 ± 17.8	24.5 ± 36.7	0.304
6 MWT			
Rest O$_2$ sat (%)	96.4 ± 1.6	93.5 ± 4.4	0.001
Lowest O$_2$ sat (%)	87.7 ± 6.4	85.2 ± 10.2	0.237
ΔO$_2$ sat (%)	8.7 ± 6.1	8.4 ± 7.4	0.816
Walk distance (meters)	469.3 ± 78.2	436.1 ± 104.1	0.136
HRCT scores	21.7 ± 9.8	28.1 ± 13.1	0.004
Bacterial colony			
Ps. aeruginosa	6	11	0.115
Others	8	4	
Normal flora/no growth	24	16	
Hospitalizations before recruitment (times/year)			
<2	35	21	0.01
$\geq$2	3	10	

Abbreviations: hs-CRP: high-sensitivity C-reactive protein, PFT: pulmonary function test, IgE: immunoglobulin E, ECP: eosinophilic cationic protein, 6 MWT: 6-minute walk test, ΔO$_2$ sat (%): oxygenation difference between rest and lowest during 6-minute walk test, and HRCT: high-resolution computed tomography.

between serum hs-CRP, rather than traditional CRP, and clinical variables including disease severity and HRCT in a group of patients with stable non-CF bronchiectasis. Our results demonstrated that hs-CRP had a good correlation with HRCT severity scores and may serve as a chronic inflammatory marker in the stable status phase of non-CF bronchiectasis patients, despite its broad clinical spectrum.

Progressive idiopathic bronchiectasis includes at least two subsets of patients [2, 3]. One subset, which constitutes the vast majority of cases, deteriorates over decades with an increased frequency of exacerbations, sputum volume, and extent of bronchiectasis. The other subset, usually those with single-lobe involvement, can be asymptomatic between exacerbations or without overt exacerbations and does not deteriorate even after decades. However, little is known about the severity and disease activity. No study has yet assessed the severity and disease activity of idiopathic bronchiectasis,

even though two long-term studies have assessed the factors influencing mortality [27, 28].

C-reactive protein is predominantly produced in the liver, and IL-1, IL-6, and TNF-α have been identified as regulators of its production [29, 30]. More sensitive immune assays for CRP (high-sensitivity CRP, hs-CRP) have become available, making possible measurement and comparison of low CRP levels in blood. These sensitive assays have revealed the relationship between hs-CRP levels and the developmentand progression of coronary heart disease [23, 24] and osteoarthritis [31]. Moreover, the significant correlations between hs-CRP and diabetes [32] and airway diseases such as chronic obstructive pulmonary disease [33] and asthma [34] have been reported. In the present study, disease severity was correlated with hs-CRP in stable bronchiectasis, demonstrating that hs-CRP may be a good biomarker in low-grade systemic inflammation in such patients.

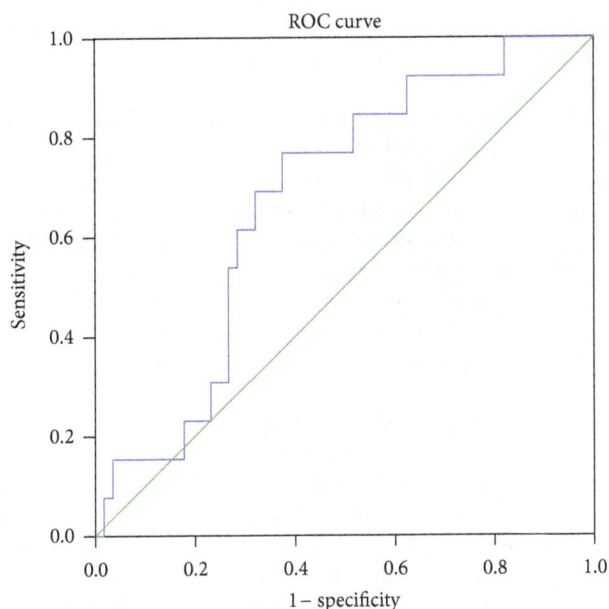

(AUC = 0.676)

hs-CRP cutoff	Sensitivity (%)	Specificity (%)
3.72	76.9	58.9
4.10	76.9	60.7
4.26	76.9	62.5
4.42	69.2	62.5
4.49	69.2	64.3
4.56	69.2	66.1

FIGURE 2: ROC curve of hs-CRP for prediction patients with repeated hospitalization (≥ 2 exacerbation-related hospitalization events).

TABLE 3: Correlations between hs-CRP, clinical variables, and HRCT score.

	hs-CRP(mg/L)	P value
Age (years)	0.124	0.312
BMI (kg/m^2)	−0.094	0.441
FVC (L)	−0.161	0.187
FEV$_1$ (L)	−0.153	0.211
FEV$_1$/FVC	−0.058	0.637
IgE (KU/L)	0.180	0.140
ECP (mcg/L)	0.087	0.479
Rest O$_2$%	−0.269	**0.025**
Lowest O$_2$%	−0.108	0.376
ΔO$_2$%	−0.003	0.982
6 MWD (m)	−0.190	0.118
HRCT score	0.473	**<0.001**

Abbreviations: BMI: body mass index, FVC: forced vital capacity, FEV$_1$: first second, 6 MWD: 6-minute walk test distance, HRCT: high-resolution computed tomography, and hs-CRP: high-sensitivity C-reactive protein.

Bronchiectasis patients in a stable phase with elevated levels of systemic markers of inflammation have been studied [17]. Other authors [35] have suggested that even in periods

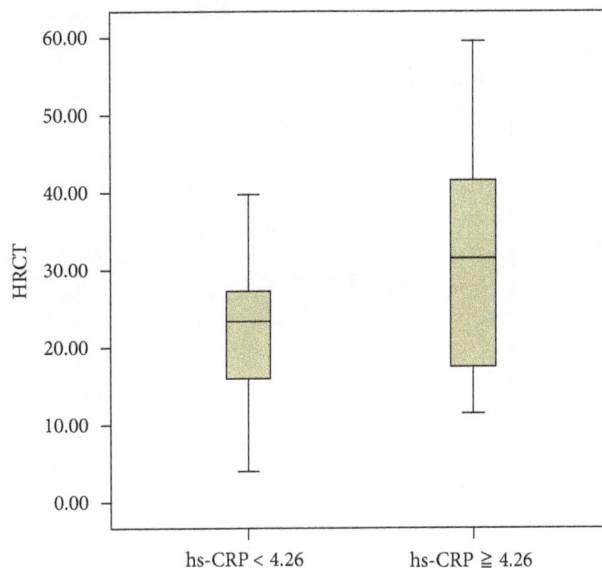

FIGURE 3: HRCT scores in higher and lower serum hs-CRP groups. HRCT scores were significantly higher in bronchiectasis patients with higher hs-CRP (mg/L). Boxes, median and interquartile range; whiskers, full range of values obtained; $P = 0.004$.

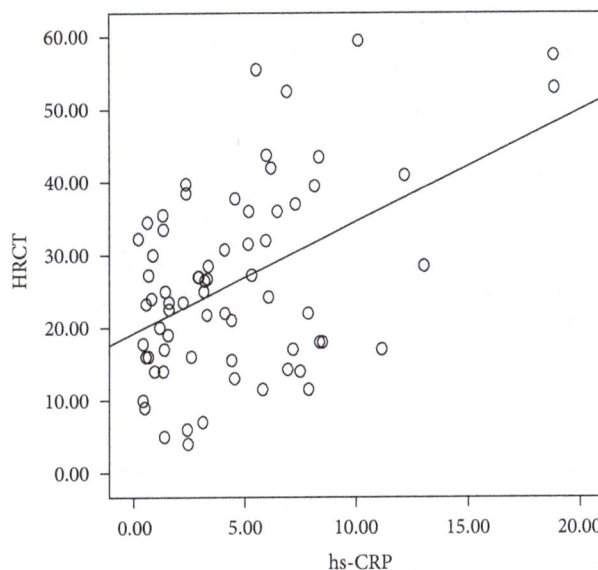

FIGURE 4: Relationship between serum high-sensitivity C-reactive protein (hs-CRP, mg/L) levels and HRCT scores in patients with stable bronchiectasis ($n = 69$, $r = 0.473$, $P < 0.001$, by Pearson's correlation).

of clinical stability, patients with non-CF bronchiectasis experience increased bronchial inflammation. During an exacerbation, particularly an infective episode, large quantities of neutrophils migrate into the airway, which can lead to increased levels of proteolytic agents. These agents participate in the destruction of the lung matrix and contribute to the development of bronchiectasis. The same authors [35] noted that, while the observed increase in inflammation during

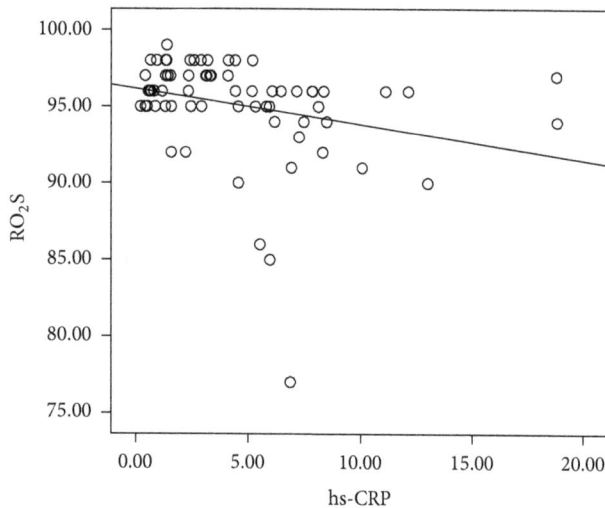

FIGURE 5: Relationship between serum high-sensitivity C-reactive protein (hs-CRP, mg/L) levels and $RO_2S\%$ (rest oxygenation saturation under room air) in patients with stable bronchiectasis ($n = 69$, $r = -0.269$, $P = 0.025$ by Pearson's correlation).

exacerbations decreases with antibiotic treatment, it does not disappear entirely. This may be the cause of the higher hs-CRP levels observed in our patients with multiple exacerbation-related hospitalizations.

Levels of CRP (not hs-CRP) have been shown to significantly correlate with HRCT bronchiectasis scores; however, a very poor correlation with lung function measures has also been reported [17]. In the current study, hs-CRP had a marginal, negative correlation with lung function measures (FVC or FEV_1). This may be because there was only low-grade inflammation in these patients and the fact that the hs-CRP assay is more sensitive than the CRP assay. Twenty-nine patients (42%) had hs-CRP levels lower than 3.0 mg/L in this study.

The 6-minute walk test, a functional assessment of patients with cardiopulmonary disease, is a good outcome predictor of obstructive airway diseases such as COPD and idiopathic pulmonary fibrosis. However, it has been reported that exercise tolerance demonstrates a stronger correlation to health-related quality of life than physiological measures of lung function or disease severity in bronchiectasis [36]. Other exercise tests have been used to assess cystic fibrosis-related bronchiectasis in children [37], and the results revealed a poor correlation between exercise test and HRCT abnormalities. In the current study, there was no difference in walking distances between the hs-CRP groups, indicating a more complicated pathogenesis and disease progression in bronchiectasis than in other obstructive airway diseases.

Resting oxygen saturation was significantly lower in the higher hs-CRP group. Furthermore, the association between the need for long-term oxygen therapy and mortality has been reported [38]. The correlation between hs-CRP and baseline oxygenation saturation (rest $O_2\%$) may reflect the underlying disease activity in these patients. Moreover, the stronger correlation between rest $O_2\%$ and HRCT ($r = -0.478$, $P < 0.001$) suggests that it can be a useful tool in assessing disease severity in stable bronchiectasis, although its role in disease progression and mortality warrants further investigations.

A high prevalence of atopy and increased serum ECP in adult patients with bronchiectasis has been reported [39, 40]. Serum ECP may be more relevant in assessing local eosinophil involvement than number of blood eosinophils. Atopic status was shown to not affect hs-CRP levels in steroid-naive or steroid-using asthma patients [34]. There was no significant difference between the hs-CRP groups in the current study, which suggests that eosinophils in the airway do not play a key role in persistent inflammation in bronchiectasis.

Bacterial infections are a major cause of morbidity and mortality in bronchiectasis patients. Acute inflammation is an important host defense against bronchial infection; however, if the infection becomes chronic, it can cause lung damage and lead to disease progression [3, 41]. The most common bacteria in the current study were *Pseudomonas aeruginosa*, which is consistent with previous reports [17]. Patients with bronchiectasis in a stable phase have raised levels of systemic markers of inflammation; however, this was not dependent on the presence of colonization in sputum in the current study.

Because there are so few randomized controlled trials of therapies for non-CF bronchiectasis and no US Food and Drug Administration approved therapies for non-CF bronchiectasis, patients must be evaluated and treated on an individual basis. Patients with mild-to-moderate bronchiectasis and infrequent exacerbations may not need maintenance therapy. According to the study of K.W. Tsang, inhaled corticosteroid (ICS) treatment is beneficial to patients with bronchiectasis, particularly those with *Pseudomonas aeruginosa* infection [42]. Twenty-three patients (35%) received regular inhaled cortical steroid/long acting β_2 agonist (LABA) treatment in the current study; however, no patient was treated with long-term macrolides to prevent exacerbations. There are 4 patients (5.8%) with diabetes mellitus and 9 patients (13.0%) with positive methacholine provocation test in the current cohort study. Therefore, the inhaled corticosteroid/long acting β_2 agonist (LABA) treatment was prescribed for our bronchiectasis patients, either with or without airway hyperreactivity/asthma. There was no significant difference between the hs-CRP groups in the present study (data not shown), which may reflect the minor role of such therapy in systemic inflammation in stable bronchiectasis. Interestingly, none of the other management strategies applied in our cohort, including therapy with inhaled and oral steroids, antibiotics, and secretion clearance maneuvers and oxygen therapy, had a significant effect on hs-CRP. Previous study showed that in patients with asthma on ICS treatment, serum hs-CRP levels did not differ from those of healthy controls and did not correlate with clinical or sputum indices. It is likely that the ICS, which has well-characterized anti-inflammatory properties, used in these patients might have reduced serum hs-CRP [34]. Similarly, there is no previous study to confirm the effects of ICS/LABA on the serum level of hs-CRP in bronchiectasis. Further research will be considered to study this important issue.

Two patients died of pneumonia and respiratory failure later within the study period, and their initial hs-CRP levels were 18.78 and 18.81 mg/L, respectively. Hence, the significance of higher hs-CRP in stable bronchiectasis needs further investigation.

There are several limitations to the current study. First, the number of patients is limited, and they were recruited from a single hospital, which may limit the generalizability of the study results. Second, evolutionary variables such as clinical evolution and the numbers of following exacerbation or hospitalization were not included in the analysis due to the short study period. Third, important transversal variables related to bronchiectasis such as systemic inflammatory diseases other than cardiovascular disorders and quality of life were not included in the analysis because the limited number of patients did not allow for the inclusion of more variables in the factorial analysis. Only four patients had type 2 diabetes mellitus and the study of osteoporosis was incomplete. Finally, the impact of nontuberculosis mycobacterial colonization or infection in these patients was not studied. Therefore, larger, multicentric studies are needed, with long-term follow-up and a larger number of patients in order to corroborate our results.

In conclusion, in patients with stable non-CF bronchiectasis, there was a good correlation between serum hs-CRP and HRCT scores. Increased HRCT scores and decreased rest oxygenation saturation were associated with higher levels of serum hs-CRP, which suggests that serum hs-CRP may be a useful biomarker that directly reflects the degree of systemic inflammation in stable non-CF bronchiectasis. However, further studies are required in order to better elucidate the clinical significance of the role of hs-CRP in bronchiectasis progression and treatment response, either in anti-inflammatory pharmacological therapy or in regular pulmonary rehabilitation programs.

Abbreviations

Hs-CRP: High-sensitivity C-reactive protein
CF: Cystic fibrosis
PFT: Pulmonary function test
IgE: Immunoglobulin E
ECP: Eosinophilic cationic protein
6 MWT: 6-minute walk test
HRCT: High-resolution computed tomography
ICS: Inhaled steroids
LABA: Long-acting beta-agonists.

Conflict of Interests

The authors declare no conflict of interests in the study itself or in the publication of the paper.

Acknowledgments

This work was supported by research Grant no. 370791 from Chang Gung Medical Foundation, Chang Gung University, Taiwan, and National Science Council, Taipei, Taiwan, NSC 100-2314-B-182-046.

References

[1] A. F. Barker, "Bronchiectasis," *The New England Journal of Medicine*, vol. 346, no. 18, pp. 1383–1393, 2002.

[2] K. W. Tsang and G. L. Tipoe, "Bronchiectasis: not an orphan disease in the East," *International Journal of Tuberculosis and Lung Disease*, vol. 8, no. 6, pp. 691–702, 2004.

[3] S. Fuschillo, A. De Felice, and G. Balzano, "Mucosal inflammation in idiopathic bronchiectasis: cellular and molecular mechanisms," *European Respiratory Journal*, vol. 31, no. 2, pp. 396–406, 2008.

[4] T. Keistinen, O. Säynäjäkangas, T. Tuuponen, and S.-L. Kivelä, "Bronchiectasis: an orphan disease with a poorly-understood prognosis," *European Respiratory Journal*, vol. 10, no. 12, pp. 2784–2787, 1997.

[5] A. E. O'Donnell, "Bronchiectasis," *Chest*, vol. 134, no. 4, pp. 815–823, 2008.

[6] H. J. Roberts and R. Hubbard, "Trends in bronchiectasis mortality in England and Wales," *Respiratory Medicine*, vol. 104, no. 7, pp. 981–985, 2010.

[7] A. E. O'Donnell, A. F. Barker, J. S. Ilowite, and R. B. Fick, "Treatment of idiopathic bronchiectasis with aerosolized recombinant human DNase I," *Chest*, vol. 113, no. 5, pp. 1329–1334, 1998.

[8] M. C. Pasteur, D. Bilton, and A. T. Hill, "British thoracic society guideline for non-CF bronchiectasis," *Thorax*, vol. 65, supplement 1, pp. i1–i58, 2010.

[9] G. C. Ooi, P. L. Khong, M. Chan-Yeung et al., "High-resolution CT quantification of bronchiectasis: clinical and functional correlation," *Radiology*, vol. 225, no. 3, pp. 663–672, 2002.

[10] H. R. Roberts, A. U. Wells, M. B. Rubens et al., "Airflow obstruction in bronchiectasis: correlation between computed tomography features and pulmonary function tests," *Thorax*, vol. 55, no. 3, pp. 198–204, 2000.

[11] R. E. Sheehan, A. U. Wells, S. J. Copley et al., "A comparison of serial computed tomography and functional change in bronchiectasis," *European Respiratory Journal*, vol. 20, no. 3, pp. 581–587, 2002.

[12] D. B. Reiff, A. U. Wells, D. H. Carr, P. J. Cole, and D. M. Hansell, "CT findings in bronchiectasis: limited value in distinguishing between idiopathic and specific types," *American Journal of Roentgenology*, vol. 165, no. 2, pp. 261–267, 1995.

[13] P. Grenier, M.-P. Cordeau, and C. Beigelman, "High-resolution computed tomography of the airways," *Journal of Thoracic Imaging*, vol. 8, no. 3, pp. 213–229, 1993.

[14] G. McGuinness and D. P. Naidich, "Bronchiectasis: CT/clinical correlations," *Seminars in Ultrasound CT and MRI*, vol. 16, no. 5, pp. 395–419, 1995.

[15] B. Schaaf, A. Wieghorst, S.-P. Aries, K. Dalhoff, and J. Braun, "Neutrophil inflammation and activation in bronchiectasis: comparison with pneumonia and idiopathic pulmonary fibrosis," *Respiration*, vol. 67, no. 1, pp. 52–59, 2000.

[16] J. C. W. Mak, S. P. Ho, R. Y. H. Leung et al., "Elevated levels of transforming growth factor-β1 in serum of patients with stable bronchiectasis," *Respiratory Medicine*, vol. 99, no. 10, pp. 1223–1228, 2005.

[17] C. B. Wilson, P. W. Jones, C. J. O'Leary et al., "Systemic markers of inflammation in stable bronchiectasis," *European Respiratory Journal*, vol. 12, no. 4, pp. 820–824, 1998.

[18] M. B. Pepys and G. M. Hirschfield, "C-reactive protein: a critical update," *Journal of Clinical Investigation*, vol. 111, no. 12, pp. 1805–1812, 2003.

[19] P. M. Ridker, "High-sensitivity C-reactive protein: potential adjunct for global risk assessment in the primary prevention of cardiovascular disease," *Circulation*, vol. 103, no. 13, pp. 1813–1818, 2001.

[20] M. J. Kaplan, "Management of cardiovascular disease risk in chronic inflammatory disorders," *Nature Reviews*, vol. 5, no. 4, pp. 208–217, 2009.

[21] B. M. Everett, T. Kurth, J. E. Buring, and P. M. Ridker, "The Relative Strength of C-Reactive Protein and Lipid Levels as Determinants of Ischemic Stroke Compared With Coronary Heart Disease in Women," *Journal of the American College of Cardiology*, vol. 48, no. 11, pp. 2235–2242, 2006.

[22] P. M. Ridker, M. J. Stampfer, and N. Rifai, "Novel risk factors for systemic atherosclerosis: a comparison of C-reactive protein, fibrinogen, homocysteine, lipoprotein(a), and standard cholesterol screening as predictors of peripheral arterial disease," *Journal of the American Medical Association*, vol. 285, no. 19, pp. 2481–2485, 2001.

[23] M. Cesari, B. W. J. H. Penninx, A. B. Newman et al., "Inflammatory markers and onset of cardiovascular events: results from the health ABC study," *Circulation*, vol. 108, no. 19, pp. 2317–2322, 2003.

[24] E. T. H. Yeh and J. T. Willerson, "Coming of age of C-reactive protein: using inflammation markers in cardiology," *Circulation*, vol. 107, no. 3, pp. 370–372, 2003.

[25] A. S. Brody, J. S. Klein, P. L. Molina, J. Quan, J. A. Bean, and R. W. Wilmott, "High-resolution computed tomography in young patients with cystic fibrosis: distribution of abnormalities and correlation with pulmonary function tests," *Journal of Pediatrics*, vol. 145, no. 1, pp. 32–38, 2004.

[26] "ATS statement: guidelines for the six-minute walk test," *American Journal of Respiratory and Critical Care Medicine*, vol. 166, no. 1, pp. 111–117, 2002.

[27] M. R. Loebinger, A. U. Wells, D. M. Hansell et al., "Mortality in bronchiectasis: a long-term study assessing the factors influencing survival," *European Respiratory Journal*, vol. 34, no. 4, pp. 843–849, 2009.

[28] Z. P. Onen, B. Eris Gulbay, E. Sen et al., "Analysis of the factors related to mortality in patients with bronchiectasis," *Respiratory Medicine*, vol. 101, no. 7, pp. 1390–1397, 2007.

[29] B. Weinhold and U. Rüther, "Interleukin-6-dependent and -independent regulation of the human C-reactive protein gene," *Biochemical Journal*, vol. 327, no. 2, pp. 425–429, 1997.

[30] N. Yoshida, S. Ikemoto, K. Narita et al., "Interleukin-6, tumour necrosis factor α and interleukin-1β in patients with renal cell carcinoma," *British Journal of Cancer*, vol. 86, no. 9, pp. 1396–1400, 2002.

[31] T. D. Spector, D. J. Hart, D. Nandra et al., "Low-level increases in serum C-reactive protein are present in early osteoarthritis of the knee and predict progressive disease," *Arthritis and Rheumatism*, vol. 40, no. 4, pp. 723–727, 1997.

[32] A. D. Pradhan, J. E. Manson, N. Rifai, J. E. Buring, and P. M. Ridker, "C-reactive protein, interleukin 6, and risk of developing type 2 diabetes mellitus," *Journal of the American Medical Association*, vol. 286, no. 3, pp. 327–334, 2001.

[33] J. P. De Torres, V. Pinto-Plata, C. Casanova et al., "C-reactive protein levels and survival in patients with moderate to very severe COPD," *Chest*, vol. 133, no. 6, pp. 1336–1343, 2008.

[34] M. Takemura, H. Matsumoto, A. Niimi et al., "High sensitivity C-reactive protein in asthma," *European Respiratory Journal*, vol. 27, no. 5, pp. 908–912, 2006.

[35] M. Gaga, A. M. Bentley, M. Humbert et al., "Increases in CD4+ T lymphocytes, macrophages, neutrophils and interleukin 8 positive cells in the airways of patients with bronchiectasis," *Thorax*, vol. 53, no. 8, pp. 685–691, 1998.

[36] A. L. Lee, B. M. Button, S. Ellis et al., "Clinical determinants of the 6-Minute Walk Test in bronchiectasis," *Respiratory Medicine*, vol. 103, no. 5, pp. 780–785, 2009.

[37] E. A. Edwards, I. Narang, I. Li, D. M. Hansell, M. Rosenthal, and A. Bush, "HRCT lung abnormalities are not a surrogate for exercise limitation in bronchiectasis," *European Respiratory Journal*, vol. 24, no. 4, pp. 538–544, 2004.

[38] M. Dupont, A. Gacouin, H. Lena et al., "Survival of patients with bronchiectasis after the first ICU stay for respiratory failure," *Chest*, vol. 125, no. 5, pp. 1815–1820, 2004.

[39] C. Kroegel, M. Schüler, M. Förster, R. Braun, and P. R. Grahmann, "Evidence for eosinophil activation in bronchiectasis unrelated to cystic fibrosis and bronchopulmonary aspergillosis: discrepancy between blood eosinophil counts and serum eosinophil cationic protein levels," *Thorax*, vol. 53, no. 6, pp. 498–500, 1998.

[40] F. Santamaria, S. Montella, M. Pifferi et al., "A descriptive study of non-cystic fibrosis bronchiectasis in a pediatric population from central and southern Italy," *Respiration*, vol. 77, no. 2, pp. 160–165, 2009.

[41] P. Cole and R. Wilson, "Host-microbial interrelationships in respiratory infection," *Chest*, vol. 95, no. 3, 1989.

[42] K. W. Tsang, K. C. Tan, P. L. Ho et al., "Inhaled fluticasone in bronchiectasis: a 12 month study," *Thorax*, vol. 60, no. 3, pp. 239–243, 2005.

A Simple Clinical Measure of Quadriceps Muscle Strength Identifies Responders to Pulmonary Rehabilitation

James R. Walsh,[1,2,3] Norman R. Morris,[1,4] Zoe J. McKeough,[5] Stephanie T. Yerkovich,[1,2] and Jenny D. Paratz[2]

[1] Queensland Lung Transplant Service, The Prince Charles Hospital, Rode Road, Chermside, QLD 4032, Australia
[2] School of Medicine, The University of Queensland, St Lucia, QLD 4072, Australia
[3] Physiotherapy Department, The Prince Charles Hospital, Rode Road, Chermside, QLD 4032, Australia
[4] School of Rehabilitation Sciences and Griffith Health Institute, Griffith University, Parklands Drive, Southport, QLD 4215, Australia
[5] Discipline of Physiotherapy, The University of Sydney, 75 East Street, Lidcombe, NSW 2141, Australia

Correspondence should be addressed to James R. Walsh; james.walsh@health.qld.gov.au

Academic Editor: Andrew Sandford

The aim was to determine if baseline measures can predict response to pulmonary rehabilitation in terms of six-minute walk distance (6MWD) or quality of life. Participants with COPD who attended pulmonary rehabilitation between 2010 and 2012 were recruited. Baseline measures evaluated included physical activity, quadriceps strength, comorbidities, inflammatory markers, and self-efficacy. Participants were classified as a responder with improvement in 6MWD (criteria of ≥25 m or ≥2SD) and Chronic Respiratory Questionnaire (CRQ; ≥0.5 points/question). Eighty-five participants with a mean (SD) age of 67(9) years and a mean forced expiratory volume in one second of 55(22)% were studied. Forty-nine and 19 participants were responders when using the 6MWD criteria of ≥25 m and ≥61.9 m, respectively, with forty-four participants improving in CRQ. In a regression model, responders in 6MWD (≥25 m criteria) had lower baseline quadriceps strength ($P = 0.028$) and higher baseline self-efficacy scores ($P = 0.045$). Independent predictors of 6MWD response (≥61.9 m criteria) were participants with metabolic disease ($P = 0.007$) and lower baseline quadriceps strength ($P = 0.016$). Lower baseline CRQ was the only independent predictor of CRQ response. A participant with relatively lower baseline quadriceps strength was the strongest independent predictor of 6MWD response. Metabolic disease may predict 6MWD response, but predictors of CRQ response remain unclear.

1. Introduction

Chronic obstructive pulmonary disease (COPD) is a major cause of morbidity and mortality [1]. International statements recommend the implementation of pulmonary rehabilitation for people with COPD who are symptomatic, have decreased functional capacity or reduced health-related quality of life [2]. There is clear evidence that pulmonary rehabilitation can improve exercise capacity, health-related quality of life, and dyspnea [3]. However, whilst the benefits are well documented, not all individuals who meet these criteria are able to access pulmonary rehabilitation [4]. There is also considerable variation in individual program response with between 33% [5] and 53% [6] of participants gaining no meaningful

improvement in six minute walk distance (6MWD) and over 50% [5, 6] of participants gaining no meaningful improvement in health-related quality of life. Therefore, a better understanding is required of which participant factors influence program response.

Despite several studies investigating the influence of participant factors on program response, the clinical utility of the findings remains unclear. Lower baseline quadriceps strength [6, 7] or greater quadriceps contractile fatigue [8] possibly best identify responders in exercise capacity. However, the measures used to assess quadriceps muscle strength and fatigue were a Cybex II dynamometer [7], a Cybex Norm Testing and Rehabilitation System [6], and a muscle stimulator [8], respectively. Therefore, it is unclear how the measures used to assess quadriceps muscle strength and fatigue can be incorporated into a routine clinical environment. Hand-held dynamometry is a more clinically accessible measure of quadriceps strength and, importantly, it has been shown to be a valid measure of muscle strength when compared to isokinetic dynamometry [9]. However, it is unknown if quadriceps strength measured via hand-held dynamometry is a factor that predicts response in exercise capacity following pulmonary rehabilitation.

There are other participant factors that have been suggested as inclusion criteria and/or identified as predictors of pulmonary rehabilitation response that require further investigation. For instance, limited physical activity has been recommended as an inclusion criterion for pulmonary rehabilitation [2]. However, the effect of preprogram physical activity level on response to pulmonary rehabilitation is not known. Moderate to severe dyspnea has been proposed previously as a general indicator [2], although, Evans et al. has subsequently reported that individuals can benefit in exercise performance regardless of the dyspnea grade [10]. One study has shown that participants with lower baseline self-efficacy have a better response in exercise capacity following pulmonary rehabilitation [6]. There are also conflicting findings on the influence of comorbidities, with a higher Charlson comorbidity index [11], metabolic syndrome [11], and osteoporosis [12] being associated with poor response in exercise capacity. Identifying a responder in quality of life also appears difficult, with only lower baseline quality of life [7], greater quadriceps contractile fatigue [8], higher 6MWD [6], and comorbidities [11] being identified as independent predictors. Furthermore, the presence of inflammatory markers, including Interleukin-6, Interleukin-8, and C Reactive Protein (CRP), has been associated with reduced quadriceps strength [13] and quality of life [14] in people with COPD and may be able to identify responders to pulmonary rehabilitation.

Therefore, the study's primary aim was to determine if the measures of quadriceps strength, physical activity or inflammatory markers, in combination with dyspnea, comorbidities, and self-efficacy, can predict responders in exercise capacity or quality of life following pulmonary rehabilitation. As the threshold used to define 6MWD appears important in identifying responders [15], a second aim was to evaluate if different methods used to define improvement in 6MWD affected the predictors of response.

2. Materials and Methods

This study used a prospective observational cohort design. Inclusion criteria were all participants with stable COPD, who completed baseline assessment at the single institution's pulmonary rehabilitation program between January 2010 and March 2012. Exclusion criteria were participants who did not complete the reassessment measures on program completion or participants who missed $\geq$ four supervised sessions. Approval was gained from the institutional ethics committees prior to recruitment (HREC/08/QPCH/116-EC28116 and 2009000403) and all participants provided informed consent.

2.1. Measurements. Demographic information and medical history were collected at initial assessment. The lung function measures of forced expiratory volume in one second (FEV_1) and diffusing capacity of the lung for carbon monoxide (DLCO) were assessed prior to program commencement according to standard methods [16]. Baseline dyspnea was assessed on initial assessment using the modified MRC dyspnea scale [17, 18]. Participant's exercise capacity and quality of life were assessed at program commencement and on completion. Exercise capacity was assessed by the 6MWD as per established guidelines [19]. The better of two 6MWD was used at baseline assessment. Quality of life was assessed using the self-reported Chronic Respiratory Questionnaire (CRQ) [20].

The following baseline participant factors were collected.

2.1.1. Quadriceps Strength. Quadriceps strength was measured at initial assessment using hand-held dynamometry (Lafayette Manual Muscle Test System) as per the published protocol [21] with an adjustable strap added. The adjustable strap was secured behind the participant's leg and held to the dynamometer to ensure an isometric contraction. Participants performed three maximal knee extension efforts on each leg with at least one minute rest between tests. In a pilot study, the test-retest reliability for this technique was $r = 0.996$ with a coefficient of variation of 2.7%. In order to normalise this measure, quadriceps strength was expressed as a percentage calculated by adding the best attempt on each leg together (kilograms) and dividing by the participant's body weight.

2.1.2. Physical Activity. Physical activity level was estimated for a cohort of the participants using the SenseWear Pro 3 Armband (SenseWear, Bodymedia Inc.). Participants were asked to wear the armband on the upper right arm for one week from program commencement using standardised protocols [22]. Minimum requirements were for the participant to wear the multisensor device for $\geq$20 hours/day on a minimum of four days.

2.1.3. Measurement of Inflammatory Markers. Plasma was obtained from peripheral blood samples at initial assessment in participants prior to exercise. The inflammatory markers of Interleukin-6, Interleukin-8, and C Reactive Protein (CRP) were used. Interleukin-6 and Interleukin-8 were measured by in-house ELISA (BD biosciences, lower limit of detection 30 pg/mL). CRP was measured by commercially available ELISA (R&D Systems, USA, lower limit of detection of 0.78 ng/mL).

2.1.4. Comorbidities. The Charlson comorbidity index was calculated at the initial assessment from the participant's medical history [23]. The participant's comorbidities were grouped into the following categories: musculoskeletal, cardiac, and metabolic disease as per the previously described method [11].

2.1.5. Self-Efficacy. Baseline self-efficacy was assessed using the COPD self-efficacy scale at initial assessment [24].

The COPD self-efficacy scale consists of 34 items and it has good test-retest reliability and internal consistency reliability [24]. Self-efficacy was calculated by averaging the total score by the number of questions answered [6].

2.2. Pulmonary Rehabilitation Program. The multidisciplinary program was a twice weekly, eight week program. The supervised exercise program included lower limb endurance training and upper and lower limb strength training [25]. The lower limb endurance training consisted of a minimum of twenty minutes of walking and/or cycling per session [25]. The prescribed walking program was commenced at 80% of each participant's average walking speed achieved during the six minute walk test [25]. The cycling program was on a bicycle ergometer with the work rate started at 80% intensity and calculated from the participant's 6MWD [26]. As a guide for training intensity, the participant's walking or cycling intensity was progressed throughout the program to target a four rating or "somewhat severe" of dyspnea or fatigue from the Borg scale [2]. Participants were prescribed a strengthening program of one to three sets/exercise, with the aim of attaining muscle fatigue between six to ten repetitions. The training load was increased when the participant was able to complete ten repetitions. All participants were given a home program and encouraged to complete at least three sessions each week of lower limb endurance and strength training [2].

2.3. Defining a Responder. Improvements in exercise capacity and quality of life were used to define a program responder. Due to the debate in defining the important difference in the 6MWD, both the smallest published criteria [27] and the coefficient of repeatability method [15] were used. Therefore, a participant was considered a responder if 6MWD increased by ≥25 m [27] or ≥2SD [15]. For the purpose of this study a responder in CRQ was defined as improvement ≥ 0.5 points/question [20, 28].

2.4. Statistical Analysis. Data were analysed using parametric and nonparametric tests as appropriate. Participants were grouped as responders or nonresponders in 6MWD and CRQ. The coefficient of repeatability was calculated from the difference between the baseline 6MWDs. Age, physical activity, dyspnea, quadriceps strength, Interleukin-8, CRP, comorbidities, self-efficacy, baseline assessment 6MWD, and CRQ were examined in a univariate model with significant outcome measures ($P < 0.1$) analysed using a multivariate binary logistic regression model. As there were two different criteria used to define a responder in 6MWD, the Receiver Operating Characteristic ROC curve was used to determine the goodness-of-fit to evaluate the sensitivity (true positive) and specificity (false positive) of the different 6MWD logistic regression models. A sample size of eighty-five participants was needed to detect a 10% difference (power of 0.9 and $P < 0.05$) in multiple factors including quadriceps strength, dyspnea, and self-efficacy score. SPSS version 21 was used to perform the statistical analysis.

3. Results

Eighty-five eligible participants, with thirty-six females, a mean ($\pm$SD) age of 67.4 ± 9.1 years, $FEV_1\%$ of $55.4 \pm 22.3\%$, and DLCO% of $54.2 \pm 19.4\%$, completed pulmonary rehabilitation and were included (Figure 1). Forty-five participants (52.9%) had a baseline mMRC dyspnea grade of ≥2. Sixty-two participants (72.9%) had ≥ one additional comorbidity. Twenty-seven participants (31.8%) were categorised with musculoskeletal disease, twenty-five participants (29.4%) with cardiac disease, and twenty-five participants (29.4%) with metabolic disease. Physical activity level was assessed in forty-six participants. Inflammatory markers were analysed in seventy-seven participants, with all participants having detectable levels of CRP but only four participants had detectable levels of Interleukin-6 and thirty-four participants had detectable levels of Interleukin-8.

Twenty-six participants (26/111) did not complete the program during the study period due to illness ($n = 15$), musculoskeletal injury ($n = 5$), transport difficulties ($n = 5$), and other commitments ($n = 7$), with participants providing multiple reasons for noncompletion. Program completers had a higher mean baseline 6MWD (406 ± 107 m versus 354 ± 133 m; $P = 0.041$) and CRQ (86.7 ± 21.5 versus 73.3 ± 29.3; $P = 0.011$) when compared to noncompleters. Program completers were not significantly different in any other baseline factor (see Table 1 in the Supplementary Material available online at http://dx.doi.org/10.1155/2014/782702).

The mean difference between the two baseline 6MWDs at initial assessment was 18.5 ± 30.9 m ($r = 0.938$) and, therefore, the coefficient of repeatability (2SD) was 61.9 m. Participant's mean overall improvement in 6MWD, from initial assessment to program completion, was 32.6 m ($P < 0.001$). Forty-nine (58%) and nineteen (22%) participants were classified as responders when using the 6MWD criteria of ≥25 m and ≥61.9 m, respectively. The mean improvement in the CRQ was 11.2 points ($P < 0.001$) with forty-four participants (52%) classified as a responder. Twenty-six (59%) and eleven (25%) participants responded in both CRQ and 6MWD when using ≥25 m and ≥61.9 m criteria, respectively.

Participant factors were evaluated for baseline differences in program response. When using the ≥25 m 6MWD criteria, responders were 11.1% lower in mean quadriceps strength ($P = 0.025$) and 0.4 points higher in the self-efficacy score ($P = 0.025$) when compared to nonresponders. Similarly, with the ≥61.9 m criteria, responders were 18.1% lower in mean quadriceps strength ($P = 0.002$) when compared to nonresponders (Table 1). In this model, there was a significant difference in baseline 6MWD between responders (359 ± 20 m) and nonresponders (420 ± 13 m; $P = 0.015$). There was also a relationship between 6MWD response and both musculoskeletal (Fisher's exact test $P = 0.048$) and metabolic disease ($P = 0.004$). No other factor, including physical activity, was significantly different in either 6MWD model. The only significant difference between responders and nonresponders in CRQ was that responders (79 ± 3) had a lower baseline CRQ when compared to nonresponders (95 ± 4; $P = 0.001$). There were no significant differences between

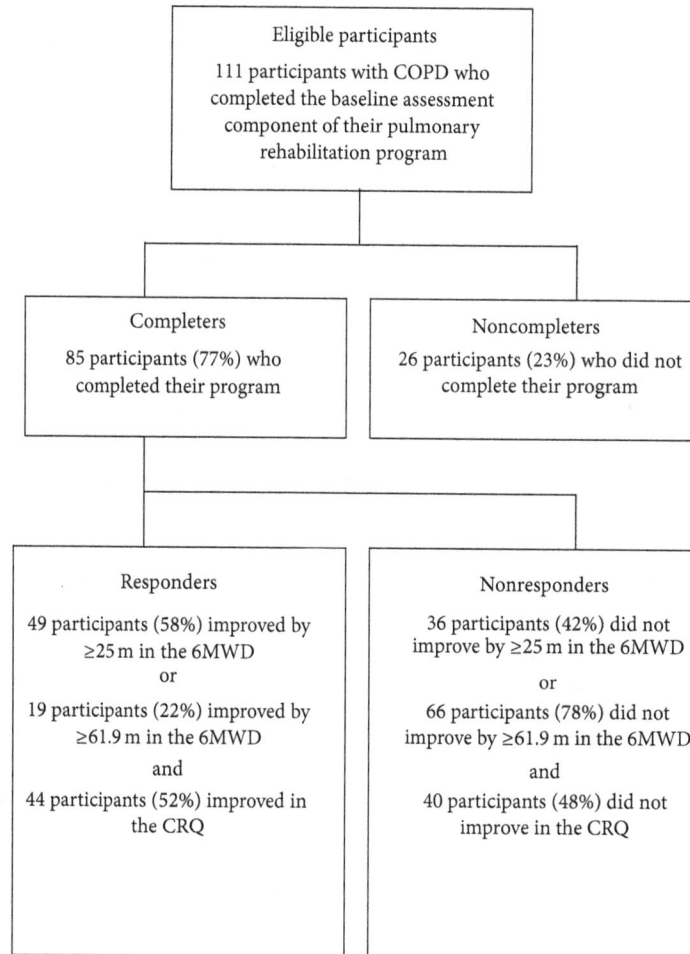

Eligible participants

111 participants with COPD who completed the baseline assessment component of their pulmonary rehabilitation program

Completers

85 participants (77%) who completed their program

Noncompleters

26 participants (23%) who did not complete their program

Responders

49 participants (58%) improved by ≥25 m in the 6MWD

or

19 participants (22%) improved by ≥61.9 m in the 6MWD

and

44 participants (52%) improved in the CRQ

Nonresponders

36 participants (42%) did not improve by ≥25 m in the 6MWD

or

66 participants (78%) did not improve by ≥61.9 m in the 6MWD

and

40 participants (48%) did not improve in the CRQ

*One participant did not complete the CRQ on program completion

FIGURE 1: Study flow chart.

TABLE 1: Baseline assessment data for responders compared to nonresponders in the six minute walk distance.

	(A) Responders	(A) Nonresponders		(B) Responders	(B) Nonresponders	
Number (%)	49 (57.6%)	36 (42.4%)		19 (22.4%)	66 (77.6%)	
Age (years)	68.0 ± 8.6	66.7 ± 9.7	$P = 0.523$	68.3 ± 8.1	67.2 ± 9.5	$P = 0.628$
FEV$_1$% predicted	57.0 ± 23.3	53.3 ± 21.3	$P = 0.458$	62.8 ± 26.6	53.2 ± 20.6	$P = 0.101$
mMRC	1.6 ± 1.1	1.7 ± 0.9	$P = 0.964$	1.8 ± 1.1	1.6 ± 1.0	$P = 0.570$
Quadriceps strength (%)	57.5 ± 21.9	68.6 ± 21.9	$P = 0.025$	48.1 ± 16.5	66.2 ± 22.4	$P = 0.002$
Physical activity level (METs)[+]	1.49 ± 0.18	1.54 ± 0.22	$P = 0.443$	1.45 ± 0.15	1.52 ± 0.20	$P = 0.307$
Interleukin-8 (pg/mL)[*]	151 ± 434	175 ± 485	$P = 0.818$	144 ± 370	167 ± 478	$P = 0.856$
C Reactive Protein (pg/mL)[*]	7217 ± 13805	10771 ± 10813	$P = 0.223$	9643 ± 18638	8684 ± 10711	$P = 0.793$
COPD self-efficacy score	3.0 ± 0.8	2.6 ± 0.7	$P = 0.060$	2.8 ± 0.5	2.8 ± 0.8	$P = 0.884$
Charlson comorbidity index	1.9 ± 1.1	2.0 ± 1.1	$P = 0.608$	2.3 ± 1.1	1.8 ± 1.1	$P = 0.126$
Metabolic disease	15/49 (31%)	10/36 (28%)	$P = 0.814$	11/19 (31%)	14/66 (28%)	$P = 0.004$
Cardiac disease	13/49 (27%)	12/36 (33%)	$P = 0.631$	5/19 (26%)	20/66 (30%)	$P = 1.000$
Musculoskeletal disease	18/49 (37%)	9/36 (25%)	$P = 0.346$	10/19 (31%)	17/66 (28%)	$P = 0.048$
Baseline 6MWD (m)	393 ± 16	423 ± 17	$P = 0.202$	359 ± 20	420 ± 13	$P = 0.015$

Part (A) responders/non-responders used the criteria of six-minute walk distance (6MWD) ≥25 m. Part (B) responders/non-responders used the criteria of 6MWD ≥61.9 m. Data expressed as the mean ± standard deviation. FEV$_1$: forced expiratory volume in one second, mMRC: modified Medical Research Council dyspnea scale, and METs: metabolic equivalent of task.
[*]Systemic inflammatory markers were assessed in 77 participants.
[+]Physical activity level was assessed in 46 participants.

TABLE 2: Baseline assessment data for responders compared to non-responders in the Chronic Respiratory Questionnaire.

	Responders	Nonresponders	
Number (%)	44 (52.3%)	40 (47.6%)	
Age (years)	66.6 ± 8.2	68.3 ± 10.3	$P = 0.385$
FEV$_1$% predicted	55.5 ± 23.0	55.0 ± 22.1	$P = 0.925$
mMRC	1.8 ± 1.1	1.6 ± 1.0	$P = 0.384$
Quadriceps strength (%)	64.8 ± 23.1	59.4 ± 22.0	$P = 0.278$
Physical activity level (METs)[+]	1.52 ± 0.25	1.49 ± 0.20	$P = 0.697$
Interleukin-8 (pg/mL)[*]	201 ± 514	120 ± 384	$P = 0.438$
C Reactive Protein (pg/mL)[*]	8765 ± 11327	8998 ± 14108	$P = 0.937$
COPD self-efficacy score	2.8 ± 0.7	2.9 ± 0.8	$P = 0.554$
Charlson comorbidity index	2.2 ± 1.2	1.7 ± 0.8	$P = 0.051$
Metabolic disease	17/44 (39%)	8/40 (20%)	$P = 0.062$
Cardiac disease	12/44 (27%)	13/40 (33%)	$P = 0.639$
Musculoskeletal disease	15/44 (34%)	12/40 (30%)	$P = 0.688$
Baseline CRQ	79 ± 3	95 ± 4	$P = 0.001$

Data expressed as the mean ± standard deviation. FEV$_1$%: forced expiratory volume in one second, mMRC: modified Medical Research Council dyspnea scale, METs: metabolic equivalent of task, and CRQ: Chronic Respiratory Questionnaire.
[*]Systemic inflammatory markers were assessed in 77 participants.
[+]Physical activity level was assessed in 46 participants.

responders and nonresponders in any other participant factor (Table 2).

Responders in 6MWD and CRQ were assessed using logistic regression models with responders (Yes = 1 and No = 0) as the dependent variable. Significant participant characteristics ($P < 0.1$) in the univariate models were assessed in a multivariate analysis. Using the 6MWD criteria of ≥25 m, the univariate analysis showed a difference between responders and nonresponders in quadriceps strength and self-efficacy. In the multivariate analysis, lower baseline quadriceps strength ($P = 0.028$) and higher self-efficacy scores ($P = 0.045$) were identified as independent predictors of 6MWD response (Table 3). Using the 6MWD criteria of ≥61.9 m, the univariate analysis indicated a difference between responders and nonresponders in quadriceps strength, baseline 6MWD, and metabolic and musculoskeletal disease. In the multivariate model, lower baseline quadriceps strength ($P = 0.016$) and metabolic disease ($P = 0.007$) were identified as independent predictors. No other participant factor contributed to either 6MWD regression model. Quadriceps strength was the only measure that was an independent predictor of response in both 6MWD models, with these findings translating to a participant 10% weaker in baseline strength increasing the odds of a favourable response in 6MWD by a factor of approximately 1.27 in the ≥25 m model and a factor of approximately 1.51 in the ≥61.9 m model. The Receiver Operating Characteristic curve was used to determine the goodness-of-fit of the 6MWD models. Using the 6MWD criteria of ≥25 m, the area under the curve was 0.608 (95% CI: 0.484–0.733; $P = 0.092$). When using the 6MWD criteria of ≥61.9 m, the area under the curve was 0.803 (95% CI: 0.688–0.917; $P ≤ 0.001$).

The CRQ univariate analysis indicated a difference between responders and nonresponders in the baseline CRQ, the Charlson comorbidity index, and participants with

metabolic disease. In the multivariate model, only baseline CRQ ($P = 0.003$) was identified as an independent predictor of response in CRQ (Table 4). No other participant factor contributed to the model.

4. Discussion

The present study investigated a more clinically accessible measure of quadriceps strength and a multisensor device to estimate physical activity level, along with assessing inflammatory markers, dyspnea, comorbidities, and self-efficacy measures to better understand predictors of response following pulmonary rehabilitation. The only predictor that consistently identified response in 6MWD following pulmonary rehabilitation, no matter what model was used to define improvement, was lower baseline quadriceps strength. Higher baseline self-efficacy scores and participants with metabolic disease were independent predictors of response in 6MWD when using ≥25 m and ≥61.9 m models, respectively. In the current study, identifying independent predictors of response in CRQ was difficult with only lower baseline CRQ scores being identified.

Not surprisingly, the method used to define the minimally important difference for 6MWD impacted on the number of participants classified as responders and nonresponders. Although there was a relatively lower number of participants being classified as a responder in 6MWD when using the ≥61.9 m criteria, this model's sensitivity was significantly stronger as demonstrated by a better goodness-of-fit in the Receiver Operating Characteristic curve analysis. Furthermore, the baseline quadriceps strength's mean difference increased between responders and nonresponders and the odds ratio also improved when using the ≥61.9 m model to define 6MWD response. Importantly, lower baseline quadriceps strength was identified as an independent predictor of

TABLE 3: Binary logistic regression models for a responder in the six-minute walk distance (6MWD).

(a) Binary logistic regression analysis—responders defined as ≥25 m increase in 6MWD

	β	SE	Wald χ^2	P	Odds ratio (Exp β)	95% CI for Exp β
Univariate analysis						
Quadriceps strength	−0.023	0.011	4.737	0.030	0.977	0.957–0.998
COPD self-efficacy score	0.565	0.304	3.450	0.063	1.760	0.969–3.196
Multivariate analysis						
Quadriceps strength	−0.024	0.011	4.822	0.028	0.976	0.955–0.997
COPD self-efficacy score	0.626	0.313	4.015	0.045	1.871	1.014–3.451

(b) Binary logistic regression analysis—responders defined as ≥61.9 m increase in 6MWD

	β	SE	Wald χ^2	P	Odds ratio (Exp β)	95% CI for Exp β
Univariate analysis						
Quadriceps strength	−0.048	0.017	8.291	0.004	0.953	0.922–0.985
Metabolic disease	−1.631	0.554	8.673	0.003	0.196	0.066–0.580
Musculoskeletal disease	−1.164	0.539	4.666	0.031	0.312	0.109–0.898
Baseline 6MWD	−0.006	0.003	4.592	0.032	0.994	0.989–1.000
Multivariate analysis						
Quadriceps strength	−0.043	0.018	5.776	0.016	0.958	0.924–0.992
Metabolic disease	−1.762	0.648	7.391	0.007	0.172	0.048–0.612
Baseline 6MWD	−0.006	0.003	3.008	0.083	0.994	0.988–1.001

Only variables with $P < 0.1$ are shown in the table.

TABLE 4: Binary logistic regression model for a responder in the Chronic Respiratory Questionnaire (CRQ).

	β	SE	Wald χ^2	P	Odds ratio (Exp β)	95% CI for Exp β
Univariate analysis						
Charlson comorbidity index	0.426	0.223	3.643	0.056	1.531	0.989–2.370
Metabolic disease	−0.924	0.502	3.384	0.066	2.519	0.941–6.738
Baseline CRQ	−0.038	0.012	9.486	0.002	0.962	0.939–0.986
Multivariate analysis						
Metabolic disease	−0.914	0.539	2.872	0.090	0.401	0.139–1.154
Baseline CRQ	−0.038	0.013	9.100	0.003	0.963	0.939–0.987

Only variables with $P < 0.1$ are shown in the table.

response regardless of the model used and these findings support the previous results by Troosters et al. ($n = 49$) [7] and Garrod et al. ($n = 51$) [6]. Furthermore, our relatively simple method of using hand-held dynamometry to assess quadriceps strength can be more easily translated into the clinical pulmonary rehabilitation environment which also broadens the applicability of our findings. Metabolic disease was associated with 6MWD response only when using ≥61.9 m criteria to define improvement. There were conflicting results with self-efficacy, as this measure was found to be an independent predictor of 6MWD response using the ≥25 m criteria, but not when using the ≥61.9 m criteria. Our conflicting results would suggest that self-efficacy is not a useful indicator of 6MWD response.

In the current study, baseline physical activity level and dyspnea grade did not identify responders to pulmonary rehabilitation, despite people with these criteria being recommended for program inclusion [2]. Our findings support those by Evans et al. which reported no significant difference in exercise performance between participants with different dyspnea grades [29]. The current study is novel in being the first to assess whether physical activity level could identify responders to pulmonary rehabilitation. While only forty-six participants had this measure assessed due, in part, to the limited availability of the multisensor devices this sample size was sufficient to detect a 10% difference in physical activity during the univariate analyses. Although improving physical activity remains an important goal of pulmonary rehabilitation [30], our findings would suggest that participants can benefit from pulmonary rehabilitation regardless of preprogram physical activity level.

Interleukin-6, Interleukin-8, and CRP also did not identify responders in 6MWD or CRQ in the current study, despite inflammatory markers being previously associated with decreased quadriceps strength [13, 31] and quality of life [14]. Spruit et al. also concluded that markers of systemic inflammation do not adequately identify 6MWD or quality of life response following pulmonary rehabilitation [14]. Although all participants in our study had detectable levels of CRP, ≤44% of participants had detectable levels of Interleukin-6 and Interleukin-8. With persistent systemic inflammation being perhaps more important given the association with mortality [32], an increased rate of COPD exacerbation [32], and an increased risk of comorbidities [33], it may have been more useful to assess participant's inflammatory markers at several time points before, during, and at the end of the pulmonary rehabilitation program. Therefore, due to the possible variation in inflammatory markers over an outpatient pulmonary rehabilitation program, one sample per participant may be inadequate to identify program response.

Similar to our cohort, previous studies have reported a large percentage of pulmonary rehabilitation participants having additional comorbidities [11, 12]. In the current study, metabolic disease was an independent predictor of 6MWD response only when using the ≥61.9 m criteria. This finding supports our previous study [34] but it is contradictory to the findings by Crisafulli et al. which found that metabolic disease was inversely related to 6MWD response [11]. This variation in findings, despite using the same classification method, may be because grouping different diseases into the categories of musculoskeletal and metabolic disease may have masked the ability of these categories to consistently identify pulmonary rehabilitation response. The Charlson comorbidity index was not identified as an independent predictor of response which supports Crisafulli et al. finding [11, 12]. The conflicting findings suggest that further investigation is required to better define the severity of comorbidities to understand the influence on pulmonary rehabilitation response.

The current study also assessed multiple factors with the aim to better understand the influence of participant factors on response in quality of life. However, lower baseline CRQ score was the only independent predictor of response in CRQ. These findings support the previous conclusions by Troosters et al. [7] but are not particularly useful in increasing the understanding of what participant factors identify a responder in CRQ.

Lower baseline quadriceps strength and participants with metabolic disease were identified as independent predictors of response in 6MWD with the threshold used to define improvement in 6MWD an important consideration. Our findings suggest that quadriceps strength becomes a better predictor of response when using a larger threshold to define improvement in 6MWD. In addition, hand-held dynamometry identified participants with weaker baseline strength that were more likely to respond in 6MWD and this result is similar to the previous findings [6, 7]. Importantly, hand-held dynamometry has been shown previously to be a valid measure of muscle strength when compared to isokinetic dynamometry [9] and in our hands has excellent test-retest reliability. However, it is unclear if participants with relatively lower baseline quadriceps strength are more likely to improve in other measures of exercise capacity or important

pulmonary rehabilitation objectives such as improving physical activity [30]. Therefore, based upon 6MWD response alone, it is difficult to recommend that participants with relatively lower baseline quadriceps strength should be preferentially considered for pulmonary rehabilitation referral. Further research should investigate whether lower baseline quadriceps strength identifies response to other program objectives such as improving physical activity and if different methods of delivering pulmonary rehabilitation improve the overall number of participants that respond to pulmonary rehabilitation.

5. Conclusions

Quadriceps strength was the strongest independent predictor of response in 6MWD following pulmonary rehabilitation with this measure becoming a better predictor of response when using a larger threshold to define improvement. Metabolic disease may be useful in predicting 6MWD response, but predictors of CRQ response remain unclear.

Abbreviations

COPD: Chronic obstructive pulmonary disease
CRP: C Reactive Protein
CRQ: Chronic Respiratory Questionnaire
DLCO: Diffusing capacity of the lung for carbon monoxide
FEV_1: Forced expiratory volume in one second
mMRC: modified Medical Research Council dyspnea scale
6MWD: Six-minute walk distance.

Conflict of Interests

The authors declare that there is no conflict of interests regarding the publication of this paper.

Acknowledgment

This paper is supported by The Prince Charles Hospital Foundation and the Queensland Health's Health Practitioner Research Scheme.

References

[1] D. M. Mannino and A. S. Buist, "Global burden of COPD: risk factors, prevalence, and future trends," *The Lancet*, vol. 370, no. 9589, pp. 765–773, 2007.

[2] L. Nici, C. Donner, E. Wouters et al., "American thoracic society/European respiratory society statement on pulmonary rehabilitation," *American Journal of Respiratory and Critical Care Medicine*, vol. 173, no. 12, pp. 1390–1413, 2006.

[3] A. L. Ries, G. S. Bauldoff, B. W. Carlin et al., "Pulmonary rehabilitation: joint ACCP/AACVPR Evidence-Based Clinical Practice Guidelines," *Chest*, vol. 131, supplement 5, pp. 4S–42S, 2007.

[4] P. Frith, J. Alison, J. Burdon et al., "Case Statement: Chronic Obstructive Pulmonary Disease (COPD): the Australian

Lung Foundation," 2001, http://www.lungfoundation.com.au/professional-resources/.

[5] B. Vagaggini, F. Costa, S. Antonelli et al., "Clinical predictors of the efficacy of a pulmonary rehabilitation programme in patients with COPD," *Respiratory Medicine*, vol. 103, no. 8, pp. 1224–1230, 2009.

[6] R. Garrod, J. Marshall, E. Barley, and P. W. Jones, "Predictors of success and failure in pulmonary rehabilitation," *European Respiratory Journal*, vol. 27, no. 4, pp. 788–794, 2006.

[7] T. Troosters, R. Gosselink, and M. Decramer, "Exercise training in COPD: how to distinguish responders from nonresponders," *Journal of Cardiopulmonary Rehabilitation*, vol. 21, no. 1, pp. 10–17, 2001.

[8] C. Burtin, D. Saey, M. Saglam et al., "Effectiveness of exercise training in patients with COPD: the role of muscle fatigue," *European Respiratory Journal*, vol. 40, no. 2, pp. 338–344, 2012.

[9] L. Noreau and J. Vachon, "Comparison of three methods to assess muscular strength in individuals with spinal cord injury," *Spinal Cord*, vol. 36, no. 10, pp. 716–723, 1998.

[10] R. A. Evans, S. J. Singh, R. Collier, J. E. Williams, and M. D. L. Morgan, "Pulmonary rehabilitation is successful for COPD irrespective of MRC dyspnoea grade," *Respiratory Medicine*, vol. 103, no. 7, pp. 1070–1075, 2009.

[11] E. Crisafulli, S. Costi, F. Luppi et al., "Role of comorbidities in a cohort of patients with COPD undergoing pulmonary rehabilitation," *Thorax*, vol. 63, no. 6, pp. 487–492, 2008.

[12] E. Crisafulli, P. Gorgone, B. Vagaggini et al., "Efficacy of standard rehabilitation in COPD outpatients with comorbidities," *European Respiratory Journal*, vol. 36, no. 5, pp. 1042–1048, 2010.

[13] S. Yende, G. W. Waterer, E. A. Tolley et al., "Inflammatory markers are associated with ventilatory limitation and muscle dysfunction in obstructive lung disease in well functioning elderly subjects," *Thorax*, vol. 61, no. 1, pp. 10–16, 2006.

[14] M. A. Spruit, R. Gosselink, T. Troosters, A. Kasran, M. van Vliet, and M. Decramer, "Low-grade systemic inflammation and the response to exercise training in patients with advanced COPD," *Chest*, vol. 128, no. 5, pp. 3183–3190, 2005.

[15] T. E. Dolmage, K. Hill, R. A. Evans, and R. S. Goldstein, "Has my patient responded? Interpreting clinical measurements such as the 6-minute-walk test," *American Journal of Respiratory and Critical Care Medicine*, vol. 184, no. 6, pp. 642–646, 2011.

[16] J. Wanger, J. L. Clausen, A. Coates et al., "Standardisation of the measurement of lung volumes," *European Respiratory Journal*, vol. 26, no. 3, pp. 511–522, 2005.

[17] J. G. W. Burdon, E. F. Juniper, and K. J. Killian, "The perception of breathlessness in asthma," *American Review of Respiratory Disease*, vol. 126, no. 5, pp. 825–828, 1982.

[18] A. D. Lopez, C. D. Mathers, M. Ezzati, D. T. Jamison, and C. J. L. Murray, "Measuring the global burden of disease and risk factors, 1990–2001," in *Global Burden of Disease and Risk Factors*, A. D. Lopez, C. D. Mathers, M. Ezzati, D. T. Jamison, and C. J. L. Murray, Eds., World Bank, Washington, DC, USA, 2006.

[19] ATS Committee on Proficiency Standards for Clinical Pulmonary Function Laboratories, "ATS statement: guidelines for the Six-Minute Walk Test," *American Journal of Respiratory and Critical Care Medicine*, vol. 166, no. 1, pp. 111–117, 2002.

[20] J. E. A. Williams, S. J. Singh, L. Sewell, G. H. Guyatt, and M. D. L. Morgan, "Development of a self-reported Chronic Respiratory Questionnaire (CRQ-SR)," *Thorax*, vol. 56, no. 12, pp. 954–959, 2001.

[21] S. D. O'Shea, N. F. Taylor, and J. D. Paratz, "Measuring muscle strength for people with chronic obstructive pulmonary disease: retest reliability of hand-held dynamometry," *Archives of Physical Medicine and Rehabilitation*, vol. 88, no. 1, pp. 32–36, 2007.

[22] H. Watz, B. Waschki, T. Meyer, and H. Magnussen, "Physical activity in patients with COPD," *European Respiratory Journal*, vol. 33, no. 2, pp. 262–272, 2009.

[23] M. E. Charlson, P. Pompei, K. A. Ales, and C. R. MacKenzie, "A new method of classifying prognostic comorbidity in longitudinal studies: development and validation," *Journal of Chronic Diseases*, vol. 40, no. 5, pp. 373–383, 1987.

[24] J. K. Wigal, T. L. Creer, and H. Kotses, "The COPD self-efficacy scale," *Chest*, vol. 99, no. 5, pp. 1193–1196, 1991.

[25] J. Alison, C. Barrack, P. Cafarella et al., "The Pulmonary Rehabilitation Toolkit on behalf of The Australian Lung Foundation," 2009, http://www.pulmonaryrehab.com.au/welcome.asp.

[26] N. Luxton, J. A. Alison, J. Wu, and M. G. Mackey, "Relationship between field walking tests and incremental cycle ergometry in COPD," *Respirology*, vol. 13, no. 6, pp. 856–862, 2008.

[27] A. E. Holland, C. J. Hill, T. Rasekaba, A. Lee, M. T. Naughton, and C. F. McDonald, "Updating the minimal important difference for six-minute walk distance in patients with chronic obstructive pulmonary disease," *Archives of Physical Medicine and Rehabilitation*, vol. 91, no. 2, pp. 221–225, 2010.

[28] H. J. Schünemann, M. Puhan, R. Goldstein, R. Jaeschke, and G. H. Guyatt, "Measurement properties and interpretability of the Chronic Respiratory disease Questionnaire (CRQ)," *Journal of Chronic Obstructive Pulmonary Disease*, vol. 2, no. 1, pp. 81–89, 2005.

[29] R. A. Evans, S. J. Singh, R. Collier, J. E. Williams, and M. D. L. Morgan, "Pulmonary rehabilitation is successful for COPD irrespective of MRC dyspnoea grade," *Respiratory Medicine*, vol. 103, no. 7, pp. 1070–1075, 2009.

[30] "Global strategy for the diagnosis, management, and prevention of chronic obstructive pulmonary disease," 2011, http://www.goldcopd.org/.

[31] M. A. Spruit, R. Gosselink, T. Troosters et al., "Muscle force during an acute exacerbation in hospitalised patients with COPD and its relationship with CXCL8 and IGF-I," *Thorax*, vol. 58, no. 9, pp. 752–756, 2003.

[32] A. Augusti, L. D. Edwards, S. I. Rennard et al., "Persistent systemic inflammation is associated with poor clinical outcomes in COPD: a novel phenotype," *PLos ONE*, vol. 7, no. 5, Article ID e37483, 2012.

[33] M. Thomsen, M. Dahl, P. Lange, J. Vestbo, and B. G. Nordestgaard, "Inflammatory biomarkers and comorbidities in chronic obstructive pulmonary disease," *American Journal of Respiratory and Critical Care Medicine*, vol. 186, no. 10, pp. 982–988, 2012.

[34] J. R. Walsh, Z. J. McKeough, N. R. Morris et al., "Metabolic disease and participant age are independent predictors of response to pulmonary rehabilitation," *Journal of Cardiopulmonary Rehabilitation and Prevention*, vol. 33, no. 4, pp. 249–256.

15

Effects of Symptom Perception Interventions on Trigger Identification and Quality of Life in Children with Asthma

Thomas Janssens[1] and Andrew Harver[2]

[1] University of Leuven, Tiensestraat 102, Box 3726, 3000 Leuven, Belgium
[2] The University of North Carolina at Charlotte, Charlotte, NC 28223, USA

Correspondence should be addressed to Thomas Janssens; thomas.janssens@ppw.kuleuven.be

Academic Editor: Akio Niimi

Background. Management of individual triggers is suboptimal in practice. In this project, we investigated the impact of symptom perception interventions on asthma trigger identification and self-reported asthma quality of life. *Methods.* Children with asthma (n = 227) participated in three asthma education sessions and then were randomized first to one of three home monitoring conditions (symptom monitoring and peak flow training with feedback, peak flow training without feedback, or no peak flow training) and then subsequently to one of three resistive load discrimination training conditions (signal detection training with feedback, signal detection training without feedback, or no training). Triggers were reported at enrollment, following home monitoring, and following discrimination training; quality of life was measured after home monitoring and after resistive load testing. *Results.* Symptom perception interventions resulted in increases in reported triggers, which increased reliably as a function of home monitoring, and increased further in participants who completed discrimination training with feedback. Increases in the number of reported asthma triggers were associated with decreases in quality of life. *Discussion.* Patients may benefit from strategies that make trigger-symptom contingencies clear. Complementary strategies are needed to address changes in the perceived burden of asthma which comes from awareness of new asthma triggers.

1. Introduction

Indoor and outdoor allergens, intense emotion, irritants, physical exercise, and respiratory infections trigger asthma symptoms [1, 2], and both national and international asthma management guidelines emphasize the relevance of trigger knowledge and avoidance to achieve asthma control [3–6]. Although asthma triggers are often discussed with health care providers, trigger management remains suboptimal in clinical practice and individuals with asthma often report not knowing their triggers [5, 7–10].

The identification of idiosyncratic triggers by patients may be complex because relevant triggers are not always easy to determine and some triggers may be identified more readily than others [11]. Theoretically, accurate identification of asthma triggers results from three interacting processes: (a) identification of potential asthma triggers, (b) perception of asthma symptoms, and (c) recognition of a contingency between triggers and symptoms [11]. Trigger knowledge and avoidance may be hampered by inconsistencies in one or more of these processes and explain, in part, why patients with more severe or poorly controlled asthma report greater numbers of relevant asthma triggers [2, 12, 13].

Interventions to improve perception of symptoms may translate into improved perception of trigger-symptom contingencies. We evaluated the impact of two types of feedback-based interventions (peak flow monitoring and discrimination training) on both the frequency and the type of self-reported asthma triggers. Providing feedback for patient estimates of peak expiratory flow rate (PEFR) has been shown to increase perceptual accuracy of airflow obstruction and to improve adherence to inhaled corticosteroids [14, 15]; and feedback training for discrimination between the presence or absence of increases in the resistance to breathing has been shown to yield improved perception of airflow obstruction [16–18]. We examined not only the effects of these interventions on self-reported triggers but also the effects of changes in the number of perceived triggers on asthma quality of life [19, 20]. We hypothesized that changes in quality of life follow changes in the identification of relevant asthma triggers.

2. Materials and Methods

2.1. Research Setting and Participants. The data reported in this paper were collected within the context of Project On TRAC (Taking Responsibility for Asthma Control), a pediatric asthma research program. Program participants were between 8 and 15 years of age, were diagnosed with asthma at least two years prior to their entry into the study, were prescribed daily controller medications, and reported at least occasional asthma symptoms and/or nighttime cough.

At an initial enrollment session, children and their families were advised about all aspects of the research protocol, each child's legal guardian provided written informed consent, and the child provided written informed assent. Institutional review boards at both UNC Charlotte (#09-09-03) and Ohio University (#03F024) approved the research protocol. In addition to an enrollment session at which both children and caregivers completed baseline measures, the program consisted of three sessions of asthma education, two cycles of home monitoring of asthma symptoms for 30 days, four resistive load detection sessions, and six-month follow-up. This report provides detailed analysis of trigger identification and associated quality of life in children ($n = 227$) who completed data collection activities at enrollment, at the end of the first cycle of home monitoring, and at the end of resistive load testing.

Children were randomized to one of three home monitoring conditions at the end of the second asthma education session: PEFR training with feedback, PEFR training without feedback, and no PEFR. All conditions involved daily use of a common asthma symptom diary that included questions on symptoms, activity limitations, nighttime awakenings, and self-efficacy, as well as an open-ended question on perceived causes of symptoms. Additionally, children assigned to both PEFR training conditions recorded both estimated and actual PEFR values with the AM2+ Asthma Monitor (Jaeger, Hoechberg, Germany); the meters were programmed to display actual PEFR values to feedback group children but not to children in the no-feedback group. Effects of home monitoring on the correspondence between estimated and actual peak flow measures, and between peak flow measures and asthma symptoms, have been presented in preliminary form [16] and are the focus of a separate manuscript.

At the end of home monitoring, children completed one of three resistive load detection conditions: signal detection training with feedback, signal detection training without feedback, and no resistive load training. Children were assigned at random to one condition following completion of the first resistive load detection session, which established the threshold resistance to breathing in all participants [17]. Children assigned to the signal detection conditions determined whether or not an increased resistance to breathing was evident on selected breaths; children assigned to the feedback

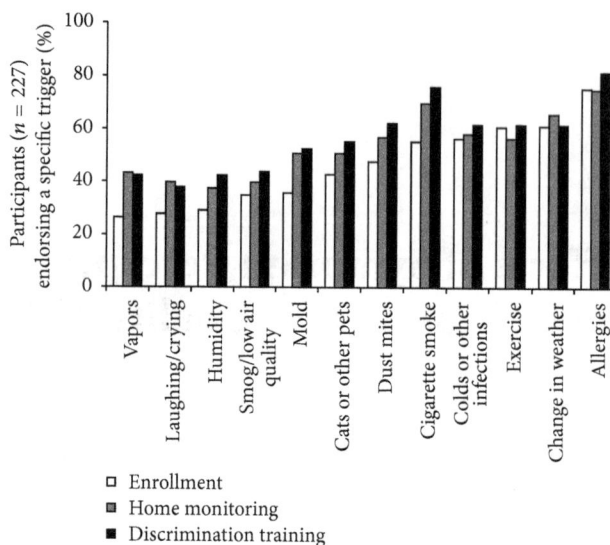

FIGURE 1: Trigger identification at enrollment, after home monitoring, and after discrimination training.

condition were given feedback regarding the accuracy of their responses whereas children assigned to the no feedback condition were kept uninformed about their performance. The effects of discrimination training on the perception of resistive loads were published previously [18].

2.2. Study Procedures. We collected participant demographic characteristics at enrollment and lung function was measured at the first asthma education session using the VMAX ENCORE 20C testing system (VIASYS Healthcare; Yorba Linda, California). Our primary outcome variables were asthma trigger identification and quality of life. At enrollment and following completion of both home monitoring and resistive load testing children were asked, "What usually triggers, or worsens, your asthma?" and they were instructed to select from a list of 12 possible triggers the ones that pertained to them and to add other items if necessary (Figure 1). Quality of life was measured with the Mini Asthma Quality of Life Questionnaire (Mini-AQLQ) [20] in children during the interview session (after home monitoring) and after resistive load testing.

At each interaction, children reported the degree to which they depended on symptoms for detecting worsening asthma (from not at all ("1") to always ("10")) and the extent to which they were able to predict an upcoming asthma attack ("yes" or "no"). We measured children's perceived asthma difficulty ranging from mild ("1") to severe ("5"), from very well managed ("1") to not managed at all ("5"), and from hardly noticeable ("1") to very troublesome ("5"). We also conducted semistructured interviews with families at the end of home monitoring, which consisted of four open-ended questions about experiences and observations made by the child and family member during the home monitoring period.

2.3. Data Analysis. Data points were entered into our statistical program (SPSS version 22; IBM Inc.; Armonk, NY)

TABLE 1: Associations between covariates and individual triggers.

Covariate	Trigger	OR	Lower 95% CI	Upper 95% CI	t	p
Age	Exercise	1.21	1.02	1.42	2.21	0.028
	Humidity	1.23	1.05	1.44	2.52	0.012
	Colds	0.83	0.72	0.96	−2.57	0.011
Asthma duration	Weather	1.14	1.03	1.25	2.58	0.011
Race (White versus Black)	Exercise	2.05	1.01	4.04	2.44	0.047
Sex (female versus male)	Cigarette smoke	2.06	1.15	3.70	2.45	0.015
SES	Allergies	1.01	1.00	1.02	2.13	0.034
	Colds	0.99	0.98	1.00	−2.03	0.044
	Mold	0.99	0.98	1.00	−2.22	0.028
	Weather	0.99	0.98	1.00	−2.66	0.008
Perceived severity	Laughing/crying	1.25	1.03	1.54	2.21	0.028
	Humidity	1.33	1.10	1.62	2.94	0.004
	Dust Mites	1.29	1.07	1.57	2.63	0.009
	Cigarette smoke	1.44	1.17	1.78	3.42	0.001
	Colds	1.02	1.01	1.42	2.07	0.04
	Mold	1.28	1.05	1.57	2.47	0.014
	Smog	1.50	1.25	1.81	4.31	<0.001
	Vapors	1.42	1.16	1.74	3.37	0.001
	Weather	1.35	1.10	1.65	2.95	0.004

OR = odds ratio (odds of reporting a trigger/odds of not reporting a trigger), adjusted for covariates; CI = confidence interval; t = t-statistic; p = probability; SES = socioeconomic status.

and reviewed for accuracy. Data are presented as mean ± standard deviation unless otherwise noted. Differences in baseline data between groups were investigated using independent sample t-tests (t) or Chi-Square tests (χ^2); and we used analyses of variance (F) to test differences among groups. The total number of identified triggers and changes in specific triggers were analyzed using generalized hierarchical linear models using a 3 (peak flow monitoring condition: PEFR with feedback, PEFR without feedback, diary only) × 3 (resistive load testing condition: training with feedback, training without feedback, no training) × 3 (time: enrollment, after monitoring, after resistive load testing) design, and an unstructured covariance matrix. Items children added to our list of possible triggers (e.g., "grass," "hay," and "going to places") were excluded from our analyses due to the low number of participants who responded ($n = 9$). Bonferroni corrections were used to control for multiple comparisons. SPSS employs Satterthwaite approximation for degrees of freedom, which we report rounded to the nearest integer.

Because the relationship between symptom perception and triggers is influenced by age, asthma duration, race, asthma control, and socioeconomic status (SES) [21, 22], we controlled for these variables in our analyses. Lung function (forced expiratory volume in one second percent predicted) and perceived asthma severity were used as indices of asthma control; levels of perceived asthma severity were related reliably to the number of reported asthma flare-ups the previous 12 months ($r(216) = 0.19$, $p = 0.005$) and to the number of school days missed the past year ($r(223) = 0.34$, $p < 0.001$). The Barratt Simplified Measure of Social Status was used to estimate SES, which is based on a weighted combination of education and occupation [23]. Caregivers reported the highest level of school completed by each parent and indicated their occupation from among clusters of related occupations that ranged from unemployed to physician, professor, or senior manager.

3. Results

3.1. Baseline Characteristics. A total of 227 participants completed both home monitoring and the resistive load training sessions. The sample included 155 boys and 72 girls, 98 were non-Hispanic Black and 112 were non-Hispanic White. Their age, on average, was 10 ± 1.6 years and children had been diagnosed with asthma for 6.6 ± 2.8 years. Average percent predicted lung function values for forced expiratory volume in one second (FEV_1), forced vital capacity (FVC), and the FEV_1/FVC ratio recorded at the first asthma education visit were 87.3 ± 19.1, 92.2 ± 17.4, and 82.5 ± 9.4, respectively.

At enrollment, participants selected, on average, 5.5 ± 2.7 triggers. The odds of identifying a trigger as relevant increased with more severe asthma for most triggers (9 of 12). Allergies were endorsed most often (75% of participants) and irritant vapors were endorsed least often (23% of participants; see Figure 1). Older participants were more likely to endorse exercise and humidity and less likely to endorse colds as relevant asthma triggers; those with higher SES were more likely to endorse allergens as asthma triggers, but less likely to endorse colds, mold, and weather changes as relevant (Table 1). Neither baseline characteristics nor the frequency of selected triggers at enrollment varied as a function of either home monitoring or discrimination training group assignment (data not shown).

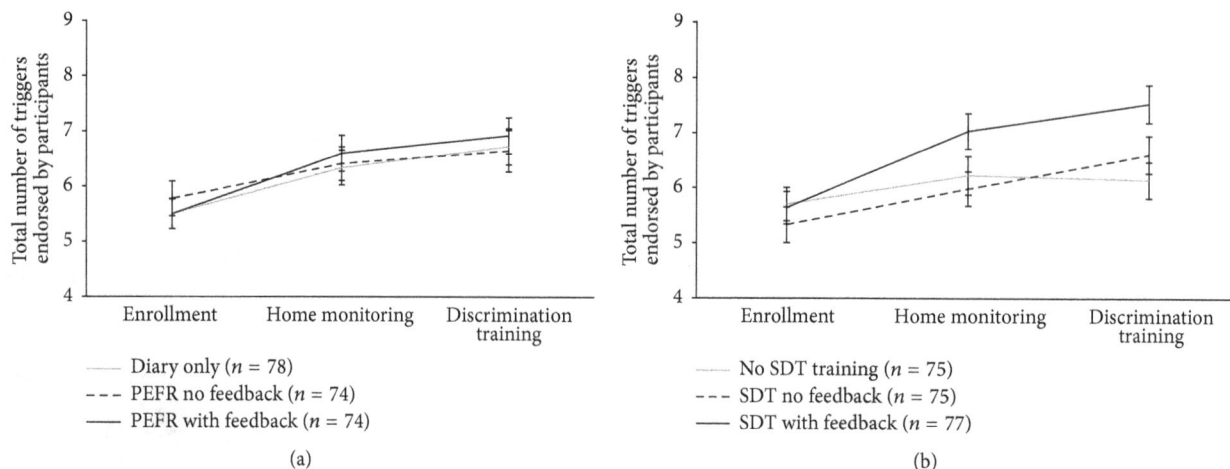

FIGURE 2: Total number of reported asthma triggers (mean ± SEM) for each home monitoring condition (a) and for each resistive load signal detection training (SDT) condition (b) at enrollment, after home monitoring, and after discrimination training.

3.2. Change in Trigger Identification. The total number of triggers endorsed by children significantly increased over time ($F(2, 223) = 20.91$, $p < 0.001$) both from enrollment to home monitoring ($t(223) = 4.72$, $p < 0.001$) and from home monitoring to discrimination training ($t(222) = 2.90$, $p = 0.012$) (Figure 2). The results of the covariate analyses demonstrated that greater numbers of new triggers were associated with lower SES ($F(1, 223) = 4.91$, $p = 0.028$), longer duration of asthma ($F(1, 223) = 6.68$, $p = 0.01$), and greater perceived asthma severity ($F(1, 223) = 20.77$, $p < 0.001$), but not with participant age, sex, race, or lung function.

Increases in the number of triggers were not differentially affected by home monitoring condition (time × monitoring, $F(4, 223) = 0.43$, $p = 0.788$). Interviews conducted at the end of the home monitoring period, however, consistently affirmed that families reported greater understanding of individual triggers. We provide the following examples of asthma trigger-related comments obtained during interviews held with families at the end of home monitoring in response to the question, "Did you learn anything from keeping the diary?"

Parent comments were as follows:

(i) We didn't know what triggered the girls' asthma so it helped us know that. That what we thought was congestion from a cold...was really from a trigger. We are on the right meds now.

(ii) Learned the triggers, looking back through the day what triggers his physical symptoms.

(iii) Helped me pin point his triggers which felt worse. Helped me to be more aware of his triggers.

(iv) She's a bit more sensitive (to triggers) than I thought she was.

(v) I think she is more aware of her triggers since the program.

(vi) Yes, we learned what his triggers were.

Child comments were as follows:

(i) How to control it more, I noticed triggers.

(ii) Playing outside in the cold, being dehydrated (triggers that he didn't know before).

(iii) Triggers: cold air, cats.

(iv) To stay away from your triggers. When outside breathe through nose instead of mouth.

(v) It made me think about the triggers.

Resistive load training, on the other hand, resulted in differential increases in reported triggers ($F(4, 223) = 3.33$, $p = 0.011$); participants who completed signal detection training with feedback subsequently reported more triggers compared to those who did not receive feedback training ($t(226) = 2.91$, $p = 0.012$).

Symptom interventions involving feedback differentially affected the perceived relevance of specific triggers (Figure 1). Participants assigned to peak flow monitoring with feedback were more likely to endorse mold as a trigger compared to other home monitoring conditions (Figure 3(a)); participants assigned to the signal detection training with feedback condition evidenced reliable increases in the identification of pets as relevant (Figure 3(b)).

3.3. Trigger Identification and Quality of Life. Regardless of feedback training experience, participants demonstrated overall improvement in quality of life, as well as improved self-reported asthma difficulty and ability to predict an asthma episode (Table 2). However, both the number of asthma triggers at enrollment and changes in asthma trigger identification had an impact on quality of life. At enrollment, participants who reported greater numbers of triggers not only evidenced a greater dependence on symptoms to manage asthma ($t(255) = 2.26$, $p = 0.025$) but also reported more severe, less well-managed, and more troublesome asthma as well as reduced asthma-related quality of life (Table 2).

TABLE 2: Self-reported asthma outcomes and associations with asthma trigger identification.

Variable	Enrollment		Home monitoring		Discrimination training				Association with trigger identification at enrollment			Change		
	Mean	SD	Mean	SD	Mean	SD	F	p	Estimate	SE	p	Estimate	SE	p
Self-reported asthma difficulty														
Severe	2.59	1.21	2.33	1.20	2.28	1.24	9.69	<0.001	0.11	0.02	<0.001	0.07	0.02	<0.001
Managed	2.71	1.07	2.37	1.11	2.20	1.04	22.99	<0.001	0.04	0.02	0.037	0.05	0.02	0.006
Troublesome	2.85	1.16	2.67	1.06	2.50	1.03	12.20	<0.001	0.10	0.02	<0.001	0.05	0.02	0.002
Depend on symptoms	6.41	2.70	5.26	2.88	5.69	3.02	13.87	<0.001	0.09	0.05	0.077	0.12	0.05	0.022
Able to predict an attack (n, %)	109	48%	111	50%	131	58%	4.62	0.01	0.082	0.05	0.079	−0.01	0.04	0.795
Asthma-related quality of life														
Symptoms			4.90	1.51	5.03	1.44	4.25	0.04	−0.14	0.03	<0.001	−0.16	0.03	<0.001
Activities			5.81	1.37	6.04	1.27	7.57	0.006	−0.15	0.03	<0.001	−0.14	0.02	<0.001
Emotions			5.29	1.53	5.57	1.49	11.58	0.001	−0.12	0.03	0.001	−0.08	0.03	0.004
Environment			4.78	1.74	5.02	1.65	8.72	0.003	−0.22	0.04	<0.001	−0.19	0.03	<0.001
Overall			5.19	1.30	5.40	1.21	12.93	<0.001	−0.15	0.03	<0.001	−0.14	0.02	<0.001

Asthma difficulty was rated from mild ("1") to severe ("5"), from very well managed ("1") to not managed at all ("5"), and from hardly noticeable ("1") to very troublesome ("5"). SD = standard deviation; F = F-test; p = probability; SE = standard error.

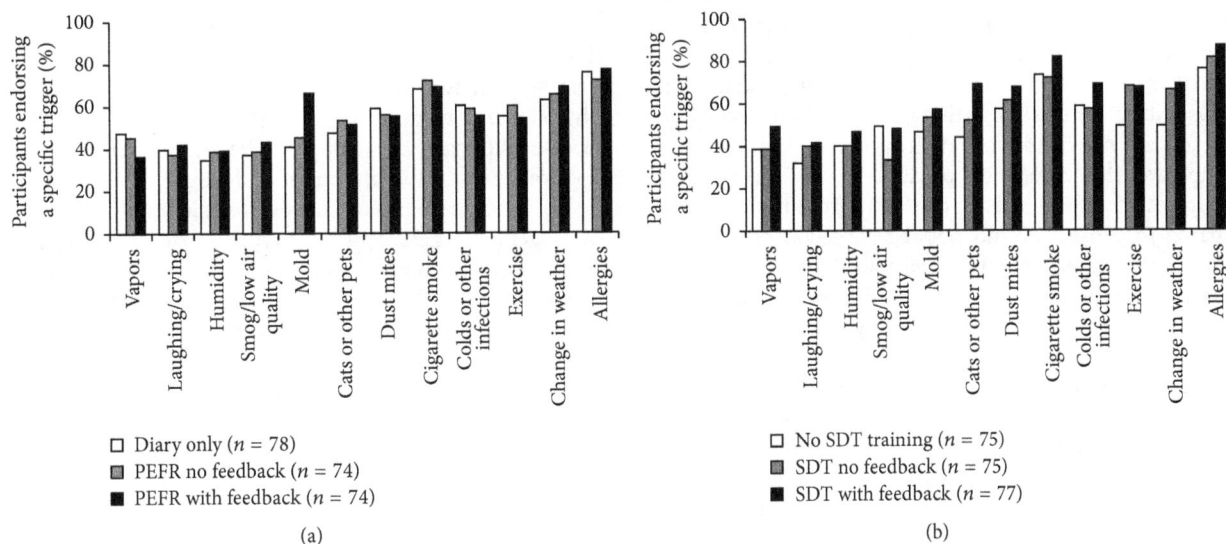

FIGURE 3: Triggers endorsed following home monitoring (a) and following resistive load signal detection training (SDT) (b).

Increases in the number of reported triggers across time were also associated with reduced asthma-related quality of life for overall mini-AQLQ scores life ($t(415) = -6.55$, $p < 0.001$) as well as for scores for each subscale (Table 2). We evaluated mini-AQLQ scores obtained after home monitoring between children who reported the same or fewer numbers of triggers compared to enrollment ($n = 103$) and those who reported one or more new triggers ($n = 124$). Reliably poorer quality of life scores were observed in

children who reported more triggers for overall mini-AQLQ scores ($t(225) = 3.05$, $p = 0.003$) as well as for the subscales symptoms ($t(225) = 3.16$, $p = 0.002$), environment ($t(225) = 3.47$, $p < 0.001$), and emotions ($t(225) = 1.99$, $p < 0.05$). Similar findings were obtained for analyses conducted between children who reported the same or fewer numbers of triggers after discrimination training compared to those after home monitoring ($n = 130$) and those who reported one or more new triggers ($n = 96$). Reliably poorer quality of life was observed in children who reported more triggers for overall mini-AQLQ scores ($t(224) = 2.14$, $p < 0.05$) as well as for the symptom subscale ($t(224) = 2.66$, $p = 0.008$).

4. Discussion

The aim of this study was to evaluate the differential impact of two symptom perception interventions on asthma trigger identification and associated asthma quality of life in children with persistent asthma. Both the number and the types of triggers reported by participants at enrollment were similar to those observed by other groups [9, 12, 24, 25] and affirmed the variability in trigger prevalence reported in previous investigations [2, 10, 12, 24]. We observed that interventions involving accurate detection of airflow obstruction were effective at increasing trigger identification. Not all triggers were endorsed equally in this regard; those that were commonly reported at enrollment (e.g., allergies, weather, colds, and smog) were less influenced by our interventions. Feedback training experiences differentially affected the perceived relevance of specific triggers including mold and pets, triggers less likely discussed in encounters with health care professionals [8].

Increases in the number of triggers endorsed as relevant were not differentially affected by home monitoring condition. We attribute this uniform effect to daily use of an asthma symptom diary by all participants. Self-management is organized around the monitoring of disease-related variables, and diaries play a key role in establishing relationships between the environment and behavior in individual patients [26]. Despite widespread use of asthma diaries, daily recordings of triggers are not commonly evident in previous work [12]. Participants who completed resistive load discrimination training with feedback subsequently reported more triggers compared to those who did not receive feedback training. Taken together, interventions aimed at facilitating perception of airflow obstruction may serve to reinforce associations among disease-related variables, including symptom-trigger contingencies, and may be beneficial in discerning problematic sources of symptoms [11, 26].

Participants who reported greater numbers of triggers also reported lower levels of asthma-related quality of life. Although these findings may appear counterintuitive, they might be expected based on earlier work. First, new triggers may result in increases in the perceived burden of asthma in accordance with other studies that showed associations between the number of perceived asthma triggers and poorer asthma outcomes [12, 27]. Our finding that increases in trigger identification were associated with an increased reliance on symptoms to guide asthma management corroborates this line of thinking. Second, patients may have concluded that changes in asthma self-management behaviors to avoid or reduce trigger exposures were ineffective [10, 15, 28]. Trigger knowledge does not automatically lead to adequate trigger avoidance or removal, as studies have shown that exposure to known allergens and other environmental triggers can remain high [5, 25]. Third, avoiding or managing new triggers may result in behavioral adjustments (e.g., staying indoors) that negatively impact health-related quality of life, effects

that have not been well documented [1, 5, 7, 11, 12, 24]. Trigger education research is needed to address effective self-management strategies that reduce the perceived burden of asthma when new asthma triggers are discovered.

Our observations are in contrast to the positive effects of extensive environmental interventions on health outcomes in children with asthma, implemented in mostly urban settings and focused primarily on minority populations [29–32]. Our sample, for example, was neither inner city nor disadvantaged; and similar proportions of black and white children were prescribed either inhaled corticosteroids with or without a long-acting beta-agonist (73% and 79%, resp.) and/or leukotriene modifiers (57% and 60%, resp.). On the other hand, covariate analyses showed that lower SES, longer asthma duration, and increased perceived asthma severity at enrollment were associated with greater increases in reported asthma triggers over time. These findings are consistent with a large body of work highlighting differences in both trigger knowledge and exposure between low-SES and high-SES individuals [33, 34]. Subsequent research may clarify the importance of trigger awareness interventions tailored to the needs of particular groups of patients.

Limitations are evident in our approach. We were unable to confirm directly the effects of existing or newly identified asthma triggers on asthma control or to differentiate between increases in the identification of previously unknown triggers from improvements in trigger identification accuracy. On the other hand, self-monitoring involving use of a daily diary appears as an especially feasible approach for confirming symptom-inducing properties of allergic as well as physical and environmental asthma triggers. Second, we assessed changes in quality of life immediately following the conclusion of symptom monitoring interventions; our design precluded assessment of possible long-term benefits of trigger awareness. Third, the types of triggers we measured were similar to those in inventories employed in previous investigations, although our inventory was relatively lacking in psychological triggers [35]. Recent efforts have been made to collect trigger data in standardized ways [11, 12], which may benefit future research on trigger identification [1] as well as routine documentation of asthma triggers in clinical practice [36]. Finally, all participants received education and completed symptom diaries, which precludes us from evaluating the independent contributions of these two activities on asthma trigger identification.

Although many asthma triggers are modifiable risk factors, trigger avoidance advice is not universal in practice and efforts to control trigger exposures are not uniformly effective [6, 8–10, 12, 24, 36]. We have demonstrated that participants randomized to symptom perception interventions that included feedback training for accurate detection of airflow obstruction report increases in the relevance of specific triggers. Such interventions may reinforce associations between disease-related variables, including symptom-trigger contingencies, and contribute to increased trigger awareness. However, the association of increased trigger reports with poorer quality of life suggests that additional actions may be required of patients to confront the burden of newly identified asthma triggers.

5. Conclusions

Effective asthma management includes not only assessment and monitoring of asthma control, education that enables patient-provider asthma partnerships, and adequate pharmacotherapy but also tailored trigger knowledge and avoidance [4]. Interventions involving accurate detection of airflow obstruction are effective at increasing trigger identification and may serve to reinforce associations between disease-related variables including symptom-trigger contingencies. Increases in the perceived burden of asthma which comes from awareness of new asthma triggers, however, may complicate management goals set by health care providers.

Disclaimer

The content is solely the responsibility of the authors and does not necessarily represent the official views of the National Heart, Lung, and Blood Institute or the National Institutes of Health.

Conflict of Interests

The authors report no conflict of interests.

Financial Support

NIH/NHLBI R01HL068706 (PI: Dr. Harver); KU Leuven, Leuven (University of Leuven); FWO (Research foundation-Flanders); European Respiratory Society (STRTF 2014-5337).

Acknowledgments

The authors thank Professor Omer Van den Bergh and the Research Group on Health Psychology, KU Leuven, Leuven, Belgium, for the support provided to Dr. Harver during the preparation of the paper. The authors also thank Dr. Van den Bergh as well as Dr. Ahmed Arif and Dr. Thomas Ritz for review of an earlier version of the paper. This project was supported by Grant no. R01HL068706 from the National Institutes of Health/National Heart, Lung, and Blood Institute (PI: Dr. Harver). Dr. Janssens is a Postdoctoral Fellow of the FWO (Research foundation, Flanders) and the recipient of a European Respiratory Society Fellowship (STRTF 2014-5337). The research was carried out primarily at The University of North Carolina at Charlotte and presented in part at the Annual Meeting of the American Thoracic Society in San Diego, CA, May 20, 2014.

References

[1] M. K. Vernon, I. Wiklund, J. A. Bell, P. Dale, and K. R. Chapman, "What do we know about asthma triggers? A review of the literature," *Journal of Asthma*, vol. 49, no. 10, pp. 991–998, 2012.

[2] T. Ritz, A. Steptoe, C. Bobb, A. H. S. Harris, and M. Edwards, "The asthma trigger inventory: validation of a questionnaire for perceived triggers of asthma," *Psychosomatic Medicine*, vol. 68, no. 6, pp. 956–965, 2006.

[3] Global Initiative for Asthma (GINA), *Global Strategy for Asthma Management and Prevention*, 2014.

[4] National Asthma Education and Prevention Program, *Expert Panel Report 3: Guidelines for the Diagnosis and Management of Asthma*, National Heart, Lung, and Blood Institute, Bethesda, Md, USA, 2007.

[5] J. A. Finkelstein, A. Fuhlbrigge, P. Lozano et al., "Parent-reported environmental exposures and environmental control measures for children with asthma," *Archives of Pediatrics and Adolescent Medicine*, vol. 156, no. 3, pp. 258–264, 2002.

[6] M. Schatz, "Predictors of asthma control: what can we modify?" *Current Opinion in Allergy and Clinical Immunology*, vol. 12, no. 3, pp. 263–268, 2012.

[7] A.-L. Caress, K. Luker, A. Woodcock, and K. Beaver, "An exploratory study of priority information needs in adult asthma patients," *Patient Education and Counseling*, vol. 47, no. 4, pp. 319–327, 2002.

[8] D. Washington, K. Yeatts, B. Sleath et al., "Communication and education about triggers and environmental control strategies during pediatric asthma visits," *Patient Education and Counseling*, vol. 86, no. 1, pp. 63–69, 2012.

[9] M. A. Rank, P. Wollan, J. T. Li, and B. P. Yawn, "Trigger recognition and management in poorly controlled asthmatics," *Allergy and Asthma Proceedings*, vol. 31, no. 6, pp. e99–e105, 2010.

[10] Ö. Göksel, G. E. Çelik, F. Öner Erkekol, E. Güllü, D. Mungan, and Z. Mısırlıgil, "Triggers in adult asthma: are patients aware of triggers and doing right?" *Allergologia et Immunopathologia*, vol. 37, no. 3, pp. 122–128, 2009.

[11] T. Janssens and T. Ritz, "Perceived triggers of asthma: key to symptom perception and management," *Clinical & Experimental Allergy*, vol. 43, no. 9, pp. 1000–1008, 2013.

[12] D. Price, P. Dale, E. Elder, and K. R. Chapman, "Types, frequency and impact of asthma triggers on patients' lives: a quantitative study in five European countries," *Journal of Asthma*, vol. 51, no. 2, pp. 127–135, 2014.

[13] M. G. E. Peterson, T. J. Gaeta, R. H. Birkhahn, J. L. Fernández, and C. A. Mancuso, "History of symptom triggers in patients presenting to the emergency department for asthma," *Journal of Asthma*, vol. 49, no. 6, pp. 629–636, 2012.

[14] B. A. Silverman, D. Mayer, R. Sabinsky et al., "Training perception of air flow obstruction in asthmatics," *Annals of Allergy*, vol. 59, no. 5, pp. 350–354, 1987.

[15] J. M. Feldman, H. Kutner, L. Matte et al., "Prediction of peak flow values followed by feedback improves perception of lung function and adherence to inhaled corticosteroids in children with asthma," *Thorax*, vol. 67, no. 12, pp. 1040–1045, 2012.

[16] H. Kotses, X. Hyseni, A. Harver, S. Walford, and S. J. Hardy, "Effects of feedback on the correspondence between estimated and actual PEFR in children with persistent asthma. Paper presented at the 2008 annual meeting of the International Society for the Advancement of Respiratory Psychophysiology, Ann Arbor, MI," *Biological Psychology*, vol. 83, p. 70, 2010.

[17] A. Harver and D. A. Mahler, "Perception of increased resistance to breathing," in *Self-Management of Asthma, Lung Biology in Health and Disease*, H. Kotses and A. Harver, Eds., pp. 147–193, Marcel Dekker, New York, NY, USA, 1998.

[18] A. Harver, H. Kotses, J. Ersek, C. T. Humphries, W. S. Ashe Jr., and H. R. Black II, "Effects of feedback on the perception of inspiratory resistance in children with persistent asthma: a signal detection approach," *Psychosomatic Medicine*, vol. 75, no. 8, pp. 729–736, 2013.

[19] W. W. Busse, W. J. Morgan, V. Taggart, and A. Togias, "Asthma outcomes workshop: overview," *The Journal of Allergy and Clinical Immunology*, vol. 129, no. 3, pp. S1–S8, 2012.

[20] E. F. Juniper, G. H. Guyatt, F. M. Cox, P. J. Ferrie, and D. R. King, "Development and validation of the mini asthma quality of life questionnaire," *European Respiratory Journal*, vol. 14, no. 1, pp. 32–38, 1999.

[21] H. L. Yoos, H. Kitzman, A. McMullen, and K. Sidora, "Symptom perception in childhood asthma: how accurate are children and their parents?" *Journal of Asthma*, vol. 40, no. 1, pp. 27–39, 2003.

[22] B. L. Wood, P. A. Cheah, J. Lim et al., "Reliability and validity of the asthma trigger inventory applied to a pediatric population," *Journal of Pediatric Psychology*, vol. 32, no. 5, pp. 552–560, 2007.

[23] W. Barratt, *The Barratt Simplified Measure of Social Status (BSMSS): Measuring SES*, vol. 2014, Indiana State University, Terre Haute, Ind, USA, 2006.

[24] M. D. Cabana, K. K. Slish, T. C. Lewis et al., "Parental management of asthma triggers within a child's environment," *Journal of Allergy and Clinical Immunology*, vol. 114, no. 2, pp. 352–357, 2004.

[25] S. T. Weiss, A. Horner, G. Shapiro, and A. L. Sternberg, "The prevalence of environmental exposure to perceived asthma triggers in children with mild-to-moderate asthma: data from the Childhood Asthma Management Program (CAMP)," *Journal of Allergy and Clinical Immunology*, vol. 107, no. 4, pp. 634–640, 2001.

[26] H. Kotses, P. Lewis, and T. L. Creer, "Environmental control of asthma self-management," *Journal of Asthma*, vol. 27, no. 6, pp. 375–384, 1990.

[27] T. Ritz, C. Bobb, and C. Griffiths, "Predicting asthma control: the role of psychological triggers," *Allergy and Asthma Proceedings*, vol. 35, no. 5, pp. 390–397, 2014.

[28] T. Janssens, G. Verleden, S. De Peuter, I. Van Diest, and O. Van den Bergh, "Inaccurate perception of asthma symptoms: a cognitive-affective framework and implications for asthma treatment," *Clinical Psychology Review*, vol. 29, no. 4, pp. 317–327, 2009.

[29] T. Bryant-Stephens, C. Kurian, R. Guo, and H. Zhao, "Impact of a household environmental intervention delivered by lay health workers on asthma symptom control in urban, disadvantaged children with asthma," *American Journal of Public Health*, vol. 99, supplement 3, pp. S657–S665, 2009.

[30] D. D. Crocker, S. Kinyota, G. G. Dumitru et al., "Effectiveness of home-based, multi-trigger, multicomponent interventions with an environmental focus for reducing asthma morbidity: a community guide systematic review," *American Journal of Preventive Medicine*, vol. 41, no. 2, pp. S5–S32, 2011.

[31] W. J. Morgan, E. F. Crain, R. S. Gruchalla et al., "Results of a home-based environmental intervention among urban children with asthma," *The New England Journal of Medicine*, vol. 351, no. 11, pp. 1068–1080, 2004.

[32] J. Postma, C. Karr, and G. Kieckhefer, "Community health workers and environmental interventions for children with asthma: a systematic review," *Journal of Asthma*, vol. 46, no. 6, pp. 564–576, 2009.

[33] P. M. Salo, S. J. Arbes Jr., P. W. Crockett, P. S. Thorne, R. D. Cohn, and D. C. Zeldin, "Exposure to multiple indoor allergens in US homes and its relationship to asthma," *Journal of Allergy and Clinical Immunology*, vol. 121, no. 3, pp. 678–684.e2, 2008.

[34] B. P. Leaderer, K. Belanger, E. Triche et al., "Dust mite, cockroach, cat, and dog allergen concentrations in homes of asthmatic children in the Northeastern United States: impact of socioeconomic factors and population density," *Environmental Health Perspectives*, vol. 110, no. 4, pp. 419–425, 2002.

[35] T. Ritz, A. Kullowatz, F. Kanniess, B. Dahme, and H. Magnussen, "Perceived triggers of asthma: evaluation of a German version of the Asthma Trigger Inventory," *Respiratory Medicine*, vol. 102, no. 3, pp. 390–398, 2008.

[36] B. P. Yawn, S. Bertram, and P. Wollan, "Introduction of asthma APGAR tools improve asthma management in primary care practices," *Journal of Asthma and Allergy*, vol. 1, pp. 1–10, 2008.

16

Factors Influencing Early Health Facility Contact and Low Default Rate among New Sputum Smear Positive Tuberculosis Patients, India

Ashok Kumar Bhardwaj,[1] **Surender Kashyap,**[2] **Pradeep Bansal,**[1] **Dinesh Kumar,**[1] **Sunil Kumar Raina,**[1] **Vishav Chander,**[1] **and Sushant Sharma**[1]

[1] *Department of Community Medicine, Dr. Rajendra Prasad Government Medical College,*
 Kangra, Himachal Pradesh 176001, India
[2] *Kalpana Chawla Government Medical College, Karnal, Haryana, India*

Correspondence should be addressed to Dinesh Kumar; dinesh9809@gmail.com

Academic Editor: Hisako Matsumoto

Early case identification and prompt treatment of new sputum smear positive case are important to reduce the spread of tuberculosis (TB). Present study was planned to study the associated factors for duration to contact the health facility since appearance of symptoms and treatment default. *Methodology.* It was prospective cohort study of TB patients already registered for treatment in randomly selected TB units (TUs) in Himachal Pradesh, India. Relative risk (RR) was calculated as risk estimate to find out the explanatory variables for early contact and default. *Results.* Total 1607 patients were recruited and 25 (1.5%) defaulted treatment. Patients from nuclear family (aRR: 1.37; 1.09–1.73), ashamed of TB (aRR: 1.32; 1.03–1.70), wishing to disclose disease status (aRR: 1.79; 1.43–2.24), but aware of curable nature (aRR: 1.67; 1.17–2.39) and preventable (aRR: 1.35; 1.07–1.70) nature of disease, contacted health facility early since appearance of symptoms. *Conclusion.* Better awareness and less misconceptions about disease influences the early contact of health facility and low default rate in North India.

1. Introduction

One-third of the world population is infected with *Mycobacterium tuberculosis* causing disease in about 10 million individuals and resulting in 1.3 million deaths per year. Asia and Africa regions together share 85.0% of the global disease burden [1]. India notified total 1.3 million cases including 0.62 million sputum smear positive cases [2]. Evidence from India showed that tuberculosis (TB) contributes about 30% of deaths due to communicable disease and 7% of total deaths [2]. Based upon World Health Organization (WHO) recommendations, the Government of India implemented Directly Observed Treatment Short Course (DOTS) strategy under Revised National Tuberculosis Program (RNTCP) [2]. Since then, treatment success rate among sputum smear positive patients improved from 25% in the year 1985 to about 90% by the year 2011 [2] as compared to the global treatment

success rate of 84% [1]. Early case detection and treatment is a public health principle for disease control. Under RNTCP, an awareness campaign for signs and symptoms of TB demands an early contact of health facility for diagnosis. Contact of patient to health facility for treatment compliance depended on the program and patient related factors [3–5]. A lot has been done for disease awareness under program; the community behavior becomes supportive toward patient. However, evidence also showed that still stigma associated with signs and symptoms of TB, availability of diagnostic, and treatment services under RNTCP. Patients tend to hesitate and choose not to disclose their disease status to their family/friends out of fear of being socially marginalized [3–6]. The nature and degree of influence of such factors on health facility contact and so compliance for DOTS have not been reported as often. Therefore, the present study was planned to understand the role of factors in contacting a health facility since the appearance of symptoms and treatment default among patients on DOTS under RNTCP, Himachal Pradesh, India.

2. Methodology

It was a prospective cohort study of two years' (2008-09) duration conducted at randomly selected tuberculosis units (TUs) in the state of Himachal Pradesh, India. As per the census of 2011, the state has population of about 7 million spread over 55, 670 km² area residing in 12 districts. Sample size of 1537 was calculated with default rate of 4.0% (based upon the selected TUs for study) at 5% significance level and 80% of study power. Sample size was revised to 1691 with 10% nonresponse rate. Interview was done to collect the data by the trained project staff using pretested and structured questionnaire.

Patients were getting DOTS for the period of six months from the DOTS providers as per the RNTCP. All new smear positive (NSP) TB cases with more than 15 years of age already on DOTS from selected TUs of study area were recruited. Once recruited every patient was contacted three times: first, as soon as they started with DOTS, second, at the end of intensive phase of DOTS, and, third, one week before completion of DOTS (i.e., at the time of administration of last dose of DOTS). A patient was considered to be a defaulter if he/she interrupted the treatment for two consecutive months or more. All the defaulted patients were contacted to assess the reason for default and were motivated to continue the DOTS. Based on review, studies differentially had used the definition for "delay in health facility contact" and no such clear definition is being used under RNTCP. Therefore, a cutoff of 30 days for deciding the early facility contact was considered after calculation of central tendency (median) of duration (days) of health facility contact since the appearance of symptoms.

RNTCP is providing DOTS to the patients through total 41 TUs in the state. Total 20 TUs were selected based upon population proportion to size (PPS) using the cluster sampling technique. Retrospective information was collected from patients already on DOTS who were interviewed about their place of residence, type of family, socioeconomic class, appearance of symptoms, time of contact to a health facility, substance abuse, disease knowledge, and misconceptions. Information about the health system related factors like distance of health facility from the place of residence and waiting time at centre and exact treatment duration explained by the DOTS provider was also asked from the patient. Prospective information in next two subsequent visits was also collected for sputum conversion, drug side effects, and family and society response towards the patient. If defaulted patient did not respond to the DOTS then patient was contacted prospectively at the place of residence by the project staff to assess the reasons for default. Data was collected on structured questionnaire and was translated into local language and back to English before the data collection. Before recruiting the patient an informed consent was taken in the first visit explaining that there would be further collection of information in the next two consecutive visits.

A prior ethical clearance from institutional ethics committee was also obtained.

Data was entered and analyzed using Epi Info software version 3.3.2 for Windows. Effect size in terms of relative risk (RR) with 95% confidence interval (CI) was also calculated. The continuous variables were recoded into categorical variable and the reference category was selected and was compared with the rest of categories. Multivariate analysis using bimodal logistic regression was carried out for control of confounding and adjusted effect size (aRR) was computed. Multivariate analysis was not carried out for defaulters and nondefaulter patients due to less (25) number of treatment defaulters.

3. Results

Total 1607 patients were enrolled from all the randomly selected TUs and followed up in the study. Patients were largely from rural (80.0%) area, male (67.9%), and of 15–44 years (62.3%) of age group. Almost half of the patients had joint family of middle socioeconomic class (65.5%) with more than three members (86.5%) in the family. Majority reported alcohol (56.9%) consumption and smoking (54.4%) at the time of interview. It was observed that only 25 (1.5%) patients defaulted (1.5%) DOTS. Comparatively, the number of defaulted patients was small to look for statistically significant difference, but most of patients (76.0%) thought that TB and its treatment affect their work performance, 56.0% hid their disease status from others, and 52.0% did not disclose their disease status to their family members. Despite this, 96.0% of defaulted patients were aware of the curable nature of disease and 84.0% knew about the duration of available treatment (data not shown).

Since appearance of symptoms, patients were put on DOTS after median (mean: 49 days; mode: 33 days) duration of 33 days. Treatment was started after more than 30 days among 55.6% of patients. Once patient contacted the health facility, treatment was started within 2.4 day. Most of the patients (62.1%) first contacted government health facility for care. Almost all (95.5%) patients were on category I treatment of DOTS.

Significantly early (within 30 day) contact to health facility was observed among patients of upper socioeconomic status (RR: 1.80; CI: 1.72–1.88), nuclear family (RR: 1.27; CI: 1.04–1.55) with family size of 3–5 (RR: 1.22; CI: 1.00–1.49), and of rural area (RR: 1.55; CI: 1.20–2.00). Early contact was observed less among patients of urban area (RR: 0.64; CI: 0.48–0.83) (Table 1). When analyzed for patient related factors, it was found that significantly more patients contacted health facility early, who felt ashamed about their disease status (RR: 1.41; CI: 1.15–1.74), but, ready to disclose their disease status (RR: 1.63; CI: 1.33–1.98), thought that treatment would be costly (RR: 2.08; CI: 1.40–3.09), and they knew disease is curable (RR: 1.96; CI: 2.43–2.69) and could be prevented by vaccine (RR: 1.29; CI: 1.05–1.59). Significantly fewer patients contacted early who wished to hide the disease from others (RR: 0.80; CI: 0.65–0.97). It was also observed that the exact treatment duration was explained by DOTS

TABLE 1: Demographic profile among TB patients with default and delay treatment, Himachal Pradesh, India, 2008-09.

Characteristics	Delay (<30 day) (713) N (%)	Delay (>30 day) (894) N (%)	Risk estimate (Unadjusted) RR (95% CI)	Risk estimate (Adjusted) aRR (95% CI)
Age group (years)				
15–24	191 (27.2)	208 (23.5)	1.23 (0.98–1.50)	Ref
25–34	156 (22.2)	172 (19.4)	1.17 (0.92–1.48)	1.05 (0.75–1.47)
35–44	111 (15.8)	152 (17.2)	0.90 (0.68–1.17)	1.39 (0.93–2.07)
45–54	92 (13.1)	137 (15.5)	0.81 (0.61–1.08)	1.46 (0.97–2.21)
55 and above	153 (21.8)	217 (24.5)	0.85 (0.67–1.07)	1.26 (0.87–1.82)
Sex				
Male	501 (70.3)	590 (66.0)	1.21 (0.98–1.50)	1.55 (1.18–2.04)
Status				
Married	479 (67.2)	622 (69.6)	0.89 (0.72–1.10)	1.05 (0.78–1.40)
Socioeconomic status				
Upper	0 (0.0)	07 (00.8)	**1.80 (1.72–1.88)***	—
Upper middle	167 (23.4)	174 (19.5)	1.26 (0.60–1.99)	0.47 (0.44–1.54)
Lower middle	310 (43.5)	402 (45.0)	0.91 (0.77–1.14)	0.54 (0.16–1.75)
Upper lower	231 (32.4)	302 (33.8)	0.93 (0.76–1.15)	0.55 (0.17–1.76)
Lower	5 (0.7)	009 (01.0)	0.69 (0.23–2.08)	Ref
Religion				
Hindus	686 (96.2)	855 (95.6)	1.15 (0.70–1.91)	1.06 (0.62–1.82)
Family				
Nuclear	361 (50.6)	399 (44.6)	**1.27 (1.04–1.55)***	**1.37 (1.09–1.73)***
Family size				
<3	75 (10.5)	141 (15.8)	**0.62 (0.46–0.84)***	Ref
>3	333 (46.7)	372 (41.6)	**1.22 (1.00–1.49)***	**0.68 (0.48–0.97)***
Place of residence				
Rural	597 (83.8)	688 (77.0)	**1.55 (1.20–2.00)***	Ref
Urban	98 (13.8)	180 (20.1)	**0.63 (0.48–0.82)***	**0.69 (0.51–0.93)***
Alcohol				
Yes	416 (58.3)	499 (55.8)	1.10 (0.90–1.35)	1.21 (0.93–1.59)
Smoking				
Yes	72 (10.1)	094 (10.5)	0.95 (0.69–1.32)	0.91 (0.63–1.30)

*Statistically significant.

provider (RR: 1.96; CI: 1.26–3.04) to patients who contacted health facility early (Table 2).

Multivariate analysis showed that significantly more patients contacted health facility early and they were males (aRR: 1.55; CI: 1.18–2.04), from nuclear family (aRR: 1.37; CI: 1.09–1.73) (Table 1), and ashamed of their disease status (aRR: 1.32; CI: 1.03–1.70), wished to disclose disease status (aRR: 1.79; CI: 1.43–2.24), thought treatment would be costly (aRR: 2.45; CI: 1.59–3.78) but were aware of curable nature (aRR: 1.67; CI: 1.17–2.39) of disease and aware of available vaccine (aRR: 1.35; CI: 1.07–1.70) for prevention and health facility (aRR: 1.72; CI: 1.08–2.74) which was more than 60 minutes away from place of residence (Table 2). Fewer patients contacted the health facility early and they were from urban area (aRR: 0.69; CI: 0.51–0.93) (Table 1), with family size of 3–5 (aRR: 0.68; CI: 0.48–0.97), 6-7 (aRR: 0.60; CI: 0.41–0.89), wished to hide status from others (aOR: 0.69; CI: 0.51–0.93), and thought that disease would affect daily work

(aRR: 0.73; CI: 0.56–0.97) performance. It was observed that the correct treatment duration was explained by the DOTS provider (aRR: 1.88; CI: 1.12–3.15) to patients who contacted health facility early (Table 2).

4. Discussion

With about 2 million deaths a year in the world and 7.0% of total deaths in India, TB is a prevalent public health problem [1, 2, 7]. In the last 50 years, reduction in disease burden in India had been observed as national TB control efforts were expanded to the entire county [7, 8]. Early diagnosis and treatment of the case to break the chain of transmission were vital for disease control. Usually patients did not report to health facility early due to perceived mild nature of symptoms, bad staff behavior, and patient dissatisfaction [9, 10]. Societal issues like expected problems related to social status, marriage, and adverse community

TABLE 2: Disease awareness among TB patients with default and delay treatment, Himachal Pradesh, India, 2008-09.

Characteristics	Delay (<30 day) (713) N (%)	Delay (>30 day) (894) N (%)	Risk estimate (Unadjusted) RR (95% CI)	Risk estimate (Adjusted) aRR (95% CI)
Stigma				
Ashamed	271 (38.0)	270 (30.2)	1.41 (1.15–1.74)*	1.32 (1.03–1.70)*
Hide from others	402 (56.4)	552 (61.7)	0.80 (0.65–0.97)*	0.70 (0.55–0.88)*
Disclose to others	384 (53.9)	373 (41.7)	1.63 (1.33–1.98)*	1.79 (1.43–2.24)*
Hereditary	300 (42.1)	362 (40.5)	1.07 (0.87–1.31)	1.03 (0.81–1.31)
Prefer to be isolated	181 (25.4)	212 (23.7)	1.09 (0.87–1.37)	1.08 (0.83–1.39)
Costly treatment	068 (09.5)	043 (04.8)	2.08 (1.40–3.09)*	2.45 (1.59–3.78)*
Effect				
Work	502 (70.4)	661 (73.9)	0.83 (0.67–1.04)	0.73 (0.56–0.97)
Marriage	218 (30.6)	270 (30.2)	1.01 (0.82–1.26)	0.99 (0.77–1.28)
Responsibility	385 (54.0)	466 (52.1)	1.07 (0.88–1.31)	0.98 (0.76–1.25)
Female infertility	145 (20.3)	149 (16.7)	1.27 (0.99–1.64)	1.22 (0.93–1.61)
Knowledge				
DOTS duration	713 (90.9)	894 (89.0)	1.22 (0.88–1.70)	0.86 (0.56–1.31)
Curable	648 (90.9)	796 (89.0)	1.96 (2.43–2.69)*	1.67 (1.17–2.39)*
Contagious	376 (52.7)	477 (53.4)	0.98 (0.81–1.20)	1.05 (0.83–1.32)
Vaccine	267 (37.4)	282 (31.5)	1.29 (1.05–1.59)*	1.35 (1.07–1.70)*
Advertisement				
Yes	642 (90.0)	781 (87.4)	1.30 (0.95–1.79)	1.18 (0.83–1.68)
Time to DOTS centre (minutes)				
<30	470 (65.9)	587 (65.7)	0.97 (0.79–1.20)	Ref
>30	205 (28.8)	264 (29.5)	1.02 (0.83–1.26)	1.72 (1.08–2.74)*
Waiting time at DOTS center (minutes)				
<30	538 (75.5)	687 (76.8)	0.93 (0.74–1.17)	Ref
>30	151 (21.2)	175 (19.6)	1.07 (0.85–1.35)	0.98 (0.75–1.27)
Provider explained				
DOTS duration	683 (95.8)	823 (92.1)	1.96 (1.26–3.04)*	1.88(1.12–3.15)*

*Statistically significant.

behavior were major reasons for stigmatizing behavior of patient [11, 12]. These factors result in late case identification and result in disease transmission in the community. Present study showed that the patients who contacted health facility early were those who felt ashamed of the disease but ready to disclose disease status to others. Few patients contacted the health facility early because they wished to hide their disease status from others and thought that the disease would affect their daily work performance. Present study observed weak evidence for disease effect on work capacity, family relations, marriage, and female infertility (Table 2).

Prior disease knowledge and awareness influence the health care seeking behavior. It was observed that patients who were on treatment were aware of infectious nature of disease and its available treatment [13]. Present study also showed that patients who contacted health facility early were aware of the preventable and curable nature of disease. In present study, correct treatment duration was explained by the DOTS provider among patients who contacted the health facility early. Present study observed average duration

of delay of 30 days which is low as compared to about 56 reported by other studies in an African country [14]. This difference amounts to perceived nature of symptoms and penetration of program in terms of availability and accessibility of management services in the country [3–6].

In India, treatment success rate approached 85.0% and met the set objective under RNTCP [15]. Poor treatment compliance could lead to high default rate and pose threat to multidrug resistant tuberculosis. However, present study had showed default rate of 1.5% similar to 1.1% as observed in North India [16]. Present study observed that defaulted patients still did not disclose their disease status to their family members and friends despite their correct knowledge about the duration of treatment and curable nature of disease. Smoking [7] and alcohol [17, 18] are known to increase the risk of mortality and high default rate among patients with substance abuse [12]. Present study observed insignificant but high prevalence of alcohol (76.0%) and smoking (12.0%). Against the reported (before the study was based upon routine health information system) default rate of 3.8% of selected TUs, present study observed low default which could be due to two prospective visits study design, in addition to the usual inbuilt patient monitoring under the program.

In the present study, disease awareness and complete information provided by the DOTS provider influenced early contact of health facility and low treatment default rate. High level of advertisement under RNTCP possibly had played a significant role in the study area. Low default rate could be attributed to study design itself as patient was approached by the study staff three times. It poses a limitation of study as it could not the controlled in study design , but it shows that additional visits to contact patient could reduce the treatment default rate. RNTCP has strengthened itself to achieve high case detection and cure rate. It will substantiate the successful efforts in the state to combat TB as one of the top ten leading killers.

Conflict of Interests

The authors declare that there is no conflict of interests regarding the publication of this paper.

Acknowledgment

The financial assistance was provided by the Central Tuberculosis Division, Ministry of Health and Family Welfare, Government of India.

References

[1] World health organization (WHO), *Global Tuberculosis Control*, World health organization, 2010.

[2] "People on health," Annual Report, Government of India, Ministry of Health and Family Welfare, New Delhi, India, 2010.

[3] K. Jaggarajamma, R. Ramachandran, N. Charles, V. Chandrasekaran, M. Muniyandi, and S. Ganapathy, "Psycho-social dysfunction: perceived and enacted stigma among tuberculosis patients registered under Revised National Tuberculosis Control Programme," *The Indian Journal of Tuberculosis*, vol. 55, no. 4, pp. 179–187, 2008.

[4] G. Sudha, C. Nirupa, M. Rajasakthivel et al., "Factors influencing the care-seeking behaviour of chest symptomatics: A community-based study involving rural and urban population in Tamil Nadu, South India," *Tropical Medicine and International Health*, vol. 8, no. 4, pp. 336–341, 2003.

[5] R. Rajeswari, V. Chandrasekaran, M. Suhadev, S. Sivasubramaniam, G. Sudha, and G. Renu, "Factors associated with patient and health system delays in the diagnosis of tuberculosis in South India," *International Journal of Tuberculosis and Lung Disease*, vol. 6, no. 9, pp. 789–795, 2002.

[6] V. K. Dhingra and S. Khan, "A sociological study on stigma among TB patients in Delhi," *Indian Journal of Tuberculosis*, vol. 57, no. 1, pp. 12–18, 2010.

[7] P. Jha, B. Jacob, V. Gajalakshmi et al., "RGI-CGHR Investigators. A nationally representative case-control study of smoking and death in India," *The New England Journal of Medicine*, vol. 358, no. 11, pp. 1137–1147, 2008.

[8] V. K. Dhingra, N. Aggarwal, S. Chandra, and R. P. Vashist, "Tuberculosis mortality trends in Delhi after implementation of RNTCP," *Indian Journal of Tuberculosis*, vol. 56, no. 2, pp. 77–81, 2009.

[9] N. Charles, B. Thomas, B. Watson, M. Raja Sakthivel, V. Chandrasekeran, and F. Wares, "Care seeking behavior of chest symptomatics: a community based study done in south india after the implementation of the RNTCP," *PLoS ONE*, vol. 5, no. 9, Article ID e12379, pp. 1–6, 2010.

[10] R. Dandona, L. Dandona, A. Mishra, S. Dhingra, K. Venkatagopalakrishna, and L. S. Chauhan, "Utilization of and barriers to public sector tuberculosis services in India," *National Medical Journal of India*, vol. 17, no. 6, pp. 292–299, 2004.

[11] V. K. Dhingra and S. Khan, "A sociological study on stigma among TB patients in Delhi," *Indian Journal of Tuberculosis*, vol. 57, no. 1, pp. 12–18, 2010.

[12] S. Atre, A. Kudale, S. Morankar, D. Gosoniu, and M. G. Weiss, "Gender and community views of stigma and tuberculosis in rural Maharashtra, India," *Global Public Health*, vol. 6, no. 1, pp. 56–71, 2011.

[13] N. Sharma, A. Nath, D. K. Taneja, and G. K. Ingle, "A qualitative evaluation of the information, education, and communication component of the tuberculosis control program in Delhi, India," *Asia-Pacific Journal of Public Health*, vol. 21, no. 3, pp. 321–332, 2009.

[14] M. Pai and D. Dowdy, "Tuberculosis: progress and challenges in product development and delivery," *The Lancet Respiratory Medicine*, vol. 2, no. 1, pp. 25–27, 2014.

[15] M. W. Borgdorff, K. Floyd, and J. F. Broekmans, "Interventions to reduce tuberculosis mortality and transmission in low- and middle-income countries," *Bulletin of the World Health Organization*, vol. 80, no. 3, pp. 217–227, 2002.

[16] G. Kaur, N. K. Goel, D. Kumar, A. K. Janmeja, H. M. Swami, and M. Kalia, "Treatment outcomes of patients placed on treatment under directly observed therapy short-course (dots)," *Lung India*, vol. 25, no. 2, pp. 75–77, 2008.

[17] V. Gajalakshmi and R. Peto, "Smoking, drinking and incident tuberculosis in rural India: population-based case-control study," *International Journal of Epidemiology*, vol. 38, no. 4, pp. 1018–1025, 2009.

[18] V. G. Rao, P. G. Gopi, J. Bhat, R. Yadav, N. Selvakumar, and D. F. Wares, "Selected risk factors associated with pulmonary tuberculosis among Saharia tribe of Madhya Pradesh, central India," *European Journal of Public Health*, vol. 22, no. 2, pp. 271–273, 2012.

Evaluation of Anthropometric and Metabolic Parameters in Obstructive Sleep Apnea

Yaşar Yildirim,[1] Süreyya Yilmaz,[2] Mehmet Güven,[1] Faruk Kılınç,[1] Ali Veysel Kara,[1] Zülfükar Yilmaz,[1] Gökhan Kırbaş,[2] Alpaslan Kemal Tuzcu,[1] and Fatma Yılmaz Aydın[1]

[1]*Department of Internal Medicine, Faculty of Medicine, Dicle University, Diyarbakır, Turkey*
[2]*Department of Pulmonology, Faculty of Medicine, Dicle University, Diyarbakır, Turkey*

Correspondence should be addressed to Yaşar Yildirim; yyil11@yahoo.com

Academic Editor: Charlie Strange

Aims. Sleep disorders have recently become a significant public health problem worldwide and have deleterious health consequences. Obstructive sleep apnea (OSA) is the most common type of sleep-related breathing disorders. We aimed to evaluate anthropometric measurements, glucose metabolism, and cortisol levels in patients with obstructive sleep apnea (OSA). *Materials and Methods.* A total of 50 patients with a body mass index ≥30 and major OSA symptoms were included in this study. Anthropometric measurements of the patients were recorded and blood samples were drawn for laboratory analysis. A 24-hour urine sample was also collected from each subject for measurement of 24-hour cortisol excretion. Patients were divided equally into 2 groups according to polysomnography results: control group with an apnea-hypopnea index (AHI) <5 ($n = 25$) and OSA group with an AHI ≥5 ($n = 25$). *Results.* Neck and waist circumference, fasting plasma glucose, HbA1c, late-night serum cortisol, morning serum cortisol after 1 mg dexamethasone suppression test, and 24-hour urinary cortisol levels were significantly higher in OSA patients compared to control subjects. Newly diagnosed DM was more frequent in patients with OSA than control subjects (32% versus 8%, $p = 0.034$). There was a significant positive correlation between AHI and neck circumference, glucose, and late-night serum cortisol. *Conclusions.* Our study indicates that increased waist and neck circumferences constitute a risk for OSA regardless of obesity status. In addition, OSA has adverse effects on endocrine function and glucose metabolism.

1. Background

Obstructive sleep apnea (OSA) is the most common type of sleep-related breathing disorders. This disorder is characterized by excessive daytime sleepiness, snoring, and episodes of apnea. Cardiovascular diseases, which are among long-term adverse effects of OSA, lead to increased mortality and morbidity [1]. The only relevant study from our country reported an OSA prevalence of 0.9–1.9% [2]. The prevalence of the disease peaks between 40 and 65 years of age and decreases after 65 years of age [3, 4]. In fact, 25% of men aged 30 to 60 years meet minimal criteria (apnea-hypopnea index greater than 5) of OSA [5]. The gold standard test for diagnosis is polysomnography (PSG).

In order to sustain life, the hypothalamus-pituitary-adrenal (HPA) axis should function to elicit the normal cortisol response to stress. In stress-free states the normal cortisol release shows a diurnal pattern; that is, the highest cortisol levels are observed early in the morning (04:00–08:00), while the lowest levels occur late at night (02:00–04:00). Patients with OSA frequently exhibit increased ventilatory effort, sleep fragmentation, and oxygen desaturation. These events produce stress in an individual's body, activating the HPA axis that increases cortisol production. Cortisol has many functions including regulation of blood glucose, vascular tone, and myocardial contractility.

OSA increases the risk of hypertension, diabetes mellitus (DM), myocardial infarction, congestive heart failure, and stroke [6]. In our study, our goal was to evaluate anthropometric measurements, glucose metabolism, and cortisol levels in patients with OSA.

2. Materials and Methods

2.1. Study Population. A total of 50 patients with a body mass index ≥30 and major OSA symptoms including snoring, daytime sleepiness, and witnessed apnea were included in this study. We conducted this study between January 2012 and September 2013 at Department of Endocrinology, Faculty of Medicine, Dicle University. We obtained approval from a local medical research ethics committee. All the following types of patients were excluded from our study: patients with previous diagnosis of OSA, continuous positive airway pressure (CPAP) treatment, or bilevel positive airway pressure (BiPAP) therapy, patients with type 2 DM, hypertension, hypothyroidism, Cushing syndrome, hyperaldosteronism, pregnancy, malignancy, congestive heart failure, psychotic disorder, chronic liver failure, nephrotic syndrome, or chronic renal failure, or patients using drugs that had a potential to impair study tests (angiotensin converting enzyme inhibitor, angiotensin receptor blocker, phenytoin, barbiturate, or oral contraceptive). All subjects entering the study gave a written informed consent prior to the study, and all study tests and examinations were performed in compliance with the Helsinki Declaration regulating biomedical research on humans.

2.2. Study Procedures. Blood samples for fasting glucose, insulin, HbA1c, adrenocorticotropic hormone (ACTH), and cortisol were drawn at 08:00 from each patient during their stay in the endocrinology department. Newly diagnosed diabetes mellitus was determined according to ADA criteria [7]. Homeostatic model assessment insulin resistance (HOMA-IR), a method used to quantify insulin resistance and beta-cell function, was measured as glucose × insulin/405. A 24-hour urine sample was also collected from each subject for measurement of 24-hour cortisol excretion.

An additional blood sample was drawn for cortisol level at 23:00. A 1 mg dexamethasone suppression test was performed on the next day. A 1 mg decort tablet was administered at 23:00 and cortisol level was measured at 08:00 the next morning. A cortisol level less than 1.8 μg/dL (50 nmol/L) suggested a suppressed cortisol level. A low dose dexamethasone suppression test with 2 mg dexamethasone was performed for 2 days in patients with high cortisol levels.

Body weight, length, waist circumference, and neck circumference were measured with a nonflexible tape and recorded in centimeters. Body mass index was calculated with the formula of body weight/height^2 (kg/m^2). Waist circumference was measured from the diameter between the costal arch and the anterior superior iliac spine at umbilicus level. Neck circumference was measured from the level of superior border of cricothyroid membrane. The same person performed all the measurements using the same tools; the results were rounded to the closest 0.5 cm to minimize measurement errors.

After completion of the procedures, each patient had a polysomnographic recording at Dicle University, Department of Chest Diseases, Center of Sleep Disorders. The polysomnographic recordings were carried out using a 32-channel E series polysomnography device (Compumedics E Series, Compumedics Limited, Abbotsford, VIC, Australia). The patients were monitored for at least 8 hours during sleep. Electroencephalography (EEG) recordings were made from 4 channels designated as C3/A2, C4/A1, O1/A2, O2/A1 according to the International 10–20 system that determines the locations of the electrodes. Left-right electrooculography (EOG), mental electromyography (EMG), and electrocardiography (ECG) recordings were also performed.

A transducer system connected to a nasal cannula was used to record respiratory events. The respiratory movements were recorded with the help of thoracic and abdominal tapes. Snoring was monitored with a microphone placed on the larynx at the anterosuperior portion of the neck. Oxygen saturation (SO$_2$) was measured with a pulse oximetry during sleep. Leg movements were recorded with a bilateral pretibial EMG. PSG recordings were scored according to the Rechtschaffen and Kales criteria as 30-second epochs. All recordings were scored manually in a digital format by a physician certified in sleep disordered breathing. Sleep stages, respiratory events, and their characteristics were recorded. Hypopnea was defined as a reduction in nasal pressure signal of ≥50% that lasted ≥10 s, resulting in a ≥3% decrease in oxygen saturation from the prevent baseline or an arousal.

The control group in this study was comprised of patients who snored and had episodes of witnessed apnea and excessive daytime sleepiness and an AHI of <5 on polysomnography. The OSA group was composed of the study subjects who snored and had a witnessed apneic episode and excessive daytime sleepiness and an AHI equal to or greater than 5.

2.3. Statistical Analysis. Data analyses were performed using Statistical Package for Social Sciences (SPSS), Version 18.0 for Windows (SPSS Inc., Chicago, IL, USA). Normally distributed variables were presented using means and standard deviations. Student's t-test was used to compare the means of the continuous variables with normal distribution for related and independent samples. The chi-square test was used to compare these proportions in different groups. The Pearson correlation was used for simple regression analysis. P values less than 0.05 were considered statistically significant.

3. Results

A total of 50 patients were enrolled in the study and patients were divided equally into 2 groups according to polysomnography results: control group (n = 25) and OSA group (n = 25). The mean age was 43.76 ± 8.36 year and the male-to-female ratio was 13 : 12 in the control group. In the OSA group, the mean age was 46.68 ± 5.75 years with a male-to-female ratio of 12 : 13. There were no differences between groups for age and gender distribution (p > 0.05).

When comparing anthropometric measurements between the control group and OSA group, neck circumference (43.28 ± 4.62 cm versus 40.28 ± 2.17 cm, p < 0.01) and waist

TABLE 1: Demographic characteristics and anthropometric measurements in control group versus OSA group.

Parameters	Control group (n = 25)	OSA group (n = 25)	p
Age (years)	43.76 ± 8.36	46.68 ± 5.75	>0.05
Gender (M/F)	13/12	12/13	>0.05
Height (cm)	164.64 ± 9.40	166.56 ± 8.76	>0.05
Weight (kg)	106.22 ± 29.20	129.72 ± 35.80	<0.05
BMI (kg/m^2)	39.87 ± 13.36	46.91 ± 12.86	>0.05
Neck circumference (cm)	40.28 ± 2.17	43.28 ± 4.62	<0.01
Waist circumference (cm)	116.28 ± 23.5	131.44 ± 20.86	<0.05
AHI	2.25 ± 0.48	24.21 ± 6.75	<0.001

BMI: body mass index.

TABLE 2: Glucose metabolism in control group versus OSA group.

Parameters	Control group (n = 25)	OSA group (n = 25)	p
Fasting glucose (mg/dL)	92.24 ± 15.17	113.44 ± 22.93	<0.01
Insulin (Uu/mL)	33.76 ± 34.07	36.72 ± 34.74	>0.05
HbA1c (%)	5.7 ± 0.60	6.80 ± 0.90	<0.01
HOMA-IR	7.95 ± 8.08	10.67 ± 10.83	>0.05
Newly diagnosed DM	8%	32%	0.034

HbA1c: hemoglobin A1c; HOMA-IR: homeostatic model assessment insulin resistance.

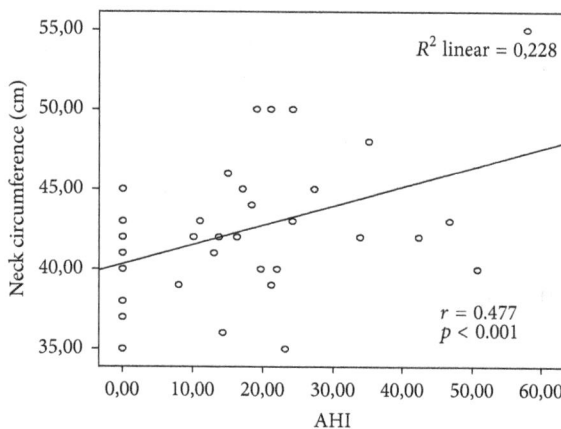

FIGURE 1: Pearson correlation analysis between AHI and neck circumference.

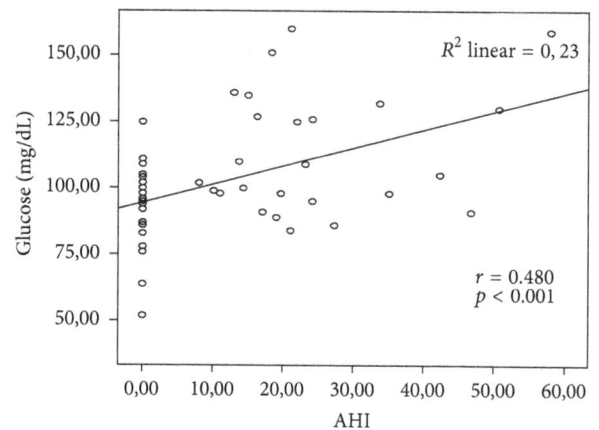

FIGURE 2: Pearson correlation analysis between AHI and glucose.

circumference (131.44 ± 20.86 cm versus 116.28 ± 23.5 cm, $p < 0.05$) were significantly higher in OSA group compared to control group. Body mass index was not significantly different between the groups (46.91 ± 12.86 kg/m^2 versus 39.87 ± 13.36 kg/m^2, $p > 0.05$). Demographic characteristics and anthropometric measurements of the groups are presented in Table 1. There was a significant positive correlation between AHI and neck circumference ($r = 0.477$, $p < 0.001$; Figure 1).

Compared to control subjects, OSA patients had significantly higher levels of fasting plasma glucose (113.44 ± 22.93 mg/dL versus 92.24 ± 15.7 mg/dL, $p < 0.01$) and HbA1c (6.80 ± 0.90% versus 5.7 ± 0.60%, $p < 0.01$). There was no significant difference between groups in insulin levels and homeostatic model assessment insulin resistance (HOMA-IR). Newly diagnosed DM was more frequent in patients with OSA than control subjects (32% versus 8%, $p = 0.034$). Results are shown in Table 2. There was a significant positive correlation between AHI and plasma glucose ($r = 0.480$, $p < 0.01$; Figure 2).

As shown in Table 3, late-night serum cortisol (6.18 ± 3.19 mcg/dL versus 3.82 ± 3.19 mcg/dL, $p < 0.05$), morning

serum cortisol after 1 mg dexamethasone suppression test (1.53 ± 1.09 mcg/dL versus 0.87 ± 0.45 mcg/dL, $p < 0.01$) and 24-hour urinary cortisol (81.96 ± 68.04 μgr/day versus 44.33 ± 42.07 μgr/day, $p < 0.05$) levels were significantly higher in the OSA group than control group. However, morning serum cortisol and adrenocorticotropic hormone (ACTH) levels were not significantly different between the groups. There was a significant positive correlation between AHI and late-night serum cortisol ($r = 0.332$, $p = 0.018$, Figure 3).

A 1 mg dexamethasone suppression test was administered to all patients. Plasma cortisol levels were not suppressed in 1 of 25 patients (4%) in the control group and in 5 out of 25 patients (20%) in the OSA group ($p = 0.189$). When a 2 mg dexamethasone suppression test was applied, plasma cortisol levels were suppressed in both group.

4. Discussion

Obstructive sleep apnea is a syndrome characterized by snoring, excessive daytime sleepiness, and oxygen desaturation as a result of repeated upper airway collapse during sleep.

The prevalence of this disorder increases with age and peaks between ages 40 and 65. The male-to-female ratio has reportedly been in the range of 2 : 1-3 : 1 for premenopausal women and 1 : 1 for postmenopausal woman. In our study the mean age of the OSA group was 46.68 ± 5.71 years. The male-to-female ratio was 1 : 1 due to relatively large proportion of postmenopausal women in the present study.

TABLE 3: ACTH and cortisol levels in control group versus OSA group.

Parameters	Control group (n = 25)	OSA group (n = 25)	p
Morning serum ACTH (pg/mL)	35.56 ± 20.82	36.72 ± 21.61	>0.05
Morning serum cortisol (mcg/dL)	12.47 ± 6.25	12.05 ± 4.57	>0.05
Late-night serum cortisol (mcg/dL)	3.82 ± 3.19	6.18 ± 3.19	**<0.05**
24-hour urinary cortisol (μgr/day)	44.33 ± 42.07	81.96 ± 68.04	**<0.05**
Morning serum cortisol after 1 mg dexamethasone suppression test (mcg/dL)	0.87 ± 0.45	1.53 ± 1.09	**<0.01**

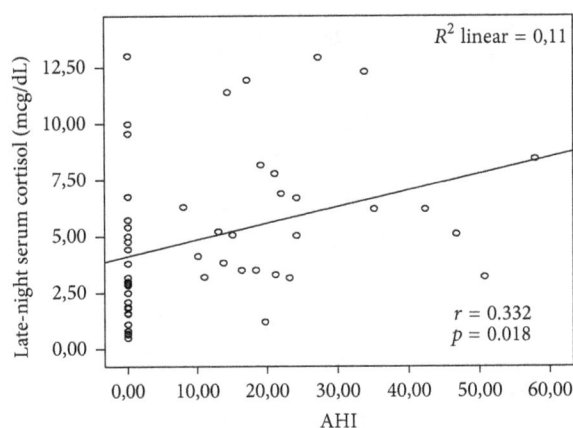

FIGURE 3: Pearson correlation analysis between AHI and late-night serum cortisol.

Obesity causes an increased tendency for OSA. As a general rule, obese OSA patients have a bigger tongue and a narrower upper airway passage. In addition, obese OSA patients have also diminished respiratory muscle strength [8]. Obesity reduces total respiratory compliance by decreasing both chest wall compliance and lung compliance. These combined effects lead to a decrease in functional residual capacity, vital capacity, and total lung capacity as well as an increased airway resistance. Abdominal obesity can reduce lung volume particularly in supine position and may reflexively affect upper airway dimensions. When lung volume regresses from total lung capacity to residual volume, the pharyngeal cross-sectional area is reduced and pharyngeal resistance increases [9].

Therefore, it is possible that obesity increases susceptibility to OSA. The risk for OSA increases 8–12 times in persons with a BMI greater than 28 [10]. This risk further increases in persons with upper body obesity and those with a BMI > 40 [11]. Neck circumference reflects upper body obesity and is considered to be a better marker than BMI for OSA [12]. A neck circumference greater than 43 cm in men and 38 cm in women increases the risk of OSA [13]. In our study, 11 out of 13 women had a neck circumference greater than

38 cm. Seven of 12 men had a neck circumference greater than 43 cm. All patients in our study had obesity (BMI > 30). Additionally, we observed that neck circumference and waist circumference were significantly higher in the OSA group compared to control group, while body mass index was not significantly different between the groups. In addition, there was a significant positive correlation between AHI and neck circumference ($r = 0.477$, $p < 0.001$). This finding supported the idea that neck circumference alone is a risk factor for OSA independent of obesity.

Repetitive respiratory difficulties during sleep cause intermittent hypoxia and alterations in intrathoracic pressure that trigger autonomic responses. Among these autonomic alterations, increased sympathetic activity plays an important role. Increased sympathetic activity, sleep fragmentation, and intermittent hypoxia contribute to metabolic dysfunction [14, 15]. Specifically, efficiency of glucose transport and insulin resistance have been linked to metabolic dysfunction. Cortisol decreases insulin sensitivity and adds to glucose intolerance at all hours of a day. Sleep deprivation itself causes HPA axis hyperactivity and negatively affects glucose tolerance [16].

In a 270-patient study, Ip et al. [17] grouped 185 patients with OSA into obese and nonobese groups and compared the two groups. They found a significant elevation in fasting insulin levels and HOMA-IR values in the OSA group with an AHI greater than 5, while they could not detect any significant difference between obese and nonobese groups in terms of insulin level and insulin resistance. We found no significant difference between the two groups with respect to HOMA-IR values that reflect insulin resistance. This may have been due to the small sample size. However, OSA patients had significantly higher levels of plasma glucose and HbA1c compared to control subjects. In addition, in the present study newly diagnosed DM was more frequent in patients with OSA than control subjects (32% versus 8%, $p = 0.034$). As patients with OSA are usually obese, their risk of having or developing insulin resistance, type 2 DM, and hypertension is increased. Nocturnal cortisol elevations in these patients further increase the already heightened risk. The prevalence of type 2 DM is around 30% in patients with OSA [18].

Cortisol release shows a diurnal variation in normal people. The HPA axis secretes cortisol in a pulsatile manner at morning hours and sets cortisol to release into blood stream at a minimum level at night. That is, the highest cortisol levels are observed early in the morning (04:00–08:00) while the lowest ones occur late at night (02:00–04:00). Daily cortisol production is at a level of 5.7 mg/m^2/day [19]. An estimated daily cortisol production of around 10–17 mg takes place in the normal healthy population and varies depending on body habitus, age, and sex [20]. In stressful conditions cortisol has a vital role for survival of an organism. It has been observed that the diurnal rhythm of cortisol is impaired in sleep disorders, certain acute and chronic abnormalities (infections, drugs, inflammatory disease, etc.), and conditions such as Cushing syndrome [21, 22]. Sleep deprivation leads to pulsatile cortisol release together with sympathetic activation in patients with OSA [23]. Sympathetic activation induces catecholamine release and especially corticotropin releasing hormone and cortisol secretion.

Various studies found no difference between OSA patients and the control group with respect to morning cortisol levels, although nocturnal cortisol levels have been found to be higher in OSA patients [24–26]. Grunstein et al. compared plasma cortisol levels at 06:00 between OSA and control groups and found no significant difference [27]. Lanfranco et al. found similar morning plasma ACTH, cortisol, and 24-hour urinary free cortisol levels in obese and nonobese OSA patients and control group [28]. We found no significant difference between the two groups with regard to morning cortisol level although nocturnal cortisol level was significantly higher in OSA group ($p < 0.05$). The severity of OSA worsens as the AHI increases. Thus, frequent awakenings and duration of hypoxia also increase. Also in our patients an increase in AHI was correlated with a nocturnal cortisol elevation ($r = 0.332$, $p = 0.018$), suggesting that stress and night wakefulness boost the activity of HPA axis and increase pulsatile cortisol release.

All of our patients underwent a 1 mg dexamethasone suppression test. The cortisol level was 0.87 ± 0.45 mcg/dL in the control group and 1.53 ± 1.09 mcg/dL in the OSA group ($p < 0.01$). This suggests that it is more difficult for OSA patients to suppress cortisol with a 1 mg dexamethasone suppression test. Patients with OSA had a higher 24-hour urinary cortisol level compared to the control group. These two findings support nocturnal cortisol elevation in patients with OSA which is in line with the two previous studies [24, 29].

Sleep disorders have recently become a significant public health problem both in our country and worldwide. As the number of people with obesity and obesity-related diseases increases, the number of patients suffering from OSA increases. Obesity, along with increased neck and waist circumferences, increases the risk of OSA. Hypoxemia and stress induced by OSA further worsen the impact of obesity on metabolic and endocrine systems.

5. Conclusions

This study reveals that recognition of newly diagnosed type 2 diabetes mellitus in 32% of OSA patients and especially increased nocturnal cortisol levels in OSA patients both point to an adverse effect of OSA on the endocrine system. One additional significant finding of our study was that increased waist and neck circumferences constituted a risk for OSA regardless of obesity status. We suggest that endocrinological and anthropometric examinations are necessary for OSAS patients. We hope that the current study will contribute significantly to the literature. A limitation of the study was the relatively small sample size; therefore further division of OSAS group could not be examined. We also believe that further studies with larger sample size are needed on this subject.

Conflict of Interests

The authors declare no conflict of interests.

References

[1] A. B. Newman, F. J. Nieto, U. Guidry et al., "Relation of sleep-disordered breathing to cardiovascular disease risk factors: the Sleep Heart Health study," *American Journal of Epidemiology*, vol. 154, no. 1, pp. 50–59, 2001.

[2] O. Köktürk, T. Tatlıcıoğlu, Y. Kemaloğlu, H. Fırat, and N. Çetin, "Habitüel horlaması olan olgularda obstrüktif sleep apne sendromu prevalansı," *Tüberküloz Toraks*, vol. 45, pp. 7–11, 1997.

[3] C. Hader, M. Hinz, A. Welz-Barth, and K. Rasche, "Sleep disordered breathing in the elderly: a three year longitudinal cohort study," *Journal of Physiology and Pharmacology*, vol. 57, supplement 4, pp. 119–129, 2006.

[4] A. I. Pack, "Advances in sleep-disordered breathing," *American Journal of Respiratory and Critical Care Medicine*, vol. 173, no. 1, pp. 7–15, 2006.

[5] T. Young, M. Palta, J. Dempsey, J. Skatrud, S. Weber, and S. Badr, "The occurrence of sleep-disordered breathing among middle-aged adults," *The New England Journal of Medicine*, vol. 328, no. 17, pp. 1230–1235, 1993.

[6] A. S. M. Shamsuzzaman, B. J. Gersh, and V. K. Somers, "Obstructive sleep apnea: implications for cardiac and vascular disease," *The Journal of the American Medical Association*, vol. 290, no. 14, pp. 1906–1914, 2003.

[7] American Diabetes Association, "Standards of medical care in diabetes—2013," *Diabetes Care*, vol. 36, supplement 1, pp. S11–S66, 2013.

[8] M. Lopata and E. Onal, "Mass loading sleep apnea and pathogenesis of obesity hypoventilation," *American Review of Respiratory Disease*, vol. 126, no. 4, pp. 640–645, 1982.

[9] R. Grunstein, "Pulmonary function, sleep apnea and obesity," in *Clinical Obesity*, P. Kopelmanand and M. Stock, Eds., pp. 248–289, Blacwell Science, London, UK, 1998.

[10] N. J. Douglas and O. Polo, "Pathogenesis of obstructive sleep apnoea/hypopnoea syndrome," *The Lancet*, vol. 344, no. 8923, pp. 653–655, 1994.

[11] S. Y. L. Kwan, J. A. Fleetham, D. A. Enarson, and M. Chan-Yeung, "Snoring, obesity, smoking and systemic hypertension in a working population in British Columbia," *The American Review of Respiratory Disease*, vol. 143, article A380, 1991.

[12] R. J. O. Davies, N. J. Ali, and J. R. Stradling, "Neck circumference and other clinical features in the diagnosis of the obstructive sleep apnoea syndrome," *Thorax*, vol. 47, no. 2, pp. 101–105, 1992.

[13] R. J. Schwab, A. N. Goldberg, and A. L. Pack, "Sleep apnea syndromes," in *Fishman's Pulmonary Diseases and Disorders*, A. P. Fishman, Ed., pp. 1617–1637, McGraw-Hill Book, New York, NY, USA, 1998.

[14] A. Omisade, O. M. Buxton, and B. Rusak, "Impact of acute sleep restriction on cortisol and leptin levels in young women," *Physiology and Behavior*, vol. 99, no. 5, pp. 651–656, 2010.

[15] L. F. Drager, J. C. Jun, and V. Y. Polotsky, "Metabolic consequences of intermittent hypoxia: relevance to obstructive sleep apnea," *Best Practice and Research: Clinical Endocrinology and Metabolism*, vol. 24, no. 5, pp. 843–851, 2010.

[16] K. Spiegel, R. Leproult, and E. Van Cauter, "Impact of sleep debt on metabolic and endocrine function," *The Lancet*, vol. 354, no. 9188, pp. 1435–1439, 1999.

[17] M. S. M. Ip, B. Lam, M. M. T. Ng, W. K. Lam, K. W. T. Tsang, and K. S. L. Lam, "Obstructive sleep apnea is independently associated with insulin resistance," *American Journal of Respiratory and Critical Care Medicine*, vol. 165, no. 5, pp. 670–676, 2002.

[18] K. Mahmood, N. Akhter, K. Eldeirawi et al., "Prevalence of type 2 diabetes in patients with obstructive sleep apnea in a multi-ethnic sample," *Journal of Clinical Sleep Medicine*, vol. 5, no. 3, pp. 215–221, 2009.

[19] A. J. L. Clark and A. Grossman, "Adrenal insufficiency," in *Endocrinology*, L. J. De Groot and J. L. Jameson, Eds., pp. 2343–2351, WB Saunders, Philadelphia, Pa, USA, 5th edition, 2006.

[20] N. V. Esteban, T. Loughlin, A. L. Yergey et al., "Daily cortisol production rate in man determined by stable isotope dilution/mass spectrometry," *Journal of Clinical Endocrinology and Metabolism*, vol. 72, no. 1, pp. 39–45, 1991.

[21] P. M. Stewart, "The adrenal cortex," in *Williams Textbook of Endocrinology*, pp. 491–551, Saunders, Philadelphia, Pa, USA, 10th edition, 2003.

[22] T. B. Carroll, D. C. Aron, J. W. Findling, and J. B. Tyrcell, "Glucocorticoids and adrenal androgens," in *Greenspan's Basic and Clinical Endocrinology*, D. G. Gardner and D. Shoback, Eds., pp. 346–395, The McGraw-Hill Companies, New York, NY, USA, 8th edition, 2007.

[23] E. Späth-Schwalbe, M. Gofferje, W. Kern, J. Born, and H. L. Fehm, "Sleep disruption alters nocturnal ACTH and cortisol secretory patterns," *Biological Psychiatry*, vol. 29, no. 6, pp. 575–584, 1991.

[24] A. N. Vgontzas, S. Pejovic, E. Zoumakis et al., "Hypothalamic-pituitary–adrenal axis activity in obese men with and without sleep apnea: effects of continuous positive airway pressure therapy," *Journal of Clinical Endocrinology and Metabolism*, vol. 92, no. 11, pp. 4199–4207, 2007.

[25] F. Dadoun, P. Darmon, V. Achard et al., "Effect of sleep apnea syndrome on the circadian profile of cortisol in obese men," *American Journal of Physiology—Endocrinology and Metabolism*, vol. 293, no. 2, pp. E466–E474, 2007.

[26] G. Carneiro, S. M. Togeiro, L. F. Hayashi et al., "Effect of continuous positive airway pressure therapy on hypothalamic-pituitary-adrenal axis function and 24-h blood pressure profile in obese men with obstructive sleep apnea syndrome," *The American Journal of Physiology—Endocrinology and Metabolism*, vol. 295, no. 2, pp. E380–E384, 2008.

[27] R. R. Grunstein, D. J. Handelsman, S. J. Lawrence, C. Blackwell, I. D. Caterson, and C. E. Sullivan, "Neuroendocrine dysfunction in sleep apnea: reversal by continuous positive airways pressure therapy," *Journal of Clinical Endocrinology and Metabolism*, vol. 68, no. 2, pp. 352–358, 1989.

[28] F. Lanfranco, L. Gianotti, S. Pivetti et al., "Obese patients with obstructive sleep apnoea syndrome show a peculiar alteration of the corticotroph but not of the thyrotroph and lactotroph function," *Clinical Endocrinology*, vol. 60, no. 1, pp. 41–48, 2004.

[29] D. E. Henley, G. M. Russell, J. A. Douthwaite et al., "Hypothalamic-pituitary-adrenal axis activation in obstructive sleep apnea: the effect of continuous positive airway pressure therapy," *Journal of Clinical Endocrinology and Metabolism*, vol. 94, no. 11, pp. 4234–4242, 2009.

18

In Situ Thrombosis of Small Pulmonary Arteries in Pulmonary Hypertension Developing after Chemotherapy for Malignancy

Kay Maeda,[1,2] **Yoshikatsu Saiki,**[2] **and Shigeo Yamaki**[1]

[1]*Japanese Research Institute of Pulmonary Vasculature, 2-2-26 Seikaen Aoba-ku, Sendai 982-0262, Japan*
[2]*Division of Cardiovascular Surgery, Tohoku University Graduate School of Medicine, 1-1 Seiryo-machi, Aoba-ku,*
 Sendai 980-8574, Japan

Correspondence should be addressed to Shigeo Yamaki; syamaki@ff.iij4u.or.jp

Academic Editor: Charlie Strange

A few reports have provided histopathological insight into pulmonary hypertension developing after antitumor chemotherapy. In general, plexogenic pulmonary arteriopathy is a commonly observed finding in patients with severe pulmonary hypertension. We herein report a novel pathological finding that may characterize the histopathological change occurring in patients with pulmonary hypertension after chemotherapy for malignancy. Lung biopsy or autopsy was performed in 7 patients with pulmonary hypertension that developed during or after chemotherapy between 2006 and 2013 to examine the pulmonary vascular changes or to determine the cause of death. Pathological findings included in situ thrombosis in the small pulmonary arteries in 4 of 7 patients. In 2 of 4 patients, pulmonary hypertension was controlled by anticoagulants and antithrombotic agents. One patient who had organized thrombi attained spontaneous remission with oxygen therapy. The other patient died of sudden cardiopulmonary arrest during chemotherapy. Autopsy showed complete occlusion of the peripheral small pulmonary arteries and veins by thrombi. These results demonstrate that in situ thrombosis in the small pulmonary arteries could cause pulmonary hypertension after chemotherapy.

1. Introduction

Pulmonary hypertensive disease can develop after chemotherapy for various malignant tumors and becomes lethal in immunocompromised patients. A few case reports have implicated a probable relationship between chemotherapy and subsequent pulmonary hypertension (PH) [1–3]. However, there have been few reports on pathological findings that are characteristic to this devastating sequela [4].

To date, we have performed a significant number of lung biopsies for diagnoses of severe PH associated with congenital and acquired heart diseases [5]. We reported distinctive pulmonary vascular changes even in relatively rare diseases associated with PH, such as chronic thromboembolic pulmonary hypertension (CTEPH), pulmonary venoocclusive disease (PVOD), idiopathic pulmonary arterial hypertension (IPAH), and portosystemic venous shunt (PSVS) [6–10]. In patients with severe PH, plexogenic pulmonary arteriopathy generally develops in the small pulmonary arteries [11].

In the present study, we demonstrate that in situ thrombosis in the small pulmonary arteries is one of the causative mechanisms for PH associated with chemotherapy.

2. Materials and Methods

Between 2006 and 2013, 7 patients who developed PH after chemotherapy for various malignancies were histopathologically examined at our research institute. Lung biopsies (3 cases) and autopsies (4 cases) were conducted to investigate the cause of unexplained PH after chemotherapy or to determine the cause of death, in detail, in terms of histopathological characteristics. The Heath-Edwards (HE) classification was used to assess the arterial changes [12].

Lung tissue was obtained from a lobe of the lung and was fixed in 10% formalin. In each case, 30 semiserial histological sections at $50\,\mu$m intervals, each $3\,\mu$m thick, were prepared as previously described [5]. Then, modified Elastica–Goldner staining was performed for the histopathological analysis

TABLE 1: Details of patients with pulmonary hypertension after chemotherapy.

Case	Age, sex	Neoplasm	Treatment for neoplasm	Period from chemotherapy to PH onset	Clinical diagnosis [cause of death]	Pathological findings	Lung specimen
1	46, M	Malignant lymphoma	Surgical resection + chemotherapy	8 years	IP	In situ thrombosis of SPA and veins	Biopsy
2	6, F	NB	Surgical resection + AutoPBSCT (2) + high-dose chemotherapy	7 days	IP, PVOD	In situ thrombosis of SPA and veins	Biopsy
3	2, F	ALL	Umbilical cord blood transplant (2) + high-dose chemotherapy	10 days	PAH, Congenital protein C deficiency	In situ thrombosis of SPA	Biopsy
4	2, M	RMS	Chemotherapy + Proton therapy	During chemotherapy	Hepatic venoocclusive disease [unknown]	In situ thrombosis of SPA and veins	Autopsy
5	5, M	Burkitt's Lymphoma	Chemotherapy	During chemotherapy	PVOD [refractory right HF]	PVOD	Autopsy
6	3, M	MB	Surgical resection + chemotherapy	9 months	s/o PAH, PVOD [IP]	IPAH, IP	Autopsy
7	2, F	AML	Allogeneic bone marrow transplant + high-dose chemotherapy	2 months	s/o PVOD, cGVHD [IP]	Plexogenic arteriopathy, IP	Autopsy

ALL = acute lymphocytic leukemia; AML = acute myelogenous leukemia; AutoPBSCT = autologous peripheral blood stem cell transplantation; cGVHD = chronic graft versus host disease; F = female; HF = heart failure; IP = interstitial pneumonia; IPAH = idiopathic pulmonary arterial hypertension; M = male; MB = medulloblastoma; NB = neuroblastoma; PAH = pulmonary arterial hypertension; PH = pulmonary hypertension; PVOD = pulmonary venoocclusive disease; RMS = rhabdomyosarcoma; SPA = small pulmonary arteries.

[13]. All protocols were conducted in compliance with the Helsinki Declaration. They were also approved by the Ethical Committee of the Japanese Research Institute of Pulmonary Vasculature and each referred hospital. Informed consent was obtained from all patients.

3. Results

The clinical and pathological characteristics of patients who developed PH after chemotherapy are presented in Table 1. Most patients (6/7) were young children (2–6 years old), including 4 lethal cases. The time interval between chemotherapy and the onset of PH varied from a few days to years. Histopathological analysis revealed that the cause of unexplained PH was in situ thrombosis in the small pulmonary arteries in 4 of 7 patients (cases 1–4). In the other 3 patients (cases 5–7), the pathological diagnoses were PVOD, IPAH, and plexogenic arteriopathy. In case 3, congenital partial protein C deficiency, which causes a clotting disorder, was detected after lung biopsy as the result of intensive examination to investigate the cause of thrombi. However, the others (cases 1, 2, and 4) had no thrombotic diathesis. The clinical findings of patients (cases 1–4), who were pathologically diagnosed with in situ thrombosis in small pulmonary arteries, are shown in Table 2.

A 46-year-old man (case 1) underwent surgery and chemotherapy for primary testicular malignant lymphoma at

the age of 38 years and remained in remission after treatment. He began to experience shortness of breath on exertion and was hospitalized due to suspicion of diffusive lung disease. Detailed examination showed no evidence of cancer recurrence. Computed tomography of the chest demonstrated ground-glass opacity. No myocardial disease was noted on the echocardiogram. Right catheterization showed tapering vascular shadows of both upper lungs, with a mean pulmonary artery pressure (PAP) of 30 mmHg. Transbronchial lung biopsy revealed mild inflammatory cell infiltration but did not yield a definite diagnosis. Therefore, video-assisted thoracic surgery was performed. Histopathology revealed long-term and extensive in situ thrombosis in the small pulmonary arteries (Figure 1(a)) and pulmonary veins (Figure 1(b)). Both the small pulmonary arteries and veins exhibited recanalization of organized fibrotic thrombi, with the lumen separated into several channels. Some small pulmonary arteries (>100 μm in diameter) showed luminal narrowing and occlusion by longitudinal smooth muscle (Figure 1(c)). There was mild inflammatory cell infiltration, but no evidence of vasculitis. Laboratory data confirmed the absence of vasculitis syndrome or coagulation disorder. The respiratory symptoms gradually improved with oxygen therapy.

A 6-year-old girl (case 2) presented with abdominal distention and abdominal pain. A biopsy specimen of the abdominal wall showed primary right adrenal neuroblastoma. Therefore, chemotherapy for neuroblastoma was initiated

TABLE 2: Clinical findings of patients with in situ thrombosis.

Case	Clinical symptoms	Computed tomography	Echocardiography	PAG	Clinical outcome
1	DOE	Ground-glass opacity Diffuse patchy nodular interstitial opacity	Normal	Tapering vascular shadow of both upper lungs, mPAP = 30 mmHg	Oxygen therapy → improved
2	Polypnoea, hypoxemia	Ground-glass opacity Pleural effusion	mPAP = 70–75, 55 mmHg (under NO), RVH	—	Diuretics → severe PH → NO, PDE5i, PGI2 → anticoagulants → improved
3	DOE, hypoxemia, polypnoea,	Ground-glass opacity	mPAP = 40–50 mmHg	—	NO, PDE5i, PGI2 → anticoagulants, antithrombotic drugs → improved
4	Hypoxemia, sudden chest-abdominal pain	—	mPAP = 50–55 mmHg	—	Oxygen → sudden cardiopulmonary arrest (death)

DOE = dyspnea on exertion; mPAP = mean pulmonary artery pressure; PAG = pulmonary angiography; PDE5i = cGMP-specific phosphodiesterase type 5 inhibitor; PGI2 = prostaglandin I2; PH = pulmonary hypertension; RVH = right ventricular enlargement.

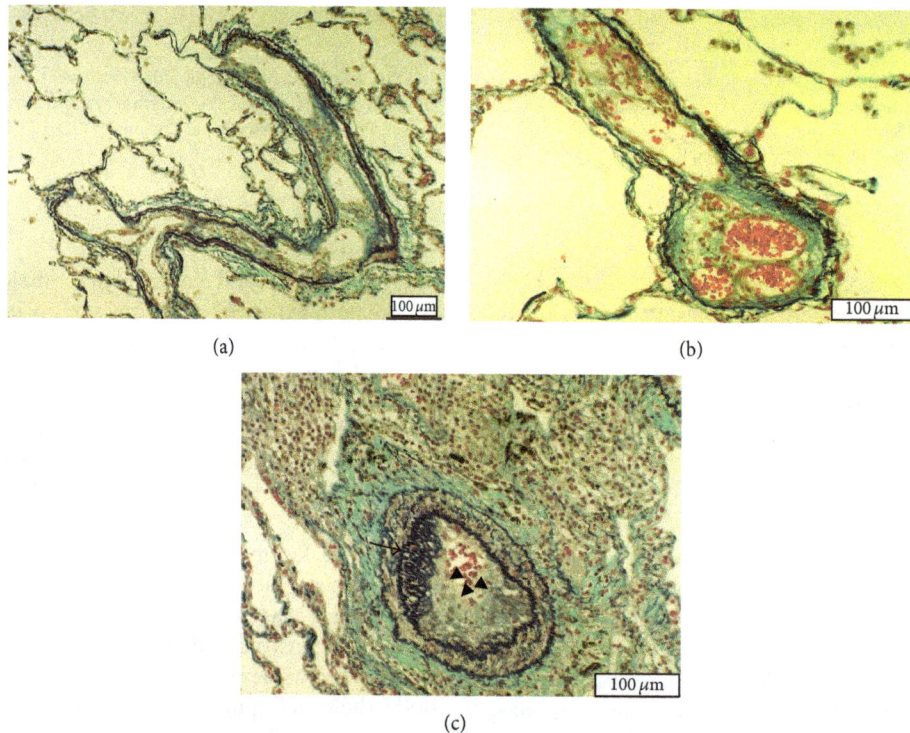

(a)

(b)

(c)

FIGURE 1: Histopathological findings of lung tissue section obtained from case 1 visualized by Elastica-Goldner staining. (a) Small pulmonary artery containing old thrombi. The lumen is separated into several channels by recanalization of organized thrombi. (b) Pulmonary vein with the recanalized thrombus separating the lumen into 3 channels. (c) Small pulmonary artery (200 μm in diameter) with moderate medial thickening and longitudinal smooth muscle proliferation inside the lumen (arrow). The thrombus is shown in the lumen (triangular arrow).

according to the protocol of the inpatient facility. After the fourth course of chemotherapy, tumorectomy was performed, followed by autologous peripheral blood stem cell transplantation (auto-PBSCT) and high-dose chemotherapy. Soon after completion of the second auto-PBSCT and

high-dose chemotherapy, the patient exhibited polypnea and hypoxemia. Chest radiographic examination revealed moderate pleural effusion. As assessed by echocardiography, mean PAP was 40 mmHg. Hypoxia was improved by the administration of diuretics. However, 1 week later, the patient

(a)

(b)

(c)

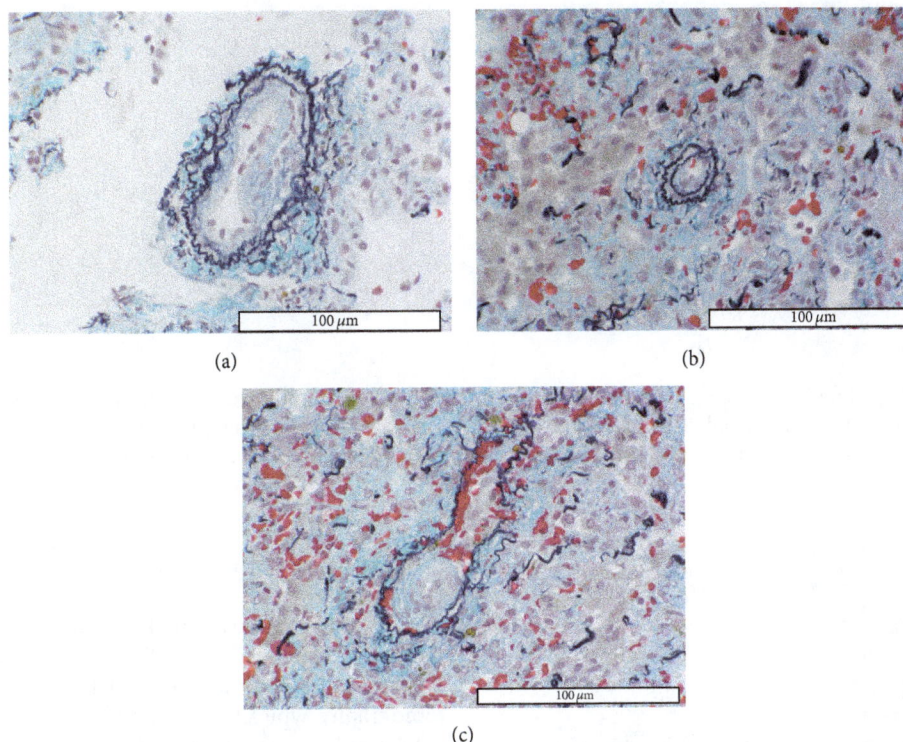

FIGURE 2: Histopathological findings in small pulmonary arteries and pulmonary veins of case 2. (a) Peripheral small pulmonary artery with newly formed eccentric intimal fibrous proliferation considered to be a thrombus, because intimal lesions usually form concentric layers in plexogenic arteriopathy. (b) The peripheral small pulmonary artery (40 μm in diameter) shows complete occlusion by a thrombus. (c) Most small pulmonary veins are almost occluded by newly formed thrombi.

exhibited polypnea, tachycardia, aggravated hypoxemia, and chest pain. Echocardiography showed PH (mean PAP = 70–75 mmHg) and right ventricular enlargement. Mean PAP decreased to 55 mmHg under nitric oxide (NO) inhalation but increased again after NO withdrawal, despite the administration of sildenafil and epoprostenol. Therefore, lung biopsy was performed for suspected PVOD. The small pulmonary arteries (>150 μm in diameter) showed no intimal proliferation but severe medial thickening (HE classification: I). Pathological findings revealed that small pulmonary arteries and veins (<30–50 μm in diameter) were almost completely occluded by newly formed thrombi not yet organized (Figures 2(a)–2(c)). The lung parenchyma presented atelectasis and cellular thickening of the alveolar wall. The patient is currently followed-up with additional administration of anticoagulants.

A 2-year-old girl (case 3) was diagnosed with acute lymphocytic leukemia (ALL) at the age of 5 months. She received high-dose chemotherapy and umbilical cord blood transplants. After the second transplant, the patient had a documented PH crisis at the age of 22 months. The respiratory symptoms were effectively relieved by NO inhalation, followed by sildenafil and beraprost administration. Echocardiography showed PH (mean PAP = 40–50 mmHg), without any myocardial disease. Therefore, PAH was suspected based on the clinical findings. Lung biopsy was performed to verify

the diagnosis. Microscopically, the small pulmonary arteries showed mild medial thickening but no intimal proliferation (HE classification: I). However, thrombi at varying stages were found in almost all peripheral small-sized pulmonary arteries (Figure 3(a)). Most thrombi were still in the process of formation (Figure 3(b)). In contrast, the pulmonary veins and respiratory system appeared normal. The detailed examination to investigate the cause of these thrombi was carried out based upon the above described lung biopsy findings, and partial congenital protein C deficiency was detected. PH was successfully controlled with anticoagulants and antithrombotic agents.

A 2-year-old boy (case 4) with rhabdomyosarcoma started receiving chemotherapy at the age of 17 months, and he developed hepatic venoocclusive disease during treatment. At the age of 24 months, he became dyspneic with hypoxemia. Mild PH was detected on the electrocardiogram and echocardiogram. After a few weeks of oxygen therapy, he experienced sudden chest-abdominal pain and died of sudden cardiopulmonary arrest at the hospital at the age of 26 months. Postmortem examination of the lungs was performed to determine the cause of death. The small pulmonary arteries (>200 μm in diameter) showed moderate medial thickening without intimal lesion (HE classification: I). Some small pulmonary arteries (<100 μm in diameter) and pulmonary veins showed intimal fibrous proliferation (Figure 4). They were

(a)

(b)

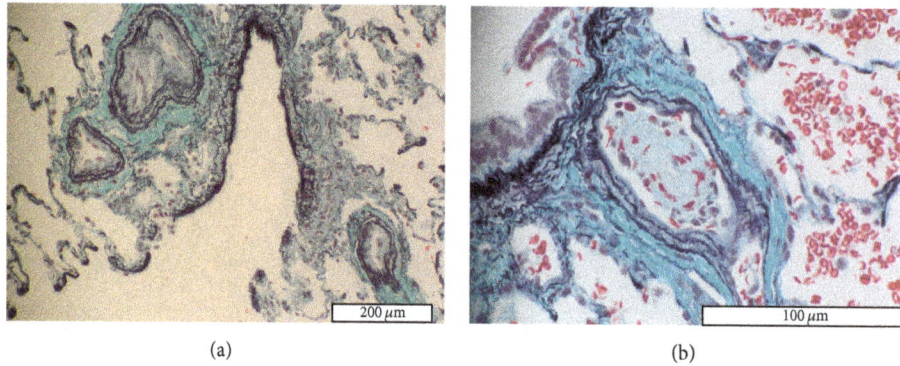

FIGURE 3: Histopathological findings in small pulmonary arteries and pulmonary veins of case 3. (a) Almost all small pulmonary arteries have mildly thickened media and are occluded by thrombi. (b) Peripheral small pulmonary artery showing almost completely occluded by a newly formed thrombus. Most thrombi shown in small pulmonary arteries are in the process of being formed.

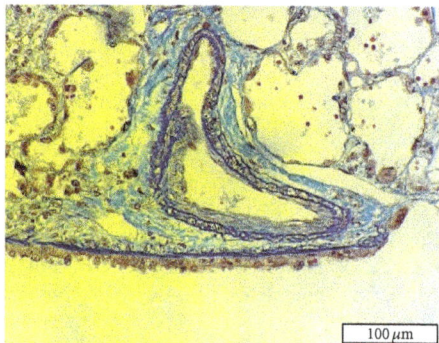

FIGURE 4: Histopathological findings in a small pulmonary artery of the right lung of case 4. This small pulmonary artery has moderate medial thickening and eccentric intimal fibrous proliferation (thrombus).

considered to be thrombi because of the eccentric intimal thickening. Small peripheral pulmonary arteries (<50 μm in diameter) showed complete occlusion by thrombi.

4. Discussion

This is the first study reporting in situ thrombosis in the small pulmonary arteries of patients who developed PH after chemotherapy. In contrast, several studies have reported PH due to PVOD after stem cell transplantation or chemotherapy [1–3]. We also diagnosed in 1 patient (case 5) that the cause of unexplained PH developing after chemotherapy was PVOD [4]. The histopathology of PVOD typically shows extensive occlusion of pulmonary veins by intimal fibrosis [14] in the form of concentric layers [6, 7]. The present cases (cases 1–4) exhibited a distinct pattern of thrombosis in pulmonary veins and small pulmonary arteries characterized by localized and eccentric intimal fibrosis. In addition, the fibrosis was associated with recanalization of the organized thrombi by separating the lumen into several channels. In contrast, plexogenic pulmonary arteriopathy, which is typically seen in PH patients, was hardly seen in all patients with in situ

thrombosis in the small pulmonary arteries even with high PAP readings.

In situ thrombosis in the small pulmonary arteries is difficult to diagnose from clinical examination due to non-specific complaints and from laboratory data. Computed tomography typically shows diffuse ground-grass opacities, patchy pulmonary opacity, atelectasis, and pleural effusion. Even with these diagnostic radiological findings, it is difficult to distinguish in situ thrombosis from other pathological conditions that can exhibit similar symptoms, such as PVOD and interstitial pneumonia. In cases 5–7, histopathological examination identified that the causes of PH were PVOD, IPAH, and interstitial pneumonia, whereas clinical findings in these cases were not distinguishable from those with in situ thrombosis. When patients undergoing antitumor chemotherapy present unexplained PH, lung disease and myocardial dysfunction should be ruled out, whereas PVOD and in situ thrombosis should be considered as differential diagnoses. Considering these facts, lung biopsy is necessary for accurate diagnosis for some patients with unexplained PH. In addition, thrombogenic factors should be investigated because some patients may develop thrombotic diathesis [15], as in case 3.

Patient 1 had mild symptoms, likely because the thrombi had developed over several years. Microscopically, organized thrombi with recanalization were found in small pulmonary arteries and veins. The direct cause of PH might be respiratory diseases, because longitudinal smooth muscles appeared under hypoxia. Therefore oxygen therapy was effective in this case. The background of organized fibrotic thrombi, which seem to have been formed a few years previously, might accelerate the bloodstream aggravation in pulmonary circulation, although the symptom was not recognized at the time of thrombosis formation. In cases 2 and 3, anticoagulants and antithrombotic agents were effective treatments for in situ thrombosis. In these cases, sudden PH resistance to pulmonary vasodilators including NO occurred, which indicated that thrombi were forming at that moment. Incidentally, histopathology revealed that small pulmonary arteries were almost completely occluded due to forming or newly formed thrombi. Thus, this wave of new thrombi caused

PH to progress rapidly. In such cases, anticoagulants and antithrombotic agents have played a crucial role in survival. Interestingly, in situ thrombosis in small pulmonary arteries is one of the pathological features of PSVS [7]. These patients with PSVS responded very well to prostaglandin E1 treatment. This study suggests that prostaglandin E1 might be an effective therapy for in situ thrombosis in the small pulmonary arteries. Possible hazard to institute anticoagulation and antithrombotic therapy may include lung hemorrhage in the presence of PVOD, which can be avoided by accurate diagnosis with lung biopsy. The most efficient therapy for PVOD is, in fact, currently lung transplant. In contrast, in situ thrombosis can possibly be treated by pharmacotherapy. Regardless, initiation of treatment should not be delayed to avoid a fatal outcome as in case 4. As early diagnosis and treatment is crucial for this disease, clinicians should keep in mind that in situ thrombosis may induce the development of PH. The lung biopsy is currently the sole diagnostic method to identify in situ thrombosis in the small pulmonary arteries.

These studies apparently have significant limitations. First, this report is consisted of small series of selected patients. However, it should be noted that in situ thrombosis in the small pulmonary arteries was detected as the possible cause of PH after chemotherapy in 4 of 7 patients. Secondly, assessment of lung biopsy was carried out only once for each patient; therefore, serial changes could not be elucidated. The precise pathogenesis of in situ thrombosis is small pulmonary arteries still remains unknown.

5. Conclusions

The present study demonstrates that in situ thrombosis in the small pulmonary arteries is one of the causative mechanisms for PH developing during chemotherapy. Further research is required to elucidate the pathogenesis of PH after chemotherapy.

Conflict of Interests

The authors declare that there is no conflict of interests regarding the publication of this paper.

Acknowledgment

The authors are grateful to the following cardiovascular institutes in Japan for the supply of materials: Departments of Pediatric Hematology and Oncology and Pediatric Cardiology, at the Okinawa Prefectural Nanbu Medical Center and Children's Medical Center; Department of Respiratory Medicine at the Miyagi Cardiovascular and Respiratory Center; Department of Pediatrics at the Tsukuba University Hospital; Department of Cardiology at the Kanagawa Children's Medical Center; Department of Pediatrics at the Miyazaki University Hospital.

References

[1] A. G. Rose, "Pulmonary veno-occlusive disease due to bleomycin therapy for lymphoma. Case reports," *South African Medical Journal*, vol. 64, no. 16, pp. 636–638, 1983.

[2] S. M. Palmer, L. J. Robinson, A. Wang, J. R. Gossage, T. Bashore, and V. F. Tapson, "Massive pulmonary edema and death after prostacyclin infusion in a patient with pulmonary veno-occlusive disease," *Chest*, vol. 113, no. 1, pp. 237–240, 1998.

[3] R. E. Waldhorn, E. Tsou, F. P. Smith, and D. M. Kerwin, "Pulmonary veno-occlusive disease associated with microangiopathic hemolytic anemia and chemotherapy of gastric adenocarcinoma," *Medical and Pediatric Oncology*, vol. 12, no. 6, pp. 394–396, 1984.

[4] D. Miyata, T. Fukushima, M. Matsunaga et al., "Fatal pulmonary veno-occlusive disease after chemotherapy for Burkitt's lymphoma," *Pediatrics International*, vol. 53, no. 3, pp. 403–405, 2011.

[5] S. Yamaki, "Pulmonary vascular disease associated with pulmonary hypertension in 445 patients: diagnosis from lung biopsy and autopsy," *General Thoracic and Cardiovascular Surgery*, vol. 61, no. 1, pp. 24–31, 2013.

[6] S. Yamaki, M. Ando, Y. Fukumoto et al., "Histopathological examination by lung biopsy for the evaluation of operability and postoperative prognosis in patients with chronic thromboembolic pulmonary hypertension," *Circulation Journal*, vol. 78, no. 2, pp. 476–482, 2014.

[7] T. Ohno, J. Muneuchi, K. Ihara et al., "Pulmonary hypertension in patients with congenital portosystemic venous shunt: a previously unrecognized association," *Pediatrics*, vol. 121, no. 4, pp. e892–e899, 2008.

[8] S. Yamaki and C. A. Wagenvoort, "Comparison of primary plexogenic arteriopathy in adults and children," *British Heart Journal*, vol. 54, no. 4, pp. 428–434, 1985.

[9] K. Maeda, S. Yamaki, H. Kado, T. Asou, A. Murakami, and S. Takamoto, "Hypoplasia of the small pulmonary arteries in hypoplastic left heart syndrome with restrictive atrial septal defect," *Circulation*, vol. 110, no. 11, supplement 1, pp. II-139–II-146, 2004.

[10] S. Yamaki, M. Kumate, S. Yonesaka, K. Maeda, M. Endo, and K. Tabayashi, "Lung biopsy diagnosis of operative indication in secundum atrial septal defect with severe pulmonary vascular disease," *Chest*, vol. 126, no. 4, pp. 1042–1047, 2004.

[11] S. Yamaki and C. A. Wagenvoort, "Plexogenic pulmonary arteriopathy. Significance of medial thickness with respect to advanced pulmonary vascular lesions," *The American Journal of Pathology*, vol. 105, no. 1, pp. 70–74, 1981.

[12] D. Heath and J. E. Edwards, "The pathology of hypertensive pulmonary vascular disease; a description of six grades of structural changes in the pulmonary arteries with special reference to congenital cardiac septal defects," *Circulation*, vol. 18, no. 4, pp. 533–547, 1958.

[13] J. Goldner, "A modification of the Masson trichrome technique for the routine laboratory purposes," *The American Journal of Pathology*, vol. 14, no. 2, pp. 237–243, 1938.

[14] C. A. Wagenvoort, N. Wagenvoort, and T. Takahashi, "Pulmonary veno-occlusive disease: involvement of pulmonary arteries and review of the literature," *Human Pathology*, vol. 16, no. 10, pp. 1033–1041, 1985.

[15] Y. Katsumura and K.-I. Ohtsubo, "Association between pulmonary microthromboembolism and coagulation variables in hypercoagulable states: an autopsy study," *Respirology*, vol. 4, no. 3, pp. 239–243, 1999.

19

Sleep Disordered Breathing in Children with Mitochondrial Disease

Ricardo A. Mosquera,[1] Mary Kay Koenig,[1] Rahmat B. Adejumo,[1] Justyna Chevallier,[1] S. Shahrukh Hashmi,[1] Sarah E. Mitchell,[2] Susan E. Pacheco,[1] and Cindy Jon[1,2]

[1]Department of Pediatrics, University of Texas Medical School, Houston, TX 77030, USA
[2]Memorial Hermann Memorial City Hospital, Pediatric Sleep Center, Houston, TX 77030, USA

Correspondence should be addressed to Ricardo A. Mosquera; ricardo.a.mosquera@uth.tmc.edu

Academic Editor: Demosthenes Bouros

A retrospective chart review study was performed to determine the presence of sleep disordered breathing (SDB) in children with primary mitochondrial disease (MD). The symptoms, sleep-related breathing, and movement abnormalities are described for 18 subjects (ages 1.5 to 18 years, 61% male) with MD who underwent polysomnography in our pediatric sleep center from 2007 to 2012. Of the 18 subjects with MD, the common indications for polysomnography were excessive somnolence or fatigue (61%, $N = 11$), snoring (44%, $N = 8$), and sleep movement complaints (17%, $N = 3$). Polysomnographic measurements showed SDB in 56% ($N = 10$) (obstructive sleep apnea in 60% ($N = 6$), hypoxemia in 40% ($N = 4$), and sleep hypoventilation in 20% ($N = 2$)). There was a significant association between decreased muscle tone and SDB (P: 0.043) as well as obese and overweight status with SDB ($P = 0.036$). SDB is common in subjects with MD. Early detection of SDB, utilizing polysomnography, should be considered to assist in identification of MD patients who may benefit from sleep-related interventions.

1. Introduction

SDB is characterized by recurrent, partial, or complete cessation in breathing that disrupts normal sleep. SDB represents a spectrum of disorders that vary from simple snoring to complete upper airway closure as seen in obstructive sleep apnea (OSA) syndrome. SDB may also include central sleep apnea (CSA), prolonged hypoxemia, and hypoventilation.

The prevalence of SDB in children varies from 1.2 to 13.9%, depending on the definition used and the method of data collection [1–4]. OSA syndrome has been estimated to be present in 1 to 2% of healthy children [5] and reports of habitual snoring vary from 4 to 34.5% in the general pediatric population [6–9].

Polysomnography identifies and quantifies sleep disturbances and is the standard method to diagnose SDB [10]. Accurate diagnosis is crucial and therapeutic interventions should be promptly initiated, as untreated SDB is associated with significant morbidity, including somatic growth impairment, poor cognitive and behavioral development, and metabolic and cardiovascular derangements [11].

Primary mitochondrial disorders (MD) are a group of inherited multisystem disorders that impair oxidative phosphorylation and create a deficiency of cellular ATP. The symptoms are varied and many organ systems are involved [12]. Approximately 45% of pediatric patients with MD first present with a neuromuscular problem [13, 14]; however, the character and degree of neuromuscular impairment are poorly defined. Fatigue and hypotonia were the most prevalent symptoms reported in children in the study done by Koene et al. [15]. The association between SDB and neuromuscular disease (NMD) has been reported; 27–62% of children with NMD have SDB [16–19]. Current guidelines recommend that sleep specialists evaluate patients with sleep disturbance and NMD with polysomnography to identify and treat SDB [20–23]. SDB in children with primary MD has not been defined. Although the exact incidence of MD remains unknown, the prevalence of MD is higher than many of the more recognized inherited NMDs, such as Duchenne's muscular dystrophy [12]. Recommendations regarding polysomnography do not exist for patients with MD, even though they may have a high potential to develop SDB. In this study, we describe the polysomnographic findings of sleep disturbances, including SDB, in 18 subjects with primary MD.

2. Material and Methods

A retrospective chart review of pediatric patients between the ages of 15 months and 18 years with primary mitochondrial disorder (MD) who were treated at the University of Texas Houston Mitochondrial Center was conducted (Table 1). Patients were diagnosed with MD using the modified Walker criteria [24]. Between 2007 and 2012, 18 subjects with MD who had complete diagnostic polysomnograms secondary to sleep complaints were identified. The modified Epworth sleepiness scale assessed sleepiness but was only documented in 3 patients [25].

Each of the 18 subjects underwent a fully attended nocturnal PSG with videographic monitoring for one night at Memorial Hermann Hospital. Prior to performing the PSG, informed consent and basic past medical history from each subject's parent/guardian were obtained. Height and weight were measured and recorded; tonsillar size and oropharyngeal dimensions using the Mallampati classification system were documented in most patients.

Sleep montage surface electrode sites included F3, F4, C3, C4, O1, O2, M1, M2, right EOG, left EOG, chin EMG, anterior tibialis EMG, and EKG. Snoring was recorded using a snore sensor and audible snoring was noted by the sleep technologist. A thermocouple and nasal pressure transducer recorded nasal and oral airflow. Thoracic and abdominal respiratory effort was measured using impedance plethysmography belts. End tidal carbon dioxide (ETCO2) was measured by capnography via nasal sensors. Oxygen saturation (SpO2) was monitored by a pulse oximeter. All signals were recorded using the Rembrandt (Embla Systems, Kanata, ON, Canada) digital acquisition system.

Each PSG was scored by a sleep technician and then interpreted by a board certified sleep physician. Stages of sleep, respiratory events, arousals, and limb movements were all scored according to the pediatric rules in the 2007 *American Academy of Sleep Medicine (AASM) Manual for the Scoring of Sleep and Associated Events* [26]. Apneas were defined as cessation of oral and nasal airflow for at least 2 breaths as compared to the patient's baseline breathing pattern. Apneas were further categorized as obstructive, central, or mixed. Obstructive apneas occurred when there was no airflow for at least 2 breaths with corresponding respiratory effort. Central apneas were identified if there was no airflow or corresponding respiratory effort for ≥20 seconds or at least 2 breaths if there was an associated arousal from sleep, awakening, or ≥3% oxygen desaturation. Mixed apneas were detected if there was no airflow without corresponding respiratory effort which resumed before the end of the apnea. Hypopneas were scored if the peak to trough airflow was decreased by ≥50% for 2 or more breath cycles and the event was accompanied by ≥3% desaturation and/or caused an arousal from sleep. Respiratory effort related arousal (RERA) was scored if there was <50% decrease in the amplitude of nasal pressure signal compared to baseline, flattening of the nasal

pressure waveform, accompanying snoring, noisy breathing, elevation in ETCO2, transcutaneous CO2, or visual evidence of increased work of breathing that persisted for ≥2 breath cycles. Periodic limb movements (PLM) were scored if four or more appeared consecutively within a 90-second interval.

The following indices were calculated with respect to the total sleep time (TST) in hours.

(i) Apnea hypopnea index (AHI) = all apneas + all hypopneas.

(ii) Obstructive AHI = obstructive apneas + mixed apneas + obstructive hypopneas.

(iii) Obstructive apnea index (AI) = obstructive and mixed apneas.

(iv) Central apnea index (CAI) = central apneas.

(v) Respiratory disturbance index (RDI) = all apneas + all hypopneas + RERA.

OSA was defined using the *International Classification of Sleep Disorders 2nd Edition (ICSD-2)* [27]. Central sleep apnea (CSA) was identified when CAI was >3 events per hour of TST [28]; sleep hypoventilation was detected when ETCO2 > 50 torr for >25% of TST [26]; hypoxemia was defined as oxygen saturation <90% for >2% of TST [29]. SDB was present if there was a respiratory disturbance index (RDI) of ≥5 events per hour of TST or presence of OSA, CSA, sleep hypoventilation, or sleep hypoxemia [30]. Periodic limb movement (PLM) index was relevant if there were >5 PLMs per hour of TST [26]. Primary snoring was diagnosed if the patient demonstrated snoring during the PSG in the absence of SDB.

Muscle tone is defined as the muscle's resistance to passive stretch during the resting state. Tone helps to maintain posture and multiple disease states can alter muscle tone. Low tone is a decreased resistance to passive motion and high tone is an increased resistance to passive motion. Tone was assessed in our study population by a board certified pediatric neurologist. The observed tone of each subject was classified into three groups: hypotonia (low tone), normal tone, and hypertonia (increased tone). Results are presented in Table 1.

Ten patients had spirometry testing (Breeze Suite 6.4, Medical Graphics Corporation, St. Paul, MN), as per American Thoracic Society guidelines [31], within a 12-month period from the polysomnography. Predicted normative values were based on Knudson et al. published data [32]. Spirometry results were interpreted by two pediatric pulmonologists, as having presence of a normal, obstructive, restrictive, or mixed restrictive/obstructive airflow pattern.

The MD patients analyzed in this study were referred to The University of Texas Medical School Houston, Division of Pulmonary Medicine by the University's Mitochondrial Center. This study was approved at inception by the Committee for the Protection of Human Subjects (CPHS# HSC-MS-13-0622).

2.1. Analysis. Frequencies with percentages were calculated for all categorical variables. Continuous variables were

TABLE 1: Patient demographics, allergic rhinitis history, adenotonsillar history, and neuromuscular tone characteristics in patients with mitochondrial disorder.

ID	Gender	Age (years) at PSG	Race/ethnicity	BMI in kg/m² (percentile)	Allergic rhinitis by history	Tonsil & adenoid history	NM Tone	Spirometry
1	F	9	W NH	17.2 (50–75%)	Y	2+	Normal	Mixed
2	M	6	W NH	15.5 (75%)	N	N	Normal	Normal
3	M	3	W NH	13.3 (90%)	N	4+, A	Hypotonia	Normal
5	M	2	W NH	12.3 (<3%)	Y	3+	Normal	—
6	F	12	W NH	26.8 (95–97%)	Y	T & A	Hypotonia	Normal
7	M	16	W NH	23.7 (75–85%)	Y	N	Hypotonia	Normal
8	M	10	W NH	18.7 (75%)	N	T & A	Normal	—
9	M	2	W NH	19.4 (>97%)	N	N	Hypertonia	—
10	F	2	W NH	15.4 (25%)	N	Y	Hypotonia	—
11	M	5	W NH	14.2 (10%)	N	Y	Normal	Normal
12	M	7	W NH	29.6 (>97%)	N	N	Hypotonia	Normal
13	F	5	W Hispanic	22.0 (>97%)	N	T & A	Hypotonia	Normal
14	M	1.5	W NH	18.8	N	N	Severe hypotonia	—
15	F	3.5	W NH	15.7 (50%)	N	N	Hypertonia	—
16	F	2	W Hispanic	16.3 (50%)	N	N	Hypertonia with cogwheel	—
17	M	16	W NH	15.8 (<3%)	N	N	Normal	—
18	M	18	W NH	22.5 (50%)	N	N	Hypotonia	Restrictive
19	F	11	W NH	18.0 (50%)	Y	N	Hypotonia	Normal

PSG: polysomnogram, W: white, NH: non-Hispanic, H: Hispanic, BMI: body mass index, T & A: posttonsillectomy, A: postadenoidectomy, NM: neuromuscular, MD: mitochondrial disorder, Y: yes, N: no or none, and ESS: Epworth sleepiness scale.

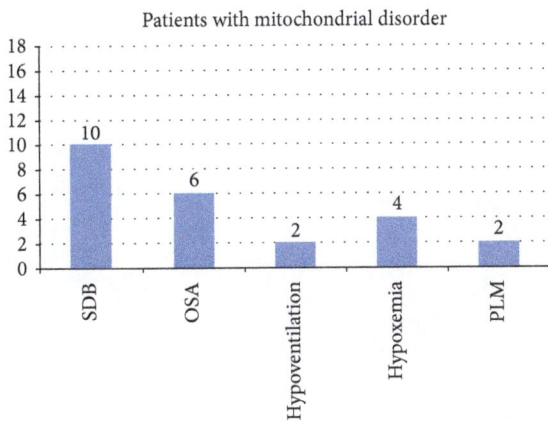

FIGURE 1: Sleep disordered breathing characteristics in 18 patients with mitochondrial disorders.

described using means (with standard deviation, SD) or medians (with interquartile ranges, IQR) for normal and non-normal data distributions, respectively. Categorical variables were compared using Fisher exact test or chi-square test, as appropriate. All statistics were performed using STATA v.12 (College Station, TX). Statistical significance was assumed at a type I error rate of 0.05.

3. Results

3.1. Symptoms. The common symptoms prompting polysomnography were parental or self-reported excessive daytime somnolence/fatigue in 11 (61%), snoring in 8 (44%), and sleep movement in 3 (17%) subjects (Table 2). Sleep movement complaints consisted of muscle jerks. Of the 8 subjects that reported snoring, only 4 were corroborated by polysomnography.

3.2. Sleep Architecture. The average total sleep time (TST) and total test time (TTT) were 6.8 hours (SD: 0.7 hours) and 8.1 hours (0.6 hours), respectively. The median sleep stage time as percentage of TST was 3.1% (IQR: 1.8–4.6) for stage N1 sleep, 53.5% (IQR: 44.1–61.8) for stage N2 sleep, 22.8% (IQR: 20.0–30.3) for stage N3 sleep, and 16.6% (1.8–22.3) for rapid eye movement (REM) sleep.

3.3. Respiratory Events. In total, 10 (56%) subjects had SDB due to either presence of OSA, CSA, hypoventilation, and hypoxemia or an RDI ≥ 5 (Figure 1). The 2 subjects with the highest RDI (47.9/hour and 10.4/hour) had a complex I mitochondrial defect. The only patient with Leigh syndrome had sleep hypoxemia.

Of the 10 subjects with MD and SDB, 6 demonstrated (60%) OSA (Figure 1) with an average obstructive AHI of 2.7/hour with an obstructive AI of 0.7/hour. There were no patients with CSA, since all patients had CAI that was less than 1.4 per hour. Four subjects with SDB (40%) were noted to have sleep hypoxemia with an average of 5.1% of TST < 90% saturation.

Based on 2007 AASM scoring criteria [26], 2 subjects with SDB (20%) demonstrated sleep hypoventilation with ETCO2 > 50 torr for >25% of TST. There were 3 other children with elevated ETCO2 (>50 torr) that was not diagnostic for sleep hypoventilation but was thought to contribute to their symptoms. Subject 13 had elevated ETCO2 for 22.8% of TST, subject 2 had elevated ETCO2 for 17.6% of TST, and subject 14's ETCO2 was elevated for 10.5% of TST.

Of the 5 patients with clinical history of allergic rhinitis, none were diagnosed with SDB. There were 5 subjects with enlarged tonsils, of which only 2 were considered to have SDB. Of the 3 subjects who had previously had an adenotonsillectomy, 2 had SDB. Of note, both of the subjects who continued with SDB after their adenotonsillectomy were obese.

Based on the Centers for Disease Control (CDC) definition of obesity (BMI of >95 percentile for age) and overweight (BMI of 85–95 percentile for age) in children, 4 (22%) of the patients were designated as obese and 1 (6%) was overweight. All of the obese and overweight patients were diagnosed with SDB. Two (11%) were noted to be underweight with BMI of <3% for age, of which 1 had SDB.

3.4. Movement Events. Two subjects (11%) were found to have elevated PLMI > 5/hour. Neither had sleep movement complaints as indicators for polysomnography.

3.5. Muscle Tone. Twelve of the 18 subjects (67%) who underwent PSG had abnormal muscle tone (Table 1). Of the 10 patients with SDB, 9 (90%) had abnormal tone. Specifically, 6 had hypotonia and 3 had hypertonia. There was a significant association between abnormal muscle tone and SDB in the study (*P* value = 0.043).

3.6. Spirometry. Ten patients had available spirometric data, of which 8 were noted to have normal airflow pattern, 1 was noted to have restrictive pattern, and 1 was noted to have mixed restrictive/obstructive airflow pattern. Of the 10 patients who underwent spirometry, 4 patients had SDB, all of which were noted to have normal airflow patterns.

4. Discussion

As expected, in the current study, we found a high incidence of SDB in children with MD undergoing nocturnal PSG. SDB was present in 56% of the subjects, compared to 1.2–13.9% in general population [1]. The most common SDB finding was OSA (60%), followed by hypoxemia (40%) and sleep hypoventilation (20%). In addition, elevated PLMI was detected in 11% of the subjects. The basis of this finding could be the result of reduced activity of respiratory muscles during sleep or an intrinsic disorder that has not been characterized in the study population. To the best of our knowledge, this is the first study that describes SDB in children with MD.

OSA was found in 60% of subjects with SDB and MD. In this study, pediatric OSA was designated using the ICSD-2 definition [27]. The authors contend that an obstructive AHI of ≥1 per hour may overestimate the incidence of OSA,

TABLE 2: Polysomnographic indications, test time, respiratory data, and limb movement description in patients with mitochondrial disorder.

ID	PSG indication	TTT	TST	Snoring	Obstructive AI	Obstructive AHI	CAI	Total AHI	RDI	% TST ETCO2 >50 torr	% TST SpO2 <90%	PLM index
1	Snoring, EDS	8.0	7.0	N	0	0	0.3	0.3	0.3	0	0	0
2	EDS, inattention at school, snoring	8.2	6.7	Y	0	0.9	0.5	1.4	1.6	17.6	0.8	5.6
3	EDS, inattention at school	9.1	5.1	N	0.2	0.2	0	0.2	6.3	0	0	0
5	Restless sleep	8.0	7.2	N	0	0	0.4	0.4	0.4	0	0.1	0
6	EDS	7.9	6.3	N	0.3	0.6	0	0.6	1.9	97.2	0.1	0
7	EDS	7.7	7.2	N	0	0.4	0.3	0.7	0.7	0	0.2	0
8	Snoring, witnessed apneas, inattention at school	8.1	6.8	N	0	0	0.3	0.3	0.3	0.4	0.1	0
9	Frequent nighttime awakening	8.2	6.9	Y	0.1	1.3	0.1	1.5	1.6	0.1	0.2	0
10	Frequent night wakening and muscle jerking episodes	7.6	6.4	N	0	0.5	1.3	1.7	2.5	0	2.7	0
11	EDS	7.4	6.6	Y	0	0.2	0.5	0.6	0.6	0	0.2	0
12	EDS, inattention at school, snoring	8.9	7.6	N	0	3.0	0.1	3.2	4.6	0.1	0	0
13	Snoring, gasping during sleep	8.9	7.9	Y	0.3	4.5	0	4.7	5.0	22.8	7.5	22.6
14	Restless sleep, muscle jerks, heavy breathing	8.6	8.1	N	0	0.6	0.7	1.4	1.6	10.5	2.9	0
15	Difficulty sleeping, EDS	7.6	7.2	Y	2.8	4.7	0.7	5.4	10.4	25.2	0.1	0
16	Snoring	7.3	5.7	N	0.9	1.1	0.2	1.2	47.9	0.4	7.4	0
17	EDS, fatigue	7.2	6.4	N	0.3	1.4	0.3	1.7	13.6	0	0.6	0
18	Snoring, morning headaches, EDS	7.2	6.4	Y	0	0.3	0.2	0.3	1.4	0	0	0
19	Snoring, morning headaches, EDS	8.5	7.8	Y	0.1	0.1	0	0.1	0.4	0	0	0.8

PSG: polysomnogram, TTT: total test time, TST: total sleep time, AI: apnea index, AHI: apnea hypopnea index, CAI: central apnea index, RDI: respiratory disturbance index, PLM: periodic limb movement, EDS: excessive daytime somnolence, Y: yes, and N: no.

especially since the threshold of clinically significant OSA in children has not been established. Recently, the Childhood Adenotonsillectomy Trial (CHAT) defined the threshold for OSA as an obstructive AI of ≥1 event per hour or obstructive AHI of ≥2 events per hour [33]. CHAT is the first large randomized controlled trial in the children designed to address the effectiveness of adenotonsillectomy in children with OSA syndrome in regard to polysomnographic, neurocognitive, and behavioral outcomes. If we applied the CHAT OSA definition to our patient population, OSA was detected in only 3 (30%) of the subjects with SDB and MD and the mean obstructive AHI changed from 2.7 per hour to 4.1 per hour. With either definition, the obstructive AHI was <5 per hour which is considered mild [10].

Sleep hypoventilation, defined according to the 2007 AASM criteria with $ETCO_2$ > 50 torr for >25% of total sleep time, was found in two subjects (22%). Elevated $ETCO_2$ (>50 torr), which did not meet the threshold for the AASM definition for sleep hypoventilation, was found in 3 subjects. Marcus et al. [34] demonstrated that children were more prone to hypoventilate than adults since a child's upper airway was more resistant to full closure with increasing applied negative pressure. Other factors may lead to hypoventilation, such as obesity, adenotonsillar enlargement, and abnormal muscle tone. Of the 5 patients with elevated $ETCO_2$, 2 were obese, none had tonsillar hypertrophy, and 4 had hypotonia. As such, abnormal muscle tone may be an important component of sleep hypoventilation in children with MD and SDB. Of note, 3 of the patients with elevated $ETCO_2$ had spirometric measurements which were normal. Interestingly, there were no subjects with CSA, despite a relatively low CSA threshold (CAI > 3).

To date, sleep hypoxemia has not been clearly defined in the pediatric population. The Centers for Medicare and Medicaid Services, a national social insurance program for Americans who are older than 65 years of age or are disabled, defines hypoxemia based on polysomnography in adults as SpO_2 < 88% for more than 10 minutes. For this study, we used the CHAT definition, which established the diagnostic threshold at SpO_2 < 90% for 2% of total sleep time [33]. Four subjects (40%) had sleep hypoxemia, one of which was placed on supplemental oxygen during the sleep study.

Oxygen is indispensable for the survival of all organisms due to its role in the production of ATP by mitochondria. Functional and quantitative mitochondrial dysfunction inherent to the MD could be potentially further deteriorated by SDB. Reactive oxygen species (ROS) are chemically reactive molecules containing oxygen formed as a natural byproduct of cellular metabolism. At physiologic levels, ROS play an important role in cell signaling and homeostasis but unregulated ROS can damage cell structures and incite apoptosis. Our cells have antioxidants to neutralize reactive oxygen species (ROS) produced during normal cellular functions. However, stressors such as infection, hypoxemia, and SDB increase ROS production. High levels of ROS can overwhelm the innate antioxidant capacity leading to mitochondrial dysfunction. During episodes of hypoxia, ROS function in signaling O2 supply increments to decrease oxygen consumption via AMPK activation and endocytosis. Hypoxia-

inducible factors orchestrate transcriptional responses also by promoting erythropoietin expression, augmentation of RBC production, and maintenance of ATP levels. Moreover, stimulation of vascular endothelial growth factor prompted by hypoxia leads to angiogenesis in undersupplied tissues. Therefore, shifts in quantity of ROS in either direction could alter the fragile homeostatic balance leading to pathologic alterations and disease [35]. OSA in itself may increase ROS, therefore worsening MD.

In this study, SDB was defined by the presence of OSA, CSA, hypoxemia, hypoventilation, and/or RDI > 5 per hour. In the literature, the prevalence of SDB in children varies from 1.2 to 13.9%, due to inconsistent definitions and the method of data collection [1–4]. The authors agree there is a wide and discrepant range of definitions for SDB which made a specific or concise cutoff difficult. Most publications agree that SDB encompasses OSA, CSA, hypoxemia, and hypoventilation. The authors chose RDI of >5/hour to capture presence of sleep disordered breathing, aside from the more well-defined OSA, CSA, hypoventilation, and hypoxemia. Tang et al. [30] showed that, using an RDI threshold of RDI ≥ 5/hour, the prevalence of SDB varied less (i.e., by <10%) when compared to using RDI ≤ 3/hour (varied by 1–74%).

There are multiple reasons for children with MD to develop SDB: neuromuscular abnormalities, tonsillar hypertrophy, obesity, allergic rhinitis, or the use of sedative medications [17, 36, 37]. We found inconsistent correlation between adenotonsillar hypertrophy, posttonsillectomy status, allergic rhinitis history, and SDB. Abnormal growth parameter was associated with SDB, especially when the BMI was >85% for age. OSA syndrome is estimated to be present in approximately 13–59% of obese children in the general population [38]. Obesity may contribute to upper airway narrowing due to fat deposition and restrictive respiratory function due to truncal adipose tissue deposition. In our dataset, there was an association between obesity and SDB ($P = 0.036$), with all 5 (27%, overall) of the obese patients having SDB. There was no association between obesity and abnormal muscle tone ($P = 0.114$) and the small sample size precluded any multivariate analysis. In addition, 2 out of the 3 SDB patients who had a positive history of adenotonsillectomy were obese. This is consistent with current findings in the general pediatric obese population that OSA may persist despite adenotonsillectomy [39, 40]. Excessive weight gain may be a contributing factor to development of SDB in our patient population. Two of the subjects were underweight with inconsistent association with SDB. Previous studies have also supported the fact that, contrary to the dogma that mitochondrial patients are typically malnourished, about one-third is obese [41].

Sedative medications were excluded as a contributing factor to the SDB in our study population as none of our study subjects were on such medications during the period preceding their sleep studies. Of note, fourteen out of our eighteen subjects that had an echocardiogram done within a year of their sleep study had no features suggestive of a cardiomyopathy.

The prevalence of SDB in MD has not been established. Untreated, SDB may lead to significant morbidity and increased mortality. The current study found a significant association between SDB and abnormal muscle tone in our subjects with MD. Predisposing factors to SDB in NMD include reduced ventilatory responses, reduced activity of respiratory muscles during sleep, and poor lung mechanics due to their underlying neuromuscular disorder. However, some patients with mitochondrial disease do not have neuromuscular disease or it is subtle.

Normally, during REM sleep atonia, the activity of the intercostal muscles is reduced but diaphragmatic muscle function remains intact. This reduction is compensated during awakening and non-REM sleep by the intercostal and accessory muscles of ventilation [42]. In neuromuscular diseases, there is a disruption of diaphragmatic ventilation [36]. Furthermore, subjects with NMD may present with a restrictive lung disorder as a consequence of chest muscle weakness, as well as obstructive respiratory function alterations, due to the weakness or collapse of the pharyngeal muscles. On the other hand, unlike the current study, in generalized myopathies, such as Duchenne's muscular dystrophy, sleep-related ventilatory deficiency is found exclusively in terminal stages of the disease [43]. Further cohort studies are necessary to establish if SDB is more prevalent in patients with MD regardless of the severity of neuromuscular weakness inherent to the pathophysiology of MD.

Ten patients had spirometry data available. Due to the retrospective nature of the study, the timing of spirometric testing was variably relative to the date of the PSG. A few of the spirometry tests were done within days of the PSG and others were within 1 year of the PSG. As such, the available spirometric measurements may not reflect the patient's true respiratory function at the time of the PSG. In addition, the younger subjects were not able to perform the technically difficult spirometric maneuvers, which limited the available data. Regardless, the 4 patients with spirometry measurements and SDB had normal airflow patterns which suggest that the SDB may predominantly be a sleep phenomenon and does not seem to translate to daytime respiratory impairment.

There is a significant overlap of symptoms between sleep disordered breathing (SDB) and mitochondrial disease (MD). Nonspecific complaints such as fatigue and lethargy, weakness, and learning disabilities found in both disorders make it almost impossible to distinguish SDB from MD without a polysomnography. The increased incidence of excessive daytime somnolence seen in study patients (61%) compared to the general population (20%) [19] suggests that although contributory, the hypersomnolence is more likely a manifestation of the MD than a pure reflection of the SDB. Modified Epworth sleepiness scale scores were found only in 3 of the patients who underwent PSG but did not have SDB. As such, objective measures of excessive daytime somnolence were not available. We can however speculate that symptoms associated with SDB aggravate the overall decreased daytime stamina seen in many patients with MD. Due to the retrospective nature of the study, the level of parent or patient reported symptoms could not be clarified or quantified. This association between SDB and mitochondrial disorder remains unclear.

In summary, we found that SDB constitutes a frequent finding in children with MD, compared to the general population. Clinical history is not a helpful screening tool in identifying SDB due to nonspecific complaints and overlap of symptoms between these two diseases. Polysomnography should be considered in all children with MD to avoid further potential deterioration caused by SDB comorbidity. Children with MD who have abnormal tone and/or are obese/overweight may be more prone to SDB and may need more careful screening for SDB. Moreover, MD may be added in spectrum of differential diagnosis in all children with nonspecific multiorgan complaints and SDB. The obvious limitation of this study is a small sample size and retrospective design of the study. Larger cohort studies are needed to further explore the association between SDB and MD in the pediatric population.

Conflict of Interests

The authors declare that there is no conflict of interests regarding the publication of this paper.

References

[1] E. O. Bixler, A. N. Vgontzas, H.-M. Lin et al., "Sleep disordered breathing in children in a general population sample: prevalence and risk factors," *Sleep*, vol. 32, no. 6, pp. 731–736, 2009.

[2] N. A. Goldstein, T. Abramowitz, J. Weedon, B. Koliskor, S. Turner, and E. Taioli, "Racial/ethnic differences in the prevalence of snoring and sleep disordered breathing in young children," *Journal of Clinical Sleep Medicine*, vol. 7, no. 2, pp. 163–171, 2011.

[3] C. L. Rosen, E. K. Larkin, H. L. Kirchner et al., "Prevalence and risk factors for sleep-disordered breathing in 8- to 11-year-old children: association with race and prematurity," *Journal of Pediatrics*, vol. 142, no. 4, pp. 383–389, 2003.

[4] K. A. Bonuck, R. D. Chervin, T. J. Cole et al., "Prevalence and persistence of sleep disordered breathing symptoms in young children: a 6-year population-based cohort study," *Sleep*, vol. 34, no. 7, pp. 875–884, 2011.

[5] N. J. Ali, D. J. Pitson, and J. R. Stradling, "Snoring, sleep disturbance, and behaviour in 4-5 year olds," *Archives of Disease in Childhood*, vol. 68, no. 3, pp. 360–366, 1993.

[6] A. M. Li, C. T. Au, H. K. So, J. Lau, P. C. Ng, and Y. K. Wing, "Prevalence and risk factors of habitual snoring in primary school children," *Chest*, vol. 138, no. 3, pp. 519–527, 2010.

[7] A. Sogut, O. Yilmaz, G. Dinc, and H. Yuksel, "Prevalence of habitual snoring and symptoms of sleep-disordered breathing in adolescents," *International Journal of Pediatric Otorhinolaryngology*, vol. 73, no. 12, pp. 1769–1773, 2009.

[8] V. Castronovo, M. Zucconi, L. Nosetti et al., "Prevalence of habitual snoring and sleep-disordered breathing in preschool-aged children in an Italian community," *The Journal of Pediatrics*, vol. 142, no. 4, pp. 377–382, 2003.

[9] J. C. Lumeng and R. D. Chervin, "Epidemiology of pediatric obstructive sleep apnea," *Proceedings of the American Thoracic Society*, vol. 5, no. 2, pp. 242–252, 2008.

[10] C. L. Marcus, L. J. Brooks, K. A. Draper et al., "Diagnosis and management of childhood obstructive sleep apnea syndrome," *Pediatrics*, vol. 130, no. 3, pp. 576–584, 2012.

[11] O. S. Capdevila, L. Kheirandish-Gozal, E. Dayyat, and D. Gozal, "Pediatric obstructive sleep apnea: complications, management,

and long-term outcomes," *Proceedings of the American Thoracic Society*, vol. 5, no. 2, pp. 274–282, 2008.

[12] M. K. Koenig, "Presentation and diagnosis of mitochondrial disorders in children," *Pediatric Neurology*, vol. 38, no. 5, pp. 305–313, 2008.

[13] A. Munnich, A. Rötig, D. Chretien et al., "Clinical presentation of mitochondrial disorders in childhood," *Journal of Inherited Metabolic Disease*, vol. 19, no. 4, pp. 521–527, 1996.

[14] M. I. Trenell, C. M. Sue, C. H. Thompson, and G. J. Kemp, "Supplemental oxygen and muscle metabolism in mitochondrial myopathy patients," *European Journal of Applied Physiology*, vol. 99, no. 5, pp. 541–547, 2007.

[15] S. Koene, S. B. Wortmann, M. C. de Vries et al., "Developing outcome measures for pediatric mitochondrial disorders: which complaints and limitations are most burdensome to patients and their parents?" *Mitochondrion*, vol. 13, no. 1, pp. 15–24, 2013.

[16] R. Arens and H. Muzumdar, "Sleep, sleep disordered breathing, and nocturnal hypoventilation in children with neuromuscular diseases," *Paediatric Respiratory Reviews*, vol. 11, no. 1, pp. 24–30, 2010.

[17] A. Culebras, "Sleep and neuromuscular disorders," *Neurologic Clinics*, vol. 14, no. 4, pp. 791–805, 1996.

[18] L. A. Corben, M. Ho, J. Copland, G. Tai, and M. B. Delatycki, "Increased prevalence of sleep-disordered breathing in Friedreich ataxia," *Neurology*, vol. 81, no. 1, pp. 46–51, 2013.

[19] M. Kaminska, R. J. Kimoff, K. Schwartzman, and D. A. Trojan, "Sleep disorders and fatigue in multiple sclerosis: evidence for association and interaction," *Journal of the Neurological Sciences*, vol. 302, no. 1-2, pp. 7–13, 2011.

[20] R. N. Aurora, R. S. Zak, A. Karippot et al., "Practice parameters for the respiratory indications for polysomnography in children," *Sleep*, vol. 34, no. 3, pp. 379–388, 2011.

[21] P. S. Roland, R. M. Rosenfeld, L. J. Brooks et al., "Clinical practice guideline: polysomnography for sleep-disordered breathing prior to tonsillectomy in children," *Otolaryngology—Head and Neck Surgery*, vol. 145, supplement 1, pp. S1–S15, 2011.

[22] S. C. Bourke and G. J. Gibson, "Sleep and breathing in neuromuscular disease," *European Respiratory Journal*, vol. 19, no. 6, pp. 1194–1201, 2002.

[23] J. F. Pagel, "Excessive daytime sleepiness," *American Family Physician*, vol. 79, no. 5, pp. 391–396, 2009.

[24] F. P. Bernier, A. Boneh, X. Dennett, C. W. Chow, M. A. Cleary, and D. R. Thorburn, "Diagnostic criteria for respiratory chain disorders in adults and children," *Neurology*, vol. 59, no. 9, pp. 1406–1411, 2002.

[25] M. C. S. Melendres, J. M. Lutz, E. D. Rubin, and C. L. Marcus, "Daytime sleepiness and hyperactivity in children with suspected sleep-disordered breathing," *Pediatrics*, vol. 114, no. 3, pp. 768–775, 2004.

[26] R. B. Berry, R. Budhiraja, D. J. Gottlieb et al., "Rules for scoring respiratory events in sleep: update of the 2007 AASM manual for the scoring of sleep and associated events," *Journal of Clinical Sleep Medicine*, vol. 8, no. 5, pp. 597–619, 2012.

[27] Diagnostic Classification Steering Committee-American Sleep Disorders Association, "The international classification of sleep disorders: diagnostic and coding manual," *Annals of Internal Medicine*, vol. 115, no. 5, p. 413, 1991.

[28] "Standards and indications for cardiopulmonary sleep studies in children. American thoracic society," *American Journal of Respiratory and Critical Care Medicine*, vol. 153, no. 2, pp. 866–878, 1996.

[29] C. L. Marcus, R. H. Moore, C. L. Rosen et al., "A randomized trial of adenotonsillectomy for childhood sleep apnea," *The New England Journal of Medicine*, vol. 368, no. 25, pp. 2366–2376, 2013.

[30] J. P. L. Tang, C. L. Rosen, E. K. Larkin et al., "Identification of sleep-disordered breathing in children: variation with event definition," *Sleep*, vol. 25, no. 1, pp. 72–79, 2002.

[31] N. Beydon, S. D. Davis, E. Lombardi et al., "An official American Thoracic Society/European Respiratory Society statement: pulmonary function testing in preschool children," *American Journal of Respiratory and Critical Care Medicine*, vol. 175, no. 12, pp. 1304–1345, 2007.

[32] R. J. Knudson, M. D. Lebowitz, C. J. Holberg, and B. Burrows, "Changes in the normal maximal expiratory flow-volume curve with growth and aging," *American Review of Respiratory Disease*, vol. 127, no. 6, pp. 725–734, 1983.

[33] S. Redline, R. Amin, D. Beebe et al., "The Childhood Adenotonsillectomy Trial (CHAT): rationale, design, and challenges of a randomized controlled trial evaluating a standard surgical procedure in a pediatric population," *Sleep*, vol. 34, no. 11, pp. 1509–1517, 2011.

[34] C. L. Marcus, J. Lutz, A. Hamer, P. L. Smith, and A. Schwartz, "Developmental changes in response to subatmospheric pressure loading of the upper airway," *Journal of Applied Physiology*, vol. 87, no. 2, pp. 626–633, 1999.

[35] L. A. Sena and N. S. Chandel, "Physiological roles of mitochondrial reactive oxygen species," *Molecular Cell*, vol. 48, no. 2, pp. 158–166, 2012.

[36] C. Guilleminault, R. Stoohs, and M. A. Quera-Salva, "Sleep-related obstructive and nonobstructive apneas and neurologic disorders," *Neurology*, vol. 42, supplement 6, no. 7, pp. 53–60, 1992.

[37] G. M. Barthlen, "Nocturnal respiratory failure as an indication of noninvasive ventilation in the patient with neuromuscular disease," *Respiration*, vol. 64, supplement 1, pp. 35–38, 1997.

[38] S. L. Verhulst, L. van Gaal, W. de Backer, and K. Desager, "The prevalence, anatomical correlates and treatment of sleep-disordered breathing in obese children and adolescents," *Sleep Medicine Reviews*, vol. 12, no. 5, pp. 339–346, 2008.

[39] E. Dayyat, L. Kheirandish-Gozal, O. S. Capdevila, M. M. A. Maarafeya, and D. Gozal, "Obstructive sleep apnea in children: relative contributions of body mass index and adenotonsillar hypertrophy," *Chest*, vol. 136, no. 1, pp. 137–144, 2009.

[40] R. Arens and H. Muzumdar, "Childhood obesity and obstructive sleep apnea syndrome," *Journal of Applied Physiology*, vol. 108, no. 2, pp. 436–444, 2010.

[41] J. Bhardwaj, D. Q. Wan, M. K. Koenig, Y. Liu, S. S. Hashmi, and J. M. Rhoads, "Impaired gastric emptying and small bowel transit in children with mitochondrial disorders," *Journal of Pediatric Gastroenterology and Nutrition*, vol. 55, no. 2, pp. 194–199, 2012.

[42] S. Happe, "Excessive daytime sleepiness and sleep disturbances in patients with neurological diseases: epidemiology and management," *Drugs*, vol. 63, no. 24, pp. 2725–2737, 2003.

[43] A. Culebras, "Sleep and neuromuscular disorders," *Neurologic Clinics*, vol. 23, no. 4, pp. 1209–1223, 2005.

20

Carbon Ion Radiotherapy for Oligo-Recurrence in the Lung

Naoyoshi Yamamoto, Mio Nakajima, Hirohiko Tsujii, and Tadashi Kamada

Research Center for Charged Particle Therapy, National Institute of Radiological Sciences, Anagawa 4-9-1, Inage-ku, Chiba 263 8555, Japan

Correspondence should be addressed to Naoyoshi Yamamoto; nao_y@nirs.go.jp

Academic Editor: Hiroshi Onishi

The clinical results after carbon ion radiotherapy for the metastatic lung tumors believed to be in the state of oligo-recurrence were evaluated. One hundred and sixteen lesions in 91 patients with lung cancer metastasis were treated with carbon ion radiotherapy at our institute from April 1997 to February 2011. Regarding the prescribed dose, total dose ranged between 40 gray equivalents (GyE) and 80 GyE, and fraction size ranged from 1 to 16 fractions. After a median followup period of 2.3 years (range, 0.3–13.1 years), the statistical overall survival rate and local control rate were 71.2% and 91.9% at 2 years after treatment, respectively. Treatment-related side effects were not a clinical problem. When classified by the primary organ, there were 49 cases of lung cancer, 20 cases of colorectal cancer, and 22 cases of others. The overall survival rate and local control rate for lung metastasis cases from lung cancer at 2 years after treatment were 81.5% and 92.4%, respectively, and 65.0% and 92.0% regarding lung metastasis from colorectal cancer. Carbon ion beam therapy for the metastatic lung tumors is a safe therapy, and the therapeutic effect is comparable to the outcome obtained from reported surgical resections.

1. Introduction

Radiotherapy is the principal treatment option for patients with early stage lung cancer and contraindications to receive surgery. The outcome from using conventional therapeutic techniques has been a 40–70% 5-year local control rate, but a local control rate equivalent to surgery is being reported due to recent advancements in irradiation techniques [1–4]. These irradiation techniques include SBRT, proton beam therapy, and carbon ion radiotherapy (CIRT).

Clinical trials for various types of tumors were initiated at the National Institute of Radiological Sciences (NIRS) from June 1994 using carbon ion beams, and dose fractionation suitable for individual diseases and irradiation techniques, such as a respiratory-gated radiotherapy and so forth, were developed. As a result, the healing of refractory cancers such as sarcoma of the bone and soft tissue, for which surgery is difficult, postoperative local recurrence of rectal cancer, and so forth, were achieved, and it was found that safe treatment is possible in a further shorter period regarding cancers of the prostate gland, the head and neck, lungs, and liver [1].

Treatment for nonsmall cell lung cancer was initiated in November 1994. Regarding peripheral stage I lung cancer, the fractionation number was gradually reduced from 9 times [5] to 4 times [6] while confirming the safety and efficacy. Currently, a clinical study is being carried out in which irradiation is completed in a day.

We herein report on our outcome from treating metastatic lung tumor believed to be in the state of oligo-recurrence [7], using carbon ion beams in which a good local control rate may be hoped for.

2. Materials and Methods

2.1. Patients. From April 1997 to February 2011, 116 lesions in 91 patients were treated with CIRT in our institute. The average age was 64.8 years old (range, 10–86 years) with a male/female ratio of 57/34. All patients were diagnosed by CT, PET, bone scintigraphy, and brain MRI before therapy. The histology and metastasis diagnosis of the tumors were determined based on the clinical course.

The conditions for applying the treatment to patients were as follows: the primary lesion is treated with no apparent local recurrence in the primary organ at the time of lung metastasis treatment, that is, the tumor is oligo-recurrence, there are no

TABLE 1: Patient characteristics.

Primary organ	Patient (n)	M/F	Age mean range	Tumor (n)	Size (mm) median range	Prescribed dose
Total	91	57/34	64.8 10–86	116	18 3–100	52.8 GyE/4 fr ($n = 54$) 60.0 GyE/4 fr ($n = 23$) Others ($n = 39$)
Lung cancer	49	35/14	69.8 39–86	58	18 3–75	52.8 GyE/4 fr ($n = 34$) 60.0 GyE/4 fr ($n = 2$) Others ($n = 22$)
Colorectal cancer	20	10/10	64.3 41–86	30	15 5–60	52.8 GyE/4 fr ($n = 6$) 60.0 GyE/4 fr ($n = 17$) Others ($n = 7$)
Other cancer	22	12/10	49.1 10–84	28	19 7–100	52.8 GyE/4 fr ($n = 14$) 60.0 GyE/4 fr ($n = 4$) Others ($n = 10$)

active lesions in organs other than the lungs, and there is one lesion in the lungs as a primary rule.

It is difficult to diagnose exactly the lung tumor as metastasis from primary lung cancer. In case, the lung tumor cannot be diagnosed as secondry primary lung cancer, we determined it as metastatic lung tumor.

Regarding the number of lesions per patient treated with carbon ion therapy, 4 lesions were treated in 2 cases, 2 lesions were treated in 19 cases, and only one lesion was irradiated in 70 patients.

The prescribed dose ranged from 40 GyE to 80 GyE, and this was divided into several fractions. The fractionation regimen of 52.8 GyE in 4 fractions was the most commonly used for the treatment of the 116 lesions, which was used on 54 tumors. This was followed by 23 lesions of 60.0 GyE in 4 fractions. In many cases, 52.8 GyE in 4 fractions was used for lung metastasis from lung cancer while 60.0 GyE in 4 fractions was used for colorectal cancer.

When classified by the primary organ, there were 49 cases of lung cancer, 20 cases of colorectal cancer, and 22 cases of other cancers. The breakdown of organs classified as other cancers included various types such as bone and soft tissue tumors, cervical cancer, thymic cancer, esophageal cancer, pharyngeal cancer, ovarian cancer, pancreatic cancer, hepatic cancer, and breast cancer, with the number of cases according to these organs being 4 cases or less.

Regarding the major axis length of the lung tumor, a small tumor was considered to be 3 mm while a large tumor was 100 mm, with a median of 18 mm. The median length of the tumor according to the primary organ was 18 mm, 15 mm, and 19 mm, respectively, regarding lung metastasis from lung cancer, lung metastasis from colorectal cancer, and other types of lung metastasis.

The patient characteristics are provided in Table 1.

Past history comprising several elements such as age, pulmonary function, cardiac function, and so forth, as investigated regarding all patients, who were either diagnosed by a surgeon as being medically unsuitable for surgery due to coexisting diseases or the patients themselves did not wish to undergo surgery.

This study was approved by the institutional review board of NIRS and was conducted in accordance with the ethical standards provided by the Declaration of Helsinki. Informed consent was obtained from all patients prior to treatment.

2.2. Treatment. Treatment was carried out within a week after treatment planning was created. In targeting, a visible legion on the CT image in the soft tissue condition was defined as the gross tumor volume (GTV). The clinical target volume (CTV) was determined by setting the margin more than 10 mm outside the GTV. To allow for the movement of the target during gated respiration, the internal margin was set by 5 mm outside the CTV. The planning target volume (PTV) was defined as CTV + internal margin. The total dose applied ranged from 40 GyE to 80 GyE to the isocenter, and 95% or more was irradiated to the PTV. Irradiation was carried out by dividing the total dosage into 1 to 16 fractions. Set-up corrections were carried out so that PTV would be less than 2 mm three dimensionally at every treatment.

2.3. Followup. Most patients underwent clinical examinations for followup, and CT scan of the thorax was carried out at our institute. Patients in which followup testing could not be carried out until completion underwent periodic CT scanning at another institute. The clinical outcomes of all patients have been confirmed.

The first followup examinations were performed 4 weeks after CIRT and in the following every 3 to 4 months. It is difficult to distinguish the change in normal tissues from radiation and tumor regrowth. We defined transitorily enlarged densities observed following approximately 3 months as locally controlled tumor. Meanwhile, local recurrence was determined from the enlarging tendency of tumors, as well as the outcome of CT image, PET scan, tumor marker, and biopsy.

3. Results

The statistical 2-year overall survival rate of 91 patients was 71.2% with a median observation period of 2.3 years (range,

(a)

(b)

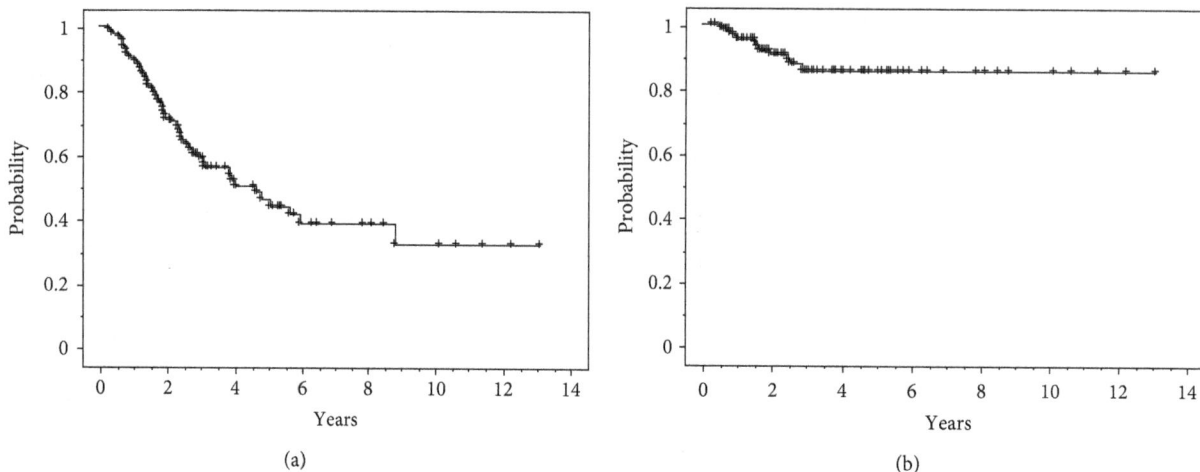

FIGURE 1: (a) Overall survival rate ($n = 91$). (b) Local control rate for lung metastases ($n = 116$).

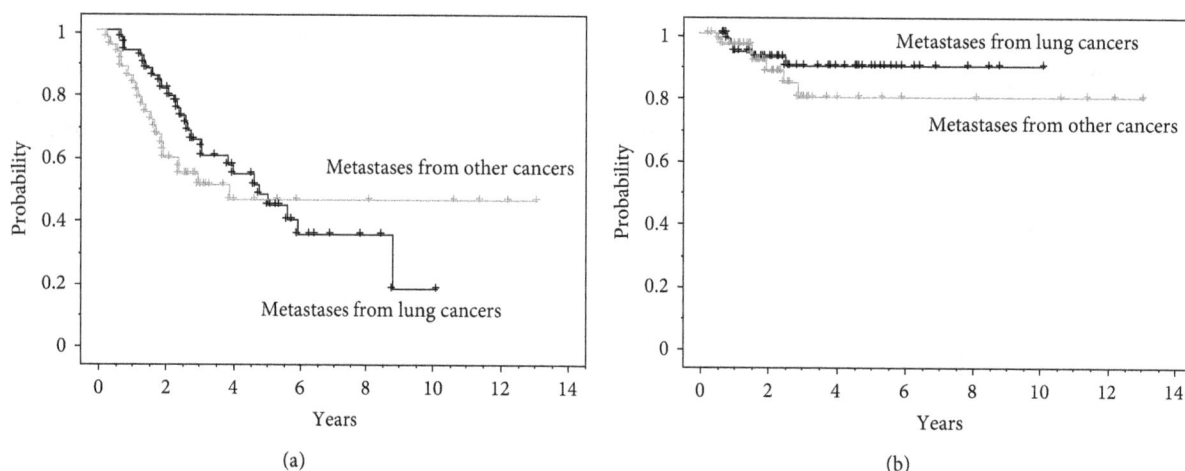

(a)

(b)

FIGURE 2: (a) Overall survival for lung metastases from lung cancer ($n = 49$) versus other cancer ($n = 42$). (b) Local control for lung metastases from lung cancers ($n = 58$) versus other cancers ($n = 58$).

0.3–13.1 years, Figure 1(a)). The local control rate of the 116 treated lesions was 91.9% at 2 years after therapy (Figure 1(b)).

The toxicities to the skin and lung caused by CIRT were assessed according to the NCI-CTC (early) and RTOG/EORTC (late). Early skin reactions were assessed for 116 lesions and late skin reactions for 114 lesions. Of the early reaction lesions, 116 were grade 1. Of the late reaction lesions, 114 were grade 1. Lung reactions were clinically assessed in the 116 lesions of 91 patients. Only five patients had grade 2 in early reaction; no adverse events greater than grade 2 were detected among early and late reactions.

Twelve of 91 patients (12 of 116 lesions) had recurrences. In fifty-five of 91 patients, new lesions appeared in other sites, for example, lung, bone, and brain. In following this treatment, 47 patients died. Regarding the cause of death, 5 of 26 patients (19.2%) of all deceased lung cancer died due to causes other than the primary disease such as pneumonia and so on; however, in metastasis from other cancers such as colorectal cancer, the cause of death in all cases was cancer death due to the primary disease.

The 2-year overall survival rate of lung metastasis cases from lung cancer was 81.5%, and the overall survival rate of lung metastasis from other than lung cancer was 59.3% (Figure 2(a)). The local control rate were 92.4% and 91.3%, respectively, (Figure 2(b)). Furthermore, the 2-year overall survival rate and local control rate of 30 lesions in 20 cases of lung metastasis from colorectal cancer was 65.0% and 92.0%.

The survival rate of 70 cases with one lesion irradiated with carbon ion beams and 21 cases in which there were several irradiated regions was compared. The 2-year cause specific survival rate was 72.4% and 75.4%, with no significant difference ($P = 0.3977$).

The effect of the tumor size on local control was investigated. When the local control rate of 116 tumors was compared regarding the length of the tumor, the local control rate was significantly superior regarding those shorter than 2 cm compared to those exceeding 2 cm (Figure 3). When lung metastasis from lung cancer was compared in the same manner, the local control rate was 100% regarding tumors that are 2 cm or smaller in length.

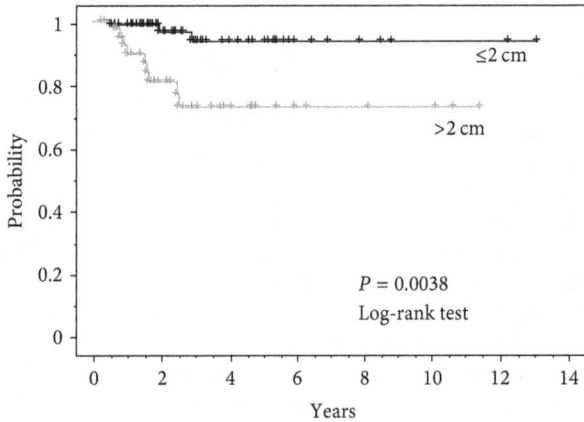

FIGURE 3: Local control for tumor diameter ≤2 cm ($n = 72$) versus >2 cm ($n = 44$) 3 y. Local control rate ≤2 cm: 93.4%, >2 cm: 72.7%.

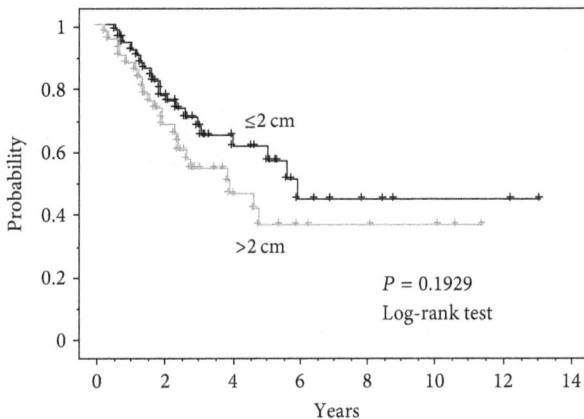

FIGURE 4: Cause specific survival for tumor diameter ≤2 cm ($n = 50$) versus >2 cm ($n = 41$) 3 y. Cause specific survival rate ≤2 cm: 70.6%, >2 cm: 54.3%.

Furthermore, the tumor size and the prognosis were investigated. The cause specific survival rate was compared regarding 50 cases in which the maximum diameter of the treated tumor was 2 cm or smaller and 41 cases in which it exceeded 2 cm. The 2-year cause specific survival rate was 77.5% regarding the group with a tumor diameter of 2 cm or smaller, and a good tendency was observed although there was no significant difference compared to those exceeding 2 cm, at 67.8% ($P = 0.1929$) (Figure 4).

Although there was no significant difference in comparing the cause specific survival rate of 10 cases in which local control was not obtained and other cases in which local control was obtained, there was no survivor of 5 years or longer regarding cases in which local control was not obtained.

The relationship between the time taken until commencing CIRT after treatment of the primary tumor and the prognosis was investigated in the cases of metastasis from lung cancer. The time taken until treatment of the primary lesion to treatment of the lung metastasis was classified into within 1 year, from 1 year to 2 years, from 2 years to 3 years, from 3 years to 5 years, and over 5 years, and the respective

cause specific survival rates were compared. There was no difference in groups that took within 1 to 5 years until treatment, though the 3-year cause specific survival rate was from 60.6% to 72.7%. While in group of over 5 years, all 7 patients are still alive (median followup period: 3.5 years) except for one case of death due to another disease.

4. Discussion

We treated metastatic lung tumors believed to be "oligo-recurrence" using carbon ion beams in which a high local control rate may be expected.

A diagnosis of metastasis was determined from the clinical course. There were many cases in which pathologic tissues were not sampled due to reasons such as the following: biopsy was difficult because the tumor was small, a malignant tumor was clearly suspected upon imaging and clinical course, diagnosis was obtained from resected lung tumors in the past by surgery. We believe that diagnosis with a malignant tumor was justifiable but discrimination with the primary lung cancer may be indicated as problematic, especially regarding cases diagnosed with lung metastasis from lung cancer. As mentioned below, this cannot be ruled out, although the possibility is low.

Regarding adverse reactions, there were no patients with grade 3 or more regarding both early-reaction NCI-CTC and late-reaction RTOG/EORTC. It is believed that the advantages of adopting respiratory-gated radiotherapy and irradiation from 4 directions are exhibited by the low frequency of normal tissue damage [8].

Considering the poor systematic medical condition of the patients, that is, the fact that many patients who are medically unsuitable for surgery are being treated and this is having a major effect on the outcome of overall survival, it was believed that the treatment outcome was generally good. The overall survival rate was favorably comparable to the outcome of CIRT for stage I lung cancer [5, 6], and we believe that this suggests that our criteria for selecting these cases was appropriate.

One lesion was determined as the subject as a general rule, but there were cases in which multiple lesions were treated as a result of clinical course. No difference was observed between the patients who treated single lesion and multiple lesions in comparison of survival. It cannot be determined that cases in which one location alone was irradiated ultimately had only one metastasis, and perhaps cases in which multiple lesions were treated were advantageous in that treatment was successfully completed.

The local control rate is discussed. It is believed that the local control rate is generally permissible. In this outcome, the local control rate for the tumors that are 2 cm or less was particularly superior. In contrast, the local control for the tumors exceeding 2 cm was by no means satisfactory compared to the outcome of the CIRT for primary lung cancer when considering that most tumors are 3 cm or smaller.

There are reports mentioning that tumor size is a prognostic factor [9]. In this study, we evaluated the overall survival concerning tumor size, not volume. Although the analysis outcome is omitted, smaller tumors have a tendency for better prognosis. One opinion is that the tumor doubling time affects the prognosis [10], thus suggesting that perhaps the same phenomenon is observed.

It is under discussion regarding whether or not the local treatment of metastatic lung tumors is effective for prolonging the prognosis. For the metastatic lesion, surgery or radiation therapy is carried out on some patients for potential effect, but the criteria for selecting cases in which an effect may be expected is not clear [11]. We determined the eligibility criteria as being the condition that is frequently used in carrying out surgical resection, that is, the primary lesion is controlled, there are no lesions in places other than the lungs, and there is only one lesion at the time of treatment as a rule. Whether or not our result is superior compared to chemotherapy and the best supportive care remains to be elucidated, but it was evaluated as being satisfactory compared to surgical resection cases due to metastasis [12] and the outcome of CIRT for stage I nonsmall cell lung cancer. In our outcome as well, there were no long-term survival cases of 5 years or more regarding cases in which local control was not achieved, although there was no significant difference, and it is believed that the prognosis is poor. However, in order to make an accurate evaluation, further analysis is necessary, including the effect of other treatments, such as chemotherapy, and the local control period.

There are reports mentioning that the period from treatment of the primary tumor is related to the prognosis after the treatment of lung metastasis [13]. The correlation between cause specific survival and the period from primary lesion treatment to metastasis treatment was investigated with lung metastasis cases from lung cancer in our cases as the subject; however, there was no clear difference. Moreover, 7 of 49 cases underwent the treatment of lung metastasis at 5 years or more after the primary lesion treatment; however, patients in all cases are still alive except for 1 case that died from another disease, so this group had good prognosis. Naturally, it cannot be denied that some primary lung cancers are mixed in from a diagnosis of metastasis.

From the results of this study, it was shown that high local control may be obtained by CIRT with suppressing adverse reactions and that an effect comparable to surgical resection may be obtained regarding metastatic lesions of a certain size. It is believed that an opportunity for treatment may be provided for oligo-recurrence cases in which resection could not be carried out in the past due to reasons such as declined pulmonary function. Furthermore, arguments that adaption may be expanded to cases that were not adaptable to treatment for multiple metastases in the past may be expected because CIRT is a low invasive remedy; however, it is believed that this must be carefully decided upon for evaluating whether or not a long-term prognosis is achieved.

In this report, the presence of metastatic lesions other than the lung or the treatment outcome thereof was not investigated. Regarding this, the treatment course of, for example, affiliated lymph node metastasis and brain metastasis in the case of lung cancer, and local lymph node metastasis, liver metastasis, in the case of colorectal cancer, must be analyzed and investigated in detail depending on the primary organ.

5. Conclusions

We herein reported on the outcome of CIRT for metastatic lung tumors diagnosed as being oligo-recurrent. Lung cancer occupied the majority regarding the breakdown of cases, with lung metastasis of colorectal cancer occupying half of the remaining cases. Lesions other than these were metastases of multiple types of cancer.

This is a safe and effective local treatment for lung metastasis patients without adaptation to surgery. Particularly regarding small tumors, the same tumor control as surgical treatment may be expected.

Considering the fact that many patients without medical adaptation to surgery are being treated, it is believed that the treatment outcome is good. And this indicates that our criteria for selecting oligo-recurrent cases were appropriate.

References

[1] H. Tsujii and T. Kamada, "A review of update clinical results of carbon ion radiotherapy," *Japanese Journal of Clinical Oncology*, vol. 42, no. 8, pp. 670–685, 2012.

[2] H. Nakayama, S. Sugahara, M. Tokita et al., "Proton beam therapy for patients with medically inoperable stage I non-small-cell lung cancer at the University of Tsukuba," *International Journal of Radiation Oncology Biology Physics*, vol. 78, no. 2, pp. 467–471, 2010.

[3] P. Baumann, J. Nyman, M. Hoyer et al., "Outcome in a prospective phase II trial of medically inoperable stage I non-small-cell lung cancer patients treated with stereotactic body radiotherapy," *Journal of Clinical Oncology*, vol. 27, no. 20, pp. 3290–3296, 2009.

[4] U. Ricardi, A. R. Filippi, A. Guarneri et al., "Stereotactic body radiation therapy for early stage non-small cell lung cancer: results of a prospective trial," *Lung Cancer*, vol. 68, no. 1, pp. 72–77, 2010.

[5] T. Miyamoto, M. Baba, N. Yamamoto et al., "Curative treatment of Stage I non-small-cell lung cancer with carbon ion beams using a hypofractionated regimen," *International Journal of Radiation Oncology Biology Physics*, vol. 67, no. 3, pp. 750–758, 2007.

[6] T. Miyamoto, M. Baba, T. Sugane et al., "Carbon ion radiotherapy for stage I non-small cell lung cancer using a regimen of four fractions during 1 week," *Journal of Thoracic Oncology*, vol. 2, no. 10, pp. 916–926, 2007.

[7] Y. Niibe and K. Hayakawa, "Oligometastases and oligo-recurrence: the new era of cancer therapy," *Japanese Journal of Clinical Oncology*, vol. 40, no. 2, pp. 107–111, 2010.

[8] S. Minohara, T. Kanai, M. Endo, K. Noda, and M. Kanazawa, "Respiratory gated irradiation system for heavy-ion radiotherapy," *International Journal of Radiation Oncology Biology Physics*, vol. 47, no. 4, pp. 1097–1103, 2000.

[9] U. Ricardi, A. R. Filippi, A. Guarneri et al., "Stereotactic body radiation therapy for lung metastases," *Lung Cancer*, vol. 75, pp. 77–81, 2012.

[10] W. L. Joseph, D. L. Morton, and P. C. Adkins, "Prognostic significance of tumor doubling time in evaluating operability in pulmonary metastatic disease," *Journal of Thoracic and Cardiovascular Surgery*, vol. 61, no. 1, pp. 23–32, 1971.

[11] M. T. Milano, A. W. Katz, A. G. Muhs et al., "A prospective pilot study of curative-intent stereotactic body radiation therapy in

patients with 5 or fewer oligometastatic lesions," *Cancer*, vol. 112, no. 3, pp. 650–658, 2008.

[12] D. Kandioler, E. Krimer, H. Tüchler et al., "Long term results after repeated surgical removal of pulmonary metastases," *The Annals of Thoracic Surgery*, vol. 65, no. 4, pp. 909–912, 1998.

[13] Y. Norihisa, Y. Nagata, K. Takayama et al., "Stereotactic body radiotherapy for oligometastatic lung tumors," *International Journal of Radiation Oncology Biology Physics*, vol. 72, no. 2, pp. 398–403, 2008.

21

Frequency and Intensive Care Related Risk Factors of Pneumothorax in Ventilated Neonates

Ramesh Bhat Yellanthoor and Vidya Ramdas

Department of Paediatrics, Kasturba Medical College, Manipal University, Manipal, Udupi District, Karnataka 576104, India

Correspondence should be addressed to Ramesh Bhat Yellanthoor; docrameshbhat@yahoo.co.in

Academic Editor: Dimitris Georgopoulos

Objectives. Relationships of mechanical ventilation to pneumothorax in neonates and care procedures in particular are rarely studied. We aimed to evaluate the relationship of selected ventilator variables and risk events to pneumothorax. *Methods.* Pneumothorax was defined as accumulation of air in pleural cavity as confirmed by chest radiograph. Relationship of ventilator mode, selected settings, and risk procedures prior to detection of pneumothorax was studied using matched controls. *Results.* Of 540 neonates receiving mechanical ventilation, 10 (1.85%) were found to have pneumothorax. Respiratory distress syndrome, meconium aspiration syndrome, and pneumonia were the underlying lung pathology. Pneumothorax mostly (80%) occurred within 48 hours of life. Among ventilated neonates, significantly higher percentage with pneumothorax received mandatory ventilation than controls (70% versus 20%; $P < 0.01$). Peak inspiratory pressure >20 cm H_2O and overventilation were not significantly associated with pneumothorax. More cases than controls underwent care procedures in the preceding 3 hours of pneumothorax event. Mean airway pressure change ($P = 0.052$) and endotracheal suctioning ($P = 0.05$) were not significantly associated with pneumothorax. Reintubation ($P = 0.003$), and bagging ($P = 0.015$) were significantly associated with pneumothorax. *Conclusion.* Pneumothorax among ventilated neonates occurred at low frequency. Mandatory ventilation and selected care procedures in the preceding 3 hours had significant association.

1. Introduction

Pneumothorax is the most common air-leak syndrome resulting in significant morbidity and mortality in neonates [1–3]. Increased mortality and chronic lung disease with pneumothorax (about 13 times) in very low birth weight (VLBW) neonates have been reported by Powers and Clemens [3]. Its relationship with underlying primary lung disorders is well recognized [1, 4, 5]. However, higher incidences of pneumothorax in ventilated neonates [3–5] with mild increase among those receiving continuous positive airway pressure (CPAP) and dramatic increase with mandatory modes of ventilation have been addressed by only few studies [1, 4]. Similarly studies addressing association of pneumothorax to various ventilation strategies are scarce. Such strategies with high incidence of pneumothorax include high peak inspiratory pressure (PIP) and mean airway pressure (MAP), active expiratory reflex, administration of bag and mask ventilation, endotracheal tube displacement, an increase in

clinical interventions [6–9], long inspiratory time [10], and high frequency ventilation [11]. Ventilator rates greater than 60/min associated with decreased risk of pneumothorax were found by Greenough et al. [9]. Maximal PIP and suction have been found to be risk factors for pneumothorax in a study by Klinger et al. [4]. A mortality of 10% to 38.6% with neonatal pneumothorax has been reported by various studies [12, 13]. Whether associated variables are causative or merely a result of an undiagnosed air leak is debatable. Studies in this regard can help define care practices or risk factors associated with pneumothorax. We aimed to study the association of ventilator mode, selected settings, and care procedures with the development of pneumothorax in ventilated neonates.

2. Methods

Newborns who were detected to have pneumothorax while receiving mechanical ventilation between May 2006 and

August 2008 were studied. Clinically suspected pneumothorax was subjected to transillumination test using cold light (Karl Storz endoscopy) and chest X-ray. Pneumothorax was defined as accumulation of air in the pleural cavity as confirmed by chest radiograph. To study the association of ventilator parameters and other potential risk events with the development of pneumothorax among the ventilated neonates, birth weight and gestational age matched controls were selected [6]. The subsequent two neonates who were ventilated following each case without developing an air leak and gestation within two weeks and birth weight within 500 g of the cases constituted the controls. A $PaCO_2$ <30 mm Hg was considered as an indicator of overventilation. To assess this, the minimum $PaCO_2$ for each case in the preceding 3–6 hours of the diagnosis of pneumothorax and the minimum $PaCO_2$ of the matched control before that same age were noted. Ventilatory details and arterial blood gases were retrieved up to the age of diagnosis in the cases. For the preceding three hours, the data regarding procedures such as endotracheal suction, reintubation, and bagging were retrieved from the neonatal case records. The three-hour period was chosen similar to the previous study [6]. Newborns were ventilated using Drager 8000 Neonatal Ventilator (Drager Ltd, Hemel Hempstead, UK), Bear Cub Infant Ventilator, or Infant Star Ventilator. Mode of ventilation and sedation with fentanyl were selected as per clinician's choice. The initial ventilation mode was intermittent mandatory ventilation/assist control (IMV/AC); subsequently it was changed to synchronised IMV (SIMV)/CPAP as guided by arterial blood gas analysis and clinical improvement. The sedation involved infusion of fentanyl, 2–4 microgram/kg/hour. Surfactant was used as an early rescue therapy only. We did not use neuromuscular blockade in any case. Any increase in the mean airway pressure (MAP) in the preceding 3 hours of pneumothorax was considered as MAP change. Ethical approval for the study from the hospital ethical committee and informed consents from parents were obtained. Data was analysed using Statistical Package for Social Sciences (SPSS) software version 11.5. Proportions were compared and analyzed using Fischer's exact test or chi-square test.

3. Results

During the study period, 10 (1.85%) neonates had pneumothorax out of 540 who received mechanical ventilation. Mean (SD) birth weight of cases was 2250 (450) g and controls were 2150 (530) g. Birth weight range was 775–3820 g among cases and 840 g–4000 g among controls. Median gestational age of cases was 36 weeks (range, 26–40 weeks) and controls 36 weeks (range 28–40 weeks). Mode of delivery by vaginal route and cesarean section were not significantly different among cases and controls. Six among cases and 10 among controls received mask or tube ventilation at birth. Among cases, 6 had hyaline membrane disease (HMD), 3 had meconium aspiration syndrome (MAS), and 1 had pneumonia. Among controls, 14 had HMD and 6 had MAS. Most of the pneumothoraces (80%) were diagnosed within the first 48 hours of life. Three pneumothoraces among

TABLE 1: Relationship of ventilator variables and overventilation to pneumothorax.

Parameter	Cases ($n = 10$)		Controls ($n = 20$)		P value
	n	%	n	%	
Mode of ventilation at pneumothorax event					
IMV	7	70	4	20	
AC	2	20	4	20	0.007
SIMV	0	0	4	20	
CPAP	1	10	8	40	
PIP >20 cm H_2O	4	40	6	30	0.58
$PaCO_2$ <30 mmHg in ABG	5	50	11	55	0.79

IMV: intermittent mandatory ventilation; AC: assist control; SIMV: synchronized intermittent mandatory ventilation; CPAP: continuous positive airway pressure; PIP: peak inspiratory pressure; ABG: arterial blood gas.

infants with HMD and two among infants with MAS were diagnosed between 24 and 72 hours. Of 10 neonates with pneumothorax receiving mechanical ventilation, 5 died. The mortality among ventilated neonates with pneumothorax was nearly twice that of neonates without pneumothorax (50% versus 26.7%).

Table 1 shows relationship of selected ventilator variables and overventilation to pneumothorax. Among neonates with pneumothorax who were on ventilator, 70% were on mandatory positive pressure ventilation as compared to 20% among controls. Pneumothorax event had significant association ($P < 0.01$) with mandatory positive pressure ventilation as compared to other modes. Peak inspiratory pressure (PIP) > 20 cm H_2O or overventilation as evidenced by $PaCO_2$ <30 mmHg was not significantly ($P = 0.58$ and 0.79, resp.) associated with occurrence of pneumothoraces.

Table 2 shows the relationship of care procedures in the preceding 3 hours of pneumothorax event. Endotracheal suctioning and mean airway pressure (MAP) change were observed in higher proportions among cases as compared to controls. However, these differences were not statistically significant. Reintubation and bagging had significant association ($P < 0.05$) with occurrence of pneumothorax.

4. Discussion

Pneumothorax in newborn results in significant morbidity and mortality [1–5, 14]. It may even increase chronic lung disease in VLBW neonates [3] and intraventricular hemorrhage in preterm neonates [12]. Hence pneumothorax warrants preventive measures. Mechanical ventilation is said to increase the pneumothorax incidence in neonates and such incidence varies widely. Watkinson and Tiron [6] reported that 8.7% ventilated neonates developed at least one pneumothorax during the first two weeks of life. A higher incidence of 10%–13.4% has been reported by studies from UK [15, 16] and of 26% by Malek et al. from Iran [17]. We observed a low pneumothorax incidence of 1.85% among ventilated neonates. However, this low incidence refers to

TABLE 2: Relationship of risk events to pneumothorax.

Risk events	Cases (n = 10)		Controls (n = 20)		OR	95% CI	P value
	n	%	n	%			
Endotracheal suctioning	6	60	6	30	3.5	0.7–17.1	0.05
Mean airway pressure change	4	40	2	10	6.0	0.8–41.4	0.052
Reintubation	6	60	2	10	13.5	1.9–93.2	0.003
Bagging	5	50	2	10	9.0	1.3–61.1	0.015

OR: odds ratio; CI: confidence interval.

pooled neonates of low and normal body weight together and symptomatic pneumothoraces only. Morley et al. [18] reported incidence of pneumothorax as 9% after CPAP. In a case-control study on VLBW infants from 1997 to 2002, pneumothorax rate was 10.9% [4].

Improvement in mechanical ventilator strategies to reduce pulmonary complications and improve long-term outcomes has been debated. Pneumothorax event, in the present study, had significant association with mandatory positive pressure ventilation than other modes. Different rates of pneumothorax with different modes of ventilation are recognised. Pneumothorax rate of about 16% among those receiving CPAP and 34% for those being ventilated was observed by Greenough and Millner [5]. An analysis of 16 trials comparing elective high-frequency ventilation with conventional ventilation [11] showed a significant increase in air leakage in the high-frequency group (29% versus 24%).

Although higher percentage of newborns among cases had PIP >20 cm H_2O than control group in the present study, this difference was not statistically significant. This is similar to a previous observation [6]. In contrast, a study on VLBW infants found maximal PIP during the 24 hours before diagnosis of pneumothorax as significant risk factor for pneumothorax [4]. Watkinson and Tiron [6] in their analysis of 606 ventilated neonates reported that overventilation defined as a $PaCO_2$ <30 mm Hg was not associated with pneumothorax. Our study agrees with this report. These findings suggest the need for further studies to resolve the controversial association of higher PIP with occurrence of pneumothorax in ventilated neonates.

A number of care procedures in neonates receiving ventilation associated with pneumothorax have been reported [6–8, 19]. They include an increase in clinical interventions such as suction procedures, chest radiography, reintubation, chest compressions, and active expiration. The number of suction procedures during the 8 hours before diagnosis of pneumothorax with an odds ratio of 1.56 (95% CI, 1.09–2.23) was previously reported [4]. McIntosh et al. [20] reported that in most cases endotracheal tube was aspirated and at least 40% of newborns were reintubated before the diagnosis of pneumothorax. On the other hand, Primhak had found that slightly elevated PIP and MAP had association with pneumothorax but finally it was longer inspiratory time which was the major risk factor responsible for pneumothorax [21]. In the present study, reintubation and bagging in the preceding three hours were significantly associated with pneumothorax. Higher percentage of cases had MAP change than controls

but it was not statistically significant. Together, these findings suggest the need for more supervision and monitoring of these potential risk procedures.

The mortality among ventilated newborns with pneumothorax was nearly twice that of neonates without pneumothorax. This increased mortality is at least partly related to pneumothorax than solely to comorbidities. Comorbidities included persistent pulmonary hypertension (PPHN) in two and one case each of sepsis, pulmonary hemorrhage, and intraventricular hemorrhage. It is likely that pneumothorax had some association with PPHN and IVH also. Identifying risk factors for pneumothorax in ventilated neonates may reduce mortality and improve long-term outcome among survivors if subsequent air leak is prevented. The findings of the present study also positively reinforce an earlier statement that an apparent need to reintubate or bagging procedures in ventilated neonates must be accompanied by a prompt search for a pneumothorax [6].

The present study had certain limitations. Firstly, it was a single centre study. The study samples were small due to low incidence of pneumothorax although a large number of neonates received mechanical ventilation. Secondly, the adequacy of sedation among study population was monitored only clinically and not objectively by any sedation score.

In conclusion, the incidence of pneumothorax among ventilated neonates in the present study is much lower than previous studies. High mortality of pneumothorax among neonates receiving mechanical ventilation remains as a cause of concern. Regardless of whether associated variables are causative or merely a result of an undiagnosed air leak, more attention to these potential care procedures is warranted.

Conflict of Interests

The authors declare that there is no conflict of interests regarding the publication of this paper.

Authors' Contribution

Ramesh Bhat Yellanthoor was involved in conceptualization, study design, treatment, data interpretation, analysis, paper writing, and draft. Vidya Ramdas was involved in data collection, treatment, data analysis, and help in paper preparation. Both authors approved the paper and Ramesh Bhat Yellanthoor would act as guarantor of the study.

Acknowledgments

Authors thank the head of the department of paediatrics and all staff members for their kind help, suggestions, and encouragement during the study.

References

[1] J. D. Miller and W. A. Carlo, "Pulmonary complications of mechanical ventilation in neonates," *Clinics in Perinatology*, vol. 35, no. 1, Article ID 27381, pp. 273–281, 2008.

[2] H. Maksić, S. Heljić, S. Maksić, and F. Jonuzi, "Pulmonary complications during mechanical ventilation in the neonatal period," *Medicinski Arhiv*, vol. 54, no. 5-6, pp. 271–272, 2000.

[3] W. F. Powers and J. D. Clemens, "Prognostic implications of age at detection of air leak in very low birth weight infants requiring ventilatory support," *Journal of Pediatrics*, vol. 123, no. 4, pp. 611–617, 1993.

[4] G. Klinger, S. Ish-Hurwitz, M. Osovsky, L. Sirota, and N. Linder, "Risk factors for pneumothorax in very low birth weight infants," *Pediatric Critical Care Medicine*, vol. 9, no. 4, pp. 398–402, 2008.

[5] A. Greenough and A. D. Millner, "Pulmonary airleaks," in *Roberton's Text Book of Neonatology*, J. M. Rennie, Ed., pp. 487–491, Elsevier Churchill Livingstone, Philadelphia, Pa, USA, 4th edition, 2005.

[6] M. Watkinson and I. Tiron, "Events before the diagnosis of a pneumothorax in ventilated neonates," *Archives of Disease in Childhood: Fetal and Neonatal Edition*, vol. 85, no. 3, pp. F201–F203, 2001.

[7] R. Niwas, A. M. Nadroo, V. G. Sutija, M. Gudavalli, and P. Narula, "Malposition of endotracheal tube: association with pneumothorax in ventilated neonates," *Archives of Disease in Childhood: Fetal and Neonatal Edition*, vol. 92, no. 3, pp. F233–F234, 2007.

[8] S. Ngerncham, P. Kittiratsatcha, and P. Pacharn, "Risk factors of pneumothorax during the first 24 hours of life," *Journal of the Medical Association of Thailand*, vol. 88, no. 8, pp. S135–S141, 2005.

[9] A. Greenough, A. D. Milner, and G. Dimitriou, "Synchronized mechanical ventilation for respiratory support in newborn infants," *Cochrane Database of Systematic Reviews*, no. 4, Article ID CD000456, 2004.

[10] C. O. Kamlin and P. G. Davis, "Long versus short inspiratory times in neonates receiving mechanical ventilation," *Cochrane Database of Systematic Reviews*, no. 4, Article ID CD004503, 2004.

[11] U. H. Thome, W. A. Carlo, and F. Pohlandt, "Ventilation strategies and outcome in randomised trials of high frequency ventilation," *Archives of Disease in Childhood: Fetal and Neonatal Edition*, vol. 90, no. 6, pp. F466–F473, 2005.

[12] A. Hill, J. M. Pariman, and J. J. Volpe, "Relationship of pneumothorax to occurrence of intraventricular hemorrhage in the premature newborn," *Pediatrics*, vol. 69, no. 2, pp. 144–149, 1982.

[13] Z. Ilçe, G. Gündogdu, C. Kara, B. Ilikkan, and S. Celayir, "Which patients are at risk? Evaluation of the morbidity and mortality in newborn pneumothorax," *Indian Pediatrics*, vol. 40, no. 4, pp. 325–328, 2003.

[14] H. Esme, Ö. Doğru, Ş. Eren, M. Korkmaz, and O. Solak, "The factors affecting persistent pneumothorax and mortality in neonatal pneumothorax," *Turkish Journal of Pediatrics*, vol. 50, no. 3, pp. 242–246, 2008.

[15] J. H. Baumer, "International randomised controlled trial of patient triggered ventilation in neonatal respiratory distress syndrome," *Archives of Disease in Childhood: Fetal and Neonatal Edition*, vol. 82, no. 1, pp. F5–F10, 2000.

[16] B. N. J. Shaw, R. W. I. Cooke, A. B. Gill, and M. Saeed, "Randomised trial of routine versus selective paralysis during ventilation for neonatal respiratory distress syndrome," *Archives of Disease in Childhood*, vol. 69, no. 5, pp. 479–482, 1993.

[17] A. Malek, N. Afzali, M. Meshkat, and N. H. Yazdi, "Pneumothorax after mechanical ventilation in newborns," *Iranian Journal of Pediatrics*, vol. 21, no. 1, pp. 45–50, 2011.

[18] C. J. Morley, P. G. Davis, L. W. Doyle, L. P. Brion, J.-M. Hascoet, and J. B. Carlin, "Nasal CPAP or intubation at birth for very preterm infants," *The New England Journal of Medicine*, vol. 358, no. 7, pp. 700–708, 2008.

[19] A. Greenough, S. Wood, C. J. Morley, and J. A. Davis, "Pancuronium prevents pneumothoraces in ventilated premature babies who actively expire against positive pressure inflation," *The Lancet*, vol. 1, no. 8367, pp. 1–3, 1984.

[20] N. McIntosh, J.-C. Becher, S. Cunningham et al., "Clinical diagnosis of pneumothorax is late: use of trend data and decision support might allow preclinical detection," *Pediatric Research*, vol. 48, no. 3, pp. 408–415, 2000.

[21] R. A. Primhak, "Factors associated with pulmonary air leak in premature infants receiving mechanical ventilation," *Journal of Pediatrics*, vol. 102, no. 5, pp. 764–767, 1983.

22

Latex Hypersensitivity among Allergic Egyptian Children: Relation to Parental/Self Reports

Zeinab A. El-Sayed, Shereen S. El-Sayed, Rehab M. Zaki, and Mervat A. Salama

Pediatric Allergy and Immunology Unit, Children's Hospital, Faculty of Medicine, Ain Shams University, Cairo, Egypt

Correspondence should be addressed to Zeinab A. El-Sayed; zeinabawad@gmail.com

Academic Editor: Hisako Matsumoto

Background. Latex allergy is one of the major health concerns and allergic reactions to latex may be serious and fatal. *Purpose.* In this study, we sought to determine the frequency of latex hypersensitivity in a group of allergic Egyptian infants and children and its relation to the history provided by the patients or caregivers. *Methods.* We consecutively enrolled 400 patients with physician diagnosed allergic diseases. The study measurements included clinical evaluation for the site and duration of allergy, history suggestive of latex allergy, family history of allergy, and skin prick testing (SPT) using a commercial latex extract. *Results.* The study revealed that 16/400 (4%) patients had positive SPT; 11 of them only had positive history of sensitivity to latex. Positive latex SPT was reported in 3.4% (11/326) of patients with bronchial asthma, 5.9% (7/118) of patients with skin allergy, and 4.5% (2/44) of patients with allergic rhinitis. SPT was positive in 7.4% (4/54) of patients with concomitant respiratory and skin allergy. Latex SPT was more specific than sensitive (97.69% and 77.77%, resp.) with a negative predictive value of 99.47%. *Conclusion.* Although underrecognized, latex is an important allergen in the pediatric age group with a sensitization frequency of 4% among allergic children. It was observed to be especially associated with multiple allergic diseases coexisting in the same patient. Pediatric allergologists should educate their patients on latex allergy and encourage the use of latex-free products.

1. Introduction

Latex as found in nature is a milky sap-like fluid found in 10% of all flowering plants [1]. Natural rubber latex (NRL) extracted from *Hevea brasiliensis* tree has been widely used in the manufacturing of gloves, balloons, and parts of medical and dental equipment [2]. Among more than 200 polypeptides identified in NRL as potential allergens, *Hevea brasiliensis* 6 [Hev 6] and Hev b1-13 are recognized as the primary allergens by the International Union of Immunological Societies [3]. Latex elongation factor Hev d1 is the relevant allergen in patients with spina bifida. Prohevein (Hev B6) behaves as a major allergen, since it reacts to IgE in most of the sera of patients with latex allergy [4]. Exposure to latex via direct skin contact or inhalation of airborne allergens from powdered gloves poses the risk of sensitizing both clinicians and their patients. The risk of developing latex hypersensitivity increases with prolonged and repeated exposure [5].

Latex sensitization is defined as the presence of immunoglobulin antibodies to NRL products without clinical manifestations [6]. Sensitization does not always lead to allergy. It remains unclear why someone who is exposed to latex does not develop a latex sensitivity whereas others who do develop this sensitivity do not manifest reactions on contact [7]. Sensitization rates to latex differ in various populations, ranging from 0.1% to 1% in the normal population and 2.6% to 16.9% in health care workers to 28% to 67% in patients with spina bifida [8].

The association of latex allergy and allergy to plant-derived foods is called latex-fruit syndrome and is attributed to the cross-reactivity between the major latex allergen hevein and hevein-like domains (HLDs) from fruit class 1 [9]. In patients with a history suggestive of latex sensitization, physicians should ask about skin and respiratory symptoms, as well as food allergies, particularly in patients with a history of atopy [10]. The skin prick test is the cheapest, practical, and the most widely used method for the diagnosis of allergic diseases [11]. The authors are not aware of previous work addressing the prevalence of skin sensitization to latex in allergic Egyptian children. Hence, this study was carried out to determine the prevalence of latex hypersensitivity among allergic children and its relation to the history provided by the patients or their caregivers.

2. Methods

2.1. Study Population. This study comprised 400 allergic infants and children enrolled consecutively from the Pediatric Allergy and Immunology Clinic, Children's Hospital, Ain Shams University, and the outpatient clinics of El-Mounira and El-Zawya hospitals over the period from March 2011 to June 2013. Patients included suffered clinical allergic disorders including bronchial asthma (BA), skin allergy, and allergic rhinitis (AR). An informed consent was obtained from the parents and caregivers prior to enrollment. Approval of the local ethics committee was obtained.

The diagnosis of BA was established according to the criteria of the American Thoracic Society [12]. The diagnosis of AR was established according to the guidelines of AR and its impact on asthma (ARIA) [13]. The diagnosis of atopic dermatitis was established according to the scoring atopic dermatitis index (SCORAD) [14] and the diagnosis of urticaria was established according to the criteria proposed by Zuberbier and Maurer [15].

2.2. Study Measurements. All patients included in the study were subjected to the following.

(1) Clinical Evaluation. Clinical history was taken for the allergic disorder and its duration, sensitivity to latex, and exposure to latex containing products including gloves. History of allergy to fruits such as banana and kiwi was also sought. Inquiry was made about the risk factors such as neural tube defects, urogenital anomalies, repeated surgical manoeuvers, and hand dermatitis.

(2) Skin Prick Testing. Skin prick tests were performed for each patient using ammoniated allergen extract for latex (Allergopharma Joachim Ganzer D-21462 Reinbek, Germany), positive control (histamine hydrochloride 10 mg/mL), and negative saline control. The procedure was first explained to each patient and/or the caregiver then consent was obtained. First generation short-acting anti-histamines were avoided for at least 72 hours and second generation antihistamines were avoided for at least 5 days before testing. The test sites were marked and labeled at least 3 cm apart, then dropped by the allergen, and gently pricked by sterile skin test lancet. Positive and negative control solutions were similarly applied. Epinephrine was ready in case any systemic reaction occurred. The test result was interpreted after 20 minutes. Largest and orthogonal diameters of any resultant wheal and flare were measured. Pseudopod formation was considered a significant positive reaction. A wheal of 3 mm or more above the negative control was taken as a positive result.

(3) Laboratory Investigations. Serum total IgE was measured by quantitative enzyme linked immunosorbent assay (ELISA) (Medix Biotech, Inc., Agenzyme Company, Industrial Road, San Carlos, CA, USA). Due to variations of serum IgE with age, the patient's serum IgE value used for data analysis was calculated as a percentage of the highest normal for age. Complete blood counts were done on Coulter Counter (Coulter Microdiff 18, Fullerton, CA, USA).

2.3. Statistical Methods. SPSS for Windows, release 15.0 (SPSS Inc., USA), was used for data entry and analysis. All numeric variables were expressed as mean ± standard deviation (SD) or median (interquartile range (IQR)) as appropriate. Comparison of continuous variables was done using Student's t-test for normally distributed variables and Mann-Whitney test for nonparametric variables. Chi-square (χ^2) and Fisher exact tests were used for categorical variables as appropriate. Spearman's correlation test was used. For all tests a probability (P) less than 0.05 was considered significant.

3. Results

The study sample comprised 212 males (53%) and 188 females (47%) (Table 1). A positive family history of allergy was found in the first and/or second degree relatives of 269 (67.2%) of the subjects. Isolated respiratory allergy was present in 282 (70.5%) of our patients; 64 (16%) suffered from isolated skin allergy, while 54 (13.5%) had both skin and respiratory allergies. AR was present in 44 patients (11%), BA in 326 (81.5%), and skin allergy in 118 (29.5%) (N.B. some cases had more than one allergic condition).

History of exposure to balloons and rubber toys was positive in 358 (89.5%) patients, to latex bottle nipples in 166 (41.5%), to erasers in 203 (50.7%), and to latex gloves in 105 (26.2%). A history of allergy to fruits, namely, banana, kiwi, and pears, was found in 225 patients (56.25%). The presence of risk factors such as neural tube defect and urogenital anomalies with repeated urinary catheterization was found in 3 (0.75%) and hand dermatitis in 6 (1.5%).

3.1. Results of Latex SPT. The result was positive in 16/400 patients (4% of the studied sample). Seven of our patients (1.75%) had positive latex allergy; that is, they had positive history of allergy to latex products concomitant with positive latex SPT (Figure 1). Among those with latex positive SPT, 11/16 had positive family history of allergy and only one patient suffered from urogenital anomalies.

Positive history of latex allergy was significantly higher among patients with positive latex SPT having a frequency of 77.8% in comparison to 22.2% in those with negative latex SPT. The odds ratio (OR) was 148 (confidence interval: 27-817). Allergy to fruits was present in 7/16 (43.7%) of the patients who reacted positively to latex SPT versus 218/384 (56.7%) of those with negative result (OR (CI): 0.592 (0.216–1.62); insignificant).

3.2. The Results of Latex SPT according to the Type of Allergic Disease. Positive SPT to latex was observed in only 3.2% (9/282) of patients with isolated respiratory allergy and 4.7% (3/64) of patients with isolated skin allergy in contrast to

TABLE 1: Demographic and clinical data of patients.

Parameter		Positive latex SPT $N = 16$ (4%)	Negative latex SPT $N = 384$ (96%)	P value
Sex	Male	8 (2%)	204 (51%)	0.806
	Female	8 (2%)	180 (45%)	
Age (years)	Range	1–17	0.5–15	0.338
	Median	5.2	4.5	
	Interquartile range (IQR)	9.7	4	
Duration of exclusive breast feeding (months)	Mean	5.33	5.7	0.257
	SD	1.29	1.4	
Site of allergy	Respiratory allergy only (BA, AR, or both)	9 (2.25%)	273 (68.25%)	0.334
	Skin allergy only	3 (0.75%)	61 (15.25%)	
	Both respiratory and skin	4 (1%)	50 (12.5%)	
Diagnosis	All BA cases	11 (2.75%)	315 (78.75%)	0.18
	All AR cases	2 (0.5%)	42 (10.5%)	0.845
	All skin allergy cases	7 (1.75%)	111 (27.75%)	0.202
Duration of illness (years)	Median (IQR)	3.25 (3)	2.5 (4)	0.251
History of latex allergy		7 (1.75%)	2 (0.5%)	0.000
Exposure to latex gloves		8 (2%)	97 (24.25%)	0.104
Positive family history of allergy		11 (2.75%)	258 (64.5%)	0.896
Fruit allergy		7 (1.75%)	218 (54.5%)	0.304
Absolute eosinophilic count $\times 10^3$/Cu·mm	Median	0.2	0.2	0.928
	IQR	0.27	0.3	
IgE% of normal for age	Median	96.3	66.67	0.477
	IQR	133.3	105.53	

BA: bronchial asthma.
AR: allergic rhinitis.

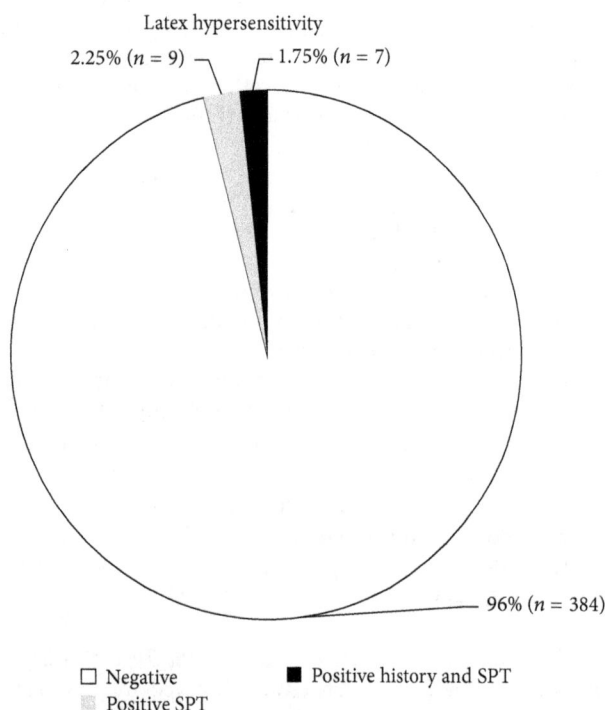

FIGURE 1: Latex sensitivity and SPT results.

7.4% (4/54) of patients with concomitant respiratory and skin allergy ($X^2 = 2.19$; $P = 0.334$).

Positive SPT to latex was seen in 3.4% (11/326) of all patients with bronchial asthma, 5.9% (7/118) of patients with skin allergy (all the 7 had urticaria), and 4.5% (2/44) of patients with AR (OR (CI): 0.48 (0.16–1.4); 1.9 (0.6–5.2); 1.16 (0.25–5.2), resp.).

The patient's age, duration of exclusive breast feeding, age of weaning, duration of the allergic disease, absolute eosinophilic count, total serum IgE, and IgE percent did not bear a statistically significant relation with positivity of latex SPT ($P = 0.33$, 0.25, 0.98, 0.25, 0.92, 0.73, and 0.477, resp.).

The sensitivity of latex SPT was 77.77% and specificity was 97.69% with positive predictive value of 43.75% and negative predictive value of 99.47% with an overall efficacy of 97.25%.

4. Discussion

Immediate hypersensitivity to natural rubber latex has increased since the early 1980s. High prevalence of latex sensitization and allergy are observed among health care workers, atopic individuals, and children who are exposed to multiple surgical maneuvers such as spina bifida and urogenital anomalies [16].

In children, latex sensitization prevalence studies are scarce and involve different population sampling and allergy testing methods, which makes it difficult to compare across studies. Aiming at determining the brunt of the problem in allergic children and its relation to positive history as reported by the patients or their caregivers, we studied the prevalence of latex sensitization in a sample of allergic Egyptian children. This might help in deciding the need for measures to reduce the problem.

In the present study, latex SPT revealed that 4% of the studied sample (16/400) was sensitized to latex. There are no reports on the size of the latex sensitization problem in Egypt. A positive history of exposure to latex products was highly encountered in our cohort of allergic children reaching as high as 89.5% for balloons and rubber toys and 26.2% for latex gloves. Latex containing products such as toys, bottle nipples, and erasers are widely used in Egypt. It is to be noted that most hospitals in Egypt are still using latex-containing medical gloves. However, few dentists and physicians became aware of this problem and started introduction of latex-free medical gloves in their private clinics. Moreover, latex allergens present in sediment and airborne particulate material, derived from tire debris due to heavy urban vehicle traffic and from latex industries in our country (such as latex paints, mattresses, and medical instruments), could be important factors in producing latex sensitization. In a study of 326 atopic children, 10 (3%) presented positive skin test to latex, but only five (1.5%) also had a positive clinical history to latex exposure [17]. The prevalence of sensitization to latex was 9% in atopic Danish children, but the prevalence of manifest type 1 latex allergy was only 1% [18]. A frequency of 4.3% was reported among 2352 Japanese children under 14 years of age with different allergic diseases [19].

Meglio and associates [20] studied a sample of 151 atopic Italian children and they found that 6 patients (3.9%) had positive SPT to latex. A lower prevalence was reported by Nettis and coworkers [21] who found that 2.8% of 1000 atopic Italian patients had latex sensitization.

The corresponding percentage in the general pediatric population is 0.3–4% as reported by some authors [6]. Moreover, Jorge and colleagues [22] studied 182 children from the outpatient clinics of two different hospitals and found that 3.8% had positive latex SPT. However, Roberts and coworkers [23] studied a sample of 1877 children at 7 years of age in the United Kingdom and they found that only 0.2% of the study population had positive latex SPT.

In the present study, 7/16 of those with positive latex SPT gave positive history of allergy to latex. This was a significant finding as compared to those with negative SPT, with a high odds ratio OR (CI): 148 (27–817). The latex SPT was specific rather than sensitive (97.6% versus 77.7%) and showed a high negative predictive value of 99.47%. In an earlier study, the sensitivity of latex SPT was 100% and the specificity was 98% [20]. In children with clinically confirmed latex allergy, sensitivity and specificity of different commercially available skin prick tests could vary. Ammoniated latex extract has shown a higher sensitivity in comparison with nonammoniated products [24].

The frequency of latex sensitization in all our asthmatic patients was 3.4% (11/326). In a sample of 1097 patients with occupational asthma, 4.9% were found sensitized to latex [25]. A higher prevalence rate of latex sensitization of 10% was recorded in adult asthmatics [26]. Sensitization to cockroach and latex was rare among Danish children with verified asthma [27].

In our series, 2/44 (4.5%) AR patients had positive latex SPT. In comparison, Airaksinen and colleagues [28] reported that 10% of the 829 individuals with suspected occupational rhinitis had positive inhalation challenge test to latex. Also, Kimata [19] studied 802 children with AR in three consecutive years between 2001 and 2003 and found that the prevalence of latex allergy was 3.1/5.1/9.1%, respectively.

Our study population included 118 patients with skin allergy (+/− other allergic diseases) where 7 of them (5.9%) had positive SPT to latex. The incidence of latex allergy among 844 patients under 14 years of age with skin allergy in 2001/2002/2003 was 6.1/11.3/15.9%, respectively, denoting a steady rise [19]. Worth mentioning is that among our 118 patients with skin allergy 101 (85.5%) had urticaria, whereas in the other studies all the patients had AEDS. Patients with contact urticaria were reported to have a significantly poorer prognosis than those with contact allergy [29]. In an Egyptian study, latex specific IgE was significantly high in asthmatic children ($n = 22$) (mean ± standard deviation: 2.09 ± 6.39) but not in those with atopic dermatitis ($n = 8$) (0.09 ± 0.16) as compared to controls [30].

The coexistence of more than one allergic disease in the same patient might increase the possibility of having latex hypersensitivity based on the finding in the present work that 7.4% (4/54) of patients with both respiratory and skin allergy had positive latex SPT in contrast to only 3.2% of patients with respiratory allergy and 4.7% of those with skin allergy.

Our study population included 3 patients with neural tube defects and urogenital anomalies necessitating frequent exposure to latex made catheters. Latex skin prick test was positive in one (25%). Spartà and associates [31] studied 85 children with urogenital defects with a median age of 10.5 years and found that 11 (12.9%) of them had positive specific IgE. In the study of El-Sayed and associates [30], latex specific IgE (mean ± standard deviation) was significantly high in children with repeated instrumentation ($n = 17$) (2.89 ± 3.66) with a frequency 52% of latex sensitization among children with spina bifida and urogenital anomalies as denoted by latex specific IgE. In Brazil, a prevalence of 25% for latex sensitization and of 20% for latex allergy was reported among 55 studied patients with meningomyelocele [32].

In the present study, half of all allergic children had history of fruit allergy (43.7% of patients with positive and 56.7% of those with negative latex SPT). Only 6 out of 222 patients with history of banana allergy (2.7%) had positive latex SPT and only 2/6 had positive history of latex allergy. The only patient who had history of kiwi allergy had positive latex SPT and denied history of latex allergy. Overall, the difference was insignificant (OR (CI): 0.59 (0.2–1.62)) perhaps indicating that history of fruit allergy should be confirmed by SPT or oral challenge before considering it as a risk factor for latex allergy. Other fruits that cross-react with latex such as avocado are not popular in Egypt. Radauer et al. [9] also found no significant correlation between latex associated plant food allergy and sensitization to hevein and HLDs which are major latex allergens.

It is concluded that latex skin sensitization was found in 4% of the studied allergic children, yet latex allergy as determined by a positive self/parental report and positive skin prick test was observed in only 1.75%. Although under-recognized, latex is an important allergen in the pediatric age group. It was observed to be especially associated with multiple allergic diseases coexisting in the same patient. Pediatric allergologists should educate their patients on latex allergy and encourage the use of latex-free products. Studies on the prevalence of latex sensitization in the general population as well as studies on environmental air pollution with latex are recommended.

Conflict of Interests

The authors declare that there is no conflict of interests regarding the publication of this paper.

References

[1] A. A. Agrawal and K. Konno, "Latex: a model for understanding mechanisms, ecology, and evolution of plant defense against herbivory," *Annual Review of Ecology, Evolution, and Systematics*, vol. 40, pp. 311–331, 2009.

[2] W. F. P. Neves-Junior, C. F. O. de Graeff, M. Ferreira, M. Mulato, M. S. Bernardes, and J. Coutinho-Netto, "Elastic properties of natural rubber tubes produced by dip-coating," *Journal of Applied Polymer Science*, vol. 100, no. 1, pp. 702–707, 2006.

[3] J. M. Rolland and R. E. O'Hehir, "Latex allergy: a model for therapy," *Clinical & Experimental Allergy*, vol. 38, no. 6, pp. 898–912, 2008.

[4] A. Sanchez Palacios, "Latex allergy: diagnosis and therapeutic aspects," *Allergologia et Immunopathologia*, vol. 29, no. 5, pp. 212–221, 2001.

[5] T. Kean and M. McNaiiy, "Latex hypersensitivity: a closer look at considerations for dentistry," *Journal of the Canadian Dental Association*, vol. 75, no. 4, pp. 279–282, 2009.

[6] R. Cremer, M. Lorbacher, F. Hering, and R. Engelskirchen, "Natural rubber latex sensitisation and allergy in patients with spina bifida, urogenital disorders and oesophageal atresia compared with a normal paediatric population," *European Journal of Pediatric Surgery*, vol. 17, no. 3, pp. 194–198, 2007.

[7] S. G. O. Johansson, J. O. Hourihane, J. Bousquet et al., "A revised nomenclature for allergy. An EAACI position statement from the EAACI nomenclature task force," *Allergy: European Journal of Allergy and Clinical Immunology*, vol. 56, no. 9, pp. 813–824, 2001.

[8] O. Gülbahar, E. Demir, N. Mete et al., "Latex allergy and associated risk factors in a group of Turkish patients with spina bifida," *Turkish Journal of Pediatrics*, vol. 46, no. 3, pp. 226–231, 2004.

[9] C. Radauer, F. Adhami, I. Fürtler et al., "Latex-allergic patients sensitized to the major allergen hevein and hevein-like domains of class I chitinases show no increased frequency of latex-associated plant food allergy," *Molecular Immunology*, vol. 48, no. 4, pp. 600–609, 2011.

[10] S. M. Pollart, C. Warniment, and T. Mori, "Latex allergy," *American Family Physician*, vol. 80, no. 12, pp. 1413–1420, 2009.

[11] G. Karakaya and A. F. Kalyoncu, "The natural course of atopy determined by skin prick tests in patients with bronchial asthma and/or rhinitis," *Allergologia et Immunopathologia*, vol. 34, no. 6, pp. 257–262, 2006.

[12] ATS (American Thoracic Society), "Guidelines for the evaluation of impairment disability in asthmatics," *The American Review of Respiratory Disease*, vol. 147, no. 4, pp. 1056–1061, 1993.

[13] J. Bousquet, N. Khaltaev, A. A. Cruz et al., "Allergic rhinitis and its impact on asthma (ARIA) 2008 update," *Allergy*, vol. 63, supplement s86, pp. 8–160, 2008.

[14] J. F. Stalder, A. Taieb, D. J. Atherton et al., "Severity scoring of atopic dermatitis: the SCORAD index. Consensus report of the European Task Force on Atopic Dermatitis," *Dermatology*, vol. 186, no. 1, pp. 23–31, 1993.

[15] T. Zuberbier and M. Maurer, "Urticaria: current opinions about etiology, diagnosis and therapy," *Acta Dermato-Venereologica*, vol. 87, no. 3, pp. 169–205, 2007.

[16] O. Bayrou, "Latex allergy," *Revue du Praticien*, vol. 56, no. 3, pp. 289–295, 2006.

[17] E. Novembre, R. Bernardini, I. Brizzi et al., "The prevalence of latex allergy in children seen in a university hospital allergy clinic," *Allergy: European Journal of Allergy and Clinical Immunology*, vol. 52, no. 1, pp. 101–105, 1997.

[18] V. B. Jensen, I. M. Jørgensen, K. B. Rasmussen, and P. Prahl, "The prevalence of latex sensitisation and allergy in Danish atopic children: evaluation of diagnostic methods," *Danish Medical Bulletin*, vol. 49, no. 3, pp. 260–262, 2002.

[19] H. Kimata, "Increased incidence of latex allergy in children with allergic diseases in Japan," *Public Health*, vol. 119, no. 12, pp. 1145–1149, 2005.

[20] P. Meglio, E. Arabito, M. Plantamura, and L. Businco, "Prevalence of latex allergy and evaluation of some risk factors in a population of atopic children," *Journal of Investigational Allergology and Clinical Immunology*, vol. 12, no. 4, pp. 250–256, 2002.

[21] E. Nettis, G. Micale, M. Fanelli et al., "Atopy and risk factors for latex sensitization in a selected population," *Allergy and Asthma Proceedings*, vol. 24, no. 3, pp. 185–191, 2003.

[22] A. Jorge, F. Lorente, and L. Taborda-Barata, "Prevalence of latex sensitization and allergy in Portuguese children," *Pediatric Allergy and Immunology*, vol. 17, no. 6, pp. 466–473, 2006.

[23] G. Roberts, G. Lack, K. Northstone, and J. Golding, "Prevalence of latex allergy in the community at age 7 years," *Clinical & Experimental Allergy*, vol. 35, no. 3, pp. 299–300, 2005.

[24] R. Bernardini, N. Pucci, C. Azzari, E. Novembre, M. De Martino, and M. Milani, "Sensitivity and specificity of different skin prick tests with latex extracts in pediatric patients with suspected natural rubber latex allergy—a cohort study," *Pediatric Allergy and Immunology*, vol. 19, no. 4, pp. 315–318, 2008.

[25] F. di Stefano, S. Siriruttanapruk, J. McCoach, M. di Gioacchino, and P. S. Surge, "Occupational asthma in a highly industrialized region of UK: report from a local surveillance scheme," *European Annals of Allergy and Clinical Immunology*, vol. 36, no. 2, pp. 56–62, 2004.

[26] O. Vandenplas, A. Larbanois, F. Vanassche et al., "Latex-induced occupational asthma: time trend in incidence and relationship with hospital glove policies," *Allergy: European Journal of Allergy and Clinical Immunology*, vol. 64, no. 3, pp. 415–420, 2009.

[27] B. Hoffmann-Petersen, A. Høst, K. Toksvig Larsen et al., "Prevalence of IgE sensitization in Danish children with suspected asthma," *Pediatric Allergy and Immunology*, vol. 24, no. 8, pp. 727–733, 2013.

[28] L. K. Airaksinen, T. O. Tuomi, M. O. Tuppurainen, A. I. Lauerma, and E. M. Toskala, "Inhalation challenge test in the diagnosis of occupational rhinitis," *The American Journal of Rhinology*, vol. 22, no. 1, pp. 38–46, 2008.

[29] K. K. B. Clemmensen, T. K. Carøe, S. F. Thomsen, N. E. Ebbehøj, and T. Agner, "Two-year follow-up survey of patients with allergic contact dermatitis from an occupational cohort: is the prognosis dependent on the omnipresence of the allergen?" *British Journal of Dermatology*, vol. 170, no. 5, pp. 1100–1105, 2014.

[30] Z. A. El-Sayed, K. S. Awwaad, M. Z. Mahran, and H. El-Sakka, "Latex hypersensitivity among Egyptian children at risk," *British Medical Journal Middle East*, vol. 6, no. 61, pp. 7–10, 1999.

[31] G. Spartà, M. J. Kemper, A. C. Gerber, P. Goetschel, and T. J. Neuhaus, "Latex allergy in children with urological malformation and chronic renal failure," *Journal of Urology*, vol. 171, no. 4, pp. 1647–1649, 2004.

[32] A. Bueno de Sá, R. Faria Camilo Araujo, S. Cavalheiro, M. Carvalho Mallozi, and D. Solé, "Profile of latex sensitization and allergies in children and adolescents with myelomeningocele in São Paulo, Brazil," *Journal of Investigational Allergology and Clinical Immunology*, vol. 23, no. 1, pp. 43–49, 2013.

23

Knowledge Level of the Primary Healthcare Providers on Chronic Obstructive Pulmonary Disease and Pulmonary Rehabilitation

Tuğba Göktalay,[1] Ayşe Nur Tuncal,[2] Seçil Sarı,[1] Galip Köroğlu,[2] Yavuz Havlucu,[1] and Arzu Yorgancıoğlu[1]

[1]*Department of Pulmonology, Celal Bayar University, Manisa, Turkey*
[2]*Public Health Directorate, Manisa, Turkey*

Correspondence should be addressed to Tuğba Göktalay; tugbagoktalay@yahoo.com

Academic Editor: Leif Bjermer

Introduction. Awareness of the healthcare providers on chronic obstructive pulmonary disease (COPD), which is an important cause of mortality and morbidity in our country and all over the world, and on pulmonary rehabilitation (PR) which plays an important role in its nonpharmacological treatment will provide effectiveness in diagnosis and treatment of COPD. The present study aimed at determining knowledge level of the healthcare providers about COPD and PR. *Materials and Methods.* In this cross-sectional study, family practitioners and staff of home-care in central county of Manisa City were applied a questionnaire in order to determine their knowledge level on COPD and pulmonary rehabilitation during the in-service training on "pulmonary rehabilitation, home-care services for the pulmonary diseases, and respiratory exercises." *Results.* 65.5% of the healthcare providers responded to the survey. Rate of those correctly knowing at least one of four items was 97.2%. No responder knew all items correctly. Average value for correct answers was 5.30 ± 2.1 (range: 1–10). The physicians, men, and those working in family health centers had higher level of knowledge on COPD compared to nonphysician healthcare providers ($p = 0.006$), women ($p = 0.002$), and those working in other practices ($p = 0.019$), respectively. *Conclusion.* Knowledge level of the primary healthcare providers on COPD and PR remains inadequate. Dynamic postgraduate training on this topic will be useful in referring the patients to centers giving service for this condition.

1. Introduction

Chronic obstructive pulmonary disease (COPD) is an important cause of mortality and morbidity in our country and all over the world. Prevalence of COPD is being anticipated to increase due to continuing risk factors and aging of the society [1]. Being a preventable and manageable condition, CODP ranks fourth in our country and third on the world in the list of causes of death [1, 2]. Main reasons for low rate of making diagnosis are that the individuals realize the symptoms late or the symptoms appear late in the course of the disease as well as low utilization of respiratory function test and uncertainty of the diagnostic criteria.

Pulmonary rehabilitation (PR) is a multidisciplinary, evidence-based therapeutic approach to the patient used in management of the symptoms that is specific to the patient.

Its main objectives are to decrease the symptoms, to increase quality of life and contribution to the daily life by optimizing the emotional status, and to reduce health-related expenses by reversing or stabilizing the systemic effects of the disease [1]. It has been used in treatment and management of the patients with COPD since the 1990s [3]. PR improves sense of dyspnea, quality of life, exercise capacity, hospital admission rate, anxiety, and depression in the patients with COPD at the level A. It has also positive effects on mortality [4, 5].

Although COPD is a disease involving the respiratory medicine experts, its symptoms and diagnostic criteria should also be known by the primary healthcare providers considering its economical burden. Early diagnosis of the disease and having the patients quit smoking, the most significant etiological factor, are important in taking measures prior to proceeding to advanced stages of the disease requiring symptomatic and expensive approaches. COPD, however, is not known adequately and underdiagnosed and undertreated [1, 2], being compatible with data from the studies from our country and world [6–8]. In the Turkish Pilot Study BOLD on COPD conducted in Adana, prevalence of COPD in the individuals older than 40 years was 19.1% while rate of the patients with COPD diagnosed by a physician was found to be 5.6% [9].

In Manisa City, in-service training was made titled "pulmonary rehabilitation, home-care services in the respiratory diseases, and respiratory exercises" on March 13, 2014, in corporation with Directorate of Public Health and Department of Chest Diseases of Medical School of Celal Bayar University. The training was performed for the family physicians and home-care service providers practicing in Manisa City. Prior to this training program, pretest was applied in order to determine knowledge level of the participants on COPD and PR. Research hypothesis was to be low knowledge level of the family physicians and home-care service (HCS) providers on COPD and PR. Aim of the present cross-sectional study was to determine knowledge level of the family physicians and home-care service (HCS) providers on COPD and PR.

2. Materials and Methods

In Manisa City, in-service training was made titled "pulmonary rehabilitation, home-care services in the respiratory diseases, and respiratory exercises" on March 13, 2014. This training activity was conducted in corporation with Directorate of Public Health and Department of Chest Diseases of Medical School of Celal Bayar University.

Prior to the training program given in two separate seasons, a survey was applied to the participants consisting of 5 items on sociodemographical characteristics and 14 items on knowledge level on the COPD and PR (Appendices A and B). The survey was used which was developed by Study Group 2 developing and administering the strategic plan in the context of the target "advocating and making the public adopt the program and the diseases" of the Action Plan and Control Program for Preventing Chronic Airway Diseases [6].

Knowledge level of the participants was evaluated based on age, sex, occupation, working years, and practice settings.

The data were analyzed by frequency and chi-square tests using SPSS software v.15.0. Chi-square test was used to compare the answers to the items based on sex, age, working years, occupational group, and practice settings. p values less than 0.05 were considered as statistically significant.

3. Results

The sample of the study included 130 individuals with 110 being invited to participate in the study. 65.5% of the participants in the training program responded to this cross-sectional study.

Of the participants to the training 72.7% were practitioners, 9.7% were specialist physicians, and 18.1% were other types of healthcare providers (nurses, dentists, and health

TABLE 1: Sociodemographical characteristics of the responders.

	n	%*
Sex ($n = 64$)		
Female	23	35,9
Male	41	64,1
Range of age ($n = 69$)		
20–30 years	4	5,8
31–40 years	9	13,0
41–50 years	40	58,0
51–60 years	15	21,7
61+	1	1,5
Average years ($n = 67$)		
Above average years (>45,6)	31	46,3
Below average years (≤45,6)	36	53,7
Working years ($n = 65$)		
1–10 years	5	7,7
11–20 years	21	32,3
21+	39	60,0
Mean working years ($n = 64$)		
Above the average (>21,4)	29	45,3
Below the average (≤21,4)	35	54,7
Occupational group ($n = 72$)		
General practitioner	52	72,2
Specialist physician	7	9,7
Other	13	18,1
Practice setting ($n = 70$)		
FHC	56	80,0
HCS	9	12,9
CODH	5	7,1

*Column percentage.

officers). Of the participants, 35.9% were female and 64.1% were male; mean age was 45.6±7.1 years (range: 25–61 years); mean number of working years was 21.4 ± 6.6 (range: 1–32 years). Of the participants, 80.0% were practicing in family health center (FHC), 12.9% in home-care services (HCS), and 7.1% in the center of oral and dental health (CODH) (Table 1).

Rate of correctly knowing at least one of four items to measure knowledge level of the responders was 97.2%. No responder knew all items correctly. Average value for correct answers was 5.30 ± 2.1 (range: 1–10). The physicians, men, and those working in family health centers had higher level of knowledge on COPD compared to nonphysician healthcare providers ($p = 0.006$), women ($p = 0.002$), and those working in other practices ($p = 0.019$), respectively.

Rate of correctly knowing the items related to knowledge level, consisting of 6 items, is given below along with frequency distribution based on sections and questions. Sociodemographical characteristics were compared to knowledge level and those found to be significant were presented separately (Table 2).

The items in the first section (questions (1) and (2)) were related to definition, risk factors, pathophysiology, and epidemiology of COPD. Rate of correctly knowing 2 items in

TABLE 2: Rate of correctly answering the questions in the sections based on sex, age, mean age, year, occupational group, and practice setting.

	Definition, risk factors, physiopathology, and epidemiology of COPD Section 1		Diagnosis and management of COPD Section 2		Basic concepts in pulmonary function test (PFT) for COPD Section 3		Patient training and pharmacological treatment in stable COPD Section 4		Nonpharmacological treatment in COPD Section 5		Approach to diagnosis and management in exacerbations of COPD Section 6	
	n	%	n	%	n	%	n	%	n	%	n	%
Sex												
Male	15	75,0*	3	75,0	7	77,8	1	33,3	5	83,3	1	100,0
Female	5	25,0	1	25,0	2	22,2	2	66,7	1	16,7	0	0,0
Mean age												
Above mean age (>45,6)	16	72,7	4	66,7	3	33,3	1	25,0	5	71,4	0	0,0
Below mean age (<45,6)	6	27,3	2	33,3	6	66,7	3	75,0	2	28,6	1	100,0
Mean number of working years												
Above mean number of working years (>21,4)	17	77,3*	4	66,7	2	25,0	1	33,3	4	57,1	0	0,0
Below mean number of working years (<21,4)	5	22,7	2	33,3	6	75,0	2	66,7	3	42,9	1	100,0
Occupational group												
Physician	5	20,8	1	16,7	1	11,1	1	25,0	0	0,0	0	0,0
Nonphysician healthcare provider	19	79,2	5	83,3	8	88,9	3	75,0	7	100,0	1	100,0
Practice setting												
FHC	19	82,6	4	66,7	7	77,8	3	75,0	7	100,0	1	50,0
HCS	4	17,4	0	0,0	0	0,0	1	25,0	0	0,0	0	0,0
CODH	0	0,0	2	33,3	2	22,2	0	0,0	0	0,0	1	50,0

*$p < 0.05$.

this section was 33.3% ($n = 24$) with those older than average age ($p = 0.022$) and those with more working years (>21.4 years) ($p = 0.008$) correctly answered this item. 73.9% of the participants correctly answered the item "what are the risk factors for COPD," which was one of the two items. 51.5% of the participants correctly answered the second item noting that "COPD ranks third in causes of death in Turkey" with men ($p = 0.009$), elders (being more than 45.6 years old) ($p = 0.019$), and those with more working years (>21.4 years) ($p = 0.022$) answering this item correctly.

The items in the second section (questions (3)–(5)) were related to diagnosis and management of COPD. Rate of knowing correctly all three items in this section was 8.3% ($n = 6$). Of the participants, 46.7% correctly knew spirometric description of COPD and 25.4% of them correctly knew that the first method was reversibility test for differential diagnosis for airway obstruction. Of the participants, 49.3% correctly knew differential diagnosis of asthma and COPD with physicians ($p = 0.045$), elder participants (>45.6 years old) ($p = 0.004$), those practicing in FHCs ($p = 0.043$), and those with more working years (>21.4 years) ($p = 0.001$) correctly knew this item.

The items in the third section (question (6)) were related to basic concepts on the PFT for COPD. The only item in this section specified that FEV1 was the concept used with priority in order to assess the response of the patients with COPD to the treatment; 14.1% of the participants ($n = 9$) correctly knew this item. No statistically significant difference was found when the items in this section were evaluated.

The items in the fourth section (questions (7)–(9)) were related to patient education and pharmacological treatment in COPD. Rate of correctly knowing three items in this section was 5.6% ($n = 4$). Of the participants, 85.7% correctly knew that the most important intervention was "quitting smoking and avoiding risk factors"; 26.9% correctly knew that "administration of pneumococcal vaccine" was not necessary to inquire; 25.0% correctly knew that, in managing COPD treatment, pulmonary rehabilitation should be started when expected postbronchodilator FEV1 was <80%. No statistically significant difference was found when the items in this section were evaluated.

The items in the fifth section (questions (10)–(12)) were related to nonpharmacological treatment of COPD. Rate of correctly knowing all three items in this section was 9.7% ($n = 7$). Of the participants, 29.0% correctly knew aims of the pulmonary rehabilitation in COPD; 31.7% correctly knew home-care criteria in COPD; and 49.2% correctly knew headings of evaluating effectivity in the pulmonary rehabilitation. No statistically significant difference was found when the items in this section were evaluated.

The items in the sixth section (questions (13) and (14)) were related to approach to diagnosis and treatment of COPD exacerbation. Rate of correctly knowing all two items in this section was 1.4% ($n = 1$). 34.4% of the participants correctly knew the approach to the treatment for the patient in question. Those with more working years (>21.4 years) correctly answered this item ($p = 0.024$). 27.6% of the participants correctly knew use of antibiotics in exacerbation of COPD.

4. Discussion

Being the fourth leading cause of death in our country, COPD is not known adequately and is underdiagnosed. Diagnosis and management of the disease are primarily done by specialists of respiratory diseases. In diagnosis of the disease selection of the patients, quality of staff, evaluation, compliance of the patient, and knowledge of the physician are also important [10]. For fighting the disease, it is also important that primary care physicians and other primary healthcare providers have adequate level of knowledge on risk factors, diagnosis and management, pharmacological and nonpharmacological therapeutic approaches, and approaches to the exacerbation.

In a survey evaluating knowledge level of 139 medical students on COPD, average number of correct answers of the students was found to be 8.35 ± 2.75 and their knowledge level was considered to be intermediate. The researchers noted that education in the medical faculty on COPD should be given meticulously [8]. Walters et al. found that attitudes of the primary care physicians had a role in delay in diagnosing COPD [11]. In a study by Başyiğit et al. evaluating effects of postgraduate training on knowledge level on COPD, the authors found that there was a significant increase in the rate for the physicians practicing in the primary care to correctly answer the questions in the COPD survey and noted that the primary care physicians had lack of information on COPD [12]. In the present study as well, knowledge level of the healthcare providers was low. Mean number of correct answers of the physicians was higher than other healthcare providers although it was still at inadequate level. Increasing level of knowledge by providing in-service training to the physicians and other healthcare providers seems to be important.

Using tobacco and its derivatives is the most important risk factor in development of COPD. Although rate of smoking reduced in our country as a consequence of efforts to fight smoking, it is still at a rate of 27% in the individuals >15 years old [13]. In the study by Yildiz et al., rate of knowing that smoking was the most important risk factor in development of COPD was 51% [6]. In the study by Başyiğit et al., all of 92 physicians practicing in the primary care answered correctly the questions related to the etiological factor [12]. In the present study, rate of accuracy we found about risk factors for COPD among the physicians and other healthcare providers practicing in the primary care was lower. This discordance was mainly attributable to the fact that all participants in the study of Başyiğit et al. were physicians. In the present study, however, accuracy rate was found to be higher in those with more working years.

Unfortunately, rate of using pulmonary function test (PFT) in diagnosing COPD is low [10, 14, 15]. When the second and third sections of our survey related to diagnosis and management of COPD were evaluated, physicians, the elder participants, those practicing in ASMs, and those with more working years were more competent in using PFT although it may be concluded that rate of using and assessing PFT was low.

Being one of the nonpharmacological therapeutic methods for COPD and playing an important role in decreasing

COPD symptoms, pulmonary rehabilitation (PR) is not known adequately by the physicians and other healthcare providers in the primary care. Pulmonary rehabilitation programs have been applied by specialists of chest diseases for almost 10 years in our country. In 2014, activities of the week of pulmonary rehabilitation were held for the first time in order to create awareness. Decramer et al. found that the specialist physicians were not attentive in COPD to the pulmonary rehabilitation, using noninvasive mechanical ventilation, and methods to quit smoking [16]. In the present study, in addition to overall lack of adequate information on COPD, rate of correct answers to the questions on nonpharmacological treatment of COPD also remained low. Nonetheless, the questions related to timing and targets of starting pulmonary rehabilitation were correctly answered with rates of 25% and 29%, respectively. Information on methods to evaluate effectiveness of pulmonary rehabilitation such as exercise capacity, quality of life, degree of the symptoms, body composition, and psychosocial status was at higher level. In the present study, however, we found that the variables of age, sex, working years, occupational group, and practice setting had no effect on it. Including nonpharmacological therapeutic approaches in the postgraduate training given to the physicians and other healthcare providers as well as specialist physicians will be useful in creating awareness and referring the patients in need to the centers providing service on this subject.

The fact that rate of responding remained at 65% is one of the limitations of the current study. The main limitation of the present study was that posttraining survey was not applied. Nevertheless, the data we obtained indicate that knowledge level of the physicians and other healthcare providers practicing in primary care on COPD was inadequate. Nonpharmacological treatment of COPD including PR is also not known sufficiently. Our findings support that postgraduate training efforts remain inadequate on COPD. As a consequence of the present study, it was concluded that postgraduate training to the primary care providers should be performed more dynamically on preventing development and progression of the disease and its early detection, effective treatment, and preventing development of complications. It was also concluded that national sources of written and visual media emphasizing importance of physical activity should be used in order to create awareness among the healthcare providers and in the society and that number of the centers giving PR should be increased.

Appendices

Assessment for COPD and pulmonary rehabilitation before education.

A. Sociodemographical Characteristics

(1) Your degree:

(a) Practitioner
(b) Specialist physician
(c) Other..........................

(2) Gender:

(a) Female
(b) Male

(3) Age: ....
(4) Your unit:

(a) Family health center
(b) Home-care services
(c) Other............................

(5) How long have you been working in the profession: for............................... years

B. Questions about COPD and Pulmonary Rehabilitation

(1) Which of the following is not a risk factor for COPD?

(a) Exposure to tobacco smoke
(b) Alpha-1 antitrypsin deficiency
(c) Biomass exposure
(d) Vitamin B12 deficiency
(e) Low birth weight

(2) What ranks COPD as a leading cause of death in Turkey?

(a) 1
(b) 2
(c) 3
(d) 4
(e) 5

(3) Which of the following is the criteria for obstruction in respiratory function test for COPD?

(a) FEV1 < 70%
(b) FVC < 70%
(c) FEV1/FVC < 70%
(d) PEF < 70%
(e) FEV1 < 70% and FVC < 70%

(4) Which of the following is correct about differential diagnosis of asthma and COPD?

(a) Asthma beginning on more than 40 years
(b) COPD being generally over 10-year history of cigarette packs
(c) COPD being a progressive lung function but may be returning to normal
(d) Developing asthma only by allergen exposure
(e) Being often observed in the sputum of asthma

(5) In a patient presenting with dyspnea and productive cough lasting for 5 years, which of the following is the method that should be performed first when airway obstruction has been found on pulmonary function test (PFT)?

    (a) Bronchodilator reversibility test

    (b) The bronchial provocation test

    (c) Chest X-ray

    (d) Complete blood analysis

    (e) Physical examination

(6) Which of the following item/items may be primarily used to evaluate the response to the treatment of COPD patients?

    (a) FEV1/FVC

    (b) FEV1

    (c) IC

    (d) FVC

    (e) The flow-volume curve

(7) Which of the following is the most significant intervention in COPD?

    (a) Quitting smoking and avoiding risk factors

    (b) Giving basic information on the disease

    (c) Teaching the principles of drug use and effective methods of inhalation

    (d) Prevention and early recognition of exacerbation

    (e) Oxygen treatment

(8) Which of the following does not need to be inquired in all patients in COPD management?

    (a) Smoking cessation

    (b) Avoiding passive smoke exposure

    (c) Avoiding occupational dust exposure

    (d) Applying the influenza vaccine

    (e) Applying pneumococcal vaccine

(9) Which of the following options is correct about the postbronchodilator predicted FEV1 evaluation in the management of COPD?

    (a) Pulmonary rehabilitation is started in the cases with FEV1 <80% of predicted value

    (b) Influenza and pneumococcal vaccines are applied in the subjects with FEV1 <50–80% of predicted value

    (c) Oxygen therapy is given in the subjects with FEV1 <50% of predicted value

    (d) Oxygen therapy is given in subjects with FEV1 <30% of predicted value

    (e) Surgical treatment is performed in the subjects with FEV1 <50% of predicted value

(10) Which of the following is not one of the aims of the pulmonary rehabilitation in COPD?

    (a) Decreasing symptoms

    (b) Improving functional capacity

    (c) Improving quality of life

    (d) Reducing health-related expenses by reversing or stabilizing the systemic effects of the disease

    (e) Reducing the annual decline in FEV1

(11) Which of the following is not criteria for home-care in COPD?

    (a) New diagnosis, comorbid disease

    (b) Any patient who cannot come to outpatient clinic but needing monitoring and/or education

    (c) Predicted FEV1 being less than 30%

    (d) Having more than one visit to the emergency service department or hospital admission over the last year

    (e) Use of long-term oxygen therapy

(12) Which of the following is not one of the headings of evaluating effectivity in the pulmonary rehabilitation?

    (a) Exercise capacity

    (b) Quality of life

    (c) Degree of the symptoms

    (d) Body composition and psychosocial status

    (e) Chest X-ray findings

(13) A patient who had had treatment for three times for exacerbation of COPD over the last year was presented to hospital with FVC of 60%, FEV1/FVC ratio of 55%, FEV1 45% of predicted and following values of arterial blood gases: pH: 7.35, PaO2: 55 mmHg, PaCO2: 50 mmHg, and SaO2: 88%. Which would be your approach to treatment of this patient?

    (a) Refer the patient to a center of higher level

    (b) Bronchodilator therapy with 3-4 L/min oxygen inhalation therapy is given

    (c) Oxygen treatment + 1 mg/kg of oral steroid is added to bronchodilator treatment

    (d) Inhaled bronchodilators are started with intervals of 4 hours

    (e) In addition to oral steroids bronchodilator + oxygen therapy, noninvasive ventilation is initiated

(14) Which of the following is wrong regarding the use of antibiotics in exacerbation?

    (a) True rate of finding atypical bacteria is 5 to 10% although they are serologically detected during exacerbation

(b) Amoxicillin should be given in the case of sputum culture revealing penicillin-sensitive *S. pneumonia* or non-beta lactamase producing bacteria

(c) The macrolides are not effective against *H. influenza*

(d) Cefuroxime axetil and cefprozil are the second-generation antibiotics most effective against *H. influenza*

(e) Fluoroquinolones are the first option to be given for intermediate exacerbations to the patients using beta-lactam antibiotics over the last three months or having penicillin allergy

Conflict of Interests

The authors declare that there is no conflict of interests regarding the publication of this paper.

References

[1] GOLD: Global Initiative for Chronic Obstructive Lung Disease, "Global strategy for the diagnosis, management, and prevention of chronic obstructive pulmonary disease," 2014, http://www.goldcopd.org/.

[2] Republic of Turkey Ministry of Health Refik Saydam Hygiene Center Presidency School of Public Health, *Turkey Burden of Disease Study 2004*, RSHMB, Ankara, Turkey, 2006.

[3] British Thoracic Society Pulmonary Rehabilitation Guideline Group, "BTS guideline on pulmonary rehabilitation in adult," *Thorax*, vol. 68, supplement 2, 2013.

[4] M. A. Spruit, S. J. Singh, C. Garvey et al., "An official American Thoracic Society/European Respiratory Society statement: key concepts and advances in pulmonary rehabilitation," *American Journal of Respiratory and Critical Care Medicine*, vol. 189, no. 12, p. 1570, 2014.

[5] A. Qaseem, T. J. Wilt, S. E. Weinberger et al., "Diagnosis and management of stable chronic obstructive pulmonary disease: a clinical practice guideline update from the American College of Physicians, American College of Chest Physicians, American Thoracic Society, and European Respiratory Society," *Annals of Internal Medicine*, vol. 155, no. 3, pp. 179–191, 2011.

[6] F. Yildiz, G. Bingöl Karakoç, R. E. Hamutçu, N. Yardim, B. Ekinci, and A. Yorgancioğlu, "The evaluation of asthma and COPD awareness in Turkey (GARD Turkey Project-National Control Program of Chronic Airway Diseases)," *Tuberculosis and Thorax*, vol. 61, no. 3, pp. 175–182, 2013.

[7] C. van Weel, "Underdiagnosis of asthma and COPD: is the general practitioner to blame?" *Monaldi Archives for Chest Disease*, vol. 57, no. 1, pp. 65–68, 2002.

[8] O. B. Ozoh, T. Awokola, and S. A. Buist, "Medical students' knowledge about the management of chronic obstructive pulmonary disease in Nigeria," *International Journal of Tuberculosis and Lung Disease*, vol. 18, no. 1, pp. 117–121, 2014.

[9] A. Kocabas, A. Hancioglu, S. Turkyilmaz et al., "Prevalence of COPD in Adana, Turkey (BOLD-Turkey Study)," *Proceedings of the American Thoracic Society*, vol. 3, article A543, 2006.

[10] C. P. van Schayck, J. M. C. Loozen, E. Wagena, R. P. Akkermans, and G. J. Wesseling, "Detecting patients at a high risk of developing chronic obstructive pulmonary disease in general practice: cross sectional case finding study," *British Medical Journal*, vol. 324, no. 7350, pp. 1370–1373, 2002.

[11] J. A. Walters, E. C. Hansen, E. H. Walters, and R. Wood-Baker, "Under-diagnosis of chronic obstructive pulmonary disease: a qualitative study in primary care," *Respiratory Medicine*, vol. 102, no. 5, pp. 738–743, 2008.

[12] I. Başyiğit, F. Yildiz, A. Başoğul, H. Boyaci, and A. Iilgazli, "The effect of postgraduate education on COPD knowledge level of primary care physicians," *Tüberküloz ve Toraks*, vol. 54, no. 1, pp. 51–55, 2006.

[13] Republic of Turkey Ministry of Health and General Directorate of Primary Health Care, *Global Adult Tobacco Survey Report on Turkey*, TUIK, Ankara, Turkey, 2008.

[14] N. F. Voelkel, "Raising awareness of COPD in primary care," *Chest*, vol. 117, no. 5, pp. 372S–375S, 2000.

[15] A. M. Lyngsø, V. Backer, V. Gottlieb, B. Nybo, M. S. Østergaard, and A. Frølich, "Early detection of COPD in primary care—the Copenhagen COPD Screening Project," *BMC Public Health*, vol. 10, article 524, 2010.

[16] M. Decramer, P. Bartsch, R. Pauwels et al., "Management of COPD according to guidelines. A national survey among Belgian physicians," *Monaldi Archives for Chest Disease*, vol. 59, no. 1, pp. 62–80, 2003.

The Role of Cardiopulmonary Exercise Test in IPF Prognosis

Christina Triantafillidou,[1,2] **Effrosyni Manali,**[1]
Panagiotis Lyberopoulos,[1] **Likourgos Kolilekas,**[1,3] **Konstantinos Kagouridis,**[1]
Sotirios Gyftopoulos,[1] **Konstantinos Vougas,**[4] **Anastasia Kotanidou,**[5] **Manos Alchanatis,**[6]
Anna Karakatsani,[1] **and Spyros A. Papiris**[1]

[1] *2nd Pulmonary Department, "Attikon" University Hospital, Athens Medical School, National and Kapodistrian University of Athens, 1 Rimini Street, 12462 Haidari, Greece*

[2] *6th Pulmonary Department, "Sotiria" Chest Diseases Hospital, 152 Mesogion Street, 11527 Athens, Greece*

[3] *7th Pulmonary Department, "Sotiria" Chest Diseases Hospital, 152 Mesogion Street, 11527 Athens, Greece*

[4] *Genomics and Proteomics Research Units, Center of Basic Research II, Biomedical Research Foundation, Academy of Athens, 11527 Athens, Greece*

[5] *Applied Biochemical Research and Training Laboratory "Marianthi Simou", Thorax Foundation and Department of Critical Care and Pulmonary Services, National and Kapodistrian University of Athens, "Evangelismos" Hospital, 3 Ploutarchou Street, 10675 Athens, Greece*

[6] *1st Pulmonary Department, "Sotiria" Chest Diseases Hospital, Athens Medical School, National and Kapodistrian University of Athens, 152 Mesogion Street, 11527 Athens, Greece*

Correspondence should be addressed to Spyros A. Papiris; papiris@otenet.gr

Academic Editor: Dimitris Georgopoulos

Background. In IPF, defects in lung mechanics and gas exchange manifest with exercise limitation due to dyspnea, the most prominent and disabling symptom. *Aim.* To evaluate the role of exercise testing through the 6MWT (6-minute walk test) and CPET (cardiopulmonary exercise testing) in the survival of patients with IPF. *Methods.* This is a prospective, observational study evaluating in 25 patients the relationship between exercise variables through both the 6MWT and CPET and survival. *Results.* By the end of the observational period 17 patients were alive (33% mortality). Observation ranged from 9 to 64 months. VE/VCO_2 slope (slope of relation between minute ventilation and CO_2 production), VO_2 peak/kg (peak oxygen consumption/kg), VE/VCO_2 ratio at anaerobic threshold, 6MWT distance, desaturation, and DLCO% were significant predictors of survival while VE/VCO_2 slope and VO_2 peak/kg had the strongest correlation with outcome. The optimal model for mortality risk estimation was VO_2 peak/kg + DLCO% combined. Furthermore, VE/VCO_2 slope and VO_2 peak/kg were correlated with distance and desaturation during the 6MWT. *Conclusion.* The integration of oxygen consumption and diffusing capacity proved to be a reliable predictor of survival because both variables reflect major underlying physiologic determinants of exercise limitation.

1. Introduction

Idiopathic pulmonary fibrosis (IPF) is an irreversibly progressive lung disease with substantial morbidity and mortality. No effective pharmacological treatment has been established so far [1]. Nonetheless, as research concerning IPF develops, we realize the heterogeneity of this disease which defines final prognosis [1]. Several retrospective longitudinal studies suggest a median survival time of 2 to 3 years from the time of diagnosis; nevertheless, more recent data suggest that this could be an underestimate [2]. Thus, defining prognosis remains difficult but it is of critical clinical importance.

Many prognostic factors of disease severity and outcome have been studied in IPF, either at baseline or at serial measurements over time [3]. Clinical predictors include age, gender, smoking status, dyspnea, pulmonary hypertension, and comorbidities such as emphysema [2, 4–7]. Imaging studies have shown that the overall extent of fibrosis on high-resolution computerized tomography also correlates with survival [2, 8]. Regarding pathologic predictors, the fibroblastic foci profusion has been shown in some studies to predict survival while not in others [9, 10]. Physiologic indices as predictors of survival are more extensively studied, especially the variables of the pulmonary function tests (PFTs). The forced vital capacity (FVC), total lung capacity (TLC), and diffusion capacity for carbon monoxide (DLCO) have consistently proved to relate with survival, while 6- and 12-month changes in FVC and DLCO are found even more reliable in estimating survival [11, 12].

In IPF, anatomic and functional derangements lead to defects in lung mechanics and gas exchange clinically manifesting with exertional dyspnea, the most prominent and disabling symptom in these patients [13]. Exercise limitation has a tremendous negative impact on the quality of life of IPF patients [14], and one would expect that it would additionally inversely influence their outcome. However, exercise testing in the staging and prognosis of the disease is less extensively studied than resting variables [15]. More precisely, the 6-minute walking test (6MWT), a practical and simple test which reflects submaximal exercise, has only recently been included in the evaluation of patients with IPF [16]. Desaturation and distance walked during the 6MWT have proved valuable in the estimation of prognosis [17, 18].

Cardiopulmonary exercise test (CPET) is a dynamic, accurate, and reliable tool for the estimation of severity and prognosis for patients with cardiovascular and respiratory diseases reflecting the abnormalities of both systems under submaximal and peak exercise performance [19]. However, it is considered to add little to resting lung function in assessing the severity and outcome in interstitial lung diseases [15, 16].

Based on our recent study showing significant associations between clinical predictors of survival such as the Medical Research Council (MRC) chronic dyspnea score and physiological variables obtained during maximal and submaximal exercise testing in IPF patients [13], we attempted in the present study to evaluate the role of exercise testing through two of the most commonly used exercise protocols, the 6MWT and CPET as a prognostic tool in IPF.

2. Materials and Methods

2.1. Study Subjects and Setting. This observational study was approved by the Institutional Ethics Committee of "Attikon" University Hospital, National and Kapodistrian University of Athens, Greece. Written informed consent was obtained from each patient. We prospectively recruited patients examined at the outpatient clinic over a period of one year. All patients fulfilled the criteria of the American Thoracic Society, European Respiratory Society, and the American College of Chest Physicians for the diagnosis of IPF [20]. These patients have already been recruited in another study by our team [13]. After completion of the study all patients were reexamined as far as diagnosis was concerned based on the recently published criteria of 2011 [1]. All patients were found to fulfill the new criteria of IPF. None of the patients were receiving treatment with oxygen. None of the patients

included had significant pulmonary hypertension (PASP > 45 mmHg, verified by cardiac ultrasound). Patients taking beta-blockers were specifically excluded from performing the CPET and by extension from the study. No case of lung transplant was recorded during the study. Secondary causes of lung fibrosis were excluded: none of the patients had a history of environmental or occupational exposure, drug toxicity, or autoimmune rheumatic disease, as documented by history, clinical and immunological tests.

2.2. Pulmonary Function Tests (PFTs). Lung function tests were done at diagnosis or at an interval of 15 days before the realization of the 6MWT and the CPET. PFTs included forced expiratory volume during the first second of expiration (FEV_1), forced vital capacity (FVC), total lung capacity (TLC), and single-breath carbon monoxide diffusing capacity (DLCO) all measured by MasterScreen Body apparatus (Erich Jaeger GmbH, Wuerzburg, Germany).

2.3. The 6-Minute Walking Test. The 6MWT was done according to the ATS guidelines [21]. The following data were collected and analyzed: distance (meters), duration (minutes), oxygen saturation at the initiation and at the end of the test, pulse at initiation and at the end of the test, the difference in oxygen saturation before and after the test, systolic and diastolic blood pressure before the test, Borg scale score before and after the test, and age (years), height (meters), and body weight of the patients (kilograms). Oxygen desaturation was defined as resting oxygen saturation minus oxygen saturation at the end of the 6MWT.

2.4. Cardiopulmonary Exercise Testing. The CPET was performed at an interval of 2-3 days after the 6MWT using a standardized protocol in accordance with the American Thoracic Society/American College of Chest Physicians (ATS/ACCP) statement [19]. All patients underwent a symptom-limited cardiopulmonary exercise test with an electromagnetically braked cycle ergometer (Ergometrics 900, Erich Jaeger GmbH, Wurzburg, Germany) using a ramp protocol. The protocol included 3 min of sitting rest, 3 min of unloaded cycling (at 60 revolutions per min plus or minus 5 revolutions per min), followed by a progressively increasing work rate in a ramp fashion, and 3 min of recovery. The work rate increment for each ramped exercise test was individualized on the basis of each patient's pretest activity level (range, 8 to 25 Watts/min). Cardiopulmonary data were collected and analyzed with an exercise metabolic unit (Oxycon Pro Erich Jaeger GmbH, Wurzburg, Germany). The following parameters were recorded: heart rate (HR), minute ventilation (VE), tidal volume (TV), peak oxygen consumption (VO_2 peak), peak oxygen consumption/kg (VO_2 peak/kg), %VO_2 predicted, slope of relation between minute ventilation and CO_2 production (VE/VCO_2 slope), VE/VCO_2 ratio at anaerobic threshold, respiratory rate (RR), oxygen pulse (O_2P), oxygen saturation at peak exercise (SpO_2 peak), anaerobic threshold (AT), breathing reserve (BR), heart rate recovery (HRR), and heart rate reserve (HRRes). AT was determined noninvasively through the plot of VCO_2 versus VO_2 (V-slope method).

2.5. Statistical Analysis. Data are presented as mean ± standard deviation (±SD). The parameters of the current study were individually evaluated for relevance to the overall survival through the Cox proportional hazards models. It must be noted that among parameters which presented an absolute correlation value greater than 90%, only one was included in the evaluation. Each of these models was evaluated by three independent and asymptotically equivalent tests, the Wald test, the likelihood ratio test, and the score (log rank) test, each calculating a P value for the null-hypothesis that the factor coefficients are equal to zero. For evaluating the models and ranking them from best to worst under the frame of the aforementioned tests, a sum-index was calculated by summing the P values of the aforementioned tests and the following selection criteria for the best model were set.

(1) The best model should minimize the sum-index.

(2) The null-hypothesis should be rejected by as many of the individual tests as possible after applying the Bonferroni correction for multiple testing which set the a-level of statistical significance at 0.0019; hence, only P values lower than that threshold were considered statistically significant.

In order to optimally model the risk through multiple regression hazard modelling, all the parameters having the null-hypothesis rejected in at least one of the tests after the Bonferroni correction were included in a multiple regression Cox proportional hazards model, and the optimum model was selected through a stepwise model selection procedure. Specifically the algorithm utilized for the stepwise procedure was bidirectional (combined forward selection and backward elimination) aiming at minimizing the Bayesian information criterion (BIC) [22] which is a robust measure of model adequacy. Statistical analysis was carried out using R. The Cox proportional hazards modelling was performed utilizing the "Survival" R-package. The stepwise model selection procedure was implemented by the "MASS" R-package. The nonparametric Spearman correlation coefficient was calculated to describe the relationships between variables of 6MWT, CPET, and pulmonary function tests by using SPSS v.13.0.0 (Chicago, IL). A P value less than 0.05 was considered significant.

3. Results

The population studied consisted of 25 patients. The demographic and clinical characteristics of the study population at the time of IPF diagnosis are given in Table 1. All patients were treatment naive when entering the study, while most of them received no treatment for IPF in the observational period as well. None of the patients included in the study were on treatment with beta-blockers. At the time of reporting seventeen patients were still alive (Figure 1). Follow-up time ranged from 9 months to 64 months. Mean survival was 48.7 ± 4.4 months (95% CI = 40–57.4) (Figure 1). All deaths were disease related. In Table 2, the results are reported for the 6MWT and the CPET. Out of 25 patients, 16 patients (64%) stopped CPET due to dyspnea and the rest 9 (36%) due to leg discomfort.

TABLE 1: Demographic and clinical data of the study population.

Variables (n)	(mean ± SD)
Age, year ($n = 25$)	67.5 (±8.3)
Gender (M/F)	17/8
Ex-smoker (n) %	13 (52%)
Non smoker (n) %	11 (44%)
Smoker (n) %	1 (4%)
PY (mean ± SD)	25.4 (±34.2)
FEV$_1$% ($n = 25$)	80.4 ± 18.8
FVC% ($n = 25$)	77.5 ± 21.8
FEV$_1$%/FVC ($n = 25$)	82 ± 0.04
TLC% ($n = 23$)	61.4 ± 13.7
DLCO% ($n = 23$)	45.6 ± 13.2
Comorbid disease ($n = 25$)	
Arterial hypertension	10 (40%)
Coronary disease	4 (16%)
Diabetes mellitus	3 (12%)
Gastroesophageal reflux symptoms	5 (20%)

M/F: male/female, PY: pack/years, FEV$_1$: forced expiratory volume at one second, FVC: forced vital capacity, TLC: total lung capacity, and DLCO: diffusing capacity for carbon monoxide. All values are shown as mean ± standard deviation (SD).

TABLE 2: Results of the CPET and the 6MWT in the study population.

	n	Mean ± SD
CPET variable		
VO$_2$ peak/kg (mL/kg/min)	25	15.5 ± 3.9
VO$_2$ at AT (mL/kg/min)	21	11.6 ± 3.5
Oxygen pulse (mL/beat)	25	9.2 ± 2.8
SpO$_2$ peak	25	87.7 ± 5.7
VE peak (L/min)	25	54.2 ± 17.5
BR peak %	25	27.3 ± 21.2
VE/VCO$_2$ slope	25	40.0 ± 13.5
VE/VCO$_2$ ratio at AT	21	37 ± 10.4
HR reserve	25	19.2 ± 18.0
HR recovery	25	14.5 ± 8.3
6MWT variable		
Distance (meters)	25	326.4 ± 153
SpO$_2$ at the initiation%	25	94.8 ± 2.2
SpO$_2$ at the end%	25	87.6 ± 5.6
Desaturation (%)	25	7.2 ± 4.3

Peak oxygen consumption/kg (VO$_2$ peak/kg), anaerobic threshold (AT), oxygen pulse (O$_2$P), oxygen saturation at peak exercise (SpO2 peak), total ventilation (VE), carbon dioxide output (VCO$_2$), breathing reserve (BR), VE/VCO$_2$ slope at anaerobic threshold (AT), and heart rate (HR). All values are shown as mean ± standard deviation.

Twenty-one patients reached anaerobic threshold. Among the 4 patients who did not reach AT, one stopped due to leg discomfort and the rest due to dyspnea. Among CPET parameters, VE/VCO$_2$ slope, VO$_2$ peak/kg, and VE/VCO$_2$ at anaerobic threshold were significant predictors of survival (Table 3). As far as 6MWT is concerned, distance walked and

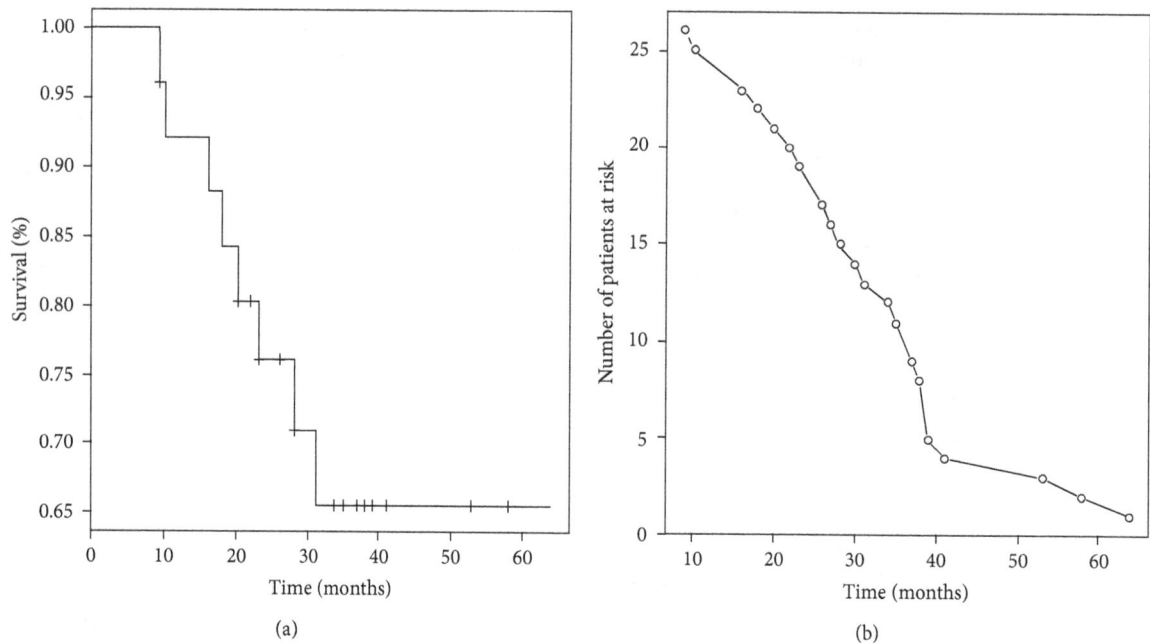

FIGURE 1: The cumulative Kaplan-Meier survival plot. (a) Survival of 25 IPF patients followed till death (uncensored: $n = 8$) or reporting of the study (censored: $n = 17$), combined by a plot (b) where the number of patients at risk is shown.

TABLE 3: Significant predictors of survival among the variables of CPET and 6MWT in IPF patients.

Variables	Wald test	Score (log rank) test	HR	CI (95%)	Sum-index
VE/VCO$_2$ slope	0.001	0.0002	1.09	1.04–1.15	0.0017
VO$_2$ peak/kg	0.001	0.0004	0.75	0.60–0.95	0.0033
DLCO%	0.002	0.0007	0.88	0.80–0.96	0.0035
Distance (meters)	0.003	0.0008	0.99	0.98–1.00	0.0047
VE/VCO$_2$ ratio at AT	0.006	0.0001	1.15	1.04–1.26	0.0074
Desaturation (%)	0.007	0.0025	1.45	1.11–1.90	0.0102

Minute ventilation (VE), carbon dioxide output (VCO$_2$), peak oxygen consumption/kg (VO$_2$ peak/kg), diffusing capacity for carbon monoxide% (DLCO%), VE/VCO$_2$ slope at anaerobic threshold (AT), and hazard ratio (HR).

oxygen desaturation were significant predictors of survival, while among PFTs parameters, only DLCO% correlated with survival (Table 3). Among all parameters, VE/VCO$_2$ slope and VO$_2$ peak/kg were the factors with the two smallest sum-indexes which reject the null-hypothesis in all the independent tests after the Bonferroni correction; thus, they were the most significant parameters predicting survival. These factors present a negative correlation of 76%. After further analysis with the stepwise model selection, the optimal model for survival prediction was identified as VO$_2$ peak/kg + DLCO% (Figure 2). Per 1-unit increase of VO$_2$ peak/kg (1 mL/kg/min) and DLCO% (1%), mortality risk is reduced by 32% and 13%, respectively (95% CI 0.60–0.95, HR = 0.75 for VO$_2$ peak/kg, 95% CI 0.80–0.96, HR = 0.88 for DLCO%). Regarding "Distance" which was the only statistically significant value of the 6MWT (after the Bonferroni correction), it must be noted that it was included in the initial model being evaluated by the stepwise model selection procedure minimizing the BIC and it was rejected along the process. Additionally, it is worth mentioning that when including

the Distance in a Cox proportional hazards model, the R-squared of this model is 0.376, while the respective R-squared of the optimum model as evaluated by the stepwise model selection procedure was 0.528 which is a clear indication that the optimum model provides a more efficient modeling of the hazard ratios than the model involving the Distance 6MWT parameter. Furthermore, according to optimum Cox proportional hazards model, a threshold VO$_2$ peak/kg of 14.2 mL/min/kg was associated with an increased risk of mortality (Figure 3). VE/VCO$_2$ slope and VO$_2$ peak/kg were also found to correlate with distance and desaturation during the 6MWT (Table 4). VO$_2$ peak/kg, distance walked, and desaturation correlated with resting functional variables such as the FEV$_1$, FVC, TLC, and DLCO, while VE/VCO$_2$ slope correlated only with DLCO (Table 5).

4. Discussion

In this study, we aimed to evaluate the role of exercise testing in the outcome of IPF patients. Therefore, we examined the

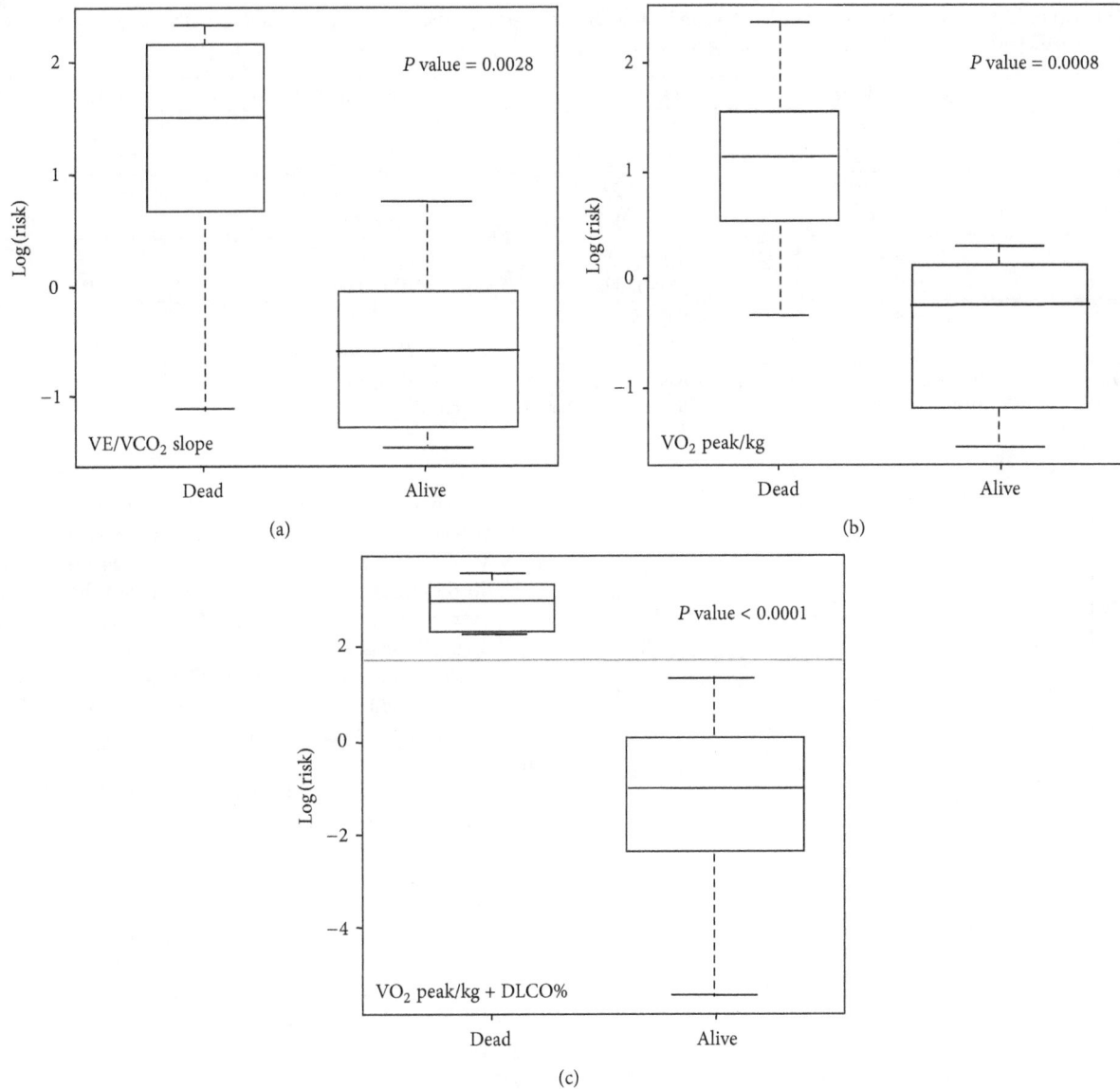

FIGURE 2: Overall death risk through the Cox proportional hazards models. In box plot (a), the Cox model includes only VE/VCO$_2$ slope, in box plot (b), the Cox model includes VO$_2$ peak/kg, and in box plot (c), the Cox model includes VO$_2$ peak/kg + DLCO%. A bidirectional stepwise model selection method minimizing the Bayesian information criterion (BIC) was utilized for selecting the optimal model which was identified as VO$_2$ peak/kg + DLCO%. Data are described using standard box plots with medians (interquartile range). Risk was found to be significantly differentiated between dead and alive with $P = 0.0028$, $P = 0.008$, and $P < 0.0001$, respectively.

TABLE 4: Relationships between the variables of 6MWT and VE/VCO$_2$ slope and VO$_2$ peak/kg by Spearman's rank correlation coefficient. P value < 0.05 is considered significant.

	VO$_2$ peak/kg	VE/VCO$_2$ slope
Distance	$r = 0.7$	$r = -0.6$
	$P < 0.0001$	$P = 0.001$
Desaturation%	$r = -0.52$	$r = 0.4$
	$P = 0.007$	$P = 0.02$

Minute ventilation (VE), carbon dioxide output (VCO$_2$), and peak oxygen consumption/kg (VO$_2$ peak/kg).

relationship between the variables of maximal-CPET and submaximal-6MWT exercise tests and survival. We found that VE/VCO$_2$ slope, VO$_2$ peak/kg, and VE/VCO$_2$ ratio at anaerobic threshold from the CPET and both distance walked and desaturation from the 6MWT are significantly correlated with survival. According to our results, the variables most strongly correlated with survival are VE/VCO$_2$ slope and VO$_2$ peak/kg, both from the CPET protocol, while the optimal model for mortality risk estimation was identified when VO$_2$ peak/kg and DLCO% were combined. In this model, a threshold VO$_2$ peak/kg of 14.2 mL/min/kg was associated with an increased risk of mortality.

The results of the present study are partly in accordance with the ones of Fell and colleagues who demonstrated that cardiopulmonary exercise testing adds significant prognostic information for patients with IPF and identified that IPF

TABLE 5: Relationships between the variables of both exercise tests and pulmonary function tests in the study population by Spearman's rank correlation coefficient. P value < 0.05 is considered significant.

	VE/VCO_2 slope	VO_2 peak/kg	Distance 6MWT	Desaturation 6MWT
$FEV_1\%$	$r = -0.26$	$r = 0.41$	$r = 0.4$	$r = -0.47$
	$P = 0.2$	$P = 0.03$	$P = 0.05$	$P = 0.01$
FVC%	$r = -0.38$	$r = 0.52$	$r = 0.48$	$r = -0.5$
	$P = 0.06$	$P = 0.007$	$P = 0.01$	$P = 0.01$
TLC%	$r = -0.36$	$r = 0.6$	$r = 0.61$	$r = -0.47$
	$P = 0.08$	$P = 0.003$	$P = 0.002$	$P = 0.02$
DLCO%	$r = -0.74$	$r = 0.64$	$r = 0.7$	$r = -0.57$
	$P < 0.001$	$P = 0.001$	$P < 0.0001$	$P = 0.004$

Minute ventilation (VE), carbon dioxide output (VCO_2), peak oxygen consumption/kg (VO_2 peak/kg), (FEV_1) forced expiratory volume at one second, (FVC) forced vital capacity, (TLC) total lung capacity, and (DLCO) diffusing capacity for carbon monoxide.

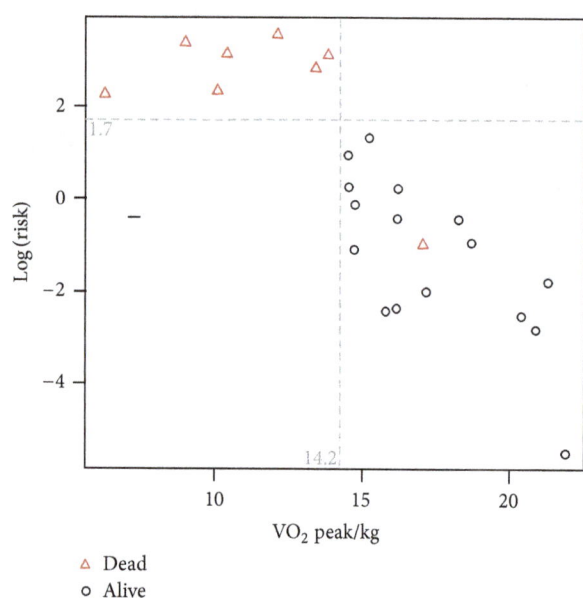

FIGURE 3: A threshold of mortality was identified. A threshold VO_2 peak/kg of 14.2 mL/min/kg was associated with an increased risk of mortality according to optimum Cox proportional hazards model.

patients with a baseline maximal oxygen uptake less than 8.3 mL/kg/min during CPET have an increased risk of death. VO_2 peak/kg did not correlate with survival when examined as a continuous variable and the baseline VO_2 peak/kg threshold with a predictive role was lower compared to the one found in the present study [23]. In addition, in their study they hypothesized that short-term longitudinal changes in VO_2 peak/kg would predict survival, but according to their results, VO_2 peak/kg did not change between baseline and 6 months. The discrepancies in the values and thresholds of the significant variables such as VO_2 peak/kg could be attributed to differences in the characteristics of the studies' populations and do not alter the similarities in the conclusions and the common clinical implication of both studies. For example, patients in the study of Fell and colleagues who were recruited from previous study protocols have a more impaired functional status as expressed by FVC values and were under

treatment with several regimens contrary to the present study where most patients are treatment naive. In a recent study which retrospectively examined the prognostic value of CPET in 63 patients with IPF, results showed that increased ventilation at anaerobic threshold (AT) as reflected by higher VE/VO_2 at AT was a major prognostic factor of death [24]. On the other hand, in the study of Gay and coworkers, VO_2 peak measurement among the factors of a composite clinical, radiographic, and physiologic scoring system for IPF patients failed to predict survival [25], while Erbes and colleagues found that gas transfer during spiroergometric exercise was not predictive of prognosis in IPF [26]. However, most of those studies were retrospective in design.

The significant correlation of CPET variables with survival indicates that exercise limitation has a tremendous effect on this group of patients. In IPF, fibrotic lung parenchymal damage leads to multiple physiologic derangements such as low tidal volume, the rapid shallow breathing pattern, and the detrimental dead space ventilation. The above disorders result in worsening gas exchange during exercise sooner or later in every patient with IPF. Exercise limitation is further aggravated by pulmonary vascular derangements, myocardial disturbances, and peripheral muscle weakness that are commonly described in IPF patients [13]. Based on the results of the present study, the physiological factors that have the most potent impact on survival are VE/VCO_2 slope and VO_2 peak/kg. In patients with chronic lung diseases, an elevated VE/VCO_2 slope is attributed to the effects of increased physiological dead space, ventilation-perfusion mismatching, and the abnormally elevated chemoreceptor and ergoreceptor sensitivity that are present at rest and deteriorate during exercise [27]. Furthermore, pulmonary hypertension that commonly develops in IPF patients has been shown to be associated with an elevated VE/VCO_2 slope [27]. In many studies, VE/VCO_2 slope has been shown to have similar or even superior ability over VO_2 peak/kg to predict serious cardiovascular events in heart failure, the disease where CPET has gained widespread use and most clinical experience exists [28].

Based on our results, the predictive role of CPET and more precisely of VO_2 peak/kg is further enforced when the model combines VO_2 peak/kg with DLCO. This finding could be explained by the fact that both values reflect very robustly and in a complementary way the pathophysiology of exercise limitation in IPF patients. Peak oxygen consumption on the one hand reflects the attainment of a limitation at some point in the oxygen conductance pathway due to the physiologic derangements already described in IPF. On the other hand, DLCO provides information regarding the above-mentioned physiologic derangements, that is, the gas transfer capability which is significantly impaired in IPF and predicts oxygen desaturation during exercise [11, 12, 29].

The evaluation of multidimensional models of survival, combining variables that independently predict mortality and share common underlying physiologic determinants, has already been studied in respiratory diseases such as COPD [30]. In IPF, most composite indices that have been identified by now usually derive from the extent of fibrosis on HRCT, pulmonary function test variables, and clinical parameters such as age and gender, thus precluding the prognostic strength of exercise data [12, 31, 32]. Only in the study of King Jr. and coworkers was PaO2 at the end of maximal exercise included among seven parameters in the new complete clinical, radiographic, and physiologic (CRP) scoring system for prediction of survival in IPF patients [12]. Nevertheless, this score is not easy to perform in everyday clinical practice and it partially depends on subjective measurements such as finger clubbing.

As far as the contribution of the 6MWT in the prognostic evaluation of IPF patients is concerned, the present data are in agreement with the conclusions of previous studies showing that a decrease in saturation of 4% or oxygen desaturation below 88% during 6MWT is a predictor of mortality for IPF patients [17]. The role of the distance walked is also highlighted, although contradictory conclusions exist on the field [18, 33]. However, the predictive role of the 6MWT seems weaker when compared to CPET when multivariable relationships are explored. This observation is in line with the conclusion of Fell and coworkers that VO_2 peak/kg threshold is a more robust predictor of survival than desaturation beyond 88% during a 6MWT [23]. Based on the results of both studies, we believe that the role of CPET in the evaluation of survival in IPF patients could be upgraded. CPET should be applied in a complementary way to the 6MWT which is much more widely performed and recommended [16].

In the present study, further evaluation of the interdependence of both maximal and submaximal exercise test variables with resting functional measurements has demonstrated a strong and significant association between them. The fact that all four pulmonary function test parameters at rest (FEV_1, FVC, TLC, and DLCO) were found to correlate significantly with indices of both 6MWT and CPET indicates that the group of patients is well selected. The restrictive defect encountered in this group of patients leads to the inability to expand tidal volume appropriately and therefore to low breathing reserve during the increased metabolic demand of exercise which is a major determinant of exercise limitation in IPF [29, 34].

Our study has a number of limitations, the most important being the relatively short observation period and in consequence the limited mortality rate. Another limitation is the moderate number of patients included mostly due to the rarity of the disease with a prevalence of 3.4 cases per 100.000 inhabitants in Greece [35]. However, it is a prospective, single centre study based on a well-selected group of IPF patients most of who are treatment naive, in contrast to the majority of already existing studies in the literature which are retrospective in design and examine patients that participate in various treatment protocols that could have an undefined impact on their survival.

5. Conclusions

In conclusion, exercise testing through two of the most commonly used protocols, the 6MWT and CPET, is shown to have a significant prognostic role for the survival of IPF patients. Most importantly, variables of cardiopulmonary exercise testing such as VE/VCO_2 slope and VO_2 peak/kg are found to be more potent than previously thought concerning the prediction of outcome in IPF, not only as thresholds but also as continuous variables. The predictive role of peak oxygen consumption is further reinforced when integrated with DLCO due to the fact that both variables share major underlying physiologic determinants of exercise limitation in IPF.

Conflict of Interests

All authors declare that they have no conflict of interests.

Authors' Contribution

Christina Triantafillidou and Effrosyni Manali have contributed equally to this work.

Acknowledgments

This work has been supported by the Thorax Foundation and by a Research Grant "Kapodistrias" of the National and Kapodistrian University of Athens, Greece. All authors would like to express their gratitude to Professor Joseph Milic-Emili for providing them with invaluable help and constant inspiration all those years.

References

[1] G. Raghu, H. R. Collard, J. J. Egan et al., "An official ATS/ERS/JRS/ALAT statement: idiopathic pulmonary fibrosis: evidence-based guidelines for diagnosis and management," *American Journal of Respiratory and Critical Care Medicine*, vol. 183, no. 6, pp. 788–824, 2011.

[2] B. Ley, H. R. Collard, and T. E. King Jr., "Clinical course and prediction of survival in idiopathic pulmonary fibrosis," *American Journal of Respiratory and Critical Care Medicine*, vol. 183, no. 4, pp. 431–440, 2011.

[3] N. P. Barlo, C. H. M. van Moorsel, J. M. M. van den Bosch, and J. C. Grutters, "Predicting prognosis in idiopathic pulmonary fibrosis," *Sarcoidosis Vasculitis and Diffuse Lung Diseases*, vol. 27, no. 2, pp. 85–95, 2010.

[4] O. Nishiyama, H. Taniguchi, Y. Kondoh et al., "A simple assessment of dyspnoea as a prognostic indicator in idiopathic pulmonary fibrosis," *European Respiratory Journal*, vol. 36, no. 5, pp. 1067–1072, 2010.

[5] N. M. Patel, D. J. Lederer, A. C. Borczuk, and S. M. Kawut, "Pulmonary hypertension in idiopathic pulmonary fibrosis," *Chest*, vol. 132, no. 3, pp. 998–1006, 2007.

[6] M. Mejía, G. Carrillo, J. Rojas-Serrano et al., "Idiopathic pulmonary fibrosis and emphysema: decreased survival associated with severe pulmonary arterial hypertension," *Chest*, vol. 136, no. 1, pp. 10–15, 2009.

[7] E. D. Manali, G. T. Stathopoulos, A. Kollintza et al., "The Medical Research Council chronic dyspnea score predicts the survival of patients with idiopathic pulmonary fibrosis," *Respiratory Medicine*, vol. 102, no. 4, pp. 586–592, 2008.

[8] D. A. Lynch, J. D. Godwin, S. Safrin et al., "High-resolution computed tomography in idiopathic pulmonary fibrosis: diagnosis and prognosis," *American Journal of Respiratory and Critical Care Medicine*, vol. 172, no. 4, pp. 488–493, 2005.

[9] C. Triantafillidou, E. D. Manali, C. Magkou et al., "Medical Research Council dyspnea scale does not relate to fibroblast foci profusion in IPF," *Diagnostic Pathology*, vol. 6, no. 1, article 28, 2011.

[10] A. G. Nicholson, L. G. Fulford, T. V. Colby, R. M. Du Bois, D. M. Hansell, and A. U. Wells, "The relationship between individual histologic features and disease progression in idiopathic pulmonary fibrosis," *American Journal of Respiratory and Critical Care Medicine*, vol. 166, no. 2, pp. 173–177, 2002.

[11] H. R. Collard, T. E. King Jr., B. B. Bartelson, J. S. Vourlekis, M. I. Schwarz, and K. K. Brown, "Changes in clinical and physiologic variables predict survival in idiopathic pulmonary fibrosis," *American Journal of Respiratory and Critical Care Medicine*, vol. 168, no. 5, pp. 538–542, 2003.

[12] T. E. King Jr., J. A. Tooze, M. I. Schwarz, K. R. Brown, and R. M. Cherniack, "Predicting survival in idiopathic pulmonary fibrosis: scoring system and survival model," *American Journal of Respiratory and Critical Care Medicine*, vol. 164, no. 7, pp. 1171–1181, 2001.

[13] E. D. Manali, P. Lyberopoulos, C. Triantafillidou et al., "MRC chronic dyspnea scale: relationships with cardiopulmonary exercise testing and 6-minute walk test in idiopathic pulmonary fibrosis patients: a prospective study," *BMC Pulmonary Medicine*, vol. 10, article 32, 2010.

[14] J. J. Swigris, W. G. Kuschner, S. S. Jacobs, S. R. Wilson, and M. K. Gould, "Health-related quality of life in patients with idiopathic pulmonary fibrosis: a systematic review," *Thorax*, vol. 60, no. 7, pp. 588–594, 2005.

[15] A. U. Wells and N. Hirani, "Interstitial lung disease guideline: the British Thoracic Society in collaboration with the Thoracic Society of Australia and New Zealand and the Irish Thoracic Society," *Thorax*, vol. 63, supplement 5, pp. v1–v58, 2008.

[16] T. Eaton, P. Young, D. Milne, and A. U. Wells, "Six-minute walk, maximal exercise tests: reproducibility in fibrotic interstitial pneumonia," *American Journal of Respiratory and Critical Care Medicine*, vol. 171, no. 10, pp. 1150–1157, 2005.

[17] V. N. Lama, K. R. Flaherty, G. B. Toews et al., "Prognostic value of desaturation during a 6 minute walk test in idiopathic interstitial pneumonia," *American Journal of Respiratory and Critical Care Medicine*, vol. 168, no. 9, pp. 1084–1090, 2003.

[18] D. J. Lederer, S. M. Arcasoy, J. S. Wilt, F. D'Ovidio, J. R. Sonett, and S. M. Kawut, "Six-minute-walk distance predicts waiting list survival in idiopathic pulmonary fibrosis," *American Journal of Respiratory and Critical Care Medicine*, vol. 174, no. 6, pp. 659–664, 2006.

[19] "ATS/ACCP Statement of cardiopulmonary testing," *American Journal of Respiratory and Critical Care Medicine*, vol. 167, no. 2, pp. 211–277, 2003.

[20] American Thoracic Society, European Respiratory Society, and American College of Chest Physicians, "Idiopathic pulmonary fibrosis: diagnosis and treatment. International consensus statement," *American Journal of Respiratory and Critical Care Medicine*, vol. 161, no. 2, pp. 646–664, 2000.

[21] R. O. Crapo, R. Casaburi, A. L. Coates et al., "ATS statement: guidelines for the six-minute walk test," *American Journal of Respiratory and Critical Care Medicine*, vol. 166, no. 1, pp. 111–117, 2002.

[22] G. Schwarz, "Estimating the dimension of a model," *Annals of Statistics*, vol. 6, no. 2, pp. 461–464, 1978.

[23] C. D. Fell, L. X. Liu, C. Motika et al., "The prognostic value of cardiopulmonary exercise testing in idiopathic pulmonary fibrosis," *American Journal of Respiratory and Critical Care Medicine*, vol. 179, no. 5, pp. 402–407, 2009.

[24] B. Wallaert, A. Guetta, L. Wemeau-Stervinou et al., "Prognostic value of clinical exercise testing in idiopathic pulmonary fibrosis," *Revue des Maladies Respiratoires*, vol. 28, no. 3, article 257, pp. 290–296, 2011.

[25] S. E. Gay, E. A. Kazerooni, G. B. Toews et al., "Idiopathic pulmonary fibrosis: predicting response to therapy and survival," *American Journal of Respiratory and Critical Care Medicine*, vol. 157, no. 4, pp. 1063–1072, 1998.

[26] R. Erbes, T. Schaberg, and R. Loddenkemper, "Lung function tests in patients with idiopathic pulmonary fibrosis: are they helpful for predicting outcome?" *Chest*, vol. 111, no. 1, pp. 51–57, 1997.

[27] G. J. Balady, R. Arena, K. Sietsema et al., "Clinician's guide to cardiopulmonary exercise testing in adults: a scientific statement from the American heart association," *Circulation*, vol. 122, no. 2, pp. 191–225, 2010.

[28] R. Poggio, H. C. Arazi, M. Giorgi, and S. G. Miriuka, "Prediction of severe cardiovascular events by VE/VCO^2 slope versus peak VO^2 in systolic heart failure: a meta-analysis of the published literature," *American Heart Journal*, vol. 160, no. 6, pp. 1004–1014, 2010.

[29] Z. Mohsenifar, S. M. Lee, P. Diaz et al., "Single-breath diffusing capacity of the lung for carbon monoxide: a predictor of PaO^2, maximum work rate, and walking distance in patients with emphysema," *Chest*, vol. 123, no. 5, pp. 1394–1400, 2003.

[30] B. R. Celli, C. G. Cote, J. M. Marin et al., "The body-mass index, airflow obstruction, dyspnea, and exercise capacity index in chronic obstructive pulmonary disease," *New England Journal of Medicine*, vol. 350, no. 10, pp. 1005–1012, 2004.

[31] B. Ley, C. Ryerson, E. Vittinghoff et al., "A multidimensional index and staging system for idiopathic pulmonary fibrosis," *Annals of Internal Medicine*, vol. 156, no. 10, pp. 684–691, 2012.

[32] A. U. Wells, S. R. Desai, M. B. Rubens et al., "Idiopathic pulmonary fibrosis: a composite physiologic index derived from disease extent observed by computed tomography," *American Journal of Respiratory and Critical Care Medicine*, vol. 167, no. 7, pp. 962–969, 2003.

[33] K. R. Flaherty, A. C. Andrei, S. Murray et al., "Idiopathic pulmonary fibrosis: prognostic value of changes in physiology and six-minute-walk test," *American Journal of Respiratory and Critical Care Medicine*, vol. 174, no. 7, pp. 803–809, 2006.

[34] D. E. O. 'Donnell, D. Ofir, and P. Laveneziana, "Patterns of cardiopulmonary response to exercise in lung diseases," *European Respiratory Monograph*, vol. 40, pp. 69–92, 2007.

[35] A. Karakatsani, D. Papakosta, A. Rapti et al., "Epidemiology of interstitial lung diseases in Greece," *Respiratory Medicine*, vol. 103, no. 8, pp. 1122–1129, 2009.

Intravenous Dexmedetomidine Provides Superior Patient Comfort and Tolerance Compared to Intravenous Midazolam in Patients Undergoing Flexible Bronchoscopy

Umesh Goneppanavar,[1] Rahul Magazine,[2] Bhavya Periyadka Janardhana,[3] and Shreepathi Krishna Achar[3]

[1]*Department of Anaesthesiology, Dharwad Institute of Mental Health and Neurosciences, Dharwad, Karnataka 580008, India*
[2]*Department of Pulmonary Medicine, Kasturba Medical College, Manipal University, Manipal, Karnataka 576104, India*
[3]*Department of Anaesthesiology, Kasturba Medical College, Manipal University, Manipal, Karnataka 576104, India*

Correspondence should be addressed to Rahul Magazine; rahulmagazine@gmail.com

Academic Editor: Dimitris Georgopoulos

Dexmedetomidine, an α_2 agonist, has demonstrated its effectiveness as a sedative during awake intubation, but its utility in fiberoptic bronchoscopy (FOB) is not clear. We evaluated the effects of midazolam and dexmedetomidine on patient's response to FOB. The patients received either midazolam, 0.02 mg/kg (group M, $n = 27$), or dexmedetomidine, 1 μg/kg (group D, $n = 27$). A composite score of five different parameters and a numerical rating scale (NRS) for pain intensity and distress were used to assess patient response during FOB. Patients rated the quality of sedation and level of discomfort 24 h after the procedure. Ease of bronchoscopy, rescue medication requirement, and haemodynamic variables were noted. Ideal or acceptable composite score was observed in 15 and 26 patients, respectively, in group M (14.48 ± 3.65) and group D (9.41 ± 3.13), $p < 0.001$. NRS showed that 11 patients in group M had severe pain and discomfort as compared to one patient with severe pain and two with severe discomfort in group D during the procedure, $p < 0.001$. Rescue midazolam requirement was significantly higher in group M ($p = 0.023$). We conclude that during FOB, under topical airway anaesthesia, IV dexmedetomidine (1 μg/kg) provides superior patient comfort and tolerance as compared to IV midazolam (0.02 mg/kg).

1. Introduction

Flexible fiberoptic bronchoscope has replaced rigid bronchoscopy as the technique of choice for evaluation of the airway. The reasons are reduced requirement of sedation, lesser complications related to the procedure, and better acceptability by the patients [1]. However, patients can still experience variable degree of pain, discomfort, and phobia, resulting in difficulty in performing the procedure and reducing its diagnostic utility [2]. Topical anaesthesia of airway alone is, often, insufficient to provide desirable patient comfort [3]. Therefore, in addition, appropriate sedation to enhance patient comfort and satisfaction is required [3–6]. Moreover, flexible bronchoscopy can cause sympathetic stimulation resulting in tachycardia, hypertension, arrhythmias,

and increased oxygen demand that can be deleterious to an already diseased heart [7]. Hence, current guidelines on flexible bronchoscopy recommend offering sedation to all patients [8].

Since the duration of the procedure is short and is performed mostly on outpatient basis, the ideal sedative should have rapid onset, short duration, rapid offset, and no adverse effects, but ensuring sedation sufficient to blunt the sympathetic responses and airway irritability. A variety of pharmacological agents including benzodiazepines, opioids, sympatholytic drugs, and propofol, alone or in combination, have been found to be useful. However, several complications are also attributed to their use, and, hence, the search is still on for a better sedative [9–14]. British Thoracic Society Guidelines have suggested the use of intravenous midazolam as 2 mg bolus prior to the procedure [8]. Midazolam is one of the most widely used drugs for sedation during bronchoscopy in view of its amnesic and anxiolytic properties along with its favourable pharmacokinetic profile such as rapid-onset and short-lasting depressant action on the central nervous system. Moreover, it has the advantage that its effect can be rapidly counteracted using flumazenil, a competitive antagonist for benzodiazepine receptors in situations of overdose. Recent evidence shows that dexmedetomidine, an α_2 agonist, can provide excellent sedation (anxiolysis, sedation, and analgesia without the risk of respiratory depression) during awake fiberoptic intubation in the management of difficult airway and also to patients in critical care units [15–19]. Dexmedetomidine has been evaluated in a few studies for its sedative effects during flexible fiberoptic bronchoscopy and has been found to be useful in enhancing patient comfort without the risk of respiratory depression [14, 20].

This study evaluated the effectiveness of midazolam or dexmedetomidine in improving patient comfort during flexible fiberoptic bronchoscopy.

2. Aims and Objective

The objective is to evaluate the effects of two intravenously administered pharmacological interventions, that is, midazolam and dexmedetomidine, on patient response to flexible bronchoscopy. Main outcome measure was a composite score of five different parameters on which patient response was assessed with the goal of identifying the drug that could provide better patient tolerance and improved fibrescopist comfort without compromising patient safety.

3. Materials and Methods

This study was prospective, randomized, and double blinded. Approval was obtained from the institutional ethics committee of our hospital. It was conducted in 54 patients who were considered appropriate for the study methodology. Written informed consent was obtained from the patients who were willing to participate in the study, after they had read and understood the patient information sheet. All patients in the age group 18 to 70 years requiring flexible bronchoscopic evaluation of the airway in the Department of Pulmonary Medicine of our institution were considered for the study. Those who were excluded from participating in the study included the ones with known or suspected allergy to any of the study drugs (dexmedetomidine, midazolam) and those with seizure disorder, moderate to severe chronic obstructive pulmonary disease, disease condition that would confuse the behaviour assessment, renal (with serum creatinine > 2 mg/dL) or hepatic impairment (elevated liver enzymes > 2 times normal) and haemodynamic instability (bradycardia with HR < 50 bpm or hypotension with SBP < 90 mmHg), or seriously ill patients with American Society of Anesthesiologists' physical status 4.

The patients were randomized into two groups, midazolam (0.02 mg/kg) and dexmedetomidine (1 μg/kg), as per a computer generated randomization table. Two drops of

oxymetazoline (0.05%) were administered into each nostril half an hour prior to beginning of the study. All patients were monitored: pulse rate, noninvasive blood pressure (NIBP), electrocardiogram, oxygen saturation with pulse oximeter, respiratory rate and sedation status using the Ramsay Sedation Score (RSS). After obtaining baseline values for these parameters, an intravenous access was established in the upper limb. The study drugs were loaded in one of the two syringes labelled A and B to help in blinding (syringe A had a volume of 10 mL and contained either dexmedetomidine 1 μg/kg diluted in normal saline or only normal saline; syringe B had a volume of 2 mL and contained either midazolam 0.02 mg/kg diluted with normal saline or normal saline). The study was begun with infusion of contents of syringe A over 10 minutes. At the beginning of the 9th minute, contents of syringe B were administered as a bolus. At the end of the 10th minute, bronchoscopy was commenced. Two mL lignocaine jelly (2%) was applied to the more patent nostril following which the fibrescope (FFB) was passed through the nostril. The throat and vocal cords were sprayed with 2 mL aliquots of 2% lignocaine solution (total 4 mL). After waiting for a minute, the fibrescope was advanced below the vocal cords where 1 mL, 2% lignocaine was sprayed. The fibrescope was advanced till carina where 1 mL, 2% lignocaine was sprayed into each main bronchus (total 2 mL). Once the patient coughing subsided, the fibrescope was advanced into either bronchi till tertiary segments were evaluated and the procedure for which the patient was scheduled was completed. In the event of patient having an RSS 1 after the topicalisation of the airway was complete, intravenous midazolam 1 mg bolus was administered (as rescue medication), which was kept in an open label syringe. At least two-minute gap between two doses of midazolam was maintained and the patient's level of sedation was constantly assessed and maintained between RSS 2 and 3.

The study involved three different observers. Observer 1 who picked up the randomization slip prepared the study drug, accordingly ensuring blinding (labelled the syringes A and B). Observer 1 did not have any further involvement with the study subject. Observer 2 performed the bronchoscopy and observer 3 assessed the patients, explained study methodology, obtained consent, administered the study drugs, and recorded the study parameters. Both observers 2 and 3 were blinded to the study drug and they were constant throughout the study.

Patient response to bronchoscopy was assessed using five different parameters which together contributed to the composite score (Table 1). For clinical and statistical purposes, the composite score was considered ideal when the score was 5–10, acceptable when the score was 11–15, and unacceptable when the score was >15. This was used as our primary outcome measure for the study. Patient response to bronchoscopy was also assessed using a numerical rating scale (for pain intensity and distress) prior to, during, and 10 min after bronchoscopy. A score of 0 on the NRS meant that the patient was comfortable and cooperative while a score of 10 was considered the worst patient response. Numerical rating scale for pain intensity and distress (assessed during procedure by observer 3 and patient response obtained at 10 min following

TABLE 1: Composite score during bronchoscopy (5–25).

Parameter	1	2	3	4	5
Sedation	Awake to voice >10 s	Light sedation, briefly awakens to voice	Moderate sedation, no eye contact	Deep sedation, response only to physical stimulation	Unarousable, no response to physical stimulation
Calmness	Alert and calm	Anxious, not aggressive	Frequent nonpurposeful movement	Pulls or removes bronchoscope; aggressive	Combative, violent
Respiratory response	Spontaneous respiration No coughing	Occasional cough	Coughing regularly	Frequent coughing or chocking	Vigorous cough preventing bronchoscopy
Physical movement	No movement	Occasional slight movement	Frequent slight movements	Vigorous movement limited to the extremities	Vigorous movement including torso and head
Facial tension	Facial muscle tone normal	Mild muscle tension evident	Tension evident in all facial muscles	Grimacing	Grimacing and crying

the procedure) is further graded for statistical analysis as mild when the score was between 0 and 3, moderate when the score was between 4 and 7, and severe when the score was between 8 and 10. Sedation state was assessed using Ramsay Sedation Score prior to, during, and 10 min after procedure. Observer 2 who performed flexible bronchoscopy on all the study subjects assessed the ease of bronchoscopy as easy, slightly difficult, or very difficult. Approximately 24 h after the procedure, all patients were asked to give their opinion regarding the quality of sedation (excellent/good/fair/poor) and level of discomfort during the procedure (none to mild, moderate, and severe). The duration of bronchoscopy, number of doses of rescue medication required, haemodynamic variables such as heart rate (HR), systolic blood pressure (SBP), diastolic blood pressure (DBP), and any change in rhythm pattern during the study period were noted. Starting just prior to bronchoscopy, the haemodynamic variables were noted every 2 minutes till the end of bronchoscopy and 10 minutes after the procedure. Patients were also monitored for any oxygen desaturation (SpO_2 < 93%) or hypoventilation (RR < 8/min).

3.1. Sample Size Estimation. A pilot study was done that included four patients in midazolam group and three patients in dexmedetomidine group. The results of pilot study showed a composite score difference of 2 between the groups. Based on this data, it was estimated that 26 patients were needed in each group to have a power of 80% at 95% confidence interval for a composite score difference of 3.

3.2. Statistical Analysis. After collecting the data, mean and standard deviation were calculated as appropriate. Continuous variables like age, height, weight, BMI, and duration of bronchoscopy between groups were compared using independent t-test. Whereas categorical data like gender, numerical rating scale, Ramsay Sedation Score, requirement of rescue medication, ease of bronchoscopy, and postprocedure patient assessment of bronchoscopy were compared between groups using either Fisher's exact test or Chi-square test, composite score was analysed using Mann-Whitney U test.

TABLE 2: Patients' characteristics and bronchoscopy data.

Characteristics and data	Group M Mean ± SD	Group D Mean ± SD	p value
Age (years)	52.52 ± 15.05	49.70 ± 13.85	0.478[#]
Gender (M/F)	24/3	20/7	0.161[*]
Height (cm)	164.89 ± 5.78	160.00 ± 5.04	0.002[#]
Weight (kg)	56.07 ± 10.84	53.26 ± 10.10	0.328[#]
BMI (kg/m^2)	20.42 ± 3.46	20.77 ± 3.40	0.713[#]
Procedures	Diagnostic (27)	Diagnostic (27)	1
Duration of bronchoscopy	8.19 ± 2.53	8.93 ± 2.96	0.327[#]

[*] Chi-square test.
[#] Independent t-test.

All the analyses were performed on SPSS version 18.0 (SPSS Inc., Chicago, IL, USA). A p value of <0.05 was considered statistically significant.

4. Results

A total of 54 patients (27 in each group) participated and all of them completed the study. The age, gender, weight, and body mass index between the groups were comparable while patients in group M were taller than those in group D. All patients underwent diagnostic evaluation of the tracheobronchial tree. The mean duration of bronchoscopy was comparable between the two groups with 8.19 ± 2.53 min in group M and 8.93 ± 2.96 in group D (Table 2).

The composite score (a reflector towards patient cooperation and tolerance to the procedure) was ideal or acceptable in 15 patients in group M and 26 patients in group D. The mean scores were 14.48 ± 3.65 in group M and 9.41 ± 3.13 in group D (p < 0.001, Table 3). Individual components of the composite score showed that >25% patients in group M had unacceptable scores (score of 4 or 5) in four out of five segments (except sedation) while most patients (>90%)

TABLE 3: Comparison of composite score (total score).

Total score	Group M (n = 27)	Group D (n = 27)
5	0	1
6–10	4	19
11–15	11	6
16–20	12	1
Mean ± SD	14.48 ± 3.65	9.41 ± 3.13

$p < 0.001$ (Mann-Whitney U test).

TABLE 4: Split-up of components of the composite score.

Component of composite score	Group M (n = 27)		Group D (n = 27)	
	Number	%	Number	%
Sedation				
1	23	85.2	22	18.5
2	4	14.8	4	70.4
3	0	0	0	11.1
4	0	0	1	0.0
5	0	0	0	0.0
Calmness				
1	1	3.7	8	29.6
2	8	29.7	13	48.2
3	11	40.7	4	14.8
4	7	25.9	2	7.4
5	0	0	0	0
Respiratory response				
1	1	3.7	5	18.5
2	4	14.8	19	70.4
3	15	55.6	3	11.1
4	6	22.2	0	0.0
5	1	3.7	0	0.0
Physical movement				
1	1	3.7	6	22.2
2	5	18.5	15	55.6
3	4	14.8	5	18.5
4	9	33.3	0	0.0
5	8	29.7	1	3.7
Facial tension				
1	0	0.0	5	18.5
2	4	14.8	17	63.0
3	8	29.6	3	11.1
4	7	25.9	0	0.0
5	8	29.6	2	7.4

in group D had ideal or acceptable scores in all segments (Table 4).

NRS showed that in group M eleven patients had severe pain and discomfort as compared to one patient with severe pain and two with severe discomfort in group D during the procedure (Table 5, p value < 0.001, Chi-square test; statistically significant). None had pain or discomfort before the beginning of the procedure in either group. One patient had moderate pain and eight patients had moderate distress 10 min following the procedure in group M while none had severe pain or distress. In contrast, group D had none experiencing moderate or severe pain while one patient had moderate discomfort 10 min following bronchoscopy. The number of patients having persistent distress following bronchoscopy was significantly higher in group M ($p = 0.024$, Table 5).

The bronchoscopy was assessed to be easy in 6, slightly difficult in 11, and very difficult in 10 patients in group M while the bronchoscopy was easy in 15, slightly difficult in 10, and very difficult in 2 patients in group D (Chi-square test, $p = 0.010$; statistically significant, Table 6). Rescue bolus midazolam requirement was significantly higher in group M where eight patients required single bolus, two patients required two boluses, and one patient required three boluses while two patients in group D required a single bolus (p value = 0.023, Fisher's exact test; statistically significant, Table 6).

A Ramsay Sedation Score of 2-3 was desired during and after the study. None in group M had deeper level of sedation than necessary at the beginning of the procedure while three patients in group D had a RSS of 4 at the beginning of bronchoscopy. An RSS score of 1 (anxious and agitated or restless or both) was found during the procedure in 11 patients in group M and in two patients in group D. One patient in group M had RSS 4 at 10 min following bronchoscopy (the same patient had received three rescue boluses of midazolam during the procedure) and four patients in group D had RSS 4 at 10 min following bronchoscopy (Table 6). All these patients were observed and monitored till they recovered from deep levels of sedation. None developed any complication.

None of the patients had any episodes of desaturation or significant bradycardia. One patient in group D had hypotension following bronchoscopy that responded to a single bolus of 250 mL crystalloid. When estimated marginal means for systolic blood pressure were compared between the two groups, the SBP was within 20% from baseline in the dexmedetomidine group at all times while there was elevation of SBP to >20% from baseline in the midazolam group at the fourth minute after starting the procedure (Figure 1). Since a significant number of procedures lasted ≤6 min, we could not compare the data beyond this time frame. However, SBP at 10 min following bronchoscopy was comparable between the groups (112 ± 18 mmHg in dexmedetomidine group versus 131 ± 19 mmHg in midazolam group, $p = 0.657$). Postoperative questionnaire of patients revealed that 7 and 21 patients in group M and group D, respectively, felt that the quality of sedation was excellent/good. Others felt that it was either fair or poor. Similarly, when asked about the amount of discomfort the patients perceived during the procedure, 12 and 23 patients in group M and group D, respectively, felt none or mild discomfort. Others felt that they experienced moderate to severe discomfort during the procedure (Table 6).

TABLE 5: Numerical rating scale for pain and distress.

	Prior to	During			10 min after bronchoscopy		
NRS pain		0–3	4–7	8–10	0–3	4–7	8–10
Group M	0	8	8	11	26	1	0
Group D	0	22	4	1	27	0	0
		p value < 0.001 (*Chi-square test; statistically significant*)			**p value = 1** (*Fisher's exact test*)		
NRS distress		0–3	4–7	8–10	0–3	4–7	8–10
Group M	0	4	12	11	19	8	0
Group D	0	19	6	2	26	1	0
		p value < 0.001 (*Chi-square test; statistically significant*)			**p value = 0.024** (*Fisher's exact test; statistically significant*)		

TABLE 6: Various other study parameters.

Ramsay sedation score			
Time in relation to bronchoscopy	RSS	Group M (*n* = 27)	Group D (*n* = 27)
Prior to	2	25	17
	3	2	7
	4	0	3
	p value = 0.024 (*Fisher's exact test; statistically significant*)		
During	1	11	2
	2	15	24
	3	1	1
	p value = 0.009 (*Fisher's exact test; statistically significant*)		
10 min after	2	2	0
	3	24	23
	4	1	3
	5	0	1
	p value = 0.356 (*Fisher's exact test*)		
Ease of bronchoscopy			
Easy		6	15
Slightly difficult		11	10
Very difficult		10	2
	p value = 0.010 (*Chi-square test; statistically significant*)		
Patient's opinion 24 h after the bronchoscopy			
Quality of sedation			
Excellent		0	5
Good		7	16
Fair		16	6
Poor		4	0
Amount of discomfort			
Nil		2	7
Mild		10	16
Moderate		10	4
Severe		5	0
Number of rescue midazolam boluses required			
1		8	2
2		1	0
3		1	0

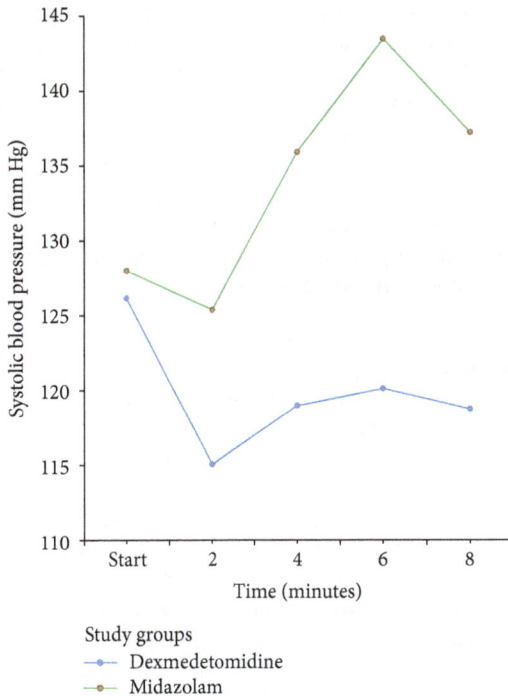

FIGURE 1: Systolic blood pressure in relation to time.

Study groups
— Dexmedetomidine
— Midazolam

5. Discussion

Flexible bronchoscopy for evaluation of tracheobronchial tree is a very commonly performed procedure by pulmonologists and in many countries it is done on outpatient basis. The protocol of our hospital was to admit the patients overnight following the procedure and this allowed us to evaluate the patients 24 h after the procedure.

In our study, we evaluated the patients using several parameters that included assessment of patient responses during bronchoscopy based on five different parameters (composite score), bronchoscopist's evaluation of the conditions for bronchoscopy, Ramsay Sedation Score, NRS for evaluating pain and distress experienced by the patient during the procedure, and patient's own evaluation of the procedural sedation 24 h following the procedure (once they were completely free of the effects of the sedative agents). Further, haemodynamic response to bronchoscopy was also evaluated. Other studies that evaluated procedural sedation with midazolam or dexmedetomidine during bronchoscopy have considered number of episodes of oxygen desaturation, number of times patient required assistance to maintain the patency of the airway, cough and satisfaction scores by patients and bronchoscopists, level of sedation, number of or type of rescue doses needed, haemodynamic responses, numerical or visual analogue scale score for assessment by patient or observer to rate the comfort or satisfaction, and postoperative patient questionnaire [9–12, 14, 15]. Strength of our study is that it was double blinded and the patient tolerance to bronchoscopy was evaluated mainly using a composite score believing that this would reflect many aspects of patient discomfort to bronchoscopy while recording only

one aspect such as cough or patient/operator evaluation of discomfort might appear too subjective and might miss out other manifestations of patient discomfort.

Analysis of various parameters in our study shows that dexmedetomidine provided superior and acceptable patient tolerance and comfort, bronchoscopy conditions, and level of sedation with an episode of hypotension (that responded to single fluid bolus) as the only adverse event while midazolam failed to provide satisfactory patient comfort or bronchoscopy conditions in a large number of patients. Other studies have found better patient acceptance and bronchoscopy conditions with midazolam, but most of them are with much higher doses of midazolam (2–2.5 mg boluses followed by 1 mg supplements or >0.03 mg/kg bolus). However, these studies have also shown that it was achieved with serious adverse effects such as oxygen desaturation [11, 12, 21, 22], inability on part of the patient to maintain the airway requiring verbal/tactile stimulation or airway manoeuvres or ventilator assistance or flumazenil for antagonizing the effects of midazolam [11, 21], considerable reduction in both the inspiratory and expiratory muscle strengths (both maximum inspiratory and expiratory pressures) [23], and hiccups [24]. This can be a very important limiting factor and deterrent for the use of higher doses of midazolam (>0.02 mg/kg or >1-2 mg bolus) when the responsibility for monitoring and managing the adverse effects rests on the pulmonologist or otorhinolaryngologist. Further, BTS Guidelines suggest that a better way to provide sedation is by incremental administration of the drug rather than a single bolus dose. Our ultimate goal is to find a suitable drug at a dose that does not produce any serious adverse effects so that the pulmonologist can safely administer and perform the bronchoscopy, as at most places the procedure is done without the presence of anaesthesiologists. Hence, we used lower dose of midazolam in our study. However, the results of our study demonstrate that, at 0.02 mg/kg, the drug does not provide suitable patient satisfaction or bronchoscopy conditions though it did not produce any serious adverse effects.

Studies have highlighted the utility of dexmedetomidine IV (1 μg/kg bolus over 10 min) as a safe and effective agent in complementing topicalisation of airway for awake fiberoptic intubation of trachea by anaesthesiologists [17–19]. Though an infusion of dexmedetomidine is usually considered during attempts at intubation, we decided to use only bolus dexmedetomidine for our study due to several reasons: (a) the procedure of flexible bronchoscopy is much less stimulating to patients than the procedure of tracheal intubation; (b) it would be convenient for the bronchoscopist to give one bolus dose and proceed to bronchoscopy; and (c) it may limit the adverse effects. As our study results demonstrate, a single bolus of dexmedetomidine at 1 μg/kg over 10 min prior to bronchoscopy was sufficient to provide safe but effective sedation. A study that included infusion of dexmedetomidine at 0.5 μg/kg/h after initial bolus showed frequent instances of hypoxaemia (14%, oxygen saturation SpO_2 < 90% for >30 s) despite nasal oxygen supplementation throughout the procedure of bronchoscopy with 6% incidence of hypotension (SBP < 90 mmHg or mean blood pressure < 60 mmHg) [20]. In another study where anaesthesiologists monitored and managed the patients using combination of propofol and dexmedetomidine for sedation during bronchoscopy, the patients were first premedicated with 0.03 mg/kg IV midazolam for topicalisation of airway and then propofol 0.5 mg/kg bolus was administered followed by dexmedetomidine bolus 0.05 mL/kg of 4 μg/kg preparation, which was further titrated as infusion at 0.4–2 μg/kg/h during the procedure. All patients received oxygen supplementation via nasal cannula. The study found one out of 35 patients having oxygen desaturation during the procedure requiring verbal/tactile stimulation to maintain the airway. However, patients appeared to be more sedated than conscious sedation during the procedure (MOAA/S scale of 4) as 27/35 could respond only to prodding and shaking and 5/35 patients were responsive only after their name was called out loudly or repeatedly or both (MOAA/S scale of 3) five minutes after the bronchoscopy. Both of these features are undesirable when an anaesthesiologist is not present for monitoring the patient [14].

Numerical rating score for pain and distress revealed unacceptable degree of pain and distress in 11 patients who received midazolam as the study drug while one patient had unacceptable pain response and two patients had unacceptable distress levels with dexmedetomidine. Further, moderate degree of distress persisted in eight patients receiving midazolam as study drug even 10 min after the bronchoscopy was over. The majority of patients receiving dexmedetomidine had adequate sedation (25/27) during the procedure while 16 patients receiving midazolam had adequate sedation. However, four patients receiving dexmedetomidine and one patient receiving midazolam (with three top up rescue doses) had unacceptably deeper level of sedation even after 10 minutes following the procedure. All these patients were followed up and found to have recovered to awake state in the following 30-minute period without any side effects.

Haemodynamic parameters were assessed during the procedure. All but one patient had <30% deviation from baseline systolic blood pressure or heart rate in either group. One patient in the dexmedetomidine group had significant reduction in the systolic blood pressure that responded to a single crystalloid bolus of 250 mL.

A study that used combination of propofol with dexmedetomidine demonstrated that there were lower instances of oxygen desaturation with this combination as compared to propofol remifentanil combination [14]. Several studies that have used higher doses of midazolam (>0.02 mg/kg) have documented risk of oxygen desaturation during the procedure despite prophylactic oxygen administration to all patients [11, 12, 21, 22]. In one study, midazolam in a dose of 0.07–0.1 mg/kg IV administered two minutes prior to bronchoscopy resulted in episodes of desaturation to 85% despite O_2 therapy, requiring administration of higher O_2 concentrations as well as requirement for flumazenil to reverse the effects of midazolam in one patient [11]. None of the patients in our study had any episode of desaturation (SpO_2 < 93%). Patient's own evaluation would probably be the best way to judge the comfort levels. Therefore, all patients were asked to give their feedback on the quality of sedation and distress experienced in a postoperative

questionnaire that was asked 24 h following the procedure (to ensure that the patient was completely out of the effects of the study drugs). This also confirmed the study findings that the majority of the patients who received dexmedetomidine as the study drug were satisfied with the quality of sedation and the majority of patients experienced nil or minimal discomfort during the procedure. These findings show that a single bolus of dexmedetomidine (1 μg/kg over 10 min) administered just prior to bronchoscopy provides acceptable sedation without any serious side effects.

5.1. Drawbacks of Our Study. One of the important drawbacks of our study probably is the timing of IV midazolam. Several studies have administered IV midazolam bolus about three minutes prior to bronchoscopy [12, 23]. It is not clear if they performed airway topicalisation prior to or following administration of midazolam. Midazolam was administered following airway topicalisation in one study [21]. During flexible bronchoscopy, maximal stimulation and patient discomfort can occur when the bronchoscope is in contact with vocal cords, trachea, carina, or bronchi as these are the most sensitive areas for foreign body sensation and are rich in irritant receptors. With our previous experience of fiberoptic bronchoscopy we felt the fiberscope will be passing through the vocal cords into the trachea approximately 2-3 min after the application of lignocaine jelly to nostril as this includes (entry of fiberscope into the nostril, its passage to nasopharynx, lignocaine spray to vocal cords and throat, and a waiting period of one minute prior to the entry of fiberscope through the vocal cords). Therefore, we injected IV midazolam bolus 2 min prior to the start of bronchoscopy anticipating that approximately 5 min would elapse by the time the fiberscope is in contact with vocal cords from the time of midazolam administration. However, the literature evidence shows that the peak effect of IV midazolam is around 5–10 min from the time of its administration [5]. Our aim was to compare the dose of midazolam recommended for sedation (0.01–0.1 mg/kg), though the dose used in our study was in the lower part of that range [5]. Further, the dose of midazolam might not be equipotent to that of dexmedetomidine. Another important limitation of the study was inability to ensure complete blinding of the individual performing bronchoscopy to group allocation as the haemodynamic profile of patients receiving dexmedetomidine was different from that of midazolam.

6. Conclusions

During flexible fiberoptic bronchoscopy under topical airway anaesthesia, IV dexmedetomidine (1 μg/kg administered 10 min prior to bronchoscopy) provides superior patient comfort and tolerance as compared to IV midazolam (0.02 mg/kg). However, monitoring of the patients in the immediate postprocedure period is essential when dexmedetomidine is used in the present dose.

Key Message

Dexmedetomidine appears to be the answer for the search for a rapid acting and short duration medication that improves patient tolerance to flexible bronchoscopy without jeopardising patient safety.

Conflict of Interests

The authors declare that there is no conflict of interests regarding the publication of this paper.

References

[1] R. P. Reddy and P. A. Vauthy, "Flexible fiberoptic bronchoscopy," *Indian Journal of Pediatrics*, vol. 54, no. 2, pp. 237–243, 1987.

[2] G. B. Diette, P. White Jr., P. Terry, M. Jenckes, R. A. Wise, and H. R. Rubin, "Quality assessment through patient self-report of symptoms prefiberoptic and postfiberoptic bronchoscopy," *Chest*, vol. 114, no. 5, pp. 1446–1453, 1998.

[3] Y. L. Ni, Y. L. Lo, T. Y. Lin, Y. F. Fang, and H. P. Kuo, "Conscious sedation reduces patient discomfort and improves satisfaction in flexible bronchoscopy," *Chang Gung Medical Journal*, vol. 33, no. 4, pp. 443–452, 2010.

[4] R. González, I. De-La-Rosa-Ramírez, A. Maldonado-Hernández, and G. Domínguez-Cherit, "Should patients undergoing a bronchoscopy be sedated?" *Acta Anaesthesiologica Scandinavica*, vol. 47, no. 4, pp. 411–415, 2003.

[5] R. J. José, S. Shaefi, and N. Navani, "Sedation for flexible bronchoscopy: current and emerging evidence," *European Respiratory Review*, vol. 22, no. 128, pp. 106–116, 2013.

[6] I. Matot and M. R. Kramer, "Sedation in outpatient bronchoscopy," *Respiratory Medicine*, vol. 94, no. 12, pp. 1145–1153, 2000.

[7] I. Matot, M. R. Kramer, L. Glantz, B. Drenger, and S. Cotev, "Myocardial ischemia in sedated patients undergoing fiberoptic bronchoscopy," *Chest*, vol. 112, no. 6, pp. 1454–1458, 1997.

[8] I. A. Du Rand, J. Blaikley, R. Booton et al., "British Thoracic Society guideline for diagnostic flexible bronchoscopy in adults," *Thorax*, vol. 68, no. 1, pp. i1–i44, 2013.

[9] K. Clarkson, C. K. Power, F. O'Connell, S. Pathmakanthan, and C. M. Burke, "A comparative evaluation of propofol and midazolam as sedative agents in fiberoptic bronchoscopy," *Chest*, vol. 104, no. 4, pp. 1029–1031, 1993.

[10] R. Rolo, P. C. Mota, F. Coelho et al., "Sedation with midazolam in flexible bronchoscopy—a prospective study," *Revista Portuguesa de Pneumologia*, vol. 18, no. 5, pp. 226–232, 2012.

[11] E. Cases Viedma, J. Pérez Pallarés, M. A. Martínez García, R. López Reyes, F. Sanchís Moret, and J. L. Sanchís Aldás, "A randomised study of midazolam for sedation in flexible bronchoscopy," *Archivos de Bronconeumología*, vol. 46, no. 6, pp. 302–309, 2010.

[12] M. Dreher, E. Ekkernkamp, J. H. Storre, H.-J. Kabitz, and W. Windisch, "Sedation during flexible bronchoscopy in patients with pre-existing respiratory failure: midazolam versus midazolam plus alfentanil," *Respiration*, vol. 79, no. 4, pp. 307–314, 2010.

[13] L. Schlatter, E. Pflimlin, B. Fehrke, A. Meyer, M. Tamm, and D. Stolz, "Propofol versus propofol plus hydrocodone for flexible bronchoscopy: a randomised study," *European Respiratory Journal*, vol. 38, no. 3, pp. 529–537, 2011.

[14] J. H. Ryu, S. W. Lee, J. H. Lee, E. H. Lee, S. H. Do, and C. S. Kim, "Randomized double-blind study of remifentanil and dexmedetomidine for flexible bronchoscopy," *British Journal of Anaesthesia*, vol. 108, no. 3, pp. 503–511, 2012.

[15] C. J. Tsai, K. S. Chu, T. I. Chen, D. V. Lu, H. M. Wang, and I. C. Lu, "A comparison of the effectiveness of dexmedetomidine versus propofol target-controlled infusion for sedation during fibreoptic nasotracheal intubation," *Anaesthesia*, vol. 65, no. 3, pp. 254–259, 2010.

[16] R. R. Riker, Y. Shehabi, P. M. Bokesch et al., "Dexmedetomidine vs midazolam for sedation of critically ill patients: a randomized trial," *The Journal of the American Medical Association*, vol. 301, no. 5, pp. 489–499, 2009.

[17] R. Avitsian, J. Lin, M. Lotto, and Z. Ebrahim, "Dexmedetomidine and awake fiberoptic intubation for possible cervical spine myelopathy: a clinical series," *Journal of Neurosurgical Anesthesiology*, vol. 17, no. 2, pp. 97–99, 2005.

[18] S. D. Bergese, K. A. Candiotti, P. M. Bokesch, A. Zura, W. Wisemandle, and A. Y. Bekker, "A phase IIIb, randomized, double-blind, placebo-controlled, multicenter study evaluating the safety and efficacy of dexmedetomidine for sedation during awake fiberoptic intubation," *American Journal of Therapeutics*, vol. 17, no. 6, pp. 586–595, 2010.

[19] S. D. Bergese, S. Patrick Bender, T. D. McSweeney, S. Fernandez, R. Dzwonczyk, and K. Sage, "A comparative study of dexmedetomidine with midazolam and midazolam alone for sedation during elective awake fiberoptic intubation," *Journal of Clinical Anesthesia*, vol. 22, no. 1, pp. 35–40, 2010.

[20] W. Liao, G. Ma, Q. G. Su, Y. Fang, B. C. Gu, and X. M. Zou, "Dexmedetomidine versus midazolam for conscious sedation in postoperative patients undergoing flexible bronchoscopy: a randomized study," *Journal of International Medical Research*, vol. 40, no. 4, pp. 1371–1380, 2012.

[21] G. Clark, M. Licker, A. B. Younossian et al., "Titrated sedation with propofol or midazolam for flexible bronchoscopy: a randomised trial," *European Respiratory Journal*, vol. 34, no. 6, pp. 1277–1283, 2009.

[22] D. Stolz, G. Kurer, A. Meyer et al., "Propofol versus combined sedation in flexible bronchoscopy: a randomised non-inferiority trial," *European Respiratory Journal*, vol. 34, no. 5, pp. 1024–1030, 2009.

[23] B. Tulek, F. Kanat, S. Tol, and M. Suerdem, "Flexible bronchoscopy may decrease respiratory muscle strength: premedicational midazolam in focus," *Multidisciplinary Respiratory Medicine*, vol. 7, no. 4, article 31, 2012.

[24] M. Arroyo-Cózar, J. Grau Delgado, and T. Gabaldón Conejos, "Hiccups induced by midazolam during sedation in flexible bronchoscopy," *Archivos de Bronconeumologia*, vol. 48, no. 3, article 103, 2012.

Hemoglobin Variant (Hemoglobin Aalborg) Mimicking Interstitial Pulmonary Disease

Vasiliki Panou,[1] **Peter-Diedrich Mathias Jensen,**[2] **Jan Freddy Pedersen,**[3]
Lars Pilegaard Thomsen,[4] **and Ulla Møller Weinreich**[1]

[1] *Department of Respiratory Diseases, Aalborg University Hospital, Mølleparkvej 4, 9000 Aalborg, Denmark*
[2] *Department of Haematology, Aalborg University Hospital, Denmark*
[3] *Department of Clinical Biochemistry, Aalborg University Hospital, Denmark*
[4] *Respiratory and Critical Care Group (RCARE), Centre for Model Based Medical Decision Support Systems,
Department of Health Science and Technology, Aalborg University, Denmark*

Correspondence should be addressed to Vasiliki Panou; vasiliki_panou@hotmail.com

Academic Editor: Luisetti Maurizio

Hemoglobin Aalborg is a moderately unstable hemoglobin variant with no affiliation to serious hematological abnormality or major clinical symptoms under normal circumstances. Our index person was a healthy woman of 58, not previously diagnosed with hemoglobinopathy Aalborg, who developed acute respiratory failure after a routine cholecystectomy. Initially she was suspected of idiopathic interstitial lung disease, yet a series of tests uncovered various abnormal physiological parameters and set the diagnosis of hemoglobinopathy Aalborg. This led us to examine a group of the index person's relatives known with hemoglobinopathy Aalborg in order to study whether the same physiological abnormalities would be reencountered. They were all subjected to spirometry and body plethysmography, six-minute walking test, pulse oximetry, and arterial blood gas samples before and after the walking test. The entire study population presented the same physiological anomalies: reduction in diffusion capacity, and abnormalities in P_aO_2 and p50 values; the latter could not be presented by the arterial blood gas analyzer; furthermore there was concordance between pulse oximetry and arterial blood gas samples regarding saturation. These data suggest that, based upon the above mentioned anomalies in physiological parameters, the diagnosis of hemoglobinopathy Aalborg should be considered.

1. Introduction

Unstable hemoglobinopathies (Hb) are a rare disease entity of mutational events in the hemoglobin which are characterized by substitutions in the primary sequence of the globin [1]. These mutations alter the tertiary or quaternary structure of the molecule and therefore cause destabilization of the hemoglobin tetramer. A wide range of hemoglobin instabilities are known from in vitro studies, and the clinical findings span from subclinical cases to cases with severe hemolytic disease, for example, beta-thalassemia major or sickle cell disease [2]. Hb present with a broad spectrum of clinical manifestations; however, patients often have very few symptoms apart from slight fatigue, because the hemoglobin is often stable under clinically stable conditions [1–4].

Hemoglobin Aalborg is a rare, unstable hemoglobin variant where a glycine residue (E18) is replaced by arginine (β74(E18)Gly->Arg). The incidence and prevalence of Hb Aalborg are not known. It has a reduced oxygen affinity, both in the absence and in the presence of organic phosphates, and a raised oxygen affinity for organic phosphates, despite the fact that the replaced amino acid residue is too far from the heme to affect it directly. The reduced oxygen affinity of the hemoglobin results from constraints on the deformability of heme T-state, which disable oxygen binding and spontaneous conversion from the T-state to the R-state in the absence of oxygen [2, 5].

Hb Aalborg is considered moderately unstable and it is not associated with any severe hematological abnormality. It may cause mild anaemia and Heinz bodies are inducible in

TABLE 1: Results of spirometry and body plethysmography, demonstrating forced expiratory volume in the 1st second in percent of expected value (FEV$_1$%), forced ventilatory capacity in percent of expected value (FVC%), the ratio between FEV$_1$ and FVC, and diffusing capacity of the lung for carbon monoxide in percent of expected value (DLCO%) and 6-minute walking tests in 7 patients with Hb Aalborg.

	Patient 1 (woman)	Patient 2 (man)	Patient 3 (woman)	Patient 4 (woman)	Patient 5 (woman)	Patient 6 (man)	Index person
FEV$_1$ (%)	106	128	94	87	117	106	117
FVC (%)	108	122	103	107	104	98	134
FEV$_1$/FVC	87	78	65	94	99	91	74
DLCO (%)	59	69	67	69	76	80	66
Walking distance (m)	417	480	562	420	568	551	273

the hemoglobin. The vast majority of patients have no or mild symptoms such as fatigue or mild dyspnea on exertion. However, conditions which stress the unstable hemoglobin, such as increased temperature or exposure to oxidant drugs, are likely to precipitate hemoglobin denaturation and significant hemolysis may occur [2, 5].

The index person of the study population was not previously diagnosed with Hb Aalborg and had no underlying chronic disease. However, acute respiratory failure occurred postoperatively in connection to an elective cholecystectomy and no cause of the acute change could be found. As the pulmonary symptoms persisted, idiopathic interstitial lung disease was suspected. The patient was subjected to thorough examination in order to elucidate the cause of the clinical symptoms. Physiological abnormalities, regarding both arterial blood samples analysis and pulse oximetry and body box examination, were observed during the diagnostic procedure.

After the diagnosis of Hb Aalborg was established, a group of family members to the index person, already diagnosed with Hb Aalborg, were also examined and underwent the same tests in order to validate the following hypothesis: "When anomalies in parameters regarding arterial blood samples analysis, pulse oximetry, and body box examination are encountered in stable state as well as on exertion, Hb Aalborg should be included in the possible, although rare, differential diagnoses." The aim of this study was therefore to investigate whether similar abnormalities in the physiological parameters could be detected in all family members. This was described by examining the following:

(i) diffusion capacity of the lung for carbon monoxide (DLCO),

(ii) the Medical Research Council (MRC) dyspnea score,

(iii) 6-minute walking test,

(iv) oxygen saturation at rest as well as after exertion.

2. Materials and Methods

In this prospective study a total of seven people were examined, who all shared the following characteristics: the patients were all heterozygote for Hb Aalborg; six were first degree relatives to the index person and did not have any underlying pulmonary disease. The group consisted of two

men and four women, aged 19–82. Two of the subjects were current smokers: patient number 2 with 13 pack-years and currently smoking 10 cigarettes per day and patient number 6 with 2.5 pack-years, currently smoking 20 cigarettes per day. The remaining four persons were never smokers. None of the participants had either significant comorbidities or respiratory complaints. Fatigue, following light physical activity, was described as the only symptom from the entire study population.

All the subjects were examined in the outpatient clinic of the Respiratory Department of Aalborg University Hospital. They were all subjected to spirometry and body plethysmography and six-minute walking test according to guidelines of the American Thoracic Society [6, 7]. The primary goal of the body plethysmography was to obtain accurate DLCO values but the static gas volumes were also measured [8]. Oxygen saturation (s_pO_2) was measured by pulse oximetry with Oximax NPB-40, Nellcor, and arterial blood gas samples were taken from arteria radialis by experienced staff, before and after the walking test, according to guidelines [9]. The arterial blood gas samples were analyzed in ABL800 FLEX Analyzer (Radiometer, Copenhagen, Denmark) in order to examine the partial oxygen pressure (p_aO_2), carbon dioxide tension (p_aCO_2), oxygen saturation fraction (s_aO_2), and total hemoglobin (ctHb). Subsequently, functional hemoglobin (ceHb) and the oxygen tension at 50% saturated hemoglobin (p50) were calculated, using the Oxygen Status Algorithm (OSA) [10].

Only descriptive statistics were performed, using Excel.

Prior to the examinations the patients were recruited according to the Helsinki Declaration and signed written consent after oral and written information about the study [11]. The project was presented to the Local Science Ethics Committee of the Region of North Jutland, Denmark, who found no need for ethical review.

3. Results

The results of the spirometry, body plethysmography, and 6 minutes' walking test are presented in Table 1. The patients had a median forced expiratory volume in 1 second of percent expected (FEV$_1$) of 106% (range 87–128), a median forced vital capacity of percent expected (FVC) of 107% (range 98–134), and a median FEV$_1$/FVC ratio of 87 (range 65–99).

TABLE 2: Oxygen saturation, measured by pulse oximetry (s_pO_2), and results from arterial blood gas analyses: arterial oxygen saturation (SaO_2), partial pressure of oxygen (PaO_2), oxygen tension at 50% saturated hemoglobin (P50), and hemoglobin, functional hemoglobin, and lactate concentration before and after 6-minute walking test in 7 patients with Hb Aalborg.

	Patient 1 (woman)	Patient 2 (man)	Patient 3 (woman)	Patient 4 (woman)	Patient 5 (woman)	Patient 6 (man)	Index person
				Before exercise			
s_pO_2 (%)	83	79	85	73	85	69	87
SaO_2 (%)	83.3	79	85.5	73.2	85	69.4	87.3
PaO_2 (mmHg)	91.5	89.25	90.75	81	114.8	100.5	102.75
P50 (mmHg)	59.6	56.85	50.63	45.23	69.68	77.25	54.9
Hemoglobin (g/dL)	0.73	0.82	0.78	0.72	0.65	0.74	0.75
Functional hemoglobin (g/dL)	0.69	0.76	0.74	0.68	0.63	0.71	0.71
Carboxyhemoglobin (g/dL)	0.0037	0.0051	0.003	0.003	0.0015	0.005	0.0033
Lactate (μg/dL)	8.11	8.11	5.41	5.41	15.3	9.91	9.91
				After exercise			
s_pO_2 (%)	87	81	81	83	85	83	83
SaO_2 (%)	87.5	81.7	81.5	83.2	85	83	82.9
PaO_2 (mmHg)	91.5	96	93.75	102.75	91.5	112.5	96.75
P50 (mmHg)	47.85	58.8	57.9	61.28	51.68	68.85	54.23
Hemoglobin (g/dL)	0.73	0.82	0.78	0.74	0.69	0.74	0.77
Functional hemoglobin (g/dL)	0.69	0.77	0.74	0.70	0.62	0.72	0.73
Carboxyhemoglobin (g/dL)	0.0037	0.0043	0.0028	0.0036	0.003	0.0043	0.003
Lactate (μg/dL)	15.32	8.11	6.31	9.91	7.21	9.91	9

The median DLCO was 69% (range 59–80) and the median walking distance was 480 m (range 273–568). All the subjects presented with FEV_1, FVC, and FEV_1/FVC ratio within the normal range but DLCO was more or less reduced in all the patients with Hb Aalborg. The static gas volumes were found within the normal range for all the subjects (data not shown).

The measurements of pulse oximetry and the results of the arterial blood gas analyses before and after exercise are presented in Table 2. Prior to the walking test, the patients had a median oxygen saturation (s_pO_2) of 83% (range 69–87) and oxygen saturation fraction of percent (s_aO_2) of 83.3% (range 69.4–87.3), a median of p_aO_2 of 91.5 mmHg (range 81–114.8), a median of p50 of 56.85 mmHg (range 45.23–77.25), a median of hemoglobin of 0.74 g/dL (range 0.65–0.82), a median of functional hemoglobin of 0.71 μg/dL (range 0.63–0.76), a median of carboxyhemoglobin of 0.0033 μg/dL (range 0.0015–0.0051), and a median of lactate of 8.11 μg/dL (range 5.41–15.3). After the walking test, a median s_pO_2 of 83% (range 81–87) and s_aO_2 of 83% (range 81.5–87.5), a median of P_aO_2 of 96 mmHg (range 91.5–112.5), a median of p50 of 57.9 mmHg (range 47.85–68.85), a median of hemoglobin of 0.74 g/dL (range 0.69–0.82), a median of functional hemoglobin of 0.72 μg/dL (range 0.62–0.77), a median of carboxyhemoglobin of 0.0036 μg/dL (range 0.0028–0.0043), and a median of lactate of 9 μg/dL (range 6.31–15.32) were observed. Carboxyhemoglobin levels were found in normal range or slightly increased for all patients but two. After the

walking test an increase in s_aO_2 and P_aO_2 was noticed in four subjects and a decrease was seen in two subjects. P50 was elevated both before and after exertion. It was increased in three subjects and decreased in four subjects following exercise.

4. Discussion

In this group of patients with Hb Aalborg the common physiological features were the low DLCO, the inability of the blood gas analyzer to present the p50 and p_aO_2 values, and low and comparable s_pO_2 and s_aO_2 levels in contrast to the high partial pressure of oxygen.

No obvious impact of exertion on the hemoglobin was seen. Elevated p50 and low saturation levels in the presence of normal partial oxygen pressure were observed both prior to and after the 6 minutes' walking test. As such our data does not suggest that exertion has an influence on the increase or decrease of these values.

DLCO may be compromised in different compartments. The oxygen supply in the alveoli may be impaired, the diffusion barrier may be the obstacle, or the blood may lack the ability to carry the oxygen to the tissues. The pathology behind this is diverse; it may be caused by anemia, interstitial lung disease, pulmonary vascular disease, increased carboxyhemoglobin, and low oxygen levels in blood [12]. Figure 1 demonstrates how anemia (Figure 1(b)), increased

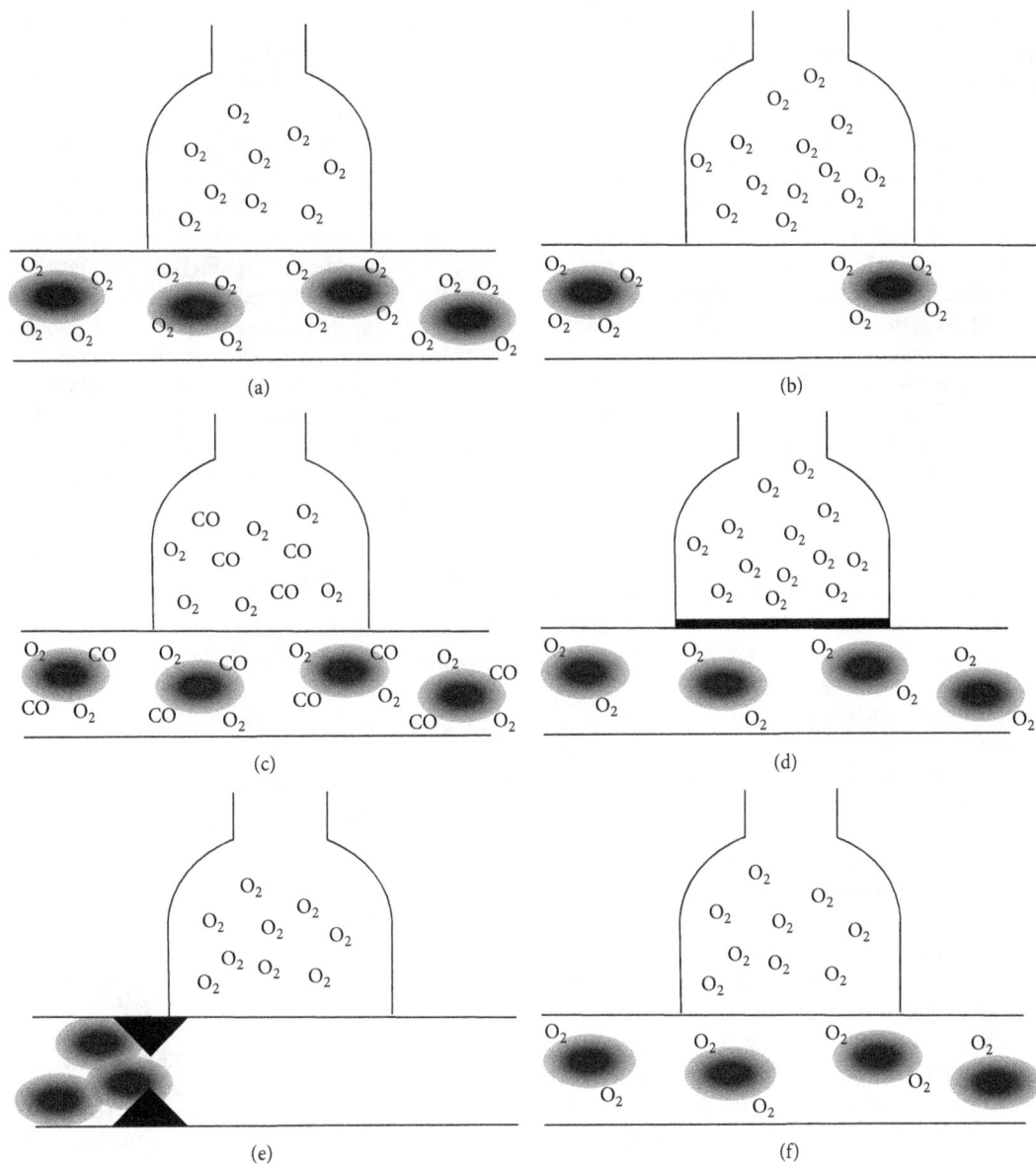

FIGURE 1: Explanations for reduction in DLCO: (a) normal physiology, (b) anemia, (c) high carboxyhemoglobin levels, (d) pulmonary disease (thickening of the alveolar membrane), (e) pulmonary vascular disease, and (f) Hb Aalborg.

carboxyhemoglobin levels (Figure 1(c)), interstitial lung disease (Figure 1(d)), which results in thickening of the alveolar membrane, and pulmonary vascular disease (Figure 1(e)) affect DLCO. However, the ability of the heme to bind the oxygen is often forgotten in this context (Figure 1(f)).

Reduced DLCO is previously described in the literature in connection with other Hb, such as sickle cell Hb and beta-thalassemia, Hb Canebiére, and Hb Louisville [13–16]. In sickle cell Hb and beta-thalassemia, DLCO is primarily reduced because of pathology in the pulmonary vascular component because of the rigidity of the hemoglobin resulting in microembolism (Figure 1(e)). With regard to beta-thalassemia, iron deposition in the lung tissue, subclinical heart failure as a result of multiple transfusions coupled with a damaged myocardium caused by iron deposition, hepatosplenomegaly and insufficient anatomical and functional

development of the lung during early infancy could also alter DLCO [17, 18]. Hb Canebiére and Hb Louisville are Hb with low oxygen affinity, similar to Hb Aalborg (Figure 1(f)) [15, 16]. The hematological changes of Hb Aalborg have been described years ago, but this is, to the authors' knowledge, the first paper to describe the effect of the condition on DLCO. In this study population no clinical explanation to the reduced DLCO was found apart from the unstable Hb Aalborg. None of the subjects in the study population were suspected to have any kind of chronic lung disease, as pulmonary comorbidity was an exclusion criterion.

Hemoglobin and p_aO_2 obtained from the arterial blood samples were normal or close to normal in the entire study population. However, the functional hemoglobin of the study objects, which was subsequently calculated, was below the normal levels, as expected for their age, origin, and sex.

This suggests that reduced DLCO is a result of the reduced quantity of the functional hemoglobin (Figure 1(f)), which is often combined with a normal hematocrit. Therefore it is essential to consider Hb, which do not affect the hematocrit but the structure of the hemoglobin, as a potential differential diagnosis to conditions where reduced DLCO is present.

The blood gas analyzer would not present p50 values, and p_aO_2 values could only be registered manually whilst the blood gas sample was being analyzed. This is due to the analyzer interpreting the simultaneous existence of normal partial pressure of oxygen and low saturation levels as a technical error (error number 1010). P50 is in the context of Hb an interesting parameter. It demonstrates the oxygen tension when 50% of the blood is oxygenated and reflects the hemoglobin's affinity for oxygen. High levels of p50 suggest that high oxygen pressure is required in order to achieve sufficient oxygen supply to the hemoglobin [19]. Increased p50 values have previously been described in Hb with low oxygen affinity, including Hb Aalborg [2, 5, 20]. However, missing data from the arterial blood gas analysis from patients with Hb Aalborg has never been reported previously. The calculated p50 values were all found to be increased.

The discordance between the high p_aO_2 and low s_aO_2 values is well known in patients with Hb Aalborg [2, 5]. There are several articles describing the presence of low saturation levels in Hb with low oxygen affinity, a finding that sometimes triggers further evaluation leading to identification of an underlying hemoglobin variant [21, 22]. The findings of this study are consistent with those of previous studies. It is, however, noticeable that, in six out of seven subjects, the exact saturation values obtained by pulse oximetry were also verified with accuracy by the blood gas sample analysis despite the low saturation levels and the already diagnosed Hb. Previous studies have demonstrated an overestimation of saturation levels when measured by pulse oximetry compared to those measured by arterial blood gas test at a saturation below 90%–92% [23, 24]. Several factors influence the accuracy of pulse oximetry in conditions of low oxygen saturation, for example, lack of reliable human calibration data during hypoxia and an increased proportion of reduced hemoglobin in hypoxic states, which can exacerbate the error of the absorption ratio [23, 24]. Whether our finding was random or represents another characteristic of Hb Aalborg remains to be clarified by future research.

A slightly decreased ratio between FEV_1 and FVC is noticed in patient number 3 but the flow-volume curve elucidates that it is due to the subject's poor technique and is not consistent with an actual obstructive pulmonary disease. Carboxyhemoglobin levels were increased in the two patients who were heavy smokers. These patients have, despite male sex and young age, low functional hemoglobin. This is possibly due to the combination of two conditions compromising oxygen DLCO: high carboxyhemoglobin levels and affected oxygen affinity of the heme (Figures 1(c) and 1(f)). Hence it is essential to stress the consequences of smoking to patients with Hb Aalborg. The index person presents a reduced walking distance at the six minutes' walking test. The index person is also the patient with the most prominent

symptoms and this reflects that the patient's hemoglobin is under condition of oxidative stress.

The participants are all members of the same family which is a limitation to this study. As such the possibility of a rare variant of Hb Aalborg with distinctive characteristics cannot be excluded. However electrophoresis of the hemoglobin confirms the features well known for Hb Aalborg.

This study describes the deductive use of test results. The above described parameter abnormalities were present in all the group members' tests on a larger or smaller scale. As a consequence, whenever p_aO_2 and p50 values cannot be measured in arterial blood gas analysis, a moderately unstable Hb, such as Hb Aalborg, should be considered a possible differential diagnosis. Furthermore, the presence of an unstable Hb should be taken into consideration when reduced DLCO of unknown origin and missing p_aO_2 and p50 values from arterial blood gas samples are encountered.

Conflict of Interests

The authors declare that there is no conflict of interests regarding the publication of this paper.

Acknowledgments

The authors would like to express their special thanks to Frøydis Slettevol for assisting in gathering the blood gas analysis data and Dan S. Karbing for his help with Figure 1.

References

[1] M. A. Lichtman, T. J. Kipps, U. Seligsohn, and K. P. J. Kaushansky, *Williams Hematology*, McGraw-Hill, New York, NY, USA, 8th edition, 2010.

[2] D. Williamson, J. Nutkins, S. Rosthoj, S. O. Brennan, D. H. Williams, and R. W. Carrell, "Characterization of Hb Aalborg, a new unstable hemoglobin variant, by fast atom bombardment mass spectrometry," *Hemoglobin*, vol. 14, no. 2, pp. 137–145, 1990.

[3] H. Lehmann and R. W. Carrell, "Variations in the structure of human haemoglobin: with particular reference to the unstable haemoglobins," *British Medical Bulletin*, vol. 25, no. 1, pp. 14–23, 1969.

[4] E. R. Huehns, "Diseases due to abnormalities of hemoglobin structure," *Annual Review of Medicine*, vol. 21, pp. 157–178, 1970.

[5] G. Fermi, M. F. Perutz, D. Williamson, and D. T. Shih, "Structure-function relationships in the low-affinity mutant haemoglobin Aalborg (Gly74 (E18)beta—Arg)," *Journal of Molecular Biology*, vol. 226, pp. 883–888, 1992.

[6] C.-P. Criée, "Whole-body plethysmography," *Medizinische Klinik*, vol. 105, no. 9, pp. 652–660, 2010.

[7] P. L. Enright, "The six-minute walk test," *Respiratory Care*, vol. 48, no. 8, pp. 783–785, 2003.

[8] N. MacIntyre, R. O. Crapo, G. Viegi et al., "Standardisation of the single-breath determination of carbon monoxide uptake in the lung," *Revue des Maladies Respiratoires*, vol. 24, no. 3, pp. S65–S82, 2007.

[9] A. J. Williams, "ABC of oxygen: assessing and interpreting arterial blood gases and acid-base balance," *The British Medical Journal*, vol. 317, no. 7167, pp. 1213–1216, 1998.

[10] M. Siggaard-Andersen and O. Siggaard-Andersen, "Oxygen status algorithm, version 3, with some applications," *Acta Anaesthesiologica Scandinavica, Supplement*, vol. 39, no. 107, pp. 13–20, 1995.

[11] "World Medical Association Declaration of Helsinki: ethical principles for medical research involving human subjects," *Journal of the American Medical Association*, vol. 310, pp. 2191–2194, 2013.

[12] P. L. Enright and J. K. Stoller, "Diffusion capacity for carbon monoxide," http://www.uptodate.com/contents/diffusing-capacity-for-carbon-monoxide#H14.

[13] R. C. Young Jr., R. E. Rachal, C. A. Reindorf et al., "Lung function in sickle cell hemoglobinopathy patients compared with healthy subjects," *Journal of the National Medical Association*, vol. 80, no. 5, pp. 509–514, 1988.

[14] G. Piatti, L. Allegra, V. Fasano, C. Gambardella, M. Bisaccia, and M. D. Cappellini, "Lung function in β-thalassemia patients: a longitudinal study," *Acta Haematologica*, vol. 116, no. 1, pp. 25–29, 2006.

[15] U. Froelund, E. Sandbakken, P. Szecsi, and H. Birgens, "Further studies on Hb canebière [β12(G4)Asn $\rightarrow$ His], a low affinity hemoglobin variant," *Hemoglobin*, vol. 34, no. 5, pp. 495–499, 2010.

[16] Y. Wu, G. V. Ramani, Q. Gai, L. C. Lemon, and M. R. Baer, "Rare hemoglobinopathy presenting as progressive dyspnea," *American Journal of Hematology*, vol. 85, no. 5, pp. 355–357, 2010.

[17] E. S. Klings, D. F. Wyszynski, V. G. Nolan, and M. H. Steinberg, "Abnormal pulmonary function in adults with sickle cell anemia," *American Journal of Respiratory and Critical Care Medicine*, vol. 173, no. 11, pp. 1264–1269, 2006.

[18] G. Piatti, L. Allegra, U. Ambrosetti, M. D. Cappellini, F. Turati, and G. Fiorelli, "β-Thalassemia and pulmonary function," *Haematologica*, vol. 84, no. 9, pp. 804–808, 1999.

[19] J. R. Kambam, L. H. Chen, and S. A. Hyman, "Effect of short-term smoking halt on carboxyhemoglobin levels and P50 values," *Anesthesia and Analgesia*, vol. 65, no. 11, pp. 1186–1188, 1986.

[20] G. Stamatoyannopoulos, A. J. Bellingham, C. Lenfant, and C. A. Finch, "Abnormal hemoglobins with high and low oxygen affinity," *Annual Review of Medicine*, vol. 22, pp. 221–234, 1971.

[21] M. Verhovsek, M. P. A. Henderson, G. Cox, H. Luo, M. H. Steinberg, and D. H. K. Chui, "Erratum to: unexpectedly low pulse oximetry measurements associated with variant hemoglobins: a systematic review," *American Journal of Hematology*, vol. 86, no. 8, pp. 722–725, 2011.

[22] C. M. Bruns, L. A. Thet, R. D. Woodson, J. Schultz, and K. M. Hla, "Hemoglobinopathy case finding by pulse oximetry," *American Journal of Hematology*, vol. 74, no. 2, pp. 142–143, 2003.

[23] J. Abdulla, L. C. Laursen, and C. B. Thomsen, "Arterial puncture or pulse oximetry?" *Ugeskrift for Læger*, vol. 161, no. 8, pp. 1110–1112, 1999.

[24] B. J. Wilson, H. J. Cowan, J. A. Lord, D. J. Zuege, and D. A. Zygun, "The accuracy of pulse oximetry in emergency department patients with severe sepsis and septic shock: a retrospective cohort study," *BMC Emergency Medicine*, vol. 10, article 9, 2010.

Higher Mobility Scores in Patients with Cystic Fibrosis Are Associated with Better Lung Function

Aneesha Thobani,[1] Jessica A. Alvarez,[1,2] Shaina Blair,[3] Kaila Jackson,[1] Eric R. Gottlieb,[4] Seth Walker,[5] and Vin Tangpricha[1,2,3,6]

[1]Division of Endocrinology, Metabolism and Lipids, Department of Medicine, Emory University School of Medicine, Atlanta, GA 30322, USA

[2]Nutrition Health Sciences Program, Graduate Division of Biological and Biomedical Sciences, Emory University, Atlanta, GA 30322, USA

[3]Emory University Cystic Fibrosis Center, Atlanta, GA 30322, USA

[4]The University of Maryland School of Medicine, Baltimore, MD 21201, USA

[5]Division of Pulmonary, Allergy and Critical Care Medicine, Department of Medicine, Emory University School of Medicine, Atlanta, GA 30322, USA

[6]Atlanta VA Medical Center, Decatur, GA 30022, USA

Correspondence should be addressed to Vin Tangpricha; vin.tangpricha@emory.edu

Academic Editor: Hartmut Grasemann

Objective. The purpose of this study was to determine whether mobility and physical activity were associated with lung function in adults with cystic fibrosis (CF). *Design*. This was a prospective cohort observational study in an urban, academic, specialized care center. Participants were ambulatory, nonhospitalized adults with CF. *Main Outcome Measures*. Mobility was assessed monthly by the Life-Space Assessment (LSA) questionnaire and quarterly by pedometer. Lung function was assessed by spirometry. *Results*. Twenty-seven subjects participated. Subjects recorded mean pedometer steps of $20,213 \pm 11,331$ over three days and FEV_1% predicted of $77.48\% \pm 22.60\%$ over one year. The LSA score at enrollment was correlated with initial pedometer steps ($r = 0.42$ and $P = 0.03$), and mean LSA score over one year was correlated with mean number of steps ($r = 0.51$ and $P = 0.007$). LSA mobility and pedometer scores were correlated with FEV_1% predicted at enrollment and throughout the study. *Conclusions*. Mobility and physical activity measured by LSA questionnaire and pedometer are positively associated with lung function in adults with CF. This study confirms the importance of mobility and physical activity and supports the utility of a simple office-based questionnaire as a measure of mobility in adults with CF.

1. Introduction

Cystic fibrosis (CF) is a hereditary, chronic respiratory illness in which patients suffer from recurrent bouts of infection causing frequent hospitalization [1–3]. Patients with CF experience a chronic decline in lung function, and those with end-stage lung disease may become candidates for lung transplant. However, patients with higher levels of physical activity may have lower rates of decline in lung function, improved airway clearance, better muscle function, and enhanced quality of life [4, 5].

Review of the Literature. The importance of physical activity in patients with CF is well supported. Physical activity may include moderate to vigorous exercise associated with structured training and athletics, as well as day-to-date activity, termed habitual physical activity (HPA) [4–6]. Physical activity is associated with increased cardiovascular endurance, muscle strength, mucus clearance, and quality of life [4]. Ideally, patients should perform a combination of aerobic and strength training since aerobic training improves peak aerobic capacity, activity levels, and quality of life, while resistance training improves weight gain, FEV_1% predicted, and strength [4]. Strength training and aerobics both increased work capacity in patients with CF and demonstrated an increase in FEV_1% predicted [6, 7]. An increased level of HPA, independent of structured exercise, is also associated with better health outcomes in patients with CF, including improved aerobic capacity and lower rates of respiratory decline [8]. There are significant barriers to physical activity, including HPA, such as muscle defects, poor health, poor nutrition, and the constraints of intensive therapy and frequent hospitalization. Patients may also self-limit their HPA due to the perception of poor health and vulnerability to infection and other adverse events [4].

A reliable patient-reported measure of HPA, independent of overall quality of life, could provide an early indication of patients who are at risk for CF-related morbidity. Physical activity questionnaires contain limited reliability and validity, as they are prone to recall bias [9]. There exist such questionnaires as the Cystic Fibrosis Questionnaire-Revised (CFQR) [10], CF Respiratory Diary [11], Cystic Fibrosis Quality of Life (CFQoL) [12], and Questions on Life Satisfaction [13], all of which are directed towards patient-reported outcomes but only target disease-specific quality of life measures, while not targeting physical activity specifically. Aside from questionnaires, there are limited tools for measuring physical activity level specifically in patients with CF. Pedometers have been used previously and are feasible for use in the CF population; steps measured with a pedometer correlate with changes in health status and can be used as an outcome measure in CF [14]. A questionnaire that produces a score consistent with pedometer steps could minimize the time and expense of assessing physical activity in patients with CF and prove useful in clinical practice.

The Life-Space Assessment (LSA) is a validated tool used to measure mobility patterns in geriatric patients [15, 16]. The LSA measures how far and how often a person travels from his or her dwelling space and the level of independence that he or she exhibits [15]. In these previous studies, the LSA was shown to be associated with physical performance, cognitive abilities, mental health, and rate of recovery following surgical and nonsurgical hospitalization [15, 17–21]. Because of the accelerated decline in function and reduced life expectancy in CF, we previously hypothesized that this instrument designed to assess changes in functional capacity might be applicable to this patient population as well. In a retrospective study, we showed that Life-Space scores were associated with FEV_1% predicted and negatively correlated with rates of hospitalization in adults with CF [16]. Thus, the LSA may be a useful tool to assess health status in CF. It was not known, however, whether Life-Space scores correlate with mobility in the CF population and whether they are predictive of future changes in lung function.

Purpose. The purpose of this study was to determine if mobility as measured by pedometers and the LSA questionnaire was associated with improved lung function in patients with CF. We hypothesized that patients who have higher mobility by both measures would have better lung function as measured by FEV_1% predicted.

2. Materials and Methods

2.1. Participants and Protocol. The study was approved by the Emory Institutional Review Board. All participants provided written informed consent for participation in this study. Participants were recruited during outpatient clinic visits at the Emory University Adult Cystic Fibrosis Center in Atlanta, Georgia, between March 2011 and May 2012. Inclusion criteria for this study were a CF diagnosis, being clinically stable, and age ≥18 years. Participants were excluded if their clinic visit indicated need for hospitalization and/or acute exacerbation. Upon enrollment, subjects completed the LSA. Subjects completed the LSA monthly, either during clinic visits or by phone interview conducted by study investigators. Demographic and clinical characteristics were extracted from subjects' medical records. Thirty-five participants were recruited for the study, out of which 27 completed the one-year follow-up visit.

2.2. Assessment of Physical Activity. Subjects were provided with a pedometer (New Lifestyles DIGI-WALKER SW-200, New-Lifestyles Inc., Lee's Summit, Montana) that they were asked to wear for three consecutive days quarterly for one year. Three days has previously been reported to provide a sufficient estimate of weekly pedometer-assessed physical activity [22]. Self-reported pedometer readings were collected by phone quarterly throughout the one-year study period. We collected information quarterly to account for potential seasonal variation in physical activity.

2.3. Life-Space Assessment. The LSA score is a measure of the frequency and independence of travel to different areas extending outward from one's dwelling space during the previous four weeks [15, 17–21]. This instrument was initially designed for the geriatric population, but we have shown that it may be appropriate for use in the CF population as well [16]. The LSA questionnaire assesses the frequency and level of independence that subjects exhibit in traveling to rooms in their homes other than the one in which they sleep (level 1); areas outside their homes in their yards or driveways (level 2); places in their neighborhoods other than their own yards or driveways (level 3); places outside of their neighborhoods but still within their towns (level 4); and places outside of their towns (level 5). For each level a subject reached, he or she was asked to report the frequency of attaining that specific level in the past four weeks (daily (score = 4), 4–6 times per week (3), 1–3 times per week (2), or less than once a week (1)). Subjects were also asked to report their levels of independence based on whether they required personal assistance (1) or equipment (1.5) or exhibited complete independence (2). The scores for each level were summed to calculate a total with a possible maximum score of 120. A higher LSA score is indicative of a larger "life-space" or zone of living for a subject. See Peel et al. 2005 [15] for an in-depth description of the LSA.

2.4. Statistical Methods. Descriptive statistics were compiled. The average number of steps by pedometer and average LSA score were recorded at time of enrollment and over the course

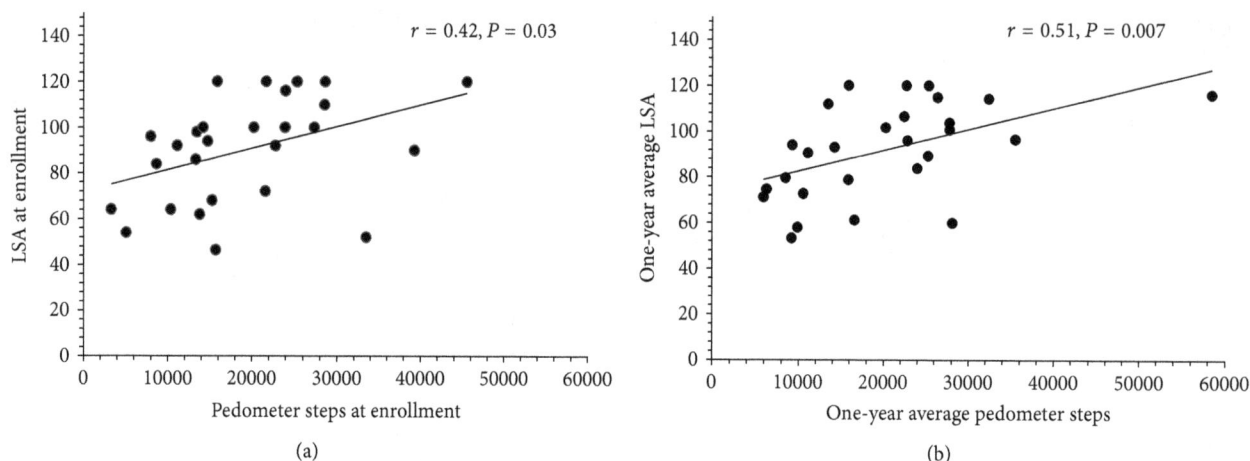

(a)   (b)

FIGURE 1: Relationship between Life-Space Assessment score and steps recorded by pedometer at enrollment (a) and over 1 year (b). The Life-Space Assessment score was positively associated with physical activity as assessed by pedometers in adult subjects with cystic fibrosis at enrollment and after 1 year of follow-up.

of the year. Pearson correlation analyses were used to assess the relationship between LSA scores and reported numbers of pedometer steps at baseline, as well as average one-year scores and steps, respectively. All statistical analyses were performed using the JMP Pro 10 software package (SAS Institute Inc., Cary, NC) and assumed a statistical significance value of $P < 0.05$.

3. Results

3.1. Study Subjects. A total of 35 subjects consented to participation in this study. Twenty-seven subjects completed the one-year follow-up study visit. Dropouts were primarily due to inconvenience of monthly phone calls or inability to be contacted by phone. The study demographics for the 27 participants are presented in Table 1. Complete pedometer data were available for 24 subjects.

3.2. Life-Space Score and Pedometer Readings. Subjects reported a mean (± SD) of 19,452 ± 10,118 steps over three days at enrollment and a mean of 20,213 ± 11,331 steps over three days recorded quarterly throughout the year. Subjects reported a mean (± SD) LSA score of 90.39 ± 22.98 out of 120 at baseline and a mean LSA score of 91.94 ± 20.64 recorded quarterly throughout the year (Table 1).

The mean LSA score at enrollment was positively correlated with number of pedometer steps at enrollment ($r = 0.42$ and $P = 0.03$). The mean LSA score over one year was positively correlated with mean number of pedometer steps recorded during the year ($r = 0.51$ and $P = 0.007$), as shown in Figure 1.

3.3. Life-Space Score and Lung Function. Participants had a mean (± SD) FEV_1% predicted of 77.48 ± 22.60%. Both enrollment and one-year average LSA were associated with lung function as measured by FEV_1% predicted ($r = 0.62$ and 0.67, resp.; $P < 0.001$ for both).

TABLE 1: Demographics of adult subjects with cystic fibrosis ($N = 27$).

Age (years)	32.15 ± 12.27
Race	
White	26 (96%)
Black	1 (4%)
Sex	
Male	13 (48%)
Female	14 (52%)
FEV_1% predicted	77.48 ± 22.60
Severity of lung disease by FEV_1%	
Very severe (<35%)	2 (7%)
Moderate to severe (35%–69%)	8 (30%)
Mild (>69%)	17 (63%)
BMI (kg/m^2)	23.46 ± 3.76
Mutation	
ΔF508 homozygous	12 (44%)
ΔF508 heterozygous	14 (52%)
Others	1 (4%)
LSA score at enrollment	90.39 ± 22.98
LSA score during study period	91.94 ± 20.64
Pedometer steps at enrollment	19452 ± 10118
Pedometer steps during study period	20213 ± 11331

Reported as mean ± SD or n (%).

3.4. Pedometer Steps and Lung Function. Both enrollment and one-year average pedometer steps were associated with FEV_1% predicted ($r = 0.39$ and 0.40, resp.; $P = 0.04$ for both).

4. Discussion

In this study we examined the relationship between the LSA score and mobility assessed with pedometer step counts and the correlation of both measures with lung function. We found a significant positive correlation between the LSA score and number of pedometer steps, both at enrollment and throughout the year. Subjects with higher LSA scores reported a greater number of steps. This study provides preliminary validation of the LSA as an instrument to assess mobility and shows that greater mobility is associated with better lung function in patients with CF.

Physical activity is associated with maintenance or improvement of health status in patients with CF [4–7]. Questionnaires have been used to assess the health status of patients with CF [23], including the Short-Form Health Survey (SF-36) [24], the Sickness Impact Profile (SIP) [25], and the Nottingham Health Profile (NHP) [26], but neither of these directly measures physical activity, and they are relatively time-consuming for physicians and other clinicians to administer. The Cystic Fibrosis Quality of Life (CFQoL) has been used to address issues specific to patients with CF [12], and of the 52 questions, some are directed towards the subjects' mobility. However, the CFQoL aims to assess the psychosocial implications of the disease and is not a validated tool for mobility and/or physical activity levels. Pedometers have been validated for the measurement of physical activity [14], but these are not readily available in most physicians' offices, and data collection requires frequent follow-up and may be a burden to patients and clinicians.

The LSA is short and concise and evaluates a subject's mobility as measured in five zones extending outwards from the closest dwelling space. It has been validated as a predictor of health in the geriatric population, and studies have shown that subjects with a higher LSA score are more mobile [15, 17–21]. LSA score is associated with standard indicators of health in patients with CF [16]. This prospective study confirms these findings and validates them as a measure of mobility in the same population.

In our study, LSA score was positively associated with the subjects' lung function as measured by FEV_1% predicted. Pedometer step counts were also associated with better lung function. Numerous reasons potentially explain our interrelationships between LSA score, pedometer step counts, and lung function. Greater step count could also reflect greater mobility, which may, in turn, indicate greater access to medical care (i.e., clinic visits), better treatment adherence, greater quality of life, and/or greater functioning in general, all of which would influence lung function [27, 28]. However, studies conducted in patients with COPD and obstructive lung disease also show that a lower number of steps is associated with severe physical inactivity and increases the risk for disability [29, 30]. We hypothesize that the same would be true in CF, which is also an obstructive lung disease characterized by progressive disability. In patients with CF, LSA score and step count may also reflect habitual physical activity, which was shown in a longitudinal study to be associated with lower rates of respiratory decline [8]. Beneficial effects of physical activity specific to CF may include serving as an adjunct to physiotherapy by agitating the characteristic mucus, strengthening the chest wall musculature, and increasing physical work capacity [4, 7]. Aerobic exercise as well as habitual physical activity may also strengthen the chest wall musculature, which could improve

pulmonary function. Strength training has been shown to increase physical work capacity, which may contribute to pulmonary rehabilitation as well [7].

A causal directionality cannot be determined with these studies. It is possible that impaired lung function precludes mobility and physical activity. Expression of defective CFTR in skeletal muscle may directly cause a reduction in work capacity and make patients with CF vulnerable to deconditioning [31]. For this reason as well, it is important to monitor physical activity in patients with CF. Some of the association may be explained simply by the fact that an individual with better lung function may be more capable of carrying out an active lifestyle and would therefore have a higher Life-Space score. Similarly, there are other psychosocial factors including perceptions of disease burden and constraints of treatment that may affect physical activity in patients with more severe disease [32]. Conversely, physical activity has been shown to affect perception of disease burden, emotional functioning, and various other subsets of quality of life scales. This in turn may improve treatment adherence. It may also increase a patient's motivation to exercise even more through positive feedback [27, 33]. Habitual physical activity may be an important mediator of quality of life because it is more accommodating to include the activities that a patient enjoys and is more sustainable than a formalized training program.

Our data suggest that LSA is an efficient and effective instrument for evaluating the health status of a patient with CF. It provides information that can be shared among the multiple clinicians that participate in the care of a patient with CF, including physicians, nurses, dietitians, respiratory therapists, and social workers. It is taken for granted that all forms of physical activity are beneficial for patients with CF, to the extent that it was considered unethical to perform a study in which some patients would be randomized not to receive exercise training [7]. If a patient visiting a CF clinic has a low Life-Space score, the clinician should investigate whether the patient is in poor health or otherwise should suggest an intervention to increase physical activity in daily life.

One limitation of this study was the small sample size. Additionally, this instrument is designed to assess habitual mobility, or "life-space," rather than vigorous exercise or habitual physical activity, which the LSA does not capture. Thus it would not be used alone to fully measure physical activity or exercise, but it provides information that is less easily reported than the type, duration, and frequency of a formalized exercise program. Although the LSA was initially developed for the geriatric population, our previous study and the association of the LSA with pedometer counts in this study validate it for the CF population as well. Insofar as measuring physical activity for the purpose of this study, it may be argued that accelerometers are preferable to pedometers. However, we believe this difference is insignificant in this study because the LSA measures only mobility, which is comparable to number of steps by pedometer. Unlike pedometers, accelerometers are able to measure the vigor of the activity, but this is not a parameter assessed by the LSA and would not contribute substantially to our analysis. Furthermore, it has also been shown in community-dwelling older adults that step counts measured by pedometers and accelerometers are closely correlated [34]. Future studies should pilot the use of the LSA questionnaire in regular clinical practice. They should also evaluate it for use in children with CF.

5. Conclusion

The Life-Space Assessment score was associated with increased mobility, as assessed by pedometers, and higher lung function in nonhospitalized adults with CF. Future investigation is warranted to determine if the LSA tool can be used to examine the impact of mobility on long-term health outcomes in the CF population.

Abbreviations

CF: Cystic fibrosis
CFQR: Cystic Fibrosis Questionnaire-Revised
CFQoL: Cystic Fibrosis Quality of Life
FEV_1% predicted: Forced expiratory volume in one second, percentage of predicted value
HPA: Habitual physical activity
LSA: Life-Space Assessment.

Conflict of Interests

The authors report no conflict of interests.

Acknowledgments

This work was made possible by a student traineeship award from the Cystic Fibrosis Foundation to Aneesha Thobani and in part by grants from the National Institutes of Health Grants UL1 TR000454 (Atlanta Clinical and Translational Science Institute), K23 AR054334 (VT), T32 DK007298, and K01 DK102851 (JAA) and the CF Center grant to Emory University. The funders had no role in study design, data collection and analysis, decision to publish, or preparation of the paper.

References

[1] F. J. Accurso, "Update in cystic fibrosis 2006," *The American Journal of Respiratory and Critical Care Medicine*, vol. 175, no. 8, pp. 754–757, 2007.

[2] E. T. Zemanick, J. K. Harris, S. Conway et al., "Measuring and improving respiratory outcomes in cystic fibrosis lung disease: opportunities and challenges to therapy," *Journal of Cystic Fibrosis*, vol. 9, no. 1, pp. 1–16, 2010.

[3] J. K. Block, K. L. Vandemheen, E. Tullis et al., "Predictors of pulmonary exacerbations in patients with cystic fibrosis infected with multi-resistant bacteria," *Thorax*, vol. 61, no. 11, pp. 969–974, 2006.

[4] D. L. Wilkes, J. E. Schneiderman, T. Nguyen et al., "Exercise and physical activity in children with cystic fibrosis," *Paediatric Respiratory Reviews*, vol. 10, no. 3, pp. 105–109, 2009.

[5] J. Schneiderman-Walker, D. L. Wilkes, L. Strug et al., "Sex differences in habitual physical activity and lung function

decline in children with cystic fibrosis," *The Journal of Pediatrics*, vol. 147, no. 3, pp. 321–326, 2005.

[6] P. A. Nixon, D. M. Orenstein, and S. F. Kelsey, "Habitual physical activity in children and adolescents with cystic fibrosis," *Medicine and Science in Sports and Exercise*, vol. 33, no. 1, pp. 30–35, 2001.

[7] D. M. Orenstein, M. F. Hovell, M. Mulvihill et al., "Strength vs aerobic training in children with cystic fibrosis: a randomized controlled trial," *Chest*, vol. 126, no. 4, pp. 1204–1214, 2004.

[8] J. E. Schneiderman, D. L. Wilkes, E. G. Atenafu et al., "Longitudinal relationship between physical activity and lung health in patients with cystic fibrosis," *The European Respiratory Journal*, vol. 43, no. 3, pp. 817–823, 2014.

[9] R. J. Shephard, "Limits to the measurement of habitual physical activity by questionnaires," *British Journal of Sports Medicine*, vol. 37, no. 3, pp. 197–206, 2003.

[10] A. L. Quittner, A. Buu, M. A. Messer, A. C. Modi, and M. Watrous, "Development and validation of the cystic fibrosis questionnaire in the United States: a health-related quality-of-life measure for cystic fibrosis," *Chest*, vol. 128, no. 4, pp. 2347–2354, 2005.

[11] C. H. Goss, T. C. Edwards, B. W. Ramsey, M. L. Aitken, and D. L. Patrick, "Patient-reported respiratory symptoms in cystic fibrosis," *Journal of Cystic Fibrosis*, vol. 8, no. 4, pp. 245–252, 2009.

[12] L. Gee, J. Abbott, S. P. Conway, C. Etherington, and A. K. Webb, "Development of a disease specific health related quality of life measure for adults and adolescents with cystic fibrosis," *Thorax*, vol. 55, no. 11, pp. 946–954, 2000.

[13] L. Goldbeck, T. G. Schmitz, G. Henrich, and P. Herschbach, "Questions on life satisfaction for adolescents and adults with cystic fibrosis: development of a disease-specific questionnaire," *Chest*, vol. 123, no. 1, pp. 42–48, 2003.

[14] B. S. Quon, D. L. Patrick, T. C. Edwards et al., "Feasibility of using pedometers to measure daily step counts in cystic fibrosis and an assessment of its responsiveness to changes in health state," *Journal of Cystic Fibrosis*, vol. 11, no. 3, pp. 216–222, 2012.

[15] C. Peel, P. S. Baker, D. L. Roth, C. J. Brown, E. V. Bodner, and R. M. Allman, "Assessing mobility in older adults: the UAB Study of Aging Life-Space Assessment," *Physical Therapy*, vol. 85, no. 10, pp. 1008–1019, 2005.

[16] E. R. Gottlieb, E. C. Smith, L. L. Wolfenden, R. M. Allman, and V. Tangpricha, "Life-space mobility is associated with frequency of hospitalization in adults with cystic fibrosis," *Clinical Respiratory Journal*, vol. 5, no. 4, pp. 245–251, 2011.

[17] C. J. Brown, D. L. Roth, R. M. Allman, P. Sawyer, C. S. Ritchie, and J. M. Roseman, "Trajectories of life-space mobility after hospitalization," *Annals of Internal Medicine*, vol. 150, no. 6, pp. 372–378, 2009.

[18] M. Crowe, R. Andel, V. G. Wadley, O. C. Okonkwo, P. Sawyer, and R. M. Allman, "Life-space and cognitive decline in a community-based sample of African American and Caucasian older adults," *Journals of Gerontology Series A: Biological Sciences and Medical Sciences*, vol. 63, no. 11, pp. 1241–1245, 2008.

[19] P. S. Baker, E. V. Bodner, and R. M. Allman, "Measuring life-space mobility in community-dwelling older adults," *Journal of the American Geriatrics Society*, vol. 51, no. 11, pp. 1610–1614, 2003.

[20] R. M. Allman, P. S. Baker, R. M. Maisiak, R. V. Sims, and J. M. Roseman, "Racial similarities and differences in predictors of mobility change over eighteen months," *Journal of General Internal Medicine*, vol. 19, no. 11, pp. 1118–1126, 2004.

[21] R. M. Allman, P. Sawyer, and J. M. Roseman, "The UAB study of aging: Background and insights into life-space mobility among older Americans in rural and urban settings," *Aging Health*, vol. 2, no. 3, pp. 417–429, 2006.

[22] C. Tudor-Locke, L. Burkett, J. P. Reis, B. E. Ainsworth, C. A. Macera, and D. K. Wilson, "How many days of pedometer monitoring predict weekly physical activity in adults?" *Preventive Medicine*, vol. 40, no. 3, pp. 293–298, 2005.

[23] J. Abbott, K. Webb, and M. Dodd, "Quality of life in cystic fibrosis," *Journal of the Royal Society of Medicine, Supplement*, vol. 90, supplement 31, pp. 37–42, 1997.

[24] J. E. Brazier, R. Harper, N. M. B. Jones et al., "Validating the SF-36 health survey questionnaire: new outcome measure for primary care," *British Medical Journal*, vol. 305, no. 6846, pp. 160–164, 1992.

[25] B. S. Gilson, J. S. Gilson, M. Bergner et al., "The sickness impact profile. Development of an outcome measure of health care," *The American Journal of Public Health*, vol. 65, no. 12, pp. 1304–1310, 1975.

[26] S. M. Hunt, S. P. McKenna, J. McEwen, J. Williams, and E. Papp, "The Nottingham health profile—subjective health status and medical consultations," *Social Science and Medicine. Part A Medical Psychology and Medical*, vol. 15, no. 3, pp. 221–229, 1981.

[27] S. A. Prasad and F. J. Cerny, "Factors that influence adherence to exercise and their effectiveness: application to cystic fibrosis," *Pediatric Pulmonology*, vol. 34, no. 1, pp. 66–72, 2002.

[28] D. M. Orenstein, P. A. Nixon, E. A. Ross, and R. M. Kaplan, "The quality of well-being in cystic fibrosis," *Chest*, vol. 95, no. 2, pp. 344–347, 1989.

[29] P. Katz, H. Chen, T. A. Omachi et al., "The role of physical inactivity in increasing disability among older adults with obstructive airway disease," *Journal of Cardiopulmonary Rehabilitation and Prevention*, vol. 31, no. 3, pp. 193–197, 2011.

[30] Z. S. Depew, P. J. Novotny, and R. P. Benzo, "How many steps are enough to avoid severe physical inactivity in patients with chronic obstructive pulmonary disease?" *Respirology*, vol. 17, no. 6, pp. 1026–1027, 2012.

[31] H. C. Selvadurai, J. Allen, T. Sachinwalla, J. Macauley, C. J. Blimkie, and P. P. van Asperen, "Muscle function and resting energy expenditure in female athletes with cystic fibrosis," *The American Journal of Respiratory and Critical Care Medicine*, vol. 168, no. 12, pp. 1476–1480, 2003.

[32] F. J. Moola, "'This is the best fatal illness that you can have': contrasting and comparing the experiences of parenting youth with cystic fibrosis and congenital heart disease," *Qualitative Health Research*, vol. 22, no. 2, pp. 212–225, 2012.

[33] A. M. Schmidt, U. Jacobsen, V. Bregnballe et al., "Exercise and quality of life in patients with cystic fibrosis: a 12-week intervention study," *Physiotherapy Theory and Practice*, vol. 27, no. 8, pp. 548–556, 2011.

[34] T. J. Harris, C. G. Owen, C. R. Victor, R. Adams, U. Ekelund, and D. G. Cook, "A comparison of questionnaire, accelerometer, and pedometer: measures in older people," *Medicine & Science in Sports and Exercise*, vol. 41, no. 7, pp. 1392–1402, 2009.

Study of Exhaled Nitric Oxide in Subjects with Suspected Obstructive Sleep Apnea: A Pilot Study in Vietnam

Sy Duong-Quy,[1,2] Thong Hua-Huy,[2] Huyen-Tran Tran-Mai-Thi,[3] Nhat-Nam Le-Dong,[4] Timothy J. Craig,[5] and Anh-Tuan Dinh-Xuan[2]

[1]*Bio-Medical Research Center, Lam Dong Medical College, Dalat, Lam Dong 063, Vietnam*
[2]*Department of Respiratory Physiology, Cochin Hospital, Paris Descartes University, Sorbonne Paris Cité, 75014 Paris, France*
[3]*Department of Technology and Biology, Dalat, Lam Dong 063, Vietnam*
[4]*Department of Pulmonology, St. Elisabeth Hospital, 5000-5999 Namur, Belgium*
[5]*Pennsylvania State University, 500 University Drive, Hershey, PA 17033, USA*

Correspondence should be addressed to Sy Duong-Quy; sduongquy.jfvp@gmail.com

Academic Editor: R. Farre

Background and Objective. The concentration of exhaled nitric oxide (eNO), reflecting the activity of inducible NO synthase in airway epithelium, has been found to increase in patients with obstructive sleep apnea (OSA). This study aimed to measure eNO concentration in patients with suspected OSA and to correlate different eNO parameters with clinical and sleep apnea characteristics. *Methods.* In this cross-sectional study, all patients underwent in-lab overnight polysomnography (PSG) and eNO measurement using a method of multiple flow rates before and after PSG (pre- and post-PSG). *Results.* According to the result of PSG, 82 persons were divided into two groups: control subjects ($n = 30$; 54 ± 14 years) and patients with OSA defined as apnea-hypopnea index (AHI) ≥ 5/hour ($n = 52$; 53 ± 12 years). Body mass index (BMI) and neck and abdomen circumferences of OSA patients were significantly higher than those from control subjects. In OSA group, post-PSG alveolar NO concentration (CANO) (5.3 ± 1.9 ppb) was significantly higher than pre-PSG CANO (4.0 ± 1.7 ppb; $P < 0.001$). Significant correlations have been found between CANO and AHI ($P < 0.001$) and between CANO and nadir SpO_2 ($P < 0.05$). The daytime CANO value of more than 4.1 ppb can be used to screen symptomatic subjects for the presence of OSA with a high specificity of 93.3%. *Conclusion.* Our findings indicate CANO as a surrogate marker for OSA in persons with suggestive symptoms.

1. Introduction

Obstructive sleep apnea (OSA) is a chronic respiratory disorder with a high and increasing prevalence [1]. OSA is characterized by intermittent upper airway collapse and reopening during sleep, leading to intermittent hypoxemia (IH) and cardiovascular comorbidities. IH during sleep increases the production of reactive oxygen species and proinflammatory mediators. Oxidative stress and inflammation generate endothelial dysfunction, cardiovascular diseases such as arterial hypertension, coronary ischemia, and lung inflammation. Therefore, noninvasive assessment of lung inflammation may be useful to predict patients with OSA and its severity [2].

In humans, nitric oxide (NO) plays an important role in modulating vascular tone and airway inflammation. In the airway, NO can be easily measured in exhaled air in order to diagnose and evaluate the severity of chronic bronchial and alveolar inflammation [3]. The exhaled fraction of NO (FENO), reflecting total NO production in the airway, has been found to increase in patients with OSA [4–10]. Bucca et al. showed that complete tooth loss favoured upper airway obstruction and inflammation, as evidenced by increased eNO concentration with offline method [5]. In overweight children, habitual snoring and OSA, but not obesity alone, are associated with increased airway inflammation [6]. Later findings showed that FENO was correlated with OSA severity and decreased after positive pressure therapy [8–10].

However, FENO does not indicate the amount of NO being released from the periphery of the lung, that is, in bronchioles, alveoli, and interstitial spaces. Measurement of exhaled NO (eNO) using the two-compartment model (alveolar and bronchial) with multiple expiratory flow rates allows the determination of maximum bronchial NO flux (J'awNO) and alveolar NO concentration (CANO) by mathematical formula [10–12]. Therefore, CANO may be used to evaluate the inflammation of distal lung due to oxidative stress [12].

This study employed a mathematical formula [13] capable of discerning between bronchial and alveolar concentration to explore which one was better correlated with clinical symptoms and sleep apnea parameters. We measured the concentration of eNO in patients with suggestive symptoms of OSA and correlated different eNO parameters with clinical symptoms and sleep apnea characteristics.

2. Patients and Methods

2.1. Patients. Subjects living in Dalat city, Vietnam, who came to the Clinical Research Center of Lam Dong Medical College for screening of OSA, were included in this cross-sectional and case-control study. Subjects with acute and chronic cardiorespiratory diseases (acute myocardial infarction, severe coronary disease, chronic heart failure, COPD, and asthma) or diseases treated with local or systemic corticosteroids (allergic rhinitis and/or conjunctivitis) were excluded from the study.

All study subjects completed a screening questionnaire about symptoms of OSA, sleep habits and quality, and snoring. Epworth score was calculated for each patient (from 0 to 24). They underwent exhaled NO measurement and overnight polysomnography (PSG). Subjects were then randomized into two groups according to the results of PSG. Subjects with OSA were defined by apnea-hypopnea index (AHI) ≥ 5/hour and classified as having mild (AHI = 5–15), moderate (AHI = 16–30), or severe (AHI > 30) OSA. Subjects with AHI < 5/hour were included in control group.

2.2. Methods

2.2.1. Polysomnography. In-laboratory overnight PSG was performed for each study subject using Alice 6 PSG (Philips, USA) as recommended [14]. The recording time was from 10 pm to 6 am of the day after. The minimum recording time for PSG was 6 hours with sleep time of at least 3 hours. Sleep G3 software was used to analyze PSG results. The recorded parameters were electroencephalography (EEG) with 4 channels: C4–A1, C3–A2, O2–A1, and O1–A2; chin electromyography (EMG); electrocardiography (ECG); nasal and buccal air flows; thorax-abdomen movements; sleeping posture; apnea-hypopnea index (times/minutes); type of apnea (central apnea, obstructive apnea, or mixed apnea); oxygen saturation (SpO_2) and minimum SpO_2 (nadir SpO_2); arousal index (times/hour); snoring (>56 dB); and sleep efficiency (%).

2.2.2. Exhaled NO. Exhaled nitric oxide was measured at multiple flow rates (50 mL/s, 100 mL/s, 150 mL/s, and 350 mL/s) before and after PSG (before PSG: 8 pm; after PSG: 6 am) using an electrochemical based analyzer (FeNO+,

Medisoft-MGCD, USA). Technical measurement of exhaled NO was conducted according to manufacturer's instructions, as recommended by the ATS/ERS guideline [15]. The maximal bronchial production rate of NO (J'awNO) and alveolar concentration of NO (CANO) were automatically determined using the two-compartment model by Tsoukias and George [13]: VNO = J'awNO + CANO × VE via Expair's software.

2.3. Statistical Analysis. Data were analyzed using IBM-SPSS 22.0 software (Chicago, Illinois, USA). Values were expressed as mean ± standard deviation and 95% CI for quantitative variables and percentage for qualitative variables. Comparisons between the OSA patients and control subjects were done using Student's t-test. Pearson's chi-squared test (or Fisher exact test) was performed for verifying the relationship between qualitative variables. Linear correlation was analyzed by Spearman's nonparametric method. The best cutoff value of CANO for OSA screening was determined by ROC curve analysis. The statistical significance was stated with $P < 0.05$.

3. Results

3.1. Characteristics of Study Subjects

3.1.1. Anthropometric and Clinical Characteristics. From March to September 2014, 82 subjects were included in the present study. They underwent polysomnography (PSG) and were divided into two groups: control subjects (AHI < 5; $n = 30$; 54 ± 14 years; male/female: 1/1) and subjects with OSA (AHI ≥ 5; $n = 52$; 53 ± 12 years; male/female: 1.2/1). All anthropometric and clinical characteristics of the study subjects are presented in Table 1. There were no significant differences between the two groups for mean age, percentage of active smokers, and Epworth scores. BMI and neck and abdomen circumferences of subjects with OSA were significantly higher than those of control subjects. The results of pulmonary function test showed no significant difference (FEV_1, FVC, FEV_1/FVC, and TLC) between the two groups (Table 1).

3.1.2. PSG Outcomes. The increases of AHI and arousal index and the decreases of mean SpO_2 and nadir SpO_2 in subjects with OSA were significantly more important than those in the control subjects (Table 1).

3.2. Exhaled Nitric Oxide Analysis. The results of exhaled NO measured before and after polysomnography (pre- and post-PSG) and PSG parameters are presented in Table 1. In the two groups, the levels of pre-PSG exhaled NO (FENO, J'awNO, and CANO) were within normal limits (9.4 ± 6.6 ppb, 26.6 ± 19.2 nL/min, and 2.2 ± 0.7 ppb, resp., for control subjects; 16.7 ± 11.4 ppb, 38.3 ± 26.1 nL/min, and 4.0 ± 1.7 ppb, resp., for patients with OSA). All the parameters of exhaled NO in subjects with OSA were significantly higher than those of the control subjects (Table 1).

TABLE 1: Clinical and functional characteristics of study subjects.

Parameters	Control group ($n = 30$)		OSA ($n = 52$)		P value
	Mean ± SD	95% CI	Mean ± SD	95% CI	
Clinical characteristics					
Age, years	54.23 ± 14.19	48.93–59.50	53.98 ± 12.81	50.72–57.13	0.936
Height, cm	158.77 ± 7.48	156.16–161.24	161.08 ± 6.90	159.32–163.07	0.171
Weight, kg	54.33 ± 7.94	51.73–56.99	62.31 ± 12.04	59.24–65.46	**0.001**
BMI, kg/m^2	21.58 ± 2.98	20.58–22.60	23.85 ± 3.43	22.96–24.78	**0.002**
Neck.$_{CIR}$, cm	32.43 ± 2.71	31.54–33.27	35.23 ± 3.92	34.23–36.23	**<0.001**
Abd.$_{CIR}$, cm	78.60 ± 8.28	75.47–81.40	86.96 ± 10.16	84.13–89.72	**<0.001**
Epworth score	10.10 ± 4.54	8.00–11.50	10.83 ± 6.05	10.00–13.00	0.539
Gender, M : F	1 : 1		1.2 : 1		NS
Smoker, %	10.0		13.5		NS
Snoring, %	76.7		76.9		NS
Lung function					
FEV$_1$, % pred.	89 ± 11	85.06–92.94	88 ± 12	84.74–91.26	0.96
FVC, % pred.	91 ± 10	87.42–94.58	89 ± 11	86.01–91.99	0.90
FEV$_1$/FVC, %	78 ± 7	75.49–80.50	79 ± 8	76.83–81.17	0.93
TLC, % pred.	94 ± 8	91.13–96.86	94 ± 8	91.83–96.17	1.00
PSG parameters					
TST, min	531.94 ± 62.43	508.35–553.04	523.74 ± 59.85	506.39–539.29	0.563
AHI, n/h	3.03 ± 1.39	2.46–3.51	25.61 ± 15.94	21.80–29.74	**<0.001**
ARI, n/h	23.37 ± 15.39	17.67–28.69	37.10 ± 18.83	31.94–42.58	**0.001**
SpO$_2$, %	92.43 ± 2.51	91.57–93.30	88.67 ± 4.20	87.52–89.73	**<0.001**
Nadir SpO$_2$, %	89.93 ± 3.29	88.80–91.03	79.83 ± 9.31	77.27–82.08	**<0.001**
Before PSG					
FENO at 50 mL/s, ppb	9.4 ± 6.6	7.5–12.0	16.7 ± 11.4	14.2–20.0	**0.003**
FENO at 100 mL/s, ppb	6.9 ± 4.0	5.7–8.3	13.1 ± 8.0	11.1–15.3	**0.002**
FENO at 150 mL/s, ppb	5.6 ± 2.6	4.7–6.6	11.3 ± 6.7	9.6–13.3	**0.001**
FENO at 350 mL/s, ppb	3.9 ± 1.6	3.3–4.5	8.6 ± 4.7	7.4–9.9	**0.001**
J'awNO, nL/min	26.6 ± 19.2	20.6–33.5	38.3 ± 26.1	31.5–45.2	**0.028**
CANO, ppb	2.2 ± 0.7	1.9–2.4	4.0 ± 1.7	3.5–4.5	**0.001**
After PSG					
FENO at 50 mL/s, ppb	12.0 ± 5.9	10.0–14.3	22.1 ± 16.8	18.2–26.9	**0.015**
FENO at 100 mL/s, ppb	8.9 ± 3.6	7.6–10.3	17.3 ± 11.3	14.7–20.5	**0.003**
FENO at 150 mL/s, ppb	7.4 ± 2.9	6.4–8.6	15.3 ± 8.5	13.0–17.9	**0.001**
FENO at 350 mL/s, ppb	5.4 ± 2.2	4.6–6.2	11.2 ± 5.3	9.8–12.7	**0.001**
J'awNO, nL/min	31.7 ± 20.6	25.0–39.0	39.1 ± 23.6	33.1–45.4	0.150
CANO, ppb	3.2 ± 1.1	2.8–3.6	5.3 ± 1.9	4.8–5.8	**0.001**

Note: OSA: obstructive sleep apnea; BMI: body mass index; Neck.$_{CIR}$: neck circumference; Abd.$_{CIR}$: abdomen circumference; M : F: male : female; FEV$_1$: forced expiratory volume in 1 second; FVC: forced vital capacity; TLC: total lung capacity; PSG: polysomnography; TST: total sleep time; AHI: apnea-hypopnea index; ARI: arousal index. FENO: fractional exhaled nitric oxide (measured at expiratory flows of 50, 100, 150, and 350 mL/s); CANO: alveolar nitric oxide concentration; J'awNO: maximal bronchial flux of nitric oxide (using the two-compartment model). 95% CI: bootstrap confidence interval is based on 1000 replications; NS: no significant difference.

Figure 1 presents the post-PSG NO profile according to the multiflow approach by Tsoukias and George [13]. As shown in this graph, the OSA patients have a significantly higher post-PSG CANO value (indicated by the slope of the regression curve) than the control group.

3.3. *Changes in Exhaled NO before and after PSG.* In the control group, there were a nonsignificant increase of J'awNO

(31.7 ± 20.6 versus 26.6 ± 19.2; $P = 0.197$) and significant nonpathological increases of FENO at 50 mL/s and CANO after PSG versus before PSG (12.0 ± 5.9 ppb and 3.2 ± 1.1 ppb versus 9.4 ± 6.6 ppb and 2.2 ± 0.7 ppb; $P < 0.01$ and $P < 0.001$; resp.). In patients with OSA, there was a significant, nonpathological increase of FENO at 50 mL/s (22.1 ± 16.8 ppb versus 16.7 ± 11.4; $P < 0.001$) and a significant and pathological increase of CANO (5.3 ± 1.9 versus 4.0 ± 1.7 ppb; $P < 0.001$) after PSG versus those before PSG while there was

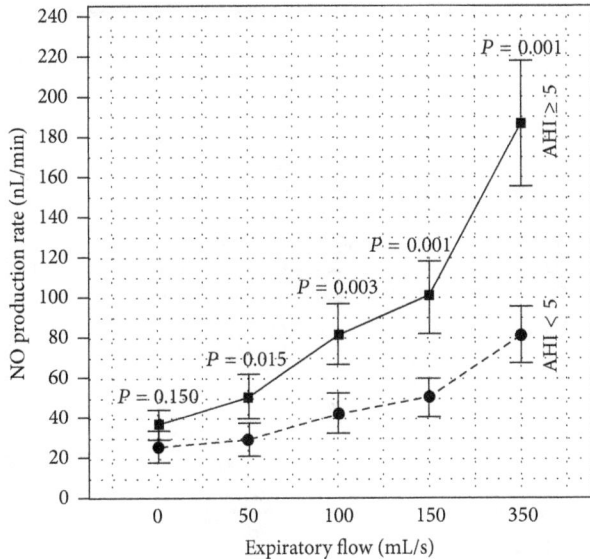

FIGURE 1: Post-PSG multiflow exhaled NO profile in two AHI groups. Note: the graph represents the mean (95% CI) of post-PSG NO production rate (VNO = FENO × Ex. flow), measured at 4 different levels of expiratory flow (50, 100, 150, and 350 mL/s). The J'awNO and CANO can be determined using the simple linear approach by Tsoukias and George [13]: VNO = J'awNO + CANO × Ex. flow. P value: significance of difference between healthy subjects (AHI < 5, circle point and dotted line) and patients with OSA (AHI ≥ 5, square point and continuous line).

TABLE 2: Correlations between AHI and snoring, Epworth score, and exhaled NO.

Parameters	AHI < 5 ($n = 30$)	AHI ≥ 5 ($n = 52$)
Snoring	$R = -0.084, P = 0.654$	$R = -0.216, P = 0.125$
Epworth score	$R = -0.085, P = 0.654$	$R = -0.021, P = 0.883$
Nadir SpO$_2$, %	$R = 0.222, P = 0.237$	$R = -0.578$, **P < 0.001**
FENO at 50 mL/s, ppb	$R = 0.074, P = 0.699$	$R = 0.373$, **P = 0.007**
J'awNO, nL/min	$R = 0.272, P = 0.146$	$R = 0.302$, **P = 0.030**
CANO, ppb	$R = 0.140, P = 0.462$	$R = 0.595$, **P < 0.0001**

Note: AHI: apnea-hypopnea index; FENO: fractional exhaled nitric oxide (measured at expiratory flows of 50, 100, 150, and 350 mL/s); CANO: alveolar nitric oxide concentration; J'awNO: maximal bronchial flux of nitric oxide (using the two-compartment model).

TABLE 3: Correlations between CANO and snoring, Epworth score, and PSG parameters.

Parameters	Control subjects ($n = 30$) CANO = 3.2 ± 1.1	OSA subjects ($n = 52$) CANO = 5.3 ± 1.9
Snoring	$R = -0.040, P = 0.833$	$R = -0.150, P = 0.287$
Epworth score	$R = -0.305, P = 0.101$	$R = -0.187, P = 0.184$
AHI, n/h	$R = 0.140, P = 0.462$	$R = 0.595$, **P < 0.0001**
SpO$_2$, %	$R = -0.166, P = 0.381$	$R = -0.153, P = 0.278$
Nadir SpO$_2$ (%)	$R = -0.215, P = 0.254$	$R = -0.374$, **P = 0.034**
Arousal index	$R = -0.102, P = 0.592$	$R = -0.207, P = 0.141$

CANO: alveolar nitric oxide concentration; PSG: polysomnography; OSA: obstructive sleep apnea; AHI: apnea-hypopnea index.

no significant difference of J'awNO (39.1 ± 23.6 ppb after PSG versus 38.3 ± 26.1 ppb before PSG; $P = 0.724$) (Table 1).

3.4. Correlation between AHI, Clinical Sleep Apnea Markers, and Exhaled NO

3.4.1. Correlations between AHI and Snoring, Epworth Score, and Exhaled NO. The correlations between AHI, snoring, Epworth score, and exhaled NO are presented in Table 2. There were no significant correlations in the control group ($P > 0.05$). In patients with OSA, there was a significant but slight correlation between AHI and FENO at 50 mL/s ($R = 0.373, P = 0.007$) and between AHI and J'awNO ($R = 0.302, P = 0.03$). Significant correlations have also been found between AHI and nadir SpO$_2$ ($R = -0.578, P < 0.001$) and between AHI and CANO ($R = 0.595, P < 0.0001$; Table 2).

3.4.2. Correlations between Post-PSG CANO and Snoring, Epworth Score, and PSG Parameters. The correlations between post-PSG CANO and snoring, Epworth score, and PSG parameters are presented in Table 3. There were no significant correlations in the control group ($P > 0.05$; Figure 2(b)). In subjects with OSA, there was a moderate and significant correlation between CANO and AHI ($R = 0.595$, $P < 0.0001$; Figure 2(a)) and a slight correlation between CANO and nadir SpO$_2$ ($R = -0.374, P = 0.034$; Figure 2(c)).

TABLE 4: Statistical parameters for the best cut-off point of CANO (4.1 ppb).

	Estimated value	95% CI Lower bound	95% CI Upper bound
Sensitivity	0.731	0.597	0.832
Specificity	0.933	0.787	0.981
PPV	0.950	0.835	0.986
NPV	0.667	0.516	0.790
LR+	10.962	2.844	42.243
LR−	0.288	0.182	0.456
Accuracy	0.805	0.706	0.876

PPV: positive predictive value; NPV: negative predictive value; LR: likelihood ratio; CI: confidence interval.

3.5. Cut-Off Point of CANO in Screening for Subjects with OSA. We performed the receiver operating characteristic (ROC) curve of post-PSG CANO for predicting the subjects with OSA (AHI ≥ 5 events/hour) and defined the best cut-off point at 4.1 ppb with highest Youden's J Index (0.664) (Figure 3). Sensibility, specificity, positive predictive value (PPV), and negative predictive value (NPV) were presented in Table 4 and Figure 3.

(a)

(b)

(c)

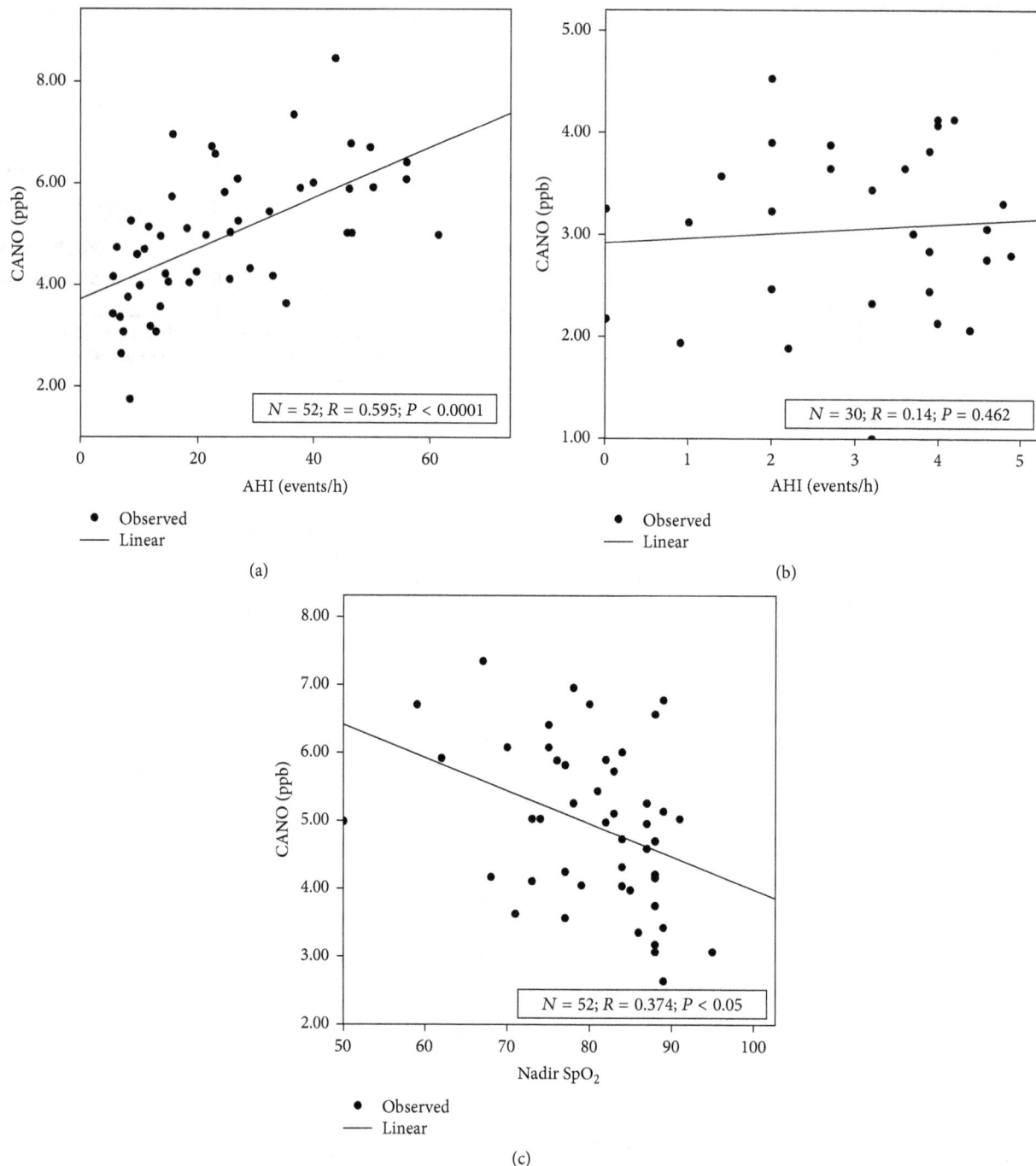

FIGURE 2: (a) Correlation between post-PSG CANO and AHI in subjects with OSA. There was a significant correlation between CANO and AHI ($R = 0.595$, $P < 0.0001$). CANO: alveolar concentration of nitric oxide; AHI: apnea-hypopnea index. (b) Correlation between post-PSG CANO and AHI in control subjects. There was no significant correlation between CANO and AHI ($R = 0.073$, $P = 0.706$). CANO: alveolar concentration of nitric oxide; AHI: apnea-hypopnea index. (c) Correlation between post-PSG CANO and nadir SpO_2 in subjects with OSA. There was a significant correlation between CANO and nadir SpO_2 ($R = -0.374$, $P = 0.034$). CANO: alveolar concentration of nitric oxide.

4. Discussion

The results of the present study showed that (1) the levels of exhaled NO (FENO, J'awNO, and CANO) during daytime were significantly higher in subjects with OSA than those without OSA; (2) FENO (at all expiratory flow rates) and CANO but not J'awNO were significantly increased on waking up (post-PSG) in both groups; and (3) significant increase of CANO in OSA subjects (as compared with control subjects) was correlated with the severity of OSA (AHI and nadir SpO_2).

In the present study, all study subjects were divided into two groups depending on apnea-hypopnea index (AHI) measuring by polysomnography (PSG): subjects without

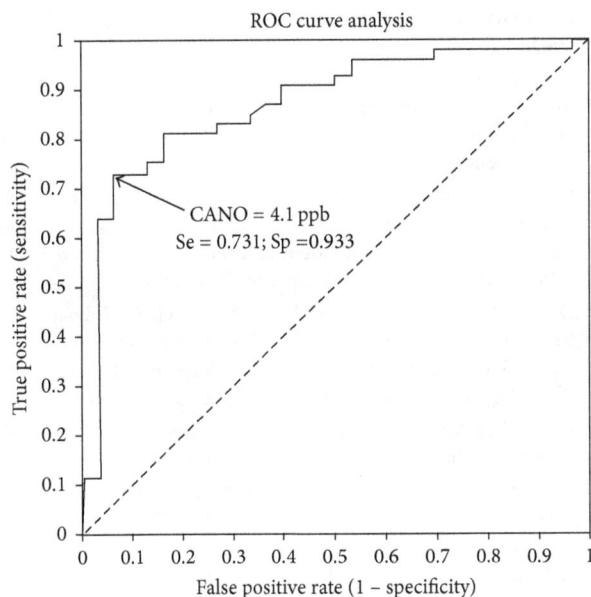

FIGURE 3: Receiver operating characteristic (ROC) curve of post-PSG CANO for predicting the subjects with OSA (AHI ≥ 5/h). CANO: alveolar nitric oxide concentration; PSG: polysomnography; post-PSG CANO: CANO measure on waking up after recording of PSG; Se: sensitivity; Sp: specificity. AUC: 0.868; best cut-off point: 4.1 ppb (Youden's J Index = 0.664) (see Table 4).

OSA (AHI < 5) and subjects with OSA (AHI ≥ 5). Similar to previous studies [4–12], subjects with OSA had some risk factors for OSA such as high weight and BMI and increased neck and abdomen circumferences. However, in the present study, snoring and Epworth score were not significantly different between subjects with or free of OSA (Table 1). In addition, there were no significant correlations between AHI and snoring and Epworth score in subjects with OSA. Our result suggests that snoring and Epworth score are less sensitive for diagnosis of OSA and for prediction of the severity of OSA. Hence, finding out a new predictive marker of OSA severity seems to be necessary.

Recent studies showed that exhaled NO (eNO), especially the measure of alveolar concentration of NO (CANO) on waking up, may be useful to diagnose and predict the severity of OSA [7, 11, 12]. The results of our study showed that the levels of eNO (FENO, J'awNO, and CANO), measured during daytime in standard conditions in subjects with OSA, were significantly higher than in subjects without OSA (Table 1) but these values were still within the normal limits for healthy subjects. Therefore, we cannot use daytime eNO to diagnose subjects with OSA. Interestingly, although FENO and CANO, but not J'awNO, were significantly increased on waking up (post-PSG) in comparison with FENO and CANO measured in daytime (pre-PSG) in subjects free of OSA (Figure 2), there was only a significant and pathological increase of CANO after PSG in subjects with OSA ($P < 0.001$; CANO > 5 ppb; Figure 1). Thus, CANO might meet the criteria for a surrogate for OSA in this symptomatic population.

The concentration of eNO is changed during daytime but it must be within normal limits for healthy subjects (circadian rhythm) [16–18]. Previous studies demonstrated that eNO measured from the upper airway was significantly increased in subjects with OSA and that was linked to overexpression of inducible NOS (iNOS) [4, 5, 7, 8], which was partially reversible after CPAP treatment [8–10]. In our study, the level of FENO on waking up (post-PSG) was significantly increased in subjects with and without OSA (Figure 1) but this level was still within normal limits of healthy adults (<25 ppb). In addition, there was no significant correlation between FENO and AHI (Table 2). Therefore, FENO on waking up can not be used to predict OSA in suspected Vietnamese subjects.

The result of the present study shows that the level of CANO on waking up in subjects with OSA was significantly higher than that when they are awake and also higher than the normal limits (CANO > 5 ppb; Figure 1). Interestingly, there were significant correlations between post-PSG CANO, AHI, and nadir SpO_2 (Tables 2 and 3 and Figures 2(a) and 2(b)), suggesting that CANO measurement on waking up may be useful to detect subjects at high risk of OSA. The result of our study showed that the specificity of CANO to diagnose OSA was best at 93.3% when the level of CANO exceeded 4.1 ppb. This result was similar to our previous study in European subjects with OSA, demonstrating the threshold of CANO at 4.5 ppb as the most relevant cut-off to specifically detect patients at high risk of OSA and nocturnal oxygen desaturation (NOD) among those with suggestive symptoms of OSA. Patients with NOD had more severe disease and might have suffered from more intense pulmonary inflammation, accounting for a higher cut-off value of CANO as compared to that found in this study. Another difference was the use of an electrochemical NO analyzer which is less expensive and more easily accessible for developing countries such as Vietnam [19].

Increased CANO in subjects with OSA has been found to be associated with oxygen desaturation during sleep [12, 20, 21]. Increasing evidence suggests the potential role of IH during sleep has been involved in an increase of CANO in OSA patients [21, 22]. IH during sleep in patients with OSA is a crucial cause of oxidative stress that activates the activity of inducible nitric oxide synthase (iNOS or NOS-2) to overproduce NO in alveolar epithelial cells. Although this study was conducted on a small number of subjects from a local population, the results of our study confirm for the first time in Vietnam that CANO is a useful biomarker in screening subjects at high risk of OSA. However, more studies in a large number of Vietnamese populations should be done to confirm the role of eNO in subjects with OSA.

5. Conclusion

Measurement of exhaled NO on waking up is useful to predict risk of OSA in subjects with suggestive symptoms. Alveolar exhaled NO (CANO) may be used as a surrogate marker for OSA.

Conflict of Interests

The authors declare that there is no conflict of interests regarding the publication of this paper.

References

[1] T. Young, M. Palta, J. Dempsey, P. E. Peppard, F. J. Nieto, and K. M. Hla, "Burden of sleep apnea: rationale, design, and major findings of the Wisconsin sleep cohort study," *Wisconsin Medical Journal*, vol. 108, no. 5, pp. 246–249, 2009.

[2] G. E. Carpagnano, D. Lacedonia, and M. P. Foschino-Barbaro, "Non-invasive study of airways inflammation in sleep apnea patients," *Sleep Medicine Reviews*, vol. 15, no. 5, pp. 317–326, 2011.

[3] P. J. Barnes, R. A. Dweik, A. F. Gelb et al., "Exhaled nitric oxide in pulmonary diseases: a comprehensive review," *Chest*, vol. 138, no. 3, pp. 682–692, 2010.

[4] C. O. Olopade, J. A. Christon, M. Zakkar et al., "Exhaled pentane and nitric oxide levels in patients with obstructive sleep apnea," *Chest*, vol. 111, no. 6, pp. 1500–1504, 1997.

[5] C. Bucca, A. Cicolin, L. Brussino et al., "Tooth loss and obstructive sleep apnoea," *Respiratory Research*, vol. 7, article 8, 2006.

[6] S. L. Verhulst, L. Aerts, S. Jacobs et al., "Sleep-disordered breathing, obesity, and airway inflammation in children and adolescents," *Chest*, vol. 134, no. 6, pp. 1169–1175, 2008.

[7] A. Depalo, G. E. Carpagnano, A. Spanevello et al., "Exhaled NO and iNOS expression in sputum cells of healthy, obese and OSA subjects," *Journal of Internal Medicine*, vol. 263, no. 1, pp. 70–78, 2008.

[8] M. Petrosyan, E. Perraki, D. Simoes et al., "Exhaled breath markers in patients with obstructive sleep apnoea," *Sleep and Breathing*, vol. 12, no. 3, pp. 207–215, 2008.

[9] A.-P. Chua, L. S. Aboussouan, O. A. Minai, K. Paschke, D. Laskowski, and R. A. Dweik, "Long-term continuous positive airway pressure therapy normalizes high exhaled nitric oxide levels in obstructive sleep apnea," *Journal of Clinical Sleep Medicine*, vol. 9, no. 6, pp. 529–535, 2013.

[10] A. M. Fortuna, R. Miralda, N. Calaf, M. González, P. Casan, and M. Mayos, "Airway and alveolar nitric oxide measurements in obstructive sleep apnea syndrome," *Respiratory Medicine*, vol. 105, no. 4, pp. 630–636, 2011.

[11] A. Foresi, C. Leone, D. Olivieri, and G. Cremona, "Alveolar-derived exhaled nitric oxide is reduced in obstructive sleep apnea syndrome," *Chest*, vol. 132, no. 3, pp. 860–867, 2007.

[12] T. Hua-Huy, N.-N. Le-Dong, S. Duong-Quy, L. Luchon, S. Rouhani, and A. T. Dinh-Xuan, "Increased alveolar nitric oxide concentration is related to nocturnal oxygen desaturation in obstructive sleep apnoea," *Nitric Oxide*, vol. 45, pp. 27–34, 2015.

[13] N. M. Tsoukias and S. C. George, "A two-compartment model of pulmonary nitric oxide exchange dynamics," *Journal of Applied Physiology*, vol. 85, no. 2, pp. 653–666, 1998.

[14] L. J. Epstein, D. Kristo, P. J. Strollo Jr. et al., "Adult Obstructive Sleep Apnea Task Force of the American Academy of Sleep Medicine. Clinical guideline for the evaluation, management and long-term care of obstructive sleep apnea in adults," *Journal of Clinical Sleep Medicine*, vol. 5, pp. 263–276, 2009.

[15] American Thoracic Society and European Respiratory Society, "ATS/ERS recommendations for standardized procedures for the online and offline measurement of exhaled lower respiratory nitric oxide and nasal nitric oxide, 2005," *American Journal of Respiratory and Critical Care Medicine*, vol. 171, pp. 912–930, 2005.

[16] M. Antosova, A. Bencova, A. Psenkova, D. Herle, and E. Rozborilova, "Exhaled nitric oxide—circadian variations in healthy subjects," *European Journal of Medical Research*, vol. 14, supplement 4, pp. 6–8, 2009.

[17] J. P. Palm, P. Graf, J. O. N. Lundberg, and K. Alving, "Characterization of exhaled nitric oxide: introducing a new reproducible method for nasal nitric oxide measurements," *European Respiratory Journal*, vol. 16, no. 2, pp. 236–241, 2000.

[18] D. J. O'Hearn, G. D. Giraud, J. M. Sippel, C. Edwards, B. Chan, and W. E. Holden, "Exhaled nasal nitric oxide output is reduced in humans at night during the sleep period," *Respiratory Physiology and Neurobiology*, vol. 156, no. 1, pp. 94–101, 2007.

[19] A. T. Dinh-Xuan, I. Annesi-Maesano, P. Berger et al., "Contribution of exhaled nitric oxide measurement in airway inflammation assessment in asthma. A position paper from the French Speaking Respiratory Society," *Revue des Maladies Respiratoires*, vol. 32, no. 2, pp. 193–215, 2015.

[20] S. Ryan, C. T. Taylor, and W. T. McNicholas, "Selective activation of inflammatory pathways by intermittent hypoxia in obstructive sleep apnea syndrome," *Circulation*, vol. 112, no. 17, pp. 2660–2667, 2005.

[21] P. Lévy, J.-L. Pépin, C. Arnaud et al., "Intermittent hypoxia and sleep-disordered breathing: current concepts and perspectives," *European Respiratory Journal*, vol. 32, no. 4, pp. 1082–1095, 2008.

[22] L. Lavie and P. Lavie, "Molecular mechanisms of cardiovascular disease in OSAHS: the oxidative stress link," *European Respiratory Journal*, vol. 33, no. 6, pp. 1467–1484, 2009.

The Epidemiology of Pulmonary Nontuberculous Mycobacteria: Data from a General Hospital in Athens, Greece, 2007–2013

Marios Panagiotou,[1] **Andriana I. Papaioannou,**[1]
Konstantinos Kostikas,[2] **Maria Paraskeua,**[1] **Ekaterini Velentza,**[3] **Maria Kanellopoulou,**[3]
Vasiliki Filaditaki,[1] **and Napoleon Karagiannidis**[1]

[1] *2nd Respiratory Medicine Department, Sismanoglio-A. Fleming General Hospital of Attiki, Sismanogliou 1, 15126 Athens, Greece*
[2] *2nd Respiratory Medicine Department, University of Athens Medical School, Attikon Hospital, Smolika 2, 16673 Athens, Greece*
[3] *Department of Biopathology, Sismanoglio-A. Fleming General Hospital of Attiki, Sismanogliou 1, 15126 Athens, Greece*

Correspondence should be addressed to Marios Panagiotou; mariopanag@googlemail.com

Academic Editor: Hisako Matsumoto

Background. The epidemiology of pulmonary nontuberculous mycobacteria (NTM) in Greece is largely unknown. *Objectives.* To determine the incidence and the demographic, microbiological, and clinical characteristics of patients with pulmonary NTM infection and pulmonary NTM disease. *Methods.* A retrospective review of the demographic, microbiological, and clinical characteristics of patients with NTM culture-positive respiratory specimens from January 2007 to May 2013. *Results.* A total of 120 patients were identified with at least one respiratory NTM isolate and 56 patients (46%) fulfilled the microbiological ATS/IDSA criteria for NTM disease. Of patients with adequate data, 16% fulfilled the complete ATS/IDSA criteria for NTM disease. The incidence of pulmonary NTM infection and disease was 18.9 and 8.8 per 100.000 inpatients and outpatients, respectively. The spectrum of NTM species was high (13 species) and predominated by *M. avium-intracellulare* complex (*M. avium* (13%), *M. intracellulare* (10%)), *M. gordonae* (14%), and *M. fortuitum* (12%). The ratio of isolation of NTM to *M. tuberculosis* in all hospitalized patients was 0.59. *Conclusions.* The first data on the epidemiology of pulmonary NTM in Athens, Greece, are presented. NTM infection is common in patients with chronic respiratory disease. However, only a significantly smaller proportion of patients fulfill the criteria for NTM disease.

1. Introduction

Nontuberculous mycobacterial (NTM) species are mycobacterial species other than those classified to the *Mycobacterium tuberculosis* complex (e.g., *M. tuberculosis* (Mtb), *M. bovis*, *M. africanum*, and *M. microti*) and *M. leprae* [1]. Despite being of the same family, NTM differ from those organisms that cause tuberculosis (TB) and leprosy in that they are widely dispersed in our environment, vary greatly in their ability to cause disease, and are not spread from person to person [2]. To date over 160 different species and subspecies of mycobacteria have been included in the List of Prokaryotic Names with Standing in Nomenclature (LPSN; http://www.bacterio.net) but the total number of mycobacterial species is constantly rising due to improved

microbiological techniques for isolating NTM from clinical specimens and, more importantly, due to advances in molecular techniques for defining new species [1]. Accordingly, a spectrum of virulence has been identified ranging from primary pathogens such as *M. kansasii* that can cause disease in presumably healthy individuals and *M. avium* that is associated with preexisting lung disease or defects of cellular immunity to species such as *M. gordonae* that are rarely associated with disease [3].

Traditionally, pulmonary diseases have been reported to account for up to 94% of cases of NTM disease [4] and pulmonary NTM disease commonly occurs in the context of chronic lung disease, such as chronic obstructive pulmonary disease (COPD), bronchiectasis, cystic fibrosis (CF), pneumoconiosis, prior TB, and esophageal motility disorders [1]. Abnormal CF genotypes and α1-antitrypsin phenotypes may predispose some patients to NTM infection [1]. Pulmonary NTM disease also occurs in women without clearly recognized predisposing factors. Bronchiectasis and NTM infection, usually *M. avium-intracellulare* complex (MAC), often coexist, making causality difficult to determine [1]. Worryingly, certain MTN species, including MAC, are associated with high failure treatment rates and increased morbidity and mortality [5]. The prolonged treatment period, drug side effects and interactions, and possibly reinfection rather than relapse have been implicated in the treatment failure [5].

Defining the epidemiology of NTM is challenging for several reasons [6]. First, humans are thought to contract the infection directly from environmental sources. There has been no published report of direct or indirect patient-to-patient respiratory spread of NTM with the sole exception of an outbreak of respiratory *M. abscessus* disease in inpatient population with cystic fibrosis [7]. Second, exposure to the omnipresent MTM is likely extremely common. Third, NTM that colonize the respiratory tract can be isolated in respiratory samples in the absence of disease [1]. Lastly, in most regions of the world, NTM disease is not reportable to public health authorities; therefore, epidemiological and surveillance data are not readily available [6]. It is therefore not surprising that, until recently, there have been virtually no population-based data for America and only limited representative population-based data for Europe available that, as Winthrop et al. [8] eloquently state, firmly document those most basic questions of epidemiology: the "who, what, where, and how much?" [9].

Despite obstacles in the study of the epidemiology of pulmonary NTM, available evidence suggests that the prevalence of pulmonary NTM disease has increased dramatically globally over the past 3 decades [6]. It is also likely that this trend will continue to rise [10] and this is believed to be multifactorial. First, an increasing proportion of the population is aging or subject to some type of immunosuppression, supported by the increase in prevalence of immune-modulating comorbidities like diabetes mellitus and chronic obstructive pulmonary disease (COPD) and in immunosuppressive medication use [11]. Second, NTM are generally free-living organisms and are ubiquitous in the human environment. NTM are present in water, biofilms, soil, and aerosols and, importantly, are natural inhabitants of the piped water supply systems [10, 12, 13]. Thus, it is likely that humans are exposed to NTM on a daily basis [10]. Simultaneously, behavioral changes such as the rising use of swimming pools and hot tub baths may increase the likelihood of exposure to NTM [14]. Third, ongoing advances in methodology in the mycobacteriology laboratory have led to enhanced isolation and more rapid and accurate identification of NTM from clinical specimens [1]. A possible alternative explanation might be the development of cross-immunity between *Mtb* and certain types of NTM. Early studies have produced immunity to *Mtb* in animals by use of *M. kansasii* and MAC [15] and therefore it is felt that there is every reason to believe that this could occur in humans also [16]. If such cross-immunity does exist, the well-known decrease of TB worldwide [17] could have led to a decrease of immunity to NTM [6]. Finally increased awareness on behalf of the physicians might have led to more thorough investigation and follow-up of patients [18].

The aim of this hospital-based study was to determine the incidence of the isolation of NTM and the frequency of various NTM species. We also evaluated the clinical and demographic characteristics of patients with NTM and attempted to identify possible differences between patients colonized with and those who were actually diseased by NTM in terms of comorbidities and use of inhaled corticosteroids.

2. Materials and Methods

2.1. Setting and Data Collection. The study included consecutive adult in- and outpatients assessed at Sismanoglio-A. Fleming General Hospital of Attiki (SGH) from January 2007 through end of May 2013 from whom at least one biological sample was tested culture-positive for NTM. SGH is a 450-bed capacity hospital with a large number of outpatient clinic visits daily and the second largest tertiary referral hospital for patients with respiratory disease in Athens, Greece. SGH has a level II mycobacteriology laboratory with extensive experience in the field also was empowered to conduct limited-scale level III (reference-level) laboratory tasks.

Initial data were gathered from the database of the Department of Biopathology of SGH and included patient identification, species of the isolated NTM, isolation source, and patient demographics as described later. Multiple identical isolates from the same site during the same hospital episode in a single individual were counted as one patient entry. Subsequently, the medical records of these patients were reviewed with the aim of identifying relevant clinical characteristics as described later.

Ethics approval for this study was granted from the Institutional Review Board.

2.2. Specimen Processing. The clinical specimens were decontam-inated using N-acetyl-L-cysteine-sodium hydroxide (NALC) in a Type 2 Biosafety Cabinet. All specimens were then inoculated into solid Löwenstein-Jensen (bioMerieux, Marcy, l' Etoile, France) and into 7H9 Middlebrook Broth Base 0.47% w/v (MGIT, Becton Dickinson, USA) media. Solid medium cultures were incubated in a 37°C incubator for 60 to 70 days and monitored every four days, whereas liquid cultures were incubated in an automated Bactec MGIT-960 (Becton Dickinson, USA) system for 45 days. Cultures exhibiting growth were subjected to light microscopy for the presence of acid-fast bacteria before being considered as positive. All positive cultures were subsequently analyzed by the GenoType Mycobacterium CM (Hain, LifeSciences, Germany) molecular genetic assay for identification of *Mtb* complex and 15 of the most common NTM species. Sporadically throughout the study period, positive cultures were analyzed with both GenoType Mycobacterium CM and GenoType Mycobacterium AS assays for identification of additional 15 less common NTM species. In this paper, NTM species identified neither by GenoType Mycobacterium CM nor by GenoType Mycobacterium AS (when used) assays are referred to as "unidentified NTM".

2.3. Definition of Pulmonary NTM Disease. Patients were considered as having pulmonary NTM disease if they met the clinical, radiological, and microbiological characteristics as defined by the 2007 American Thoracic Society and Infectious Disease Society of America (ATS/IDSA) statement: Diagnosis, Treatment, and Prevention of Nontuberculous Mycobacterial Diseases [1].

2.4. Definition of Pulmonary NTM Infection (Colonization). We defined NTM-infected (colonized) subjects as those who had at least one positive culture for NTM without fulfilling the complete diagnostic criteria and without any record of treatment for NTM disease.

2.5. Patient Characteristics. Demographic variables included age (at specimen's collection date), sex, ethnicity, and country of residence.

Clinical characteristics included the principal working diagnosis at the time of the specimen collection and the underlying medical conditions. The underlying conditions evaluated included chronic lung disease such as COPD, asthma, bronchiectasis, and old TB. Other conditions associated with immunosuppression including diabetes mellitus, HIV infection, autoimmune diseases, malignancy, chronic liver disease, and chronic renal disease were also logged. Finally we recorded the smoking status and long-term use of inhaled corticosteroids (ICS) and systemic corticosteroids (CS) prior to the diagnosis (7.5 mg or more of prednisone or equivalent daily for a period of two weeks or longer).

2.6. Statistical Analysis. Categorical variables are presented as n (%), whereas numerical variables are presented as mean ± SD. Comparisons between groups were performed using chi-square tests for categorical data and unpaired t-tests or Mann-Whitney U tests for normally distributed or skewed numerical data, respectively.

The incidence of pulmonary infection and disease caused by NTM for the duration of our study was calculated as the total number of patients with pulmonary NTM infection and disease divided by the total number of patients who attended SGH, including inpatients and outpatients.

All tests were two-tailed and P values <0.05 were considered statistically significant. Data were analyzed using SPSS 17.0 for Windows (SPSS Inc., Chicago, IL, USA).

3. Results

3.1. Study Population. A total of 132 patient entries with at least one positive culture for NTM from any site per hospital episode were identified. The majority of the identified subjects (95%) were inpatients in the respiratory medicine departments. Eight entries (6%) referred to NTM isolates in gastric fluid, ascitic fluid, urine, and lymph nodes samples and they were excluded from the analysis. Double entries were identified in four patients: two were tested positive twice for the same respiratory NTM species and two were tested positive twice for different respiratory species (all on separate hospital episodes). Therefore, we report on a total of 120 patients who had NTM species isolated from the respiratory

TABLE 1: (a) Study population; demographic characteristics (120 Patients). (b) Study population; clinical Characteristics (74 patients).

(a)

Gender	
Females	76 (63%)
Males	44 (37%)
Total age (years)	69.9 ± 15.4
Age group	
<20 years	0 (0%)
20–40 years	10 (8%)
40–60 years	12 (10%)
>60 years	98 (82%)
Ethnicity	
Greek	110 (92%)
Others (including Middle East, East Europe, and Balkans)	10 (8%)
Residence	
Greece	120 (100%)

(b)

	All	Colonized ($n = 62$)	Diseased ($n = 12$)	P value
Chronic lung disease				
COPD	32 (43%)	26 (42%)	6 (50%)	0.606
Bronchiectasis	25 (33%)	22 (35%)	3 (25%)	0.635
Asthma	5 (6%)	4 (6.4%)	1 (8.3%)	0.892
Cystic fibrosis	1 (1.3%)	1 (1.6%)	0 (0%)	0.683
Old TB	13 (17%)	8 (13%)	5 (41%)	0.030
Use of CS				
Inhaled CS	23 (32%)	20 (32%)	3 (25%)	0.528
Systemic CS	10 (14%)	10 (16%)	0 (0%)	0.140
Smoking habit				
Current or ex-smokers	44 (59%)	37 (59%)	7 (58%)	0.221
Never being smokers	30 (41%)	25 (40%)	5 (42%)	0.223
Others				
HIV	0	0	0	N/A
Autoimmune disease	1 (1.3%)	1 (1.6%)	0 (0%)	0.683

Data are presented as mean ± standard deviation (SD) for numerical variables or as number (%) for categorical variables.
COPD: chronic obstructive pulmonary disease, HIV: human immunodeficiency virus, and CS: corticosteroid.

system and they were included in the microbiological and epidemiological analysis. We were able to retrieve the medical records of 74 (61%) out of 120 patients; thus the analysis on clinical characteristics is relevant to only this subgroup of patients (Figure 1). The demographic and clinical characteristics of the patients are summarized in Table 1.

The study population consisted of 63% men, with a median age of 69.9 years, with the majority being born in

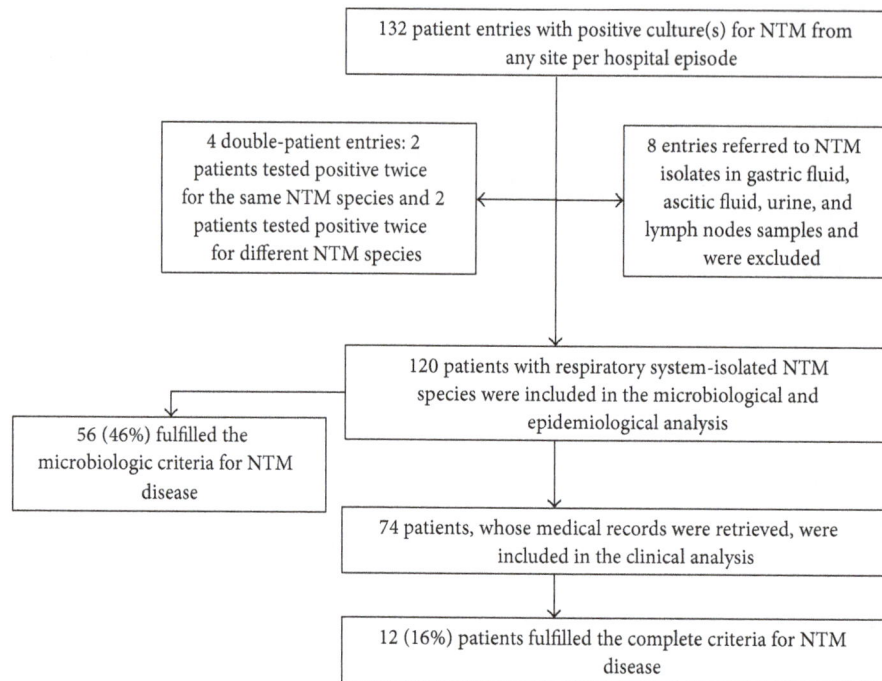

FIGURE 1: Flowchart of the study population.

Greece. The prevalence of NTM isolation increased with age, ranging from 0% in patients younger than 20 years to 82% in patients aged >60 years.

Out of the 74 patients included in the clinical analysis, 66% ($n = 49$) had a diagnosis of a chronic respiratory disease, including COPD (43%, $n = 32$), bronchiectasis (33%, $n = 25$), asthma (6%, $n = 5$), and cystic fibrosis (1%, $n = 1$). Seventeen percent ($n = 13$) of the subjects had a previous TB infection and 16% ($n = 12$) had lung cancer. Thirty-one percent ($n = 23$) were current users of ICS and 13% ($n = 10$) were current systemic CS users. Fifty-eight ($n = 43$) were current or ex-smokers. None of the patients was positive for HIV infection. Sixteen percent ($n = 12$) of patients fulfilled the complete criteria [1] for pulmonary NTM disease; all of them had an underlying chronic lung disease. However, the diagnosis of NTM disease was missed in 25% ($n = 3$) of them. No statistically significant differences were identified between colonized and diseased patients in terms of demographic and clinical characteristics.

3.2. Mycobacteriology Data. One hundred and twenty-two NTM isolates were identified. Only ten percent ($n = 13$) of all respiratory specimens were AFB smear-positive, whereas, by definition, all were culture-positive. The spectrum of NTM species was high (13 species), the most common being the slowly growing *MAC* (*M. avium* ($n = 16, 13\%$), *M. intracellulare* ($n = 12, 10\%$)) and *M. gordonae* ($n = 17, 14\%$) and the rapidly growing *M. fortuitum* ($n = 15, 12\%$). Unidentified NTM species accounted for 30% ($n = 37$) of isolates (Table 2 and Figure 2). The pathogens accounted for the twelve cases of NTM disease including *M. avium* ($n = 3$), *M. intracellulare* ($n = 3$), *M. abscessus* ($n = 1$), *M. gordonae* ($n = 1$), *M. fortuitum* ($n = 1$), *M. xenopi* ($n = 1$), and unidentified NTM

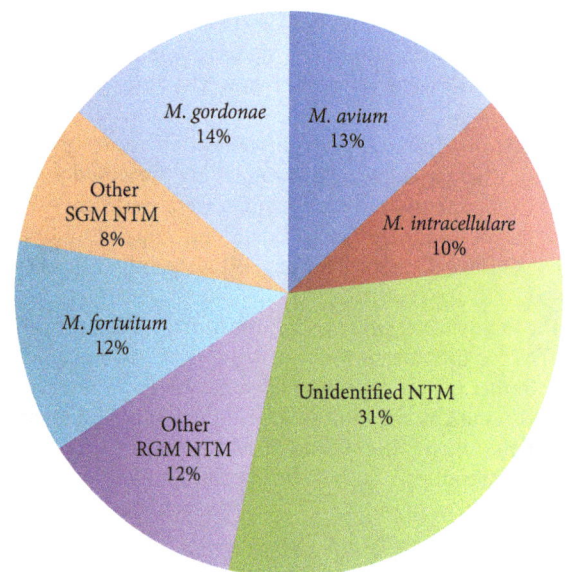

FIGURE 2: Diversity of isolated nontuberculous mycobacteria (NTM). RGM: rapidly growing, SGM: slowly growing.

($n = 2$). Fifty-six patients (46%) fulfilled the microbiological criteria of the ATS/IDSA for NTM disease.

In an attempt to identify the frequency of NTM isolates compared to that of *Mtb* we also extracted the number of isolates for *Mtb*. Within the study period, 225 patients were culture-positive for *Mtb*, rendering a ratio of NTM-to-*Mtb* isolation of 0.59. One patient (1%) was tested positive for *Mtb* and also fulfilled the microbiological criteria of the

TABLE 2: NTM isolates from all sites.

	2007	2008	2009	2010	2011	2012	2013	Total number (% of total)
Rapidly growing NTM								
M. fortuitum	6	2	6	0	1	0	0	15 (12.2)
M. peregrinum	2	1	1	0	2	0	0	6 (4.9)
M. chelonae	2	0	0	0	0	1	0	3 (2.4)
M. abscessus	0	0	0	0	1	0	1	2 (1.6)
M. smegmatis	0	1	0	1	0	0	0	2 (1.6)
M. mucogenicum	0	1	0	0	0	0	0	1 (0.8)
M. fortuitum mageritense	0	0	1	0	0	0	0	1 (0.8)
Slowly growing NTM								
M. gordonae	2	2	0	3	5	2	3	17 (13.9)
M. avium	1	3	2	2	5	3	0	16 (13.1)
M. intracellulare	2	1	2	2	2	3	0	12 (9.8)
M. lentiflavum	1	0	3	1	0	1	0	6 (4.9)
M. xenopi	2	0	1	0	0	0	0	3 (2.4)
M. scrofulaceum	1	0	0	0	0	0	0	1 (0.8)
Unidentified NTM	7	3	9	4	6	6	2	37 (30.3)
Total per year	**26**	**14**	**25**	**13**	**22**	**16**	**6**	**122 (100.0)**

ATS/IDSA for NTM disease. He was put on standard anti-TB treatment.

3.3. Incidence of NTM Pulmonary Infection. During the 65-month study period, 138.951 inpatients and 492.845 outpatients where treated at SGH. Accordingly, the incidence of NTM pulmonary infection and disease for the study period was 18.9/100.000 and 8.8/100.000 patients, respectively.

4. Discussion

During the 65-month period of our study, a total of 120 patients were identified with at least one positive culture for respiratory NTM isolate and 56 patients fulfilled the microbiological criteria of the ATS/IDSA for NTM disease. The predominant NTM species were MAC (*M. avium* (13%), *M. intracellulare* (10%)), *M. gordonae* (14%), and *M. fortuitum* (12%). Of patients with adequate data, 16% fulfilled the complete clinical, radiological, and microbiological criteria of the ATS/IDSA for NTM disease. In approximately 25% of patients the diagnosis of NTM disease was missed. The incidence of pulmonary NTM infection and disease for the study period was 18.9 and 8.8 per 100.000 inpatients and outpatients, respectively.

To our knowledge, this is the first study on the epidemiology of NTM performed in Athens, Greece. Two additional studies on the incidence of NTM in Greece were found in the literature: one conducted in Larissa, central Greece [19], and one in Crete island [20]. Notably, all three are hospital-based studies, which highlights the lack of large-scaled epidemiological studies for NTM in Greece. Finally, data from the Greek National Reference Laboratory for Mycobacterium on NTM isolates in 2008 are reported elsewhere [21]. Also data on environmental sources of NTM in Greece are scarce

although, in line with global evidence [10, 12, 13], unpublished data suggest that the municipal water systems are an important reservoir for infection [22]. Unfortunately, the only other study that has reported on the incidence of pulmonary NTM disease to date was based on different methodology (reporting a 3-year incidence rate of 0.7 per 100 000 *general* population in central Greece for 2000–2003) [19]. The latter, along with the fact that NTM infection is not notifiable in Greece, does not allow any comparisons or conclusions to be drawn regarding trends and/or geographical variations in the epidemiology of pulmonary NTM in Greece.

In our study, 94% percent of the isolates stemmed from respiratory specimens. This is similar to other studies reporting that around 90% of all NTM isolates were of respiratory origin [4, 23, 24]. However, it is well established that isolation of NTM in microbiological samples most commonly represents simple exposure rather than disease. Therefore, laboratory-based studies tracking the incidence of NTM isolation in the population cannot distinguish between diseased and nondiseased persons [9]. However, access to patient clinical and radiographic records is laborious and not always feasible [25], and this represents a major obstacle for large-scale epidemiological studies of NTM disease. Thus, it is of no surprise that only few population-based studies attempted to look into the epidemiology of NTM disease outside the boundaries of the laboratory records. A national-scaled study that attempted to record the clinical significance of pulmonary NTM infections in New Zealand in 2004 by contacting the requesting clinician reported a specific incidence for pulmonary NTM disease of 1.17 per 100,000 population [26]. More recently, a population-based study evaluated the burden of hospitalization associated with pulmonary NTM infections in Germany in 2005–2011. The cases were identified using discharge diagnosis codes. The average annual age-adjusted rate was 0.91 hospitalization per 100,000 population [27]. Another population-based study in British Columbia, Canada from 2000–2006, combined laboratory data and data from the pharmacy department (but not patient records) to estimate the median incidence rates for all-NTM-colonized patients and all-NTM-treated patients being 4.7 and 1.6 per 1000 000 population, respectively [28].

As an alternative method for the epidemiological analysis of the NTM many laboratory-based studies relied upon the microbiological criteria of the ATS/IDSA case definition (validated positive predictive value 85% [8]) in order to estimate disease prevalence. This method assumes that for patients meeting the microbiological criteria, they have coexistent radiographic abnormalities and symptoms compatible with NTM disease. Although the accuracy of this approach is unknown, it is likely to be a reasonable assumption, as most patients undergoing bronchoscopic or sputum evaluation are doing so because of radiographic or symptomatic findings. One such study, which was carried out in all NTM isolates between 1987 and 2000, in the Southwest Region of Ireland reported a mean incidence of disease-causing NTM of as low as 0.4/100 000/years [29]. A population-based study conducted at Oregon, USA, for 2005-2006 reported the estimated annual pulmonary NTM disease prevalence to be 5.6/100,000 statewide but as high as 15.5/100,000 for those over 50 years of age [23]. Subsequently, the same research team undertook a new study to review the clinical records of a significant subset of these patients [8]. That was the first study to determine pulmonary NTM disease prevalence within a population and the first to systematically examine both the clinical and epidemiologic features of pulmonary NTM disease from a general population. They reported an upper limit 2-year prevalence estimate of 11.2/100,000 in the general population, which was—as one might have expected—lower than the prevalence of the microbiologically only defined NTM disease. Notably, the upper limit 2-year prevalence estimate in those at least 50 years old was 25.7/100,000, thus providing further evidence that NTM disease involves older population [8].

In line with aforementioned evidence, we report a higher number of patients who fulfilled the microbiological criteria of the ATS/IDSA for NTM disease compared to those who fulfilled the complete microbiological, radiological, and clinical criteria for NTM disease. Specifically, of patients with adequate data, only 37.5% of those who fulfilled the microbiological criteria of NTM infection also fulfilled the complete criteria for NTM disease. Another single-centered retrospective analysis reported similar proportion of patients (33%) who fulfilled all ATS/IDSA criteria for NTM disease out of the total number of patients with pulmonary NTM isolates [24].

In the present study, no statistically significant trends were observed in the yearly incidence of NTM from 2007 to 2013. However, a unifying finding in all the aforementioned studies was that the prevalence of pulmonary NTM infection and/or disease steadily increased during the study time period [24, 27, 29, 30]. For example, the annual number of all pulmonary NTM infection-associated hospitalization processes in Germany ranged from 665 in 2005 to 1,039 in 2011, with an average annual increase of 4.9% [27]. Also, the isolation prevalence of all MTN species in Ontario, Canada, was 9.1/100 000 in 1997, rising to 14.1/100 000 by 2003 and to 19/100,000 by 2007 (P < 0.0001) with a mean annual increase of about 8.5% [24, 31]. This increasing frequency was regarded as genuine rather than being based on physicians simply ordering more tests because the increase in isolation prevalence had not been accompanied by an increase in negative cultures [18]. In Taiwan, a three-year hospital-based study that retrospectively reviewed patient records reported a statistically significant rising incidence (per 100,000 inpatients and outpatients) of patients with pulmonary NTM disease (1.06 in 2005 and 2.00 in 2008) [32]. In USA, a comparison of skin test surveys revealed that, in 1999-2000, an estimated one in six persons demonstrated *M. intracellulare* sensitization compared to one in nine persons in 1971-1972 [33].

Virtually all studies from industrialized countries (including US, Canada, and Germany) that drew comparisons between the incidence and/or prevalence of pulmonary NTM disease and TB reported significantly higher rates for NTM [8, 24, 28, 34] or at least an increase in the ratio of NTM isolation prevalence to TB case prevalence increased during the study period [3, 24, 27]. However, incidence of TB may still outrange that of pulmonary NTM infection in most European countries [19, 27]. An analysis of data collected annually through the Greek national mandatory notification system for the period 2004–2010 shows that an average of 600 cases of TB are reported each year in Greece [35]. The estimated TB incidence is about 5 cases per 100,000 population, which ranks Greece as a low-burden country. Within our study period, the ratio of isolation of NTM to *Mtb* in all hospitalized patients was 0.59.

The distribution of NTM species worldwide varies by geographic region [21, 36]. MAC, which accounted for 23% of all NTM isolates and 50% of NTM pulmonary disease in our study, is the predominant pathogen in most regions worldwide [13, 21, 37–39]. Specifically, in a modern registry of 20182 patients, from 30 countries across six continents, *M. avium* predominated in North and South America and Europe, while *M. intracellulare* was most frequently isolated in South Africa and Australia [21]. *M. kansasii* is relatively more common in the middle USA, Brazil, England and Wales, Eastern Europe and the metropolitan centres of Paris, London and Tokyo, and the Johannesburg region of South Africa; *M. xenopi* is more common in the northern USA, Ontario-Canada, UK, and some European countries including Hungary, Croatia, and Northern Italy; *M. malmoense* is common in UK and northern Europe but is uncommon in the USA and *M. simiae* is more common in arid regions of the southwestern USA, Cuba, and Israel [21, 30, 36]. Finally, rapidly growing mycobacteria (RGM), accounting for 10–20% of all NTM isolates worldwide in 2008, proved more prevalent in East Asia [21]. Interestingly, RGM made up 25% of all NTM isolates in our study and they were also the prevalent NTM species (46%) in Greece in 2008 [21]. Accordingly, it is possible that regional variations in environmental conditions may favor differences in the predominant NTM populations in the water and soil reservoirs to which susceptible patients are exposed [36]. It should be mentioned that all the identified NTM isolates were considered to be clinically significant in our study. *M. gordonae*, which is usually regarded as a nonpathogenic commensal, was also considered as ample evidence suggesting that it is still capable of causing clinically significant disease in both immunocompetent and immunosuppressed individuals [40, 41].

In terms of gender distribution of pulmonary NTM disease, there has been a gradual shift since early epidemiological data [1, 36]. Although reports from 50 years ago described lung disease most commonly in older smoking male with emphysema, in today's clinics, approximately 80% of patients with NTM disease are middle aged or elderly females with midlung bronchiectasis and other pulmonary abnormalities [36]. In the population-based Oregon, USA, study, females accounted for 60.5% of the pulmonary MAC disease, with a rate of 5.7 cases per 100,000 persons, compared with 3.7 cases per 100,000 persons among males [23]. Also, the New Zealand national-scaled study found the majority (79%) of cases of NTM disease to be females [26]. In recent studies, male sex has been associated with an elevated risk of sensitization (but not isolation) to NTM species [33]. Only one modern study reported moderately increased incidence of (microbiologically only confirmed) NTM disease in males and identified male gender as a risk factor for NTM disease in the Saudi Arabia population [42]. Although the increasing rates of smoking in women may partially account for this shift, it does not explain the also raising frequency of pulmonary NTM in nonsmoker females [36]. Notably, our data showing that NTM-diseased men outnumbered women by far (63% men and 37% women) are not in accordance with this gender shift in the epidemiology of pulmonary NTM. Similarly, the other studies on Greek populations reported that the incidence of pulmonary NTM in men was either higher [19] or equal [20] to that of women. This discordance with the international data is not well understood and it may well be due to the small size of the studies.

In our study, no statistically significant differences were identified between colonized and diseased patients in terms of demographics and other well-documented risk factors for pulmonary NTM disease, including chronic lung disease, nonpulmonary comorbidities, immunosuppression [1], and the use of corticosteroids [43]. This probably reflects the small population size rather than diversion of our population from the worldwide situation. Of interest is also the fact that approximately 30% of diseased patients had no identified coexisting conditions. Similar rates of absence of coexisting conditions among patients with pulmonary NTM disease have been reported in other recent studies [30], which might reflect a shift in the epidemiology of NTM disease in current years.

Finally, we identified a clinically significant minority (25%) of patients who fulfilled the full criteria for pulmonary NTM in whom the diagnosis was missed during their hospital admission. This group of patients did fulfill the complete criteria for NTM disease but, since the microbiological confirmation was not available before their discharge day, they were treated and discharged under the diagnosis of nonspecific lower respiratory tract infection. It is unknown whether

they were tracked at a later stage and put on treatment for NTM disease. Indeed, the microbiology cultures for NTM may take prolonged time (up to several days or weeks) to turn positive. By that time, many patients have been discharged from the hospital and may later not attend their follow-up to system or they may simply be lost in the system. Also, physicians are often reassured by the negativity of fast acid smear in that they will not chase the culture results vigorously and in timely fashion. In our study, culture positivity of the specimens was associated with AFB smear positivity in only 10% of the cases. Consequently, patients may lose their opportunity to be diagnosed with pulmonary NTM disease and receive appropriate treatment. Nevertheless, this finding suggests that NTM disease might be underdiagnosed and thus contributes to the universally reported wide gap in the percentage of the patients with NTM infection and disease.

One study limitation was the fact that only 61% of patient records were retrieved and evaluated. This is of course a universal issue in retrospective record-based studies [8] but it still decreased our study power. Additionally, the population seen in our hospital is not representative of the wider population. Our hospital is considered one of the major respiratory hospitals in Athens; therefore, our patient sample is predominated by those with respiratory disease who, in turn, are more likely to harbor a NTM infection and/or disease. Additionally, our study design allowed for the estimation of the incidence of the *hospital* rather than the *general* population of pulmonary NTM. The latter was not feasible due to this being a single-center study and also because the catchment area of our center extends well beyond the city of Athens, thus serving a wider and difficult-to-estimate population from Greek islands and mainland Greece. Finally, the high incidence of unidentified NTM species in our study may be due to the use of a single molecular genotyping assay (GenoType Mycobacterium CM) that allows the identification of 15 of the most common NTM species. GenoType Mycobacterium AS assay, which allows the identification of 15 additional (although less common) NTM species, was employed only sporadically throughout the study period and also in-house diagnostic assays for NTM were not available. Undoubtedly, the use of more powerful assays would have increased the diversity of NTM isolates.

5. Conclusions

The first data on the epidemiology of NTM in Athens, the capital city of Greece, are presented from the database of a tertiary referral hospital for patients with respiratory disease. From 2007 to 2013, 120 respiratory isolates were identified mostly from patients with chronic respiratory disease. However, only a smaller proportion of patients fulfill the criteria for disease. It is not clear whether the latter truly reflects a low penetration of the disease or underdiagnosis and/or methodological issues. In this study, the diagnosis of pulmonary NTM disease was missed in a clinically significant minority of patients. Increased awareness on behalf of the physicians is required regarding the significant morbidity and mortality of the untreated NTM disease. Moreover full application of the validated clinical, radiological, and microbiological guidelines is imperative in order to correctly identify the cases of NTM disease. This study aspires to increase physicians' insight into the challenges in the management of patients with potential NTM disease and stimulate further and larger-scale research for better determination of the epidemiology of NTM in Greece and worldwide.

Conflict of Interests

The authors declare that there is no conflict of interests regarding the publication of this paper.

References

[1] D. E. Griffith, T. Aksamit, B. A. Brown-Elliott et al., "An official ATS/IDSA statement: diagnosis, treatment, and prevention of nontuberculous mycobacterial diseases," *The American Journal of Respiratory and Critical Care Medicine*, vol. 175, no. 4, pp. 367–416, 2007.

[2] D. Schraufnagel, "Nontuberculous (environmental) mycobacterial disease," in *Breathing in America: Diseases, Progress, and Hope*, The American Thoracic Society, 2010.

[3] S. M. Arend, D. van Soolingen, and T. H. Ottenhoff, "Diagnosis and treatment of lung infection with nontuberculous mycobacteria," *Current Opinion in Pulmonary Medicine*, vol. 15, no. 3, pp. 201–208, 2009.

[4] R. J. O'Brien, L. J. Geiter, and D. E. Snider Jr., "The epidemiology of nontuberculous mycobacterium diseases in the United States: results from a national survey," *The American Review of Respiratory Disease*, vol. 135, no. 5, pp. 1007–1014, 1987.

[5] S. K. Field, D. Fisher, and R. L. Cowie, "Mycobacterium avium complex pulmonary disease in patient without HIV infection," *Chest*, vol. 126, no. 2, pp. 566–581, 2004.

[6] B. A. Kendall and K. L. Winthrop, "Update on the epidemiology of pulmonary nontuberculous mycobacterial infections," *Seminars in Respiratory and Critical Care Medicine*, vol. 34, no. 1, pp. 87–94, 2013.

[7] M. L. Aitken, A. Limaye, P. Pottinger et al., "Respiratory outbreak of Mycobacterium abscessus subspecies massiliense in a lung transplant and cystic fibrosis center," *The American Journal of Respiratory and Critical Care Medicine*, vol. 185, no. 2, pp. 231–232, 2012.

[8] K. L. Winthrop, E. McNelley, B. Kendall et al., "Pulmonary nontuberculous mycobacterial disease prevalence and clinical features: an emerging public health disease," *The American Journal of Respiratory and Critical Care Medicine*, vol. 182, no. 7, pp. 977–982, 2010.

[9] K. L. Winthrop, "Pulmonary disease due to nontuberculous mycobacteria: an epidemiologists view," *Future Microbiology*, vol. 5, no. 3, pp. 343–345, 2010.

[10] J. O. Falkinham III, "Nontuberculous mycobacteria in the environment," *Clinics in Chest Medicine*, vol. 23, no. 3, pp. 529–551, 2002.

[11] K. L. Winthrop, E. Chang, S. Yamashita, M. F. Iademarco, and P. A. LoBue, "Nontuberculous mycobacteria infections and antitumor necrosis factor-α therapy," *Emerging Infectious Diseases*, vol. 15, no. 10, pp. 1556–1561, 2009.

[12] C. F. von Reyn, R. D. Waddell, T. Eaton et al., "Isolation of Mycobacterium avium complex from water in the United States, Finland, Zaire, and Kenya," *Journal of Clinical Microbiology*, vol. 31, no. 12, pp. 3227–3230, 1993.

[13] P. C. A. M. Buijtels, M. A. B. van der Sande, C. S. de Graaff et al., "Nontuberculous mycobacteria, Zambia," *Emerging Infectious Diseases*, vol. 15, no. 2, pp. 242–249, 2009.

[14] H. Fjällbrant, M. Akerstrom, E. Svensson, and E. Andersson, "Hot tub lung: an occupational hazard," *European Respiratory Review*, vol. 22, no. 127, pp. 88–90, 2013.

[15] C. H. Ahn, J. R. Lowell, G. D. Onstad, E. H. Shuford, and G. A. Hurst, "A demographic study of disease due to Mycobacterium kansasii or M intracellulare-avium in Texas," *Chest*, vol. 75, no. 2, pp. 120–125, 1979.

[16] G. P. Youmans, "The pathogenic "atypical" mycobacteria," *Annual Review of Microbiology*, vol. 17, pp. 473–494, 1963.

[17] "Global tuberculosis report," 2013, http://apps.who.int/iris/bitstream/10665/91355/1/9789241564656_eng.pdf.

[18] N. R. Anthonisen, "Nontuberculous mycobacteria," *Canadian Respiratory Journal*, vol. 18, no. 1, pp. 9–10, 2011.

[19] I. Gerogianni, M. Papala, K. Kostikas, E. Petinaki, and K. I. Gourgoulianis, "Epidemiology and clinical significance of mycobacterial respiratory infections in Central Greece," *International Journal of Tuberculosis and Lung Disease*, vol. 12, no. 7, pp. 807–812, 2008.

[20] Z. Gitti, E. Mantadakis, S. Maraki, and G. Samonis, "Clinical significance and antibiotic susceptibilities of nontuberculous mycobacteria from patients in Crete, Greece," *Future Microbiology*, vol. 6, no. 9, pp. 1099–1109, 2011.

[21] W. Hoefsloot, J. van Ingen, C. Andrejak et al., "The geographic diversity of nontuberculous mycobacteria isolated from pulmonary samples: an NTM-NET collaborative study," *The European Respiratory Journal*, vol. 42, no. 6, pp. 1604–1613, 2013.

[22] K. Girzi, A. Skouroglou, and B. Krikelis, "Detection of atypical mycobacteria in water supply in hospital wards, schools, nurseries-kindergartens and swimming pools," *Public Health and Environment*. In press.

[23] P. M. Cassidy, K. Hedberg, A. Saulson, E. Mcnelly, and K. L. Winthrop, "Nontuberculous mycobacterial disease prevalence and risk factors: a changing epidemiology," *Clinical Infectious Diseases*, vol. 49, no. 12, pp. e124–e129, 2009.

[24] T. K. Marras, P. Chedore, A. M. Ying, and F. Jamieson, "Isolation prevalence of pulmonary non-tuberculous mycobacteria in Ontario, 1997–2003," *Thorax*, vol. 62, no. 8, pp. 661–666, 2007.

[25] C. Andréjak, V. Ø. Thomsen, I. S. Johansen et al., "Nontuberculous pulmonary mycobacteriosis in Denmark: incidence and prognostic factors," *The American Journal of Respiratory and Critical Care Medicine*, vol. 181, no. 5, pp. 514–521, 2010.

[26] J. Freeman, A. J. Morris, T. Blackmore, D. Hammer, S. Munroe, and L. Mcknight, "Incidence of nontuberculous mycobacterial disease in New Zealand, 2004," *New Zealand Medical Journal*, vol. 120, no. 1256, Article ID U2580, 2007.

[27] F. C. Ringshausen, R.-M. Apel, F.-C. Bange et al., "Burden and trends of hospitalisations associated with pulmonary non-tuberculous mycobacterial infections in Germany, 2005–2011," *BMC Infectious Diseases*, vol. 13, no. 1, article 231, 2013.

[28] E. Hernández-Garduño, M. Rodrigues, and R. K. Elwood, "The incidence of pulmonary non-tuberculous mycobacteria in British Columbia, Canada," *International Journal of Tuberculosis and Lung Disease*, vol. 13, no. 9, pp. 1086–1093, 2009.

[29] M. P. Kennedy, T. M. O'Connor, C. Ryan, S. Sheehan, B. Cryan, and C. Bredin, "Nontuberculous mycobacteria: incidence in Southwest Ireland from 1987 to 2000," *Respiratory Medicine*, vol. 97, no. 3, pp. 257–263, 2003.

[30] K. G. de Mello, F. C. Mello, L. Borga et al., "Clinical and therapeutic features of pulmonary nontuberculous mycobacterial disease, Brazil, 1993–2011," *Emerging Infectious Diseases*, vol. 19, no. 3, pp. 393–399, 2013.

[31] M. Al Houqani, F. Jamieson, P. Chedore, M. Mehta, K. May, and T. K. Marras, "Isolation prevalence of pulmonary nontuberculous mycobacteria in Ontario in 2007," *Canadian Respiratory Journal*, vol. 18, no. 1, pp. 19–24, 2011.

[32] C.-Y. Chen, H.-Y. Chen, C.-H. Chou, C.-T. Huang, C.-C. Lai, and P.-R. Hsueh, "Pulmonary infection caused by nontuberculous mycobacteria in a medical center in Taiwan, 2005–2008," *Diagnostic Microbiology and Infectious Disease*, vol. 72, no. 1, pp. 47–51, 2012.

[33] K. Khan, J. Wang, and T. K. Marras, "Nontuberculous mycobacterial sensitization in the United States: national trends over three decades," *The American Journal of Respiratory and Critical Care Medicine*, vol. 176, no. 3, pp. 306–313, 2007.

[34] D. R. Prevots, P. A. Shaw, D. Strickland et al., "Nontuberculous mycobacterial lung disease prevalence at four integrated health care delivery systems," *The American Journal of Respiratory and Critical Care Medicine*, vol. 182, no. 7, pp. 970–976, 2010.

[35] "Epidemiological data on tuberculosis in Greece, 2004–2010," http://www2.keelpno.gr/blog/?p=736&lang=en.

[36] J. L. Cook, "Nontuberculous mycobacteria: opportunistic environmental pathogens for predisposed hosts," *The British Medical Bulletin*, vol. 96, no. 1, pp. 45–59, 2010.

[37] E. Hernández-Garduño and R. K. Elwood, "Demographic risk factors of pulmonary colonization by non-tuberculous mycobacteria," *International Journal of Tuberculosis and Lung Disease*, vol. 14, no. 1, pp. 106–112, 2010.

[38] H. D. S. P. Pedro, M. I. F. Pereira, M. D. R. A. Goloni, S. Y. M. Ueki, and E. Chimara, "Nontuberculous mycobacteria isolated in São José do Rio Preto, Brazil between 1996 and 2005," *Jornal Brasileiro de Pneumologia*, vol. 34, no. 11, pp. 950–955, 2008.

[39] S. W. Ryoo, S. Shin, M.-S. Shim et al., "Spread of nontuberculous mycobacteria from 1993 to 2006 in Koreans," *Journal of Clinical Laboratory Analysis*, vol. 22, no. 6, pp. 415–420, 2008.

[40] A. Asija, A. Prasad, and E. Eskridge, "Disseminated mycobacterium gordonae infection in an immunocompetent host," *The American Journal of Therapeutics*, vol. 18, no. 3, pp. e75–e77, 2011.

[41] S. A. Mazumder, A. Hicks, and J. Norwood, "Mycobacterium gordonae pulmonary infection in an immunocompetent adult," *North American Journal of Medical Sciences*, vol. 2, no. 4, pp. 205–207, 2010.

[42] B. Varghese, Z. Memish, N. Abuljadayel, R. Al-Hakeem, F. Alrabiah, and S. A. Al-Hajoj, "Emergence of clinically relevant non-tuberculous mycobacterial infections in Saudi Arabia," *PLoS Neglected Tropical Diseases*, vol. 7, no. 5, Article ID e2234, 2013.

[43] C. Andréjak, R. Nielsen, V. Ø. Thomsen, P. Duhaut, H. T. Sørensen, and R. W. Thomsen, "Chronic respiratory disease, inhaled corticosteroids and risk of non-tuberculous mycobacteriosis," *Thorax*, vol. 68, no. 3, pp. 256–262, 2013.

30

The Interpretation of Dyspnea in the Patient with Asthma

Marc H. Lavietes

New Jersey Medical School, 100 Bergen Street, No. 1354, Rutgers, Newark, NJ 07103, USA

Correspondence should be addressed to Marc H. Lavietes; lavietmh@njms.rutgers.edu

Academic Editor: Andrew Sandford

Physicians have noted dyspnea in severely ill asthmatic patients to be associated with fright or panic; in more stable patients dyspnea may reflect characteristics including lung function, personality and behavioral traits. This study evaluates the symptom of dyspnea in 32 asthmatic patients twice: first when acutely ill and again after an initial response to therapy. Spirometry was performed, dyspnea quantified (Borg scale), and panic assessed with a specialized measure of acute panic (the acute panic inventory (API)) in the 32 patients before and again after treatment. After treatment, questionnaires to evaluate somatization and panic disorder were also administered. When acutely ill, both the API and all spirometric measures (PEFR; FEV1; IC) correlated with dyspnea. Multiple linear regression showed that measures of the API, the peak expiratory flow rate, and female sex taken together accounted for 41% of dyspnea in acute asthma. After treatment, the API again predicted dyspnea while spirometric data did not. Those subjects who described themselves as having chronic panic disorder reported high grades of dyspnea after treatment also. We conclude that interpretations of the self-report of asthma differ between acutely ill and stable asthmatic patients.

1. Introduction

Dyspnea is a cardinal symptom of asthma. The notion that fear or panic may contribute to the sensation of dyspnea accompanying acute bronchospasm has been recognized by clinicians and is discussed in the psychiatric literature [1]. Similarly, physicians caring for outpatient asthmatics have long recognized that both personality traits and psychological state as well as pulmonary dysfunction may influence the self-report of dyspnea in stable patients [2–4]. This study examines the following hypothesis: the genesis of dyspnea experienced by acutely ill asthmatic patients and that of stable asthmatic patients may differ.

2. Materials and Methods

We studied 32 English-speaking acutely ill asthmatic patients twice: once immediately upon their arrival in the emergency room and again after stabilization. Subjects older than 50 years or younger than 18 were excluded as were pregnant women and those with coexisting chronic heart or lung disease.

Spirometry was first performed upon arrival at the emergency service before administration of any therapy. We used a pneumotachograph affixed to a portable computer (Respitech, Lancaster, Pa). The procedure was repeated (as many as six times) until reproducible expiratory flow and inspiratory capacity measures were obtained. Acceptable forced vital capacity measurements could not be obtained from many subjects with severe airway obstruction and are thus not reported. Dyspnea was assessed with the modified Borg scale [5]. Patients were specifically asked to rank "how much discomfort do you feel with your breathing" on the zero through ten scale. Finally the 17-item acute panic inventory (API), a concise validated screening tool for panic, was administered [6]. Item number five of this inventory focuses specifically upon dyspnea and was thus omitted from the inventory as used in this study [6, 7].

When stable (as promptly as within 2 hours of presentation in some cases but many days later in others) patients reviewed and signed a consent form. Both the protocol in its entirety and the form were approved by our Institutional Review Board. This form encompassed both the initial and follow-up studies. In addition to repeating the three tests performed in the emergency room, subjects completed two additional questionnaires: one: the Barsky somatosensory amplification scale (SSAS), a test of somatization [8]; two: the Spitzer binary assessment (SPTZ) (Y/N) for a clinical diagnosis of panic disorder [9].

We computed from the spirometry tracing peak expiratory flow rate (PEFR), forced expiratory volume in one second (FEV1), and inspiratory capacity (IC). Data with normal distributions are presented as means and standard deviations. Data with skewed distributions are presented as three values: medians and both upper and lower extremes. Bivariate regression analysis was performed with a nonparametric method. Multiple linear regression was then used to evaluate predictors of the Borg scale jointly. We used stepwise, forward, backward, and Mallows' Cp selection methods to construct a parsimonious model. All methods yielded the same model. Since age and BMI were considered potential confounders and had not been selected via the model selection procedure, they were added to the final model. Categorical variables were compared with a one-way analysis of variance. Finally data obtained upon entrance to the study were compared with data obtained at follow-up by paired t-test. The SAS 9.3 statistical package was used. All testing was two-sided at the 0.05 significance level.

3. Results and Discussion

We studied 18 M and 14 F subjects. Their mean (SD) age was 38 ± 7; their weight (BMI) was $30 \pm 9 \, \text{kg/m}^2$. Their median initial Borg score was 5.0 (0.5; 8.0). Initial lung function data showing severe airway obstruction appear in Table 1. Lung functions and their correlations with dyspnea during acute illness appear in Table 1 also. Measures of all lung functions as well as panic (API) correlated closely with acute dyspnea. Note that only 6 of the 32 subjects responded "yes" regarding a positive clinical history of panic attacks. Borg scale scores for "yes" and "no" responders were similar. The best fit multiple linear regression model appears in Table 2. Spearman's r for this model was 0.64. Measures of PEFR and API taken together with the categorical variable sex accounted for 41% of the variability within the Borg scale response. While sex was not predictive of dyspnea in the bivariate analysis, it was in the multivariable analysis with women having higher Borg scores than men.

The median Borg score after treatment was 1 (0, 7). The differences between pre- and postvalues for the API and all lung functions (Tables 1 and 3) were significant at the $p < 0.001$ level. Correlations of dyspnea measured after treatment with independent variables appear in Table 3. Lung function and dyspnea did not correlate. Both the API and the binary assessment for the clinical diagnosis of panic correlated with dyspnea in the stable subjects. By contrast, correlation between dyspnea and either the SSAS or the BMI did not reach statistical significance. Only the API however correlated with dyspnea when all variables were entered into the multiple linear regression model.

Dyspnea in acute asthma reflects both uncoupling of inspiratory effort from inspiratory flow (airway narrowing) and hyperinflation. Both uncoupling and hyperinflation are

Table 1: Bivariate analysis using Spearman correlation to measure association of dyspnea (dependent variable) with lung function and psychometric data obtained in the emergency department (independent variables) obtained simultaneously.

Independent variable	Mean (+SD)	Spearman r	p
FEV1, % predicted	41 + 22	−0.47	0.006
IC, % predicted	57 + 27	−0.37	0.036
PEFR, % predicted	38 + 23	−0.45	0.009
API	9 (1, 32)	0.55	0.001
SPTZ		0.16	0.370

API = acute panic inventory; FEV1 = forced expiratory volume, one second; PEFR = peak expiratory flow rate; IC = inspiratory capacity; SPTZ = Spitzer binary assessment, administered after treatment only. Group data for API scores are expressed as median (maximum, minimum). For all other variables, group data are expressed as mean + SD.

Table 2: Multiple linear regression model to predict correlation with the Borg scale score.

Characteristic	Parameter estimate	95% CI	p
Intercept	5.45	(2.24, 8.67)	
Sex (M/F)	1.88	(0.59, 3.17)	0.01
Age	−0.03	(−0.09, 0.02)	0.24
BMI (kg/m^2)	0.01	(−0.05, 0.07)	0.75
PEFR, % predicted	−0.05	(−0.08, −0.03)	<0.001
API	0.11	(0.06, 0.16)	<0.001

For definition of abbreviations, see Table 1.

Table 3: Bivariate analysis, data obtained after treatment, when stable.

Independent variable	Mean (+SD)	Spearman r	p
FEV1, % predicted	65 + 24	0.11	0.561
IC, % predicted	87 + 22	0.04	0.821
PEFR, % predicted	58 + 25	−0.01	0.979
API	2 (0, 21)	0.59	0.004
SPTZ	6 Y/26 N	0.53	0.002

For definition of abbreviations, see Table 1.

promptly relieved by treatment. Subsequently in stable subjects, lung function is no longer a major determinant of dyspnea.

Anxiety, as measured by the API, is a major determinant of dyspnea in the acutely ill subject. As such it is likely to be a component of acute panic. The API is a simple, brief screening tool designed to evaluate anxiety in severely ill, unstable subjects. To this end, some of our patients when acutely ill resembled panic disorder patients. Many reported difficulty working, speaking, and concentrating. Some described sweatiness and shaking. Two reported extreme symptoms such as the need to urinate or defecate. It is likely that an occasional patient presents with both severe bronchoconstriction and panic, too agitated to participate in a study. We did not encounter such a patient. The fact that only 6 subjects responded "yes" regarding a positive clinical history of panic and that this "yes" response was not linked to high Borg scores in the emergency setting suggests that panic disorder per se is not common in these patients and plays no role in their dyspnea during acute illness.

The API as a measure of anxiety remained a strong predictor of dyspnea after treatment. In addition, panic disorder as assessed by the SPTZ questionnaire correlated with dyspnea when dyspnea was measured after treatment. The observation that the SPTZ correlates with dyspnea in the treated but not the acutely ill asthmatic patient is of interest. The SPTZ is not a definitive diagnostic tool. It is a self-assessment screening tool that identifies patients who believe they qualify for the diagnosis of panic. In the context of this study, the SPTZ identifies patients who see themselves as being emotionally labile and, as such, would be likely to exaggerate unpleasant sensations such as dyspnea. Taken together, these data support two notions: one: the panic experienced in acute asthma does not necessarily reflect a generalized panic disorder; two: the mechanisms producing dyspnea in acute versus stable asthma differ.

Note that preexisting psychological conditions may predispose to asthma or perpetuate the condition. This study does not address preexisting psychological conditions but supports the notion that only panic and airway obstruction account for the dyspnea reported during an acute, untreated asthma attack. By contrast, other psychological factors, not examined here, may be more important in determining the degree of dyspnea in the stabilized asthmatic patient [10–12]. Lastly sex differences in exertional dyspnea, noted previously, are explained by differences in respiratory reserve between men and women [13].

3.1. Limitations of This Study. This study population is limited to inner city patients. The absence of suburban and rural subjects or subjects with varied socioeconomic and ethnic backgrounds is a major limitation to a generalized interpretation of the results. Both cultural differences in the perception of symptoms and varied accessibility to health care between persons of differing socioeconomic backgrounds are well known [14, 15]. Lastly a measure of airway inflammation, known to modify dyspnea perception in asthma but not obtained here, could have enhanced the prediction of dyspnea in our subjects [16].

4. Conclusion

We conclude that the self-report of dyspnea and spirometry obtained simultaneously provide complementary information for the routine assessment of stable asthmatic patients.

Disclosure

The author is responsible for the content and writing of the paper.

Conflict of Interests

The author reports no conflict of interests.

Acknowledgments

The author thanks Dr. Soyeon Kim for her assistance with the statistical analysis and Dr. Norma MT Braun and Dr. Monroe Karetzky for critical review of the final paper. Dr. Neil Cherniack played an integral role in the development of this project but passed away before its completion.

References

[1] R. Ley, "Dyspneic—fear and catastrophic cognitions in hyperventilatory panic attacks," *Behaviour Research and Therapy*, vol. 27, no. 5, pp. 549–554, 1989.

[2] M. H. Lavietes, J. Matta, L. A. Tiersky, B. H. Natelson, L. Bielory, and N. S. Cherniack, "The perception of dyspnea in patients with mild asthma," *Chest*, vol. 120, no. 2, pp. 409–415, 2001.

[3] M. H. Lavietes, J. Ameh, and N. S. Cherniack, "Dyspnea and symptom amplification in asthma," *Respiration*, vol. 75, no. 2, pp. 158–162, 2008.

[4] A. Chetta, G. Gerra, A. Foresi et al., "Personality profiles and breathlessness perception in outpatients with different gradings of asthma," *American Journal of Respiratory and Critical Care Medicine*, vol. 157, no. 1, pp. 116–122, 1998.

[5] T. D. Bradley, D. A. Chartrand, J. W. Fitting, K. J. Killian, and A. Grassino, "The relation of inspiratory effort sensation to fatiguing patterns of the diaphragm," *American Review of Respiratory Disease*, vol. 134, no. 6, pp. 1119–1124, 1986.

[6] M. Sajatovic and L. F. Ramirez, *Rating Scales in Mental Health*, Lexi-Comp, Hudson, Ohio, USA, 2001.

[7] D. J. Dillon, J. M. Gorman, M. R. Liebowitz, A. J. Fyer, and D. F. Klein, "Measurement of lactate-induced panic and anxiety," *Psychiatry Research*, vol. 20, no. 2, pp. 97–105, 1987.

[8] A. J. Barsky, G. Wyshak, and G. L. Klerman, "The somatosensory amplification scale and its relationship to hypochondriasis," *Journal of Psychiatric Research*, vol. 24, no. 4, pp. 323–334, 1990.

[9] R. L. Spitzer, K. Kroenke, and J. B. W. Williams, "Validation and utility of a self-report version of PRIME-MD: the PHQ Primary Care study," *The Journal of the American Medical Association*, vol. 282, no. 18, pp. 1737–1744, 1999.

[10] J. W. Smoller, M. H. Pollack, M. W. Otto, J. F. Rosenbaum, and R. L. Kradin, "Panic anxiety, dyspnea, and respiratory disease. Theoretical and clinical considerations," *American Journal of Respiratory and Critical Care Medicine*, vol. 154, no. 1, pp. 6–17, 1996.

[11] W. M. Brunner, P. J. Schreiner, A. Sood, and D. R. Jacobs, "Depression and risk of incident asthma in adults: the CARDIA study," *American Journal of Respiratory and Critical Care Medicine*, vol. 189, no. 9, pp. 1044–1051, 2014.

[12] F. Di Marco, P. Santus, and S. Centanni, "Anxiety and depression in asthma," *Current Opinion in Pulmonary Medicine*, vol. 17, no. 1, pp. 39–44, 2011.

[13] J. A. Guenette, D. Jensen, K. A. Webb, D. Ofir, N. Raghavan, and D. E. O'Donnell, "Sex differences in exertional dyspnea in patients with mild COPD: physiological mechanisms," *Respiratory Physiology and Neurobiology*, vol. 177, no. 3, pp. 218–227, 2011.

[14] G. K. Fritz, E. L. McQuaid, S. J. Kopel et al., "Ethnic differences in perception of lung function: a factor in pediatric asthma disparities?" *American Journal of Respiratory and Critical Care Medicine*, vol. 182, no. 1, pp. 12–18, 2010.

[15] R. T. Cohen, J. C. Celedón, V. J. Hinckson et al., "Health-care use among Puerto Rican and African American children with asthma," *Chest*, vol. 130, no. 2, pp. 463–471, 2006.

[16] M. P. Foschino Barbaro, D. Lacedonia, G. P. Palladino et al., "Dyspnea perception in asthma: role of airways inflammation, age and emotional status," *Respiratory Medicine*, vol. 105, no. 2, pp. 195–203, 2011.

31

Accuracy of the Hospital Anxiety and Depression Scale for Identifying Depression in Chronic Obstructive Pulmonary Disease Patients

Christoph Nowak,[1,2] Noriane A. Sievi,[1] Christian F. Clarenbach,[1] Esther Irene Schwarz,[1] Christian Schlatzer,[1] Thomas Brack,[3] Martin Brutsche,[4] Martin Frey,[5] Sarosh Irani,[6] Jörg D. Leuppi,[7] Jochen Rüdiger,[4] Robert Thurnheer,[8] and Malcolm Kohler[1]

[1]Division of Pulmonology, University Hospital of Zurich, 8091 Zurich, Switzerland
[2]Medical Sciences Department, Uppsala University, 75237 Uppsala, Sweden
[3]Division of Pulmonology, Cantonal Hospital of Glarus, 8750 Glarus, Switzerland
[4]Division of Pulmonology, Cantonal Hospital of St. Gallen, 9007 St. Gallen, Switzerland
[5]Division of Pulmonology, Clinical Barmelweid, 5017 Barmelweid, Switzerland
[6]Division of Pulmonology, Cantonal Hospital of Aarau, 5000 Aarau, Switzerland
[7]University Clinic of Internal Medicine, Cantonal Hospital Baselland and University of Basel, 4031 Basel, Switzerland
[8]Division of Pulmonology, Cantonal Hospital of Münsterlingen, 8596 Münsterlingen, Switzerland

Correspondence should be addressed to Christoph Nowak; nowakchr@googlemail.com

Academic Editor: Denis Caillaud

Psychological morbidity is common in chronic respiratory diseases. The diagnostic accuracy of the Hospital Anxiety and Depression Scale (HADS) and risk factors for comorbid depression in chronic obstructive pulmonary disease (COPD) are addressed. Consecutive COPD patients (GOLD stage I–IV, 40–75 years old) were enrolled in a multicentre, cross-sectional cohort study. Diagnosis of depression was ascertained through clinical records. Lung function, HADS score, 6-minute walking test (6-MWT), MRC dyspnoea score, and COPD Assessment Test (CAT) were evaluated. Two hundred fifty-nine COPD patients (mean age 62.5 years; 32% female; mean FEV1 48% predicted) were included. Patients diagnosed with depression (29/259; 11.2%) had significantly higher HADS-D and HADS-Total scores than nondepressed patients (median (quartiles) HADS-D 6 [4; 9] versus 4 [2; 7], median HADS-Total 14 [10; 20] versus 8 [5; 14]). Receiver-operating characteristic plots showed moderate accuracy for HADS-D, AUC 0.662 (95%CI 0.601–0.719), and HADS-Total, AUC 0.681 (95%CI 0.620–0.737), with optimal cut-off scores of >5 and >9, respectively. Sensitivity and specificity were 62.1% and 62.6% for HADS-D compared to 75.9% and 55.2% for HADS-Total. Age, comorbidities, sex, and lower airflow limitation predicted depression. The HADS exhibits low diagnostic accuracy for depression in COPD patients. Younger men with comorbidities are at increased risk for depression.

1. Introduction

Depression is a common comorbidity in chronic obstructive pulmonary disease (COPD) patients [1]. Impaired lung function is a risk factor for depression with up to 4 in 10 respiratory patients affected [2]. Mood and anxiety disorders in patients with COPD are likely underdiagnosed [3], emphasising the need for a reliable and accurate instrument in the recognition of depression. The Hospital Anxiety and Depression Scale (HADS [4]) was originally designed by Zigmond and Snaith in 1983 as a short, easy-to-use, 14-item screening tool for depression and anxiety symptoms in the hospital outpatient setting [5]. It is composed of two 7-item subscales (HADS-D and HADS-A for depression and anxiety, resp.) both ranging from 0 to 21 with higher scores indicating more severe distress. Items enquire about symptoms over the preceding week and are self- or clinician-rated on a 4-point Likert scale. The developers suggested categorising subjects according to subscale score into noncases (0 to 7), possible cases (8 to 10), and probable cases (>10) of clinical depression [4].

A 1997 review found both subscales to be reliable and valid measures for assessing anxiety and depression symptoms in medical patients in European, American, and Asian cohorts [6]. An updated analysis in 2002 found similar results in general medical, psychosomatic, and psychiatric patients with an optimal cut-off score of ≥8 for both subscales to define patients with probable diagnosis of depression or anxiety [7]. However, classifying patients as either depressed/anxious or not according to HADS threshold scores is controversial, especially so in chronic disease. A range of cut-offs has been used, for example, HADS-D >4 in coronary heart disease [8], HADS-D >7 in cancer [9], and HADS-D >11 in end-stage renal disease [10]. Its original purpose as a screening tool notwithstanding, in these studies, categorisation according to HADS scores is often implicitly used to diagnose depression.

The HADS has frequently been used in patients with COPD, among other reasons to assess psychological health status [11], quality of life [12], and effectiveness of pulmonary rehabilitation [13]. In spite of its widespread use, the HADS' diagnostic accuracy in COPD patients has only been examined in a small sample for anxiety [14]: in 55 COPD patients, of whom 14 were clinically diagnosed with an anxiety disorder, the optimal HADS-A cut-off score of ≥4 achieved moderate diagnostic power. However, no validation of the HADS for diagnosing depression in COPD patients has yet been attempted although the aforementioned results indicate that optimal cut-off scores for chronic disease patients are likely to differ from those originally suggested for the general patient population.

The aim of the current cross-sectional study was to validate the use of the HADS in screening patients with COPD for the presence of clinically diagnosed depression. We furthermore explored the role of patient and disease-specific predictors for depression. Data were extracted from the baseline assessment of an ongoing longitudinal COPD cohort study in Switzerland.

2. Patients and Methods

2.1. Study Subjects. Inclusion criteria were an objective diagnosis of COPD according to GOLD guidelines [15] and age between 40 and 75 years. Exclusion criteria were mental or physical disability precluding informed consent or protocol compliance, as well as acute or recent (within the preceding six weeks) exacerbation of COPD.

2.2. Study Design. The Obstructive Pulmonary Disease Outcomes Cohort of Switzerland (TOP DOCS) is an ongoing prospective observational cohort study coordinated by the University Hospital of Zurich, Switzerland, involving patients with mild to very severe (GOLD stage I to IV) COPD examined annually for at least three years each. Recruitment involves seven hospitals in Switzerland. A range

of demographic, COPD-specific, physiologic, and quality of life-related variables are recorded. At baseline patients attending participating clinics consented and were enrolled in a nonselective, consecutive manner. The study was approved by the Ethics Committee of the Canton of Zurich, Switzerland (*Kantonale Ethikkommission Zürich*), registration reference KEK-ZH-Nr. 2011-0106.

2.3. Measurements. Patients' characteristics and clinical information were ascertained through self-report questionnaires, investigator-led interviews, and clinical records. Apart from details extracted from detailed clinical records, all assessments were conducted by either trained pulmonologists or dedicated study investigators.

Information about the presence or absence of an active diagnosis of unipolar depression according to ICD-10 [16] was extracted from patients' clinical records and double-checked by personal communication with patients' physicians. Most diagnoses had been made by primary care physicians (who are required to apply ICD-10 coding criteria to receive reimbursement from patients' health insurance providers). Whilst this precluded the uniform use of rigorous psychiatric interviews, the approach is an adequate reflection of clinical reality.

The German language version of the HADS [4] was administered as a self-rated questionnaire for patients to fill in either during the recruitment visit or as soon as possible thereafter. Both the HADS-A and HADS-D 7-item components were administered (each ranging from 0 to 21 with higher scores indicating increased symptoms) to evaluate patients' perceived psychological distress.

Forced expiratory volume in one second (FEV1) and maximum forced vital capacity (FVC) were assessed according to the criteria for reproducibility of the American Thoracic Society [17]. COPD-specific assessments included the 6-minute walking test (6-MWT; maximum distance in meters walked in six minutes) [18], Medical Research Council (MRC) Dyspnoea score (ranging in ascending severity from 0 to 4) [19], COPD assessment test (CAT; an 8-item health-related quality of life questionnaire ranging from 0 to 40 with higher scores indicating more severe impairment) [20], and BODE index (the composite of body mass index (BMI, body weight in kilograms divided by body height in meters squared), FEV1% predicted, 6-MWT, and MRC Dyspnoea scale; ranging from 0/low risk to 10/high risk) [21].

2.4. Analysis. Receiver operating characteristic (ROC) curves [22] and area under the curve (AUC) statistics were compared for HADS-D and HADS-total [23]. DeLong et al.'s [24] approach for estimating ROC parameters, Hilgers' [25] nonparametric 95% confidence interval (CI) estimation method for criterion values, and Youden's [26] index J (the maximum vertical distance between the diagonal guessing line and the ROC curve) were estimated alongside likelihood ratios (LR). A clinical diagnosis of depression at the time of assessment was the reference standard. Multivariable logistic regression models for depression with stepwise predictor selection were constructed including HADS, age,

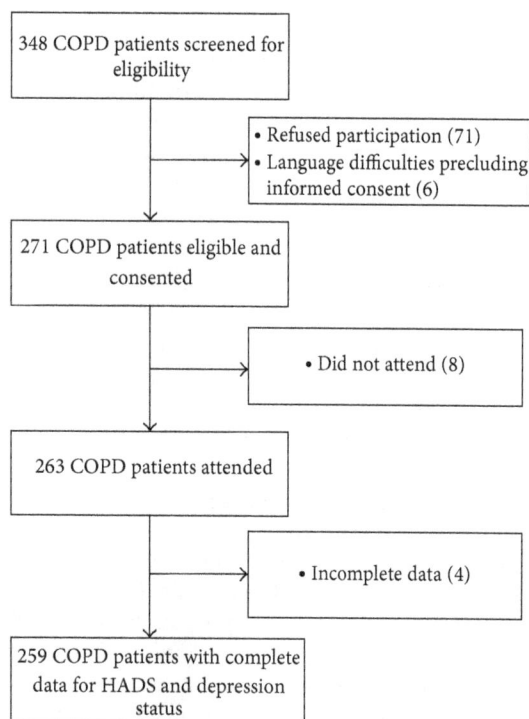

FIGURE 1: Flowchart of chronic obstructive pulmonary disease (COPD) patients in the study.

TABLE 1: Sample characteristics.

Variable	Not depressed ($n = 230$)	Depressed ($n = 29$)	P value[†]
Female, n (%)	70 (30.4%)	14 (48.3%)	0.085
Age, mean (SD)	62.7 (7.5)	60.0 (8.3)	0.057
BMI, mean (SD)	26.4 (6.1)	26.1 (5.9)	0.808
Comorbidities, mean (SD)	2.4 (2.2)	3.1 (1.6)	0.061
Diabetes mellitus, n (%)	32 (13.9%)	1 (3.4%)	0.195
OSA, n (%)	21 (9.1%)	5 (17.2%)	0.298
Arterial hypertension, n (%)	109 (47.4%)	15 (51.7%)	0.808
Malignancy, n (%)	27 (11.7%)	3 (10.3%)	0.931
GOLD stage, n (%)[††]			
I	17 (7.4%)	2 (6.9%)	
II	74 (32.2%)	16 (55.2%)	0.035
III	87 (37.8%)	10 (34.5%)	
IV	52 (22.6%)	1 (3.5%)	
CAT, mean (SD)	15.7 (7.1)	17.4 (7.4)	0.213
BODE index, mean (SD)	3.4 (2.4)	2.8 (2.3)	0.203
MRC-dyspnoea, mean (SD)	1.7 (1.1)	1.8 (1.0)	0.736
FEV1%, mean (SD)	46.6 (20.7)	54.5 (21.2)	0.044
6-MWT (meters), mean (SD)	412 (131)	410 (124)	0.916

[†]Frequencies and means were compared using χ^2-tests and independent t-tests, respectively.

[††]χ^2-test for the frequency distribution across GOLD stages I/II/III/IV in depressed versus nondepressed patients.

6-MWT: 6-minute walking test; BMI: body mass index; CAT: chronic obstructive pulmonary disease assessment test; CPAP: continuous positive airway pressure; FEV1%: percentage of predicted forced expiratory volume in one second; GOLD: global initiative for chronic obstructive pulmonary disease; MRC-dyspnoea: Medical Research Council dyspnoea scale; OSA: obstructive sleep apnoea.

gender, BMI, FEV1%, number of comorbidities, 6-MWT, and MRC-dyspnoea (chosen as established risk factors for depression in COPD [3, 27, 28]). CAT score was added to control for nonspecific COPD-related quality of life impairment and antidepressant use was included to adjust for treatment-related confounding. Model assumptions were tested via Kolmogorov-Smirnov tests and residual plots. Independent sample t-tests, Mann-Whitney U tests, and Chi-Square statistics were Bonferroni-corrected for multiple testing (nominal $P < 0.05$). Analyses were performed using MedCalc for Windows, version 12.6.1 (MedCalc Software, Ostend, Belgium).

3. Results

Figure 1 depicts the flow of all 263 participants enrolled between October 2009 and June 2013 from screening to analysis. Four patients were excluded due to missing data, leaving 259 COPD patients who provided complete information for HADS score and depression status. The prevalence of active depression according to ICD-10 was 11.2% (29/259). Among depressed patients, 35% (10/29) had been prescribed an antidepressant. Patient characteristics are displayed in Table 1. There were no significant differences between depressed and nondepressed patients with respect to demographic and disease-related characteristics although there was a trend for worse airflow limitation and more severe GOLD stage in nondepressed patients.

Patients with a preexisting diagnosis of depression had significantly higher HADS-D scores than nondepressed patients: median ± quartiles 6 (4; 9) for depressed versus 4 (2; 7) for nondepressed subjects ($P = 0.004$). The same held true for the HADS-total score: median ± quartiles 14 (10; 20) for depressed versus 8 (5; 14) for nondepressed patients ($P = 0.002$).

Figure 2 depicts the ROC curve for the HADS-D subscale. The overall discriminant performance was low but significantly different from random chance, AUC 0.66 (95% CI 0.60–0.72). Youden's index J identified a threshold of HADS-D >5 as the optimal cut-off score to diagnose depression ($J = 0.25$). A cut-off >5 yielded a sensitivity of 62.1% (95% CI 42.3%–79.3%), a specificity of 62.6% (95% CI 56.0%–68.9%), a positive LR of 1.66 (95% CI 1.2–2.3), and a negative LR of 0.61 (95% CI 0.4–1.0). Using a cut-off value of 5 on the HADS-D applied on the background of an observed prevalence for depression of 11.2% yielded a positive predictive value of 17.3% and a negative predictive value of 92.9%. Thus, in 100 hypothetical patients with a HADS-D >5, 17 will qualify for a diagnosis of depression, whilst among 100 patients with a score ≤5, on average 93 will be correctly identified as nondepressed. The comparison between HADS-D and HADS-total ROC plots is shown in Figure 3. There was no significant difference in overall performance between both scores, AUC$_{HADS-D}$ 0.662 versus AUC$_{HADS-total}$ 0.681 (95% CI for the difference 0–0.070). The optimal cut-off score for

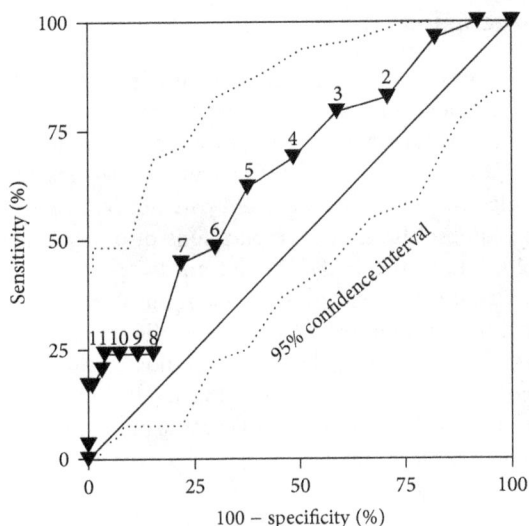

FIGURE 2: Receiver operating characteristic (ROC) curve for the HADS-depression subscale. Solid triangles indicate different cut-off scores for diagnosing depression.

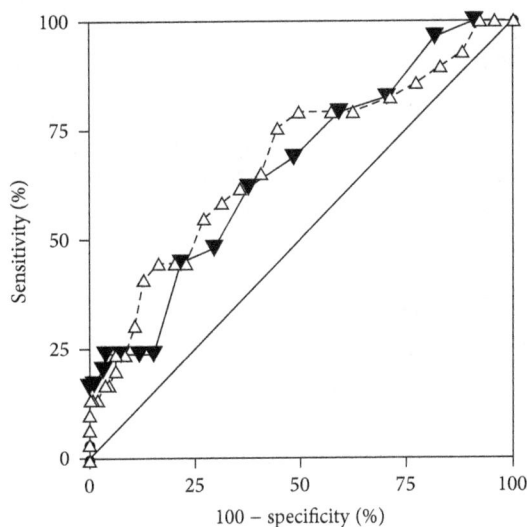

FIGURE 3: Comparative receiver operating characteristic (ROC) curves for HADS-depression (solid triangles) and HADS-total (white triangles).

diagnosing depression on the HADS-total was >9, Youden's $J = 0.311$, sensitivity 75.9% (95% CI 56.5%–89.7%), and specificity 55.2% (95% CI 48.5%–61.8%).

The stepwise logistic regression model identified four significant predictors (model fit $P < 0.001$). An increasing likelihood of suffering from depression was predicted by lower age ($P = 0.010$), higher number of comorbidities ($P = 0.004$), male gender ($P = 0.016$), and higher percentage of predicted FEV1 ($P = 0.047$). This model correctly classified 89.6% of cases. Controlling for antidepressant medication use did not alter the results. Thus, younger men with additional comorbidities had the highest risk of depression.

4. Discussion

In this cross-sectional multicentre cohort study involving patients with mild to very severe COPD, we found low accuracy of both the HADS-D and HADS-total in identifying patients with a preexisting diagnosis of depression. As the optimal cut-off HADS-D >5 yielded a positive predictive value of only 17.3% and a negative predictive value of 92.9%, the test seems to more accurately identify the absence rather than presence of depression. Its usefulness as a general measure of psychological distress notwithstanding, the validity of the HADS-D as a tool for classifying COPD patients into depressed and nondepressed categories—as commonly applied in previous studies—is questionable. This lack of discriminant power may be explained in part by the original validation of the questionnaire, which was aimed at a general medical case mix in an outpatient setting, rather than at secondary/tertiary care patients with chronic debilitating ailments. Yet, despite caveats mentioned by the HADS' developers [5], over the last three decades it has been applied to the evaluation of depression and anxiety symptoms in a large variety of clinical contexts outwith its original target group. Relying on a one-week retrospective questionnaire-based approach to classify patients as depressed or not for ensuing subgroup analyses (e.g., to predict physical activity [29]) is not appropriate. Moreover, the original purpose of the HADS as a screening rather than diagnostic tool should forbid reliance on its results as the sole indicator of clinically significant depression—a labelling approach applied in previous research. This study reemphasizes that the HADS should not be used to diagnose depression or reliably subgroup patient samples.

Our results on depression in COPD patients are in line with findings from a recent meta-analysis in cancer and palliative care patients [30], which reported a weighted combined sensitivity of 71.6% with a specificity of 82.6% of the HADS for identifying depression. Restricting analyses to trials using HADS-D >7 as cut-off yielded a sensitivity of 68.3% with a specificity of 85.7%. The authors of the meta-analysis promote the use of the HADS as a screening rather than diagnostic tool. High subscale correlations may favour using the HADS as a general measure of psychological distress rather than specifically detecting depression and anxiety [31–33]. Furthermore, studies vary substantially in cut-offs used to identify mental morbidity, casting doubt on the HADS' usefulness as a screening tool [34]. Using recommended cut-off scores may underestimate psychiatric morbidity in cancer patients [35].

A review incorporating all studies (2000 to 2010) investigating the HADS' factor structure found heterogeneous results: only half of the included trials confirmed the two-factor model (depression and anxiety), whilst others identified between one and four underlying constructs [31]. For example, an established alternative model suggests three factors labelled, respectively, "negative affectivity," "anhedonic depression," and "autonomic anxiety" [32]. Yet, a 2013 meta-confirmatory factor analysis favoured the depression/anxiety two-dimensional structure [33]. Given the confusing theory underpinning the HADS, its use as a measure of any specific psychiatric disorder should best be avoided.

Consequently, the inconsistency of the HADS' factor structure across samples [31], the discrepancy between its wordings based on colloquial British expressions, and its international application [36], compounded by the exclusion of somatic items, have led to calls for abandoning the 30-year-old HADS in favour of more accurate instruments [37]. Others continue to promote the HADS as a valid, cross-culturally appropriate tool for assessing psychological distress [38]. Future studies should make an effort to validate psychiatric diagnoses in line with the best clinical practice.

The prevalence of depression according to ICD-10 in our cohort (11.2%) was lower than in other studies with reported rates of up to 42% [27]. However, considering only studies based on a definition of depression according to established classification systems yields a lower estimate of about 20% [39]. Another explanation for the low prevalence of depression may be the homogeneous composition of our cohort composed of well looked-after patients recruited from established high-quality care centres in Switzerland. The observed higher rate of diagnosed depression in younger patients with better airway function could be due to a lower threshold for seeking professional help for psychological issues in more recent generations. Less physically limited patients may be more inclined to recognising and addressing ailments other than pulmonary disease. Alternatively, clinicians' thresholds for diagnosing depression could be different in these patients. Many factors may contribute to emotional morbidity in COPD patients, including social isolation and dependence on others for activities of daily living [28]. Crucially, however, feelings of low mood and the general psychological impact of chronic disease must not be equated with a psychiatric diagnosis of a depressive disorder. The HADS gauges psychological impairment but is not suited as a diagnostic tool. Investigators need to be cautious about labelling subjects inappropriately. As confirmed by our results, overreliance on a self-report questionnaire is prone to erroneous categorisation of patients.

There are some limitations to our study. The recruitment context of specialist pulmonary care necessitated the evaluation of preexisting rather than newly diagnosed depression. Whilst recorded diagnoses of depression were double-checked with patients' registered clinicians, short-term variations in mood may have hampered the HADS' ability to detect long-term impairment. Yet, as many clinical trials have used the HADS to label patients as depressed or not irrespective of any reference standard, our findings carry significant implications for the planning of future trials. The comparatively low prevalence of depression, potentially contributed to by underdiagnosis, may have limited the statistical power. Nonetheless, our large nonselective sample is representative of the COPD patient population in Switzerland and is consequently characterised by a high socioeconomic status and low proportion of ethnic minorities—both factors that have been linked to low rates of depression [40].

5. Conclusions

In this large cross-sectional study of stable COPD patients, the HADS questionnaire had a low accuracy in identifying a diagnosis of depression. This is the first study to address HADS-D test accuracy in COPD patients. Depression rates were highest among young male patients with additional comorbidities. The clinical implications of our findings are twofold. Firstly, the HADS should not be used as a stand-alone diagnostic tool for depression in COPD patients. It provides an appropriate scale to evaluate psychological distress but does not allow for diagnostic classification. Secondly, clinicians' awareness of the significant prevalence of psychological comorbidities in chronic pulmonary disease patients needs to be improved.

Ethical Approval

The study was approved by the Ethics Committee of the Canton of Zurich, Switzerland (*Kantonale Ethikkommission Zürich*), registration reference KEK-ZH-Nr. 2011-0106.

Disclaimer

Professor Malcolm Kohler is the guarantor of this work and, as such, had full access to all of the data in the study and takes responsibility for the integrity of the data and the accuracy of the data analysis.

Conflict of Interests

All of the authors report no conflict of interests—financial or otherwise—in relation to this paper.

Authors' Contribution

Christoph Nowak drafted the paper, implemented the data analysis, and edited the paper. Malcolm Kohler and Christian F. Clarenbach made substantial contributions to conception and design, acquisition of data, interpretation of results, and critical paper review for important intellectual content and provided final approval of the version to be published. Noriane A. Sievi, Esther Irene Schwarz, Christian Schlatzer, Thomas Brack, Martin Brutsche, Martin Frey, Sarosh Irani, Jörg D. Leuppi, Jochen Rüdiger, and Robert Thurnheer made substantial contributions to conception and design, acquisition of data, and paper revision.

Acknowledgments

The study was supported by *Lunge Zürich, Lungenliga St. Gallen, Lungenliga Thurgau, Lungenliga Glarus, Lungenliga Aagau*, the *Gottfried und Julia Bangerter-Rhyner-Stiftung*, and the *Freiwillige Akademische Gesellschaft Basel*.

References

[1] P. J. Barnes and B. R. Celli, "Systemic manifestations and comorbidities of COPD," *European Respiratory Journal*, vol. 33, no. 5, pp. 1165–1185, 2009.

[2] P. A. Cafarella, T. W. Effing, Z.-A. Usmani, and P. A. Frith, "Treatments for anxiety and depression in patients with chronic obstructive pulmonary disease: a literature review," *Respirology*, vol. 17, no. 4, pp. 627–638, 2012.

[3] J. Maurer, V. Rebbapragada, S. Borson et al., "Anxiety and depression in COPD: current understanding, unanswered questions, and research needs," *Chest*, vol. 134, no. 4, pp. 43S–56S, 2008.

[4] A. S. Zigmond and R. P. Snaith, "The hospital anxiety and depression scale," *Acta Psychiatrica Scandinavica*, vol. 67, no. 6, pp. 361–370, 1983.

[5] R. P. Snaith and A. S. Zigmond, "The hospital anxiety and depression scale," *British Medical Journal*, vol. 292, no. 6516, article 344, 1986.

[6] C. Herrmann, "International experiences with the hospital anxiety and depression scale—a review of validation data and clinical results," *Journal of Psychosomatic Research*, vol. 42, no. 1, pp. 17–41, 1997.

[7] I. Bjelland, A. A. Dahl, T. T. Haug, and D. Neckelmann, "The validity of the hospital anxiety and depression scale: an updated literature review," *Journal of Psychosomatic Research*, vol. 52, no. 2, pp. 69–77, 2002.

[8] M. Haddad, P. Walters, R. Phillips et al., "Detecting depression in patients with coronary heart disease: a diagnostic evaluation of the PHQ-9 and HADS-D in primary care, findings from the UPBEAT-UK study," *PLoS ONE*, vol. 8, no. 10, Article ID e78493, 2013.

[9] L. Castelli, L. Binaschi, P. Caldera, A. Mussa, and R. Torta, "Fast screening of depression in cancer patients: the effectiveness of the HADS," *European Journal of Cancer Care*, vol. 20, no. 4, pp. 528–533, 2011.

[10] W. L. Loosman, C. E. H. Siegert, A. Korzec, and A. Honig, "Validity of the hospital anxiety and depression scale and the beck depression inventory for use in end-stage renal disease patients," *British Journal of Clinical Psychology*, vol. 49, no. 4, pp. 507–516, 2010.

[11] M. D. Eisner, P. D. Blanc, E. H. Yelin et al., "Influence of anxiety on health outcomes in COPD," *Thorax*, vol. 65, no. 3, pp. 229–234, 2010.

[12] T. Hajiro, K. Nishimura, M. Tsukino, A. Ikeda, H. Koyama, and T. Izumi, "Comparison of discriminative properties among disease-specific questionnaires for measuring health related quality of life in patients with chronic obstructive pulmonary disease," *The American Journal of Respiratory and Critical Care Medicine*, vol. 157, no. 3 I, pp. 785–790, 1998.

[13] P. Ergün, D. Kaymaz, E. Günay et al., "Comprehensive outpatient pulmonary rehabilitation: treatment outcomes in early and late stages of chronic obstructive pulmonary disease," *Annals of Thoracic Medicine*, vol. 6, no. 2, pp. 70–76, 2011.

[14] G. Cheung, C. Patrick, G. Sullivan, M. Cooray, and C. L. Chang, "Sensitivity and specificity of the Geriatric Anxiety Inventory and the Hospital Anxiety and Depression Scale in the detection of anxiety disorders in older people with chronic obstructive pulmonary disease," *International Psychogeriatrics*, vol. 24, no. 1, pp. 128–136, 2012.

[15] K. F. Rabe, S. Hurd, A. Anzueto et al., "Global strategy for the diagnosis, management, and prevention of chronic obstructive pulmonary disease: GOLD executive summary," *American Journal of Respiratory and Critical Care Medicine*, vol. 176, no. 6, pp. 532–555, 2007.

[16] World Health Organization, *ICD-10. International Statistical Classification of Diseases and Related Health Problems*, 10th Revision, WHO, Geneva, Switzerland, 2010.

[17] J. Wanger, J. L. Clausen, A. Coates et al., "Standardisation of the measurement of lung volumes," *European Respiratory Journal*, vol. 26, no. 3, pp. 511–522, 2005.

[18] ATS Committee on Proficiency Standards for Clinical Pulmonary Function Laboratories, "ATS statement: guidelines for the six-minute walk test," *American Journal of Respiratory and Critical Care Medicine*, vol. 166, no. 1, pp. 111–117, 2002.

[19] C. M. Fletcher, P. C. Elmes, A. S. Fairbairn, and C. H. Wood, "The significance of respiratory symptoms and the diagnosis of chronic bronchitis in a working population," *British Medical Journal*, vol. 2, no. 5147, pp. 257–266, 1959.

[20] P. W. Jones, G. Harding, P. Berry, I. Wiklund, W.-H. Chen, and N. K. Leidy, "Development and first validation of the COPD Assessment Test," *European Respiratory Journal*, vol. 34, no. 3, pp. 648–654, 2009.

[21] B. R. Celli, C. G. Cote, J. M. Marin et al., "The body-mass index, airflow obstruction, dyspnoea, and exercise capacity index in chronic obstructive pulmonary disease," *The New England Journal of Medicine*, vol. 350, no. 10, pp. 1005–1012, 2004.

[22] K. H. Zou, A. J. O'Malley, and L. Mauri, "Receiver-operating characteristic analysis for evaluating diagnostic tests and predictive models," *Circulation*, vol. 115, no. 5, pp. 654–657, 2007.

[23] K. Hajian-Tilaki, "Receiver operating characteristic (ROC) curve analysis for medical diagnostic test evaluation," *Caspian Journal of Internal Medicine*, vol. 4, no. 2, pp. 627–635, 2013.

[24] E. R. DeLong, D. M. DeLong, and D. L. Clarke-Pearson, "Comparing the areas under two or more correlated receiver operating characteristic curves: a nonparametric approach," *Biometrics*, vol. 44, no. 3, pp. 837–845, 1988.

[25] R. A. Hilgers, "Distribution-free confidence bounds for ROC curves," *Methods of Information in Medicine*, vol. 30, no. 2, pp. 96–101, 1991.

[26] W. J. Youden, "Index for rating diagnostic tests," *Cancer*, vol. 3, no. 1, pp. 32–35, 1950.

[27] L. van Ede, C. J. Yzermans, and H. J. Brouwer, "Prevalence of depression in patients with chronic obstructive pulmonary disease: a systematic review," *Thorax*, vol. 54, no. 8, pp. 688–692, 1999.

[28] K. Hill, R. Geist, R. S. Goldstein, and Y. Lacasse, "Anxiety and depression in end-stage COPD," *European Respiratory Journal*, vol. 31, no. 3, pp. 667–677, 2008.

[29] H. Q. Nguyen, V. S. Fan, J. Herting et al., "Patients with COPD with higher levels of anxiety are more physically active," *Chest*, vol. 144, no. 1, pp. 145–151, 2013.

[30] A. J. Mitchell, N. Meader, and P. Symonds, "Diagnostic validity of the Hospital Anxiety and Depression Scale (HADS) in cancer and palliative settings: a meta-analysis," *Journal of Affective Disorders*, vol. 126, no. 3, pp. 335–348, 2010.

[31] T. D. Cosco, F. Doyle, M. Ward, and H. McGee, "Latent structure of the hospital anxiety and depression scale: a 10-year systematic review," *Journal of Psychosomatic Research*, vol. 72, no. 3, pp. 180–184, 2012.

[32] M. Dunbar, G. Ford, K. Hunt, and G. Der, "A confirmatory factor analysis of the Hospital Anxiety and Depression scale: comparing empirically and theoretically derived structures,"

British Journal of Clinical Psychology, vol. 39, no. 1, pp. 79–94, 2000.

[33] S. Norton, T. Cosco, F. Doyle, J. Done, and A. Sacker, "The hospital anxiety and depression scale: a meta confirmatory factor analysis," *Journal of Psychosomatic Research*, vol. 74, no. 1, pp. 74–81, 2013.

[34] A. Vodermaier and R. D. Millman, "Accuracy of the hospital anxiety and depression scale as a screening tool in cancer patients: a systematic review and meta-analysis," *Supportive Care in Cancer*, vol. 19, no. 12, pp. 1899–1908, 2011.

[35] R. Morse, K. Kendell, and S. Barton, "Screening for depression in people with cancer: the accuracy of the hospital anxiety and depression scale," *Clinical Effectiveness in Nursing*, vol. 9, no. 3-4, pp. 188–196, 2005.

[36] G. A. Maters, R. Sanderman, A. Y. Kim, and J. C. Coyne, "Problems in cross-cultural use of the hospital anxiety and depression scale: "no butterflies in the desert"," *PLoS ONE*, vol. 8, no. 8, Article ID e70975, 2013.

[37] J. C. Coyne and E. van Sonderen, "No further research needed: abandoning the Hospital and Anxiety Depression Scale (HADS)," *Journal of Psychosomatic Research*, vol. 72, no. 3, pp. 173–174, 2012.

[38] S. Norton, A. Sacker, and J. Done, "Further research needed: a comment on Coyne and van Sonderen's call to abandon the Hospital Anxiety and Depression Scale," *Journal of Psychosomatic Research*, vol. 73, no. 1, pp. 75–76, 2012.

[39] A. M. Yohannes, T. G. Willgoss, R. C. Baldwin, and M. J. Connolly, "Depression and anxiety in chronic heart failure and chronic obstructive pulmonary disease: prevalence, relevance, clinical implications and management principles," *International Journal of Geriatric Psychiatry*, vol. 25, no. 12, pp. 1209–1221, 2010.

[40] I. Tarricone, E. Stivanello, F. Poggi et al., "Ethnic variation in the prevalence of depression and anxiety in primary care: a systematic review and meta-analysis," *Psychiatry Research*, vol. 195, no. 3, pp. 91–106, 2012.

Patients with MAC Lung Disease Have a Low Visceral Fat Area and Low Nutrient Intake

Kentaro Wakamatsu,[1] Nobuhiko Nagata,[2] Sanae Maki,[1] Hisamitsu Omori,[3]
Hiroyuki Kumazoe,[1] Kayoko Ueno,[4] Yuko Matsunaga,[1] Makiko Hara,[1] Koji Takakura,[1]
Nagisa Fukumoto,[1] Nobuhisa Ando,[1] Mami Morishige,[1] Takashi Akasaki,[1]
Ichiro Inoshima,[1] Shinji Ise,[1] Miiru Izumi,[1] and Masayuki Kawasaki[1]

[1]*Department of Respiratory Medicine, National Hospital Organization, Omuta Hospital, 1044-1 Tachibana, Omuta 837-0911, Japan*
[2]*Department of Respiratory Medicine, Fukuoka University Chikushi Hospital, Japan*
[3]*Faculty of Life Sciences, Kumamoto University, Japan*
[4]*Department of Nutrition, National Hospital Organization Omuta National Hospital, Japan*

Correspondence should be addressed to Kentaro Wakamatsu; wakamatsu-k@oomuta-h.com

Academic Editor: Andrew Sandford

Objective. This study aimed to examine the nutritional status and nutrient intake of patients with MAC lung disease with a focus on visceral fat area. *Patients and Methods.* Among 116 patients of our hospital with nontuberculous mycobacteriosis who were registered between May 2010 and August 2011, 103 patients with MAC lung disease were included in this study. In all patients, nutritional status and nutrient intake were prospectively examined. *Results.* Patients were 23 men and 80 women (mean age, 72.3 ± 10.9 years). BMI (kg/m^2) at the time of registration was 20.4 ± 2.7 in men and 19.2 ± 2.9 in women. Visceral fat area (cm^2) was significantly lower in women (35.7 ± 26.6) than in men (57.5 ± 47.4) ($p = 0.0111$). The comparison with general healthy adults according to age revealed a markedly reduced visceral fat area among patients with MAC lung disease. With respect to nutrient intake, energy adequacy (86.1 ± 15.7%), protein adequacy (82.4 ± 18.2%), lipid adequacy (78.1 ± 21.8%), and carbohydrate adequacy (89.6 ± 19.2%) ratios were all low at the time of registration. BMI was significantly correlated with protein adequacy ($p = 0.0397$) and lipid adequacy ($p = 0.0214$) ratios, while no association was found between visceral fat area and nutrient intake. *Conclusion.* Patients with MAC lung disease had a low visceral fat area and low nutrient intake.

1. Introduction

Mycobacterium avium complex (MAC) lung disease is often observed in slim middle-aged and older women [1–4], and slenderness has been reported to serve as a prognostic factor [4, 5]. Although it is unclear how weight loss is involved with the etiology and pathology of MAC lung disease, the abnormal production of inflammatory cytokines due to fluctuations in adipocyte-derived adipokines, which is caused by a decrease in fat cells (particularly visceral fat cells) due to weight loss, has been suggested as one of the contributory factors [6]. In this context, it will be meaningful to investigate the association between weight loss and visceral fat area in patients with MAC lung disease, but no report exists with

regard to weight loss and visceral fat area in patients with MAC lung disease. Moreover, while it is predicted that weight loss in patients with MAC lung disease is attributable to emaciation from the illness itself as well as low nutrient intake, no published reports pertaining to nutrient intake exist. Accordingly, this study aimed to examine the nutritional status and nutrient intake of patients with MAC lung disease with a focus on visceral fat area.

2. Patients and Methods

At our hospital, 116 outpatients and inpatients with NTM disease were registered between May 2010 and September 2013. Among these, 103 patients with MAC lung disease were included in this study. All patients met the diagnostic criteria of "An Official ATS/IDSA Statement: Diagnosis, Treatment, and Prevention of Nontuberculous Mycobacterial Diseases" [7] based on imaging and bacteriological examination findings, agreed with the study content, and provided written consent to participate in this study. We first compared nutritional status and nutritional intake between FC and NB dis. and found no differences between them. Accordingly, these two groups were combined.

Patients currently under treatment were defined as those undergoing a combination therapy that included clarithromycin or new quinolone antibacterial agents. Assessment of nutritional status included body mass index (BMI), lymphocyte count, serum albumin, serum prealbumin, serum cholinesterase, serum transferrin, total cholesterol, visceral fat area assessed by abdominal CT, and waist circumference. Measurements of visceral fat area and waist circumference were obtained from abdominal CT scans taken at the level of umbilicus using image analysis software (Fat Pointer; version 1.10, Hitachi Medical Corporation, Tokyo, Japan). Furthermore, BMI, waist circumference, and visceral fat area were compared with data of general adult participants of health checkups in 2008 FY (649 patients; 418 men, 231 women) from the Japanese Red Cross Kumamoto Hospital.

Information regarding dietary content and intake was obtained through interviews by nutritionists. Preliminarily, dietary and intake survey by nutritionists was done twice during a month period in ten patients with MAC lung disease, respectively, and we confirmed the reproducibility of results of the survey. Calorie intake, protein, lipid, and carbohydrate adequacy ratios (actual intake amount of each nutrient/average intake among Japanese people determined based on the 2010 National Nutrition Survey × 100) were determined.

Data were expressed as mean ± standard deviation (SD), since a test of normality showed that all data were normally distributed. t-tests were used for comparisons with data of general adults regarding visceral fat area. $p < 0.05$ was considered statistically significant.

This study was conducted with the approval from the Ethics Board of the National Hospital Organization Omuta National Hospital.

3. Results

3.1. Patient Characteristics.
Our patients were predominantly female (24 men and 79 women), with an age range of 46–91 years and mean age of 71.3 ± 10.9 years at the time of registration. Disease duration (from the date of confirmed diagnosis to the point of registration) ranged from 0.93 to 311.8 months, with a mean duration of 78.5 ± 65.0 months. Detected bacterial strains were *M. intracellulare* in 59 patients, *M. avium* in 35, and *M. intracellulare* + *M. avium* in 9. Twenty-six patients had fibrocavitary (FC) disease, and 77 patients had nodular bronchiectatic (NB) disease (Table 1).

3.2. Nutritional Status of Patients with MAC Lung Disease.
In both men and women, BMI, waist circumference, and visceral fat area at registration were significantly lower compared

to data of health checkup participants according to age. In particular, visceral fat area was markedly lower than that of health checkup participants (Table 2).

There was no significant difference in BMI between men and women, but women had a significantly lower visceral fat area. With respect to disease type, significantly more men had FC disease. In blood examination, serum prealbumin levels were low in both men (18.4 ± 4.8 mg/dL) and women (16.4 ± 4.4 mg/dL) compared to normal value of Japanese. However serum albumin, cholinesterase, transferrin, and total cholesterol levels were all within the normal ranges (Table 1).

As for associations between visceral fat area and patient characteristics and laboratory findings, BMI, waist circumference, white blood cell count, and lymphocyte count were significantly correlated in men, but only BMI and waist circumference were significantly correlated in women (Table 3).

3.3. Nutrient Intake of Patients with MAC Lung Disease.
With respect to nutrient intake, energy adequacy (86.1 ± 15.7%), protein adequacy (82.4 ± 18.2%), lipid adequacy (78.1 ± 21.8%), and carbohydrate adequacy (89.6±19.2%) ratios were low at the time of registration (Table 4). BMI was significantly correlated with protein adequacy ($p = 0.0397$) and lipid adequacy ($p = 0.0214$) ratios (Table 5). However visceral fat area was not significantly correlated with intake of each nutrient (Table 6).

4. Discussion

One of the clinical characteristics of MAC lung disease is its high prevalence among slim women. Kim et al. performed a prospective examination of 63 patients with NTM lung disease and reported that, compared with the background-matched control group, BMI was significantly lower [1]. Kartalija et al. also reported similar results in a prospective examination of 103 patients with NTM lung disease [2]. Moreover, in Japan, Okumura et al. reported that, in 273 patients with MAC lung disease, two-thirds were female and had a BMI lower than the standard BMI, irrespective of disease type (i.e., FC or NB) [3]. In the present study, most of our patients were women and had a BMI lower than that of general healthy controls. Although it is unclear how weight loss is involved with the etiology and pathology of MAC lung disease, the abnormal production of inflammatory cytokines due to fluctuations in adipocyte-derived adipokines, which is caused by a decrease in fat cells (particularly visceral fat cells) due to weight loss, has been suggested as one of the contributory factors [6]. Moreover, while it is predicted that weight loss in patients with MAC lung disease is attributable to emaciation from the illness itself as well as low nutrient intake, no published reports pertaining to nutrient intake exist. To our knowledge, this study is the first to examine visceral fat area and nutrient intake in patients with MAC lung disease.

In the present study, BMI, waist circumference, and particularly visceral fat area were significantly lower in both men and women compared with general healthy adults. Moreover, in this study, visceral fat area was strongly correlated with

TABLE 1: Baseline characteristics of patients with MAC lung disease ($n = 103$).

	Normal ranges	Total (mean ± SD)	Female (mean ± SD)	Male (mean ± SD)	p
Patient number		103	79	24	
Age (years)		72.3 ± 10.9	72.7 ± 11.1	71.2 ± 10.4	0.5628
Disease duration (months)		78.5 ± 65.0	78.7 ± 62.7	77.9 ± 73.6 months	0.9562
Smoking history Current/former/never		0/5*/98	0/0/79	0/5*/19	0.0005
Diabetes mellitus		9	4	5	0.0301
Emphysema		5**	0	5**	0.0005
Type of bacteria		*M. intracellulare* 59 (57%) *M. avium* 35 (34%) Both 9 (9%)	*M. intracellulare* 44 (56%) *M. avium* 28 (35%) Both 7 (9%)	*M. intracellulare* 15 (63%) *M. avium* 7 (29%) Both 2 (8%)	
Radiographic features					
FC dis.		26	14	12	0.0023
NB dis.		77	65	12	
Number of patients treated		71	53	18	0.4649
Height (cm)		154.0 ± 8.9	150.9 ± 7.1	164.2 ± 6.3	<0.0001
Weight (kg)		46.3 ± 9.3	43.8 ± 8.1	54.8 ± 7.8	<0.0001
BMI (kg/m^2)		19.4 ± 2.9	19.2 ± 2.9	20.4 ± 2.7	0.0780
Visceral fat (cm^2)		41.0 ± 33.9	35.7 ± 26.6	57.5 ± 47.4	0.0111
Waist (cm)		73.3 ± 8.4	72.5 ± 8.3	75.9 ± 8.5	0.0939
WBC (/μL)	3100–8800	4968.6 ± 1559.1	4751.3 ± 1431.8	5675.0 ± 1769.1	0.0143
Lymphocytes (/μL)	837–4136	1404.9 ± 526.2	1352.8 ± 456.8	1574.4 ± 691.6	0.0807
Alb (g/dL)	4.0–5.0	4.1 ± 0.3	4.1 ± 0.3	4.1 ± 0.3	0.3883
Ch-E (IU/L)	214–466	309.8 ± 74.0	309.5 ± 72.4	310.9 ± 80.6	0.9363
T-chol (mg/dL)	128–219	186.6 ± 28.0	190.9 ± 27.6	173.0 ± 25.1	0.0080
Transferrin (mg/dL)	190–320	212.0 ± 49.6	211.7 ± 43.1	213.1 ± 67.7	0.9013
Prealbumin (mg/dL)	22.0–40.0	16.9 ± 4.5	16.4 ± 4.4	18.4 ± 4.8	0.0662

Each parameter is displayed as mean ± standard deviation, except for patient number, comorbidity, type of bacteria, radiographic features, and number of patients treated.
FC dis.: fibrocavitary disease, NB dis.: nodular bronchiectatic disease, BMI: body mass index, WBC: white blood cell, Alb: albumin, Ch-E: cholinesterase, and T-chol: total cholesterol.
*Three with FC dis. and two with NB dis.
**Three with FC dis. and two with NB dis.

TABLE 2: Visceral fat, body mass index, and waist circumference of patients with MAC lung disease according to age ($n = 103$).

	Age (years)	Visceral fat (cm^2)			BMI (kg/m^2)			Waist (cm)		
		Patients Mean ± SD	Healthy persons Mean ± SD	p value	Patients Mean ± SD	Healthy persons Mean ± SD	p value	Patients Mean ± SD	Healthy persons Mean ± SD	p value
F	40~59	33.7 ± 28.0 ($n = 13$)	69.5 ± 35.4 ($n = 99$)	0.0007	20.4 ± 1.8 ($n = 13$)	23.4 ± 3.8 ($n = 99$)	0.0050	73.9 ± 7.7 ($n = 13$)	83.5 ± 8.8 ($n = 99$)	0.0003
	60~69	33.1 ± 18.7 ($n = 14$)	88.4 ± 46.6 ($n = 43$)	<0.0001	19.2 ± 2.9 ($n = 17$)	23.0 ± 3.2 ($n = 43$)	<0.0001	75.1 ± 6.3 ($n = 14$)	84.5 ± 8.9 ($n = 43$)	0.0006
	70~79	34.5 ± 30.5 ($n = 20$)	108.8 ± 44.1 ($n = 32$)	<0.0001	18.4 ± 2.6 ($n = 22$)	23.2 ± 2.7 ($n = 32$)	<0.0001	70.6 ± 8.2 ($n = 20$)	86.5 ± 7.3 ($n = 32$)	<0.0001
	80~	39.1 ± 27.4 ($n = 25$)	130.3 ± 51.8 ($n = 8$)	<0.0001	19.2 ± 3.5 ($n = 27$)	24.1 ± 2.7 ($n = 8$)	0.0009	71.8 ± 9.6 ($n = 25$)	89.6 ± 8.6 ($n = 8$)	<0.0001
M	50~59	57.5 ± 42.8 ($n = 3$)	114.6 ± 43.3 ($n = 119$)	0.0258	21.7 ± 2.5 ($n = 4$)	24.5 ± 2.6 ($n = 119$)	0.0435	77.8 ± 14.0 ($n = 3$)	87.7 ± 7.1 ($n = 119$)	0.0217
	60~69	75.8 ± 58.2 ($n = 6$)	126.8 ± 56.1 ($n = 82$)	0.0346	19.7 ± 3.6 ($n = 6$)	24.4 ± 2.7 ($n = 82$)	0.0001	76.4 ± 11.0 ($n = 6$)	88.4 ± 8.4 ($n = 82$)	0.0014
	70~79	39.7 ± 40.0 ($n = 8$)	126.8 ± 45.2 ($n = 32$)	<0.0001	20.4 ± 2.8 ($n = 8$)	24.1 ± 2.1 ($n = 32$)	0.0002	75.0 ± 6.6 ($n = 8$)	86.9 ± 5.8 ($n = 32$)	<0.0001
	80~	63.1 ± 50.5 ($n = 6$)	123.4 ± 50.5 ($n = 10$)	0.0368	20.1 ± 1.9 ($n = 6$)	23.8 ± 3.0 ($n = 10$)	0.0185	75.8 ± 7.1 ($n = 6$)	87.9 ± 9.0 ($n = 10$)	0.0141

Data are presented as mean ± standard deviation.
F: female, M: male, and BMI: body mass index.

TABLE 3: Correlation analyses between visceral fat area and each parameter in patients with MAC lung disease.

Parameter	Female		Male	
	r	p value	r	p value
Age	0.0325	0.7864	−0.0290	0.8955
Disease duration	0.0010	0.9935	0.3908	0.0652
BMI	0.5996	<0.0001	0.7534	<0.0001
Waist	0.7120	<0.0001	0.8425	<0.0001
WBC	0.0571	0.6364	0.5196	0.0110
Lymphocyte	0.0654	0.5882	0.6337	0.0012
Albumin	0.1447	0.2287	0.3879	0.0674
Ch-E	−0.0545	0.6519	0.2396	0.2709
T-chol	−0.1602	0.1819	0.1181	0.5916
Transferrin	0.0115	0.9241	−0.0547	0.8041
Prealbumin	0.1019	0.3977	0.5789	0.0038
CRP	−0.1876	0.1145	0.0905	0.6813

BMI: body mass index, WBC: white blood cell, Ch-E: cholinesterase, T-chol: total cholesterol, and CRP: C-reactive protein.

TABLE 4: Intake (%) of energy and each nutrient in patients with MAC lung disease.

	Total Mean ± SD
Energy (%)	86.1 ± 15.7
Protein (%)	82.4 ± 18.2
Lipid (%)	78.1 ± 21.8
Carbohydrate (%)	89.6 ± 19.2

Data are presented as mean ± standard deviation.
Intake (%) of energy and each nutrient was calculated by dividing the actual intake by the average intake among Japanese people determined based on the 2010 National Nutrition Survey × 100.

TABLE 5: Correlation analyses between body mass index and intake (%) of energy and each nutrient in patients with MAC lung disease.

Parameter	r	p value
Energy (%)	0.1961	0.0568
Protein (%)	0.2114	0.0397
Lipid (%)	0.2359	0.0214
Carbohydrate (%)	0.1092	0.2920

Intake (%) of energy and each nutrient was calculated by dividing the actual intake by the average intake among Japanese people determined based on the 2010 National Nutrition Survey × 100.

TABLE 6: Correlation analyses between visceral fat area and intake (%) of energy and each nutrient in patients with MAC lung disease.

Parameter	r	p-value
Energy (%)	−0.0242	0.8243
Protein (%)	0.0401	0.7123
Lipid (%)	−0.0103	0.9248
Carbohydrate (%)	−0.0025	0.9818

Intake (%) of energy and each nutrient was calculated by dividing the actual intake by the average intake among Japanese people determined based on the 2010 National Nutrition Survey × 100.

BMI and waist circumference, but not with patient characteristics or disease duration. Tasaka et al. showed a negative correlation between adiponectin and BMI and reported that, compared to healthy individuals, MAC patients had significantly higher levels of adiponectin according to weight [8]. The anti-inflammatory activities of adiponectin extend to inhibition of IL-6 production accompanied by induction of the anti-inflammatory cytokines IL-10 and IL-1 receptor antagonist and increased adiponectin leads to increased susceptibility to infections [9]. A decrease in visceral fat is possibly associated with the development of MAC lung disease, because Staiger et al. reported that a strong association exists between adiponectin and visceral fat [10].

That many patients with MAC lung disease are slim has been consistently shown as well as our patients; however, it is unclear why patients with NTM disease tend to be slim. The present study provides some insight in this regard, as it clearly showed that patients with MAC lung disease have low energy, protein, fat, and carbohydrate intake, which could partially explain why these patients are slim. BMI was significantly correlated with intake of protein and lipid intake. However, no significant correlation was found between visceral fat area and intake of each nutrient. These results suggest that the presence of factors other than nutrient intake might be related to reduced visceral fat. Nutrient intake might be related to subcutaneous fat and muscle mass. Decreased subcutaneous fat is considered to result in decrease of leptin, which may enhance the susceptibility to MAC. Although the present study had a cross-sectional design and thus did not examine prognoses, a number of previous studies have shown that low BMI is a prognostic factor for MAC lung disease [4, 5]. Future tasks may include an investigation of possible effects of nutritional guidance on the prognosis and course of disease in patients with MAC lung disease.

Other characteristics from the nutritional aspect included a decreased serum prealbumin level, but albumin levels were within the normal range. No study has examined serum prealbumin level in patients with MAC lung disease. Decreased serum prealbumin level might be associated with the pathological conditions of patients with MAC lung disease; however, the underlying mechanisms are unclear.

There are several limitations to this study. First, this was a single-facility study with a small number of male patients. Moreover, patient data were not from their first visit (i.e., varying duration of time had elapsed after diagnosis in each case). Furthermore, the control data used for comparison were data of those who had participated in health checkups and thus may not necessarily be considered data of the general healthy population. Though we have compared visceral fat and nutritional status between patients with MAC lung disease and healthy controls, comparison between MAC lung and nonpathogen related inflammatory lung diseases would make the argument more compelling. In addition, a thin population would be a better control group rather than general population as we used in the study. Previous studies used general population as control [1, 2]. Though we have compared nutritional intake of patients with MAC lung disease with average intake among Japanese people determined based on the 2010 National Nutrition Survey, comparison with healthy controls might be more appropriate. A multicenter study is warranted, and it will be necessary to perform an investigation regarding visceral fat area and patient prognosis, as well as a prospective study in which dietary intervention is performed with a focus on lipid and protein intake.

In conclusion, this study revealed that patients with MAC lung disease have a low visceral fat area and low nutrient intake, although no significant correlation was found between them. This suggests that factors other than nutrient intake may underlie the reduced visceral fat area.

Abbreviations

MAC: Mycobacterium avium complex
NTM: Nontuberculous mycobacteriosis
BMI: Body mass index
CT: Computed tomography
FC dis.: Fibrocavitary disease
NB dis.: Nodular bronchiectatic disease
SD: Standard deviation
WBC: White blood cell
Alb: Albumin
Ch-E: Cholinesterase
T-chol: Total cholesterol
CRP: C-reactive protein.

Conflict of Interests

None of the authors have a financial relationship with a commercial entity that has an interest in the subject of this paper.

References

[1] R. D. Kim, D. E. Greenberg, M. E. Ehrmantraut et al., "Pulmonary nontuberculous mycobacterial disease: prospective study of a distinct preexisting syndrome," *American Journal of Respiratory and Critical Care Medicine*, vol. 178, no. 10, pp. 1066–1074, 2008.

[2] M. Kartalija, A. R. Ovrutsky, C. L. Bryan et al., "Patients with nontuberculous mycobacterial lung disease exhibit unique body and immune phenotypes," *American Journal of Respiratory and Critical Care Medicine*, vol. 187, no. 2, pp. 197–205, 2013.

[3] M. Okumura, K. Iwai, H. Ogata et al., "Clinical factors on cavitary and nodular bronchiectatic types in pulmonary *Mycobacterium avium* complex disease," *Internal Medicine*, vol. 47, no. 16, pp. 1465–1472, 2008.

[4] M. Hayashi, N. Takayanagi, T. Kanauchi, Y. Miyahara, T. Yanagisawa, and Y. Sugita, "Prognostic factors of 634 HIV-negative patients with *Mycobacterium avium* complex lung disease," *American Journal of Respiratory and Critical Care Medicine*, vol. 185, no. 5, pp. 575–583, 2012.

[5] Y. Yamazaki, K. Kubo, A. Takamizawa, H. Yamamoto, T. Honda, and S. Sone, "Markers indicating deterioration of pulmonary *Mycobacterium avium—intracellulare* infection," *American Journal of Respiratory and Critical Care Medicine*, vol. 160, no. 6, pp. 1851–1855, 1999.

[6] E. D. Chan and M. D. Iseman, "Slender, older women appear to be more susceptible to nontuberculous mycobacterial lung disease," *Gender Medicine*, vol. 7, no. 1, pp. 5–18, 2010.

[7] D. E. Griffith, T. Aksamit, B. A. Brown-Elliott et al., "An official ATS/IDSA statement: diagnosis, treatment, and prevention of nontuberculous mycobacterial diseases," *American Journal of Respiratory and Critical Care Medicine*, vol. 175, no. 4, pp. 367–416, 2007.

[8] S. Tasaka, N. Hasegawa, T. Nishimura et al., "Elevated serum adiponectin level in patients with *Mycobacterium avium-intracellulare* complex pulmonary disease," *Respiration*, vol. 79, no. 5, pp. 383–387, 2010.

[9] G. Fantuzzi, "Adipose tissue, adipokines, and inflammation," *Journal of Allergy and Clinical Immunology*, vol. 115, no. 5, pp. 911–919, 2005.

[10] H. Staiger, O. Tschritter, J. Machann et al., "Relationship of serum adiponectin and leptin concentrations with body fat distribution in humans," *Obesity Research*, vol. 11, no. 3, pp. 368–372, 2003.

33

Drug Resistance among Pulmonary Tuberculosis Patients in Calabar, Nigeria

Akaninyene Otu,[1] **Victor Umoh,**[1] **Abdulrazak Habib,**[2] **Soter Ameh,**[3]
Lovett Lawson,[4] **and Victor Ansa**[1]

[1] *Department of Internal Medicine, University of Calabar Teaching Hospital, PMB 1278, Cross River State, Nigeria*
[2] *Department of Medicine, Aminu Kano Teaching Hospital, PMB 3452, Kano, Nigeria*
[3] *Department of Community Medicine, University of Calabar Teaching Hospital, PMB 1278, Cross River State, Nigeria*
[4] *Zankli Medical Centre, Plot 1021 Shehu YarAdua Way, Abuja, Nigeria*

Correspondence should be addressed to Akaninyene Otu; akanotu@yahoo.com

Academic Editor: S. L. Johnston

Background. This study aimed to determine the pattern of drug susceptibility to first-line drugs among pulmonary TB patients in two hospitals in Calabar, Nigeria. *Methods.* This was a descriptive cross-sectional study carried out between February 2011 and April 2012. Sputum samples from consecutive TB patients in Calabar were subjected to culture on Lowenstein-Jensen (LJ) slopes followed by drug susceptibility testing (DST). The DST was performed on LJ medium by the proportion method. *Results.* Forty-two of the 100 *Mycobacterium tuberculosis* strains were found to be resistant to at least one drug. Resistance to only one drug (monoresistance) was found in 17 patients. No strains with monoresistance to rifampicin were found. Resistance to two drugs was found in 22 patients, while one patient was resistant to both three and four drugs. MDR TB was seen in 4% (4/100). The independent variables of HIV serology and sex were not significantly associated with resistance ($P > 0.05$). *Conclusion.* There was a high prevalence of anti-TB drug resistance in Calabar.

1. Introduction

Tuberculosis (TB), an ancient infectious disease caused by *Mycobacterium tuberculosis*, is the leading cause of death due to an infectious agent globally. It is both preventable and treatable [1, 2]. The World Health Organization (WHO) records an average of nine million new TB cases annually and about 5000 TB deaths daily [1]. TB and human immunodeficiency virus (HIV) coinfection and the exponential increase in drug resistance are greatly responsible for the resurgence of TB [3]. Other identified factors include neglect of TB control by governments, poor management of programmes, poverty, population growth, and rapid uncontrolled urbanization [4].

Drug-resistant TB is a case of TB (usually pulmonary) excreting bacilli resistant to one or more anti-TB drugs [5]. Acquired drug resistance results from exposure to a single drug due to irregular drug supply, inappropriate prescription, or poor adherence to treatment. This suppresses the growth of bacilli susceptible to that drug while permitting multiplication of drug-resistant organisms. Primary or initial drug resistance occurs when such drug resistant bacilli are transmitted to other people [5].

Resistance to one anti-TB drugs is known as mono resistance. Poly resistance is resistant to two or more anti-TB drugs, but not to both isonazid & rifampicin. Multidrug-resistant TB (MDR TB) is resistant to at least isoniazid and rifampicin, the two key first-line anti-TB drugs in short course chemotherapy [5]. These forms of TB do not respond to the standard six-month treatment with anti-TB drugs [6].

Drug resistance poses a major challenge to the control of TB. It requires a longer duration of therapy with close monitoring and specialized treatment facilities. Patients remain infectious for longer periods and drug-resistant TB causes accelerated disease leading to substantial mortality. The average treatment duration is longer than that of drug susceptible TB. This makes adherence to treatment more challenging to achieve. Treatment of drug-resistant TB employs second-line medications which are less effective and display cross-resistance and high toxicity profiles. Injectable drugs are also utilized for long durations with the attendant side effects. Also, these second-line medications are very expensive and not readily available at primary care level.

Mycobacterium tuberculosis divides slowly both in vitro and in vivo and is inherently resistant to many conventional antibiotics. For successful treatment of TB, the antibiotics should penetrate macrophages and caseous material and be effective against dormant bacilli which could be reactivated later on [7]. Rifampicin, isoniazid, and pyrazinamide are bactericidal agents which have good sterilizing activity. Ethambutol and streptomycin are less effective than other first-line agents [8]. Resistance to first-line anti-TB drugs has been linked to mutations in at least 10 genes: *katG*, *inhA*, *ahpC*, *kasA*, and *ndh* for isoniazid resistance; *rpoB* for rifampicin resistance; *embB* for ethambutol resistance; *pncA* for pyrazinamide resistance; *rpsL* and *rrs* for streptomycin resistance [9].

Nigeria has the tenth largest burden of TB cases in the world [10]. The 2010 WHO estimates for Nigeria put the prevalence of TB at about 320000 (199 per 100000) cases with an incidence of 210000 (133 per 100000) and a mortality of 33000 (21 per 100000). The case detection rate (CDR) was low at 40%, while the treatment success rate (TSR) among new smear-positive cases for 2009 was 83% [10]. The 2011 WHO report states that Nigeria has an estimated MDR-TB rate of 2.2% and 9.4% among new and retreatment TB cases, respectively. Nigeria is therefore ranked the 15th among the 27 high burden countries for MDR-TB [10].

TB drug resistance is not a new occurrence in Nigeria. It was described as early as 1976 by Fawcett in Zaria [11]. Since then, there have been other reports on TB drug resistance in various parts of the country. Kehinde and colleagues at University College Hospital Ibadan, Nigeria, in 2005, tested 56 culture positive specimens of *Mycobacterium tuberculosis* for sensitivity to first-line anti-TB drugs. Thirty (53.6%) of the culture-positive isolates were resistant to both isoniazid and rifampicin, while 26 (46.4%) were susceptible [12]. Lawson and colleagues in 2011 reported DST for streptomycin, isoniazid, rifampicin, and ethambutol performed on 428 culture-positive samples on BACTEC-MGIT 960. Eight percent of the specimens cultured were MDR TB with varying levels of resistance to individual and multiple first-line drugs. HIV status was documented in 71%. There was no association between MDR-TB and HIV coinfection ($P = 0.9$) and gender ($P > 0.2$) [13]. A study by Idigbe et al. among 48 HIV seropositive and 50 HIV seronegative prison inmates in Lagos, Nigeria, who had TB showed similar results of significant difference in initial TB drug-resistance rates between the seropositive and seronegative inmates [14].

Despite these researches, there are no studies reflecting the prevalence of TB drug resistance in the southeastern part of Nigeria. TB culture and drug-resistance testing are not routinely carried out as part of the laboratory workup of persons with TB in Nigeria as sputum microscopy for acid fast bacilli is the mainstay. This present study aimed to determine the prevalence and pattern of drug resistance to first-line anti-TB drugs among newly diagnosed pulmonary TB patients in health institutions in Calabar, Nigeria.

2. Materials and Methods

2.1. Study Area. The study took place in two health facilities in Calabar: the University of Calabar Teaching Hospital (UCTH) and the Lawrence Henshaw Hospital (LHH). Calabar is the state capital of Cross River State. Cross River State is one of the states in the southeastern part of Nigeria. According to the national census figures, Cross River State has a total population of 2,888,966 with 1,492,465 males and 1,396,501 females [15].

2.2. Study Participants. Participants were consecutive patients seen in TB clinics or admitted into the medical wards of UCTH and the LHH with a diagnosis of pulmonary TB but who were yet to start anti-TB chemotherapy. The diagnosis of pulmonary TB was made using Ziehl-Neelsen (ZN) staining of sputum to identify acid-fast bacilli (AFB). A positive test was considered to be the identification of at least 10–99 AFB per 100 oil immersion fields.

2.3. Ethical Considerations. This research received ethical approval from the Health Research and Ethics Committee of the Cross River State Ministry of Health, Nigeria. High ethical standards were maintained throughout the entire duration of the study. A signed informed consent was obtained from each participant after detailed explanation of the study objectives to them. The participants were free to withdraw from the study at any point they felt like.

2.4. Inclusion Criteria. Participants included in the study were those who gave consent and were ≥15 yrs of age with a diagnosis of pulmonary TB as confirmed by at least two out of three sputum samples positive for AFB.

2.5. Exclusion Criteria. Pulmonary TB patients who were currently receiving anti-TB chemotherapy, patients with extra pulmonary TB, and those who could not expectorate were also excluded.

2.6. Procedure. Three sputum samples were collected from each participant. Either two on-the-spot samples with one early morning specimen (from out-patients) or three early morning samples (from admitted patients) were obtained. Sputum samples were analysed for AFB by ZN method. Only intending participants with at least two sputum samples positive for AFB were admitted into the study. This conformed with the WHO's standard definition of a smear-positive TB case which stipulates at least two initial sputum smear examinations (direct smear microscopy) positive for acid-fast bacilli [16, 17].

The sputum samples were then transported from Calabar to Zankli Medical Centre, Abuja in cold boxes. Zankli is widely recognised reference centre for the isolation of *Mycobacterium tuberculosis* in Nigeria [18]. At Zankli, the samples were mixed with equal volume of 4% sodium hydroxide for digestion and decontamination. Digested specimens were washed in sterile distilled water by centrifugation at 3000 g for 15 minutes. The centrifugation process was repeated for bacilli sedimentation, and 0.1-0.2 mL of homogenate was inoculated on paired Lowenstein-Jensen (LJ) egg-based slopes. All the cultures were incubated at 37°C with weekly examination for growth of *Mycobacterium* spp. until eight weeks. All isolates showing positive reaction for catalase and nitrate reductase assays were subcultured on LJ slopes to obtain pure and confluent growth required for drug susceptibility testing (DST). A total of 120 patients were recruited with two ZN positive samples. Only one sputum sample was cultured and analysed for drug susceptibility per participant. However, 100 isolates were eventually identified as *Mycobacterium tuberculosis* following culture on LJ slopes. Twenty samples were no longer viable as they did not yield any growth following culture on LJ slopes.

DST for these 100 pulmonary isolates using isoniazid, rifampicin, ethambutol, and streptomycin was performed on LJ medium by the proportion method. The LJ media were prepared for each of the four drugs, with final concentrations of 0.2 μg isoniazid, 2 μg ethambutol, 40 μg rifampicin, and 4 μg streptomycin. Bacterial suspensions were inoculated by concentrations (S1–S4) into drug-free and drug-containing slopes. Susceptibility or resistance was recorded when the proportion of bacteria in drug-containing medium to that of drug-free medium is <1 or ≥1, respectively.

Data generated from the study was entered and analysed using the Statistical Package for Social Sciences (SPSS) IBM version 19.0.

3. Results

The mean age of the final study population was 34 ± 11. There were 53 males and 47 females and they were predominantly Christians (99%). Most (96%) of the participants had received some form of education, and, majority (52%) were from the Efik tribe. Trading was the commonest occupation among the participants as shown in Table 1. Fifty of the 100 participants were HIV seropositive.

Forty-two of the 100 patients evaluated were found to be resistant to at least one drug (42%; 95% CI: 32.3–51.7%). Figures 1 and 2 show the patterns of resistance to one or more anti-TB drugs. Resistance to only one drug (monoresistance) was found in 17 patients and was as follows: isoniazid (H): 2% (2/100); ethambutol (E): 8% (8/100); streptomycin (S): 7% (7/100). No strain with monoresistance to rifampicin was found. With respect to resistance to two drugs, 3% (3/100) were resistant to R + H; 1% (1/100) was resistant to R + E; 2% (2/100) were resistant to H + S; 7% (7/100) were resistant to H + E; 9% (9/100) were resistant to S + E. Resistance to three drugs H+E+S was seen in 1% (1/100) and 1% (1/100) was resistant to all four drugs. MDR-TB was seen in 4% (4/100).

The drug with the highest resistance profile was ethambutol occurring in 28/42 (66.6%). This was followed by streptomycin resistance in 20/42 (47.6%) and isoniazid resistance in 16/42 (38%) of the resistant cases. Resistance to rifampicin was recorded in 14/42 (33.3%) of the resistant cases.

TABLE 1: Demographics of subjects.

Characteristics	Number $n = 100$
Age (years)	
Mean (SD)	34 (11.1)
Sex	
Male	53
Female	47
Religion	
Christian	99
Muslim	1
Educational status	
None	4
Primary	25
Secondary	52
Tertiary	19
Tribe	
Efik	52
Ekoi	7
Ibibio	27
Annang	5
Ibo	8
Others	1
Occupation	
Civil servant	8
Banker	1
Student	16
Manual worker	22
Petty trader	27
Retired	1
Unemployed	9
Others	16

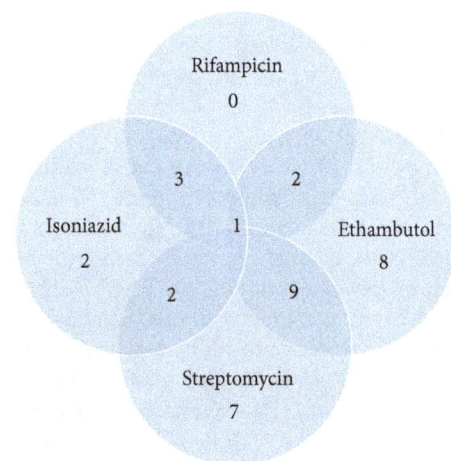

FIGURE 1: Resistance to one or more drugs in cultures of all TB subjects.

The independent variables were then cross-tabulated against the dependent variable (resistance to anti-TB drugs) to identify statistically significant associations. The independent variables tested were HIV serology and sex. These two variables were not significantly associated with resistance ($P > 0.05$) as shown in Table 2.

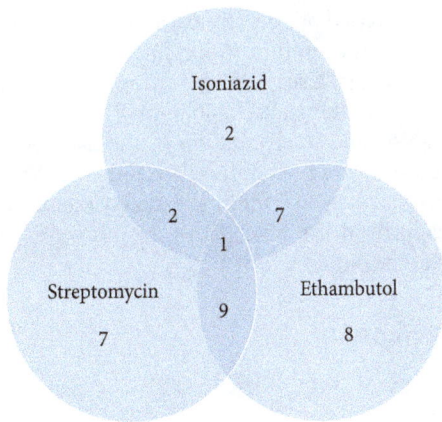

FIGURE 2: Resistance to isoniazid, ethambutol, and streptomycin.

TABLE 2: Demographic, clinical characteristics of TB participants according to general resistance to anti-TB drugs.

Variable	Number of resistant participants	Crude OR (95%)	P value
Sex			
Male	23	0.6 (0.3–1.3)	0.3
Female	19		
HIV serology			
Positive	22	1.2 (0.5–2.6)	0.9
Negative	20		

4. Discussion

This study found drug resistance in 42% of the pulmonary TB patients tested in Calabar, Southeastern Nigeria. Monoresistance rates in this present study were high for ethambutol (8%) and streptomycin (7%), but rifampicin monoresistance was not demonstrated.

Drug-resistant TB ultimately develops from the inadequate treatment of active pulmonary TB. This may result from poor prescribing practices among medical doctors with poor drug selection and insufficient treatment duration [19]. Systemic problems, through inadequate public health resources and unpredictable drug supplies, also play a role [20]. Erratic or selective compliance to treatment and default among clients is another key factor as it causes Mycobacterium tuberculosis to be exposed to sublethal doses for insufficient durations. This could thus result in treatment failure and foster emergence of drug-resistant TB and may increase the cost of treatment [21].

This low level of resistance to rifampicin in the present study is in keeping with findings of Idigbe et al. who reported a 2% resistance to rifampicin in contrast to 38% resistance to isoniazid seen in Lagos, Nigeria [17]. The high susceptibility of the Mycobacterium tuberculosis strains to rifampicin may be linked to its high bactericidal activity. Thus, the isolates showed a higher resistance rates to the less effective ethambutol and streptomycin. The low frequency of resistance to rifampicin is also generally ascribed to the new history of use of rifampicin, especially in African countries.

The high prevalence of anti-TB drug resistance in this study was mirrored by Idigbe and colleagues who reported that 56% of the TB patients studied in Lagos, Nigeria, were resistant to at least one anti-TB drug tested [22]. Similarly, Lawson et al. found lower monoresistance rates of 31% in Abuja, Nigeria, using automated BACTEC liquid culture media [18]. In Jos, Nigeria, Ani and colleagues described a monoresistance prevalence of 15% and multidrug resistance of 31% among follow-up TB patients [23]. All these studies highlight the growing threat posed by drug-resistant TB in Nigeria.

In other parts of Africa, the situation does not appear to be very different. Desta in Ethiopia found even higher rates of TB drug resistance of 58.7% [24]. Another study in Ethiopia also reported high resistance rates of 21.4% to at least one anti TB drug [25]. Kabedi et al. recorded a very high rate of primary drug resistance in a cross-sectional study in Kinshasa, Congo [26]. The primary resistance of Mycobacterium tuberculosis to first-line drugs among the subjects studied was 43.5%.

Outside of Africa, drug-resistance rates have been similarly high. A report of National Baseline Survey of drug-resistant TB (2007-2008) in China showed that resistance to at least one anti-TB drug among new cases with smear positive pulmonary TB was 35.2% [27]. Borann in Cambodia also reported high resistance to at least one anti-TB drug of 52% [28]. Dam in India also reported a high resistance to first-line anti-TB drugs (isoniazid, rifampicin, streptomycin, and ethambutol) of 39.2%. This was demonstrated among treatment failure pulmonary TB patients [29].

The high TB drug resistance rates in Calabar, Nigeria, thus reflect the rising trend in other parts of the country and indeed the world at large. Identification of the magnitude of the problem in Nigeria still remains a challenge as there is inadequate laboratory capacity to perform diagnostic testing among TB patients. Thus, the estimated numbers of drug-resistant TB cases in Nigeria have been based on mathematical modelling rather than empirical studies. Only few centres in Nigeria offer automated BACTEC TB culture and DST. The six zonal reference TB culture laboratories are yet to be fully operational [18]. This falls short of the WHO recommendation of one TB culture facility per five million population [30]. These shortcomings in the Nigerian system have militated against the effective control of drug resistant TB in Nigeria.

Several biological mechanisms linking drug-resistant TB to HIV infection have been suggested [31]. Drug malabsorption in HIV-infected patients, especially rifampicin and ethambutol, can lead to drug resistance and has been shown to lead to treatment failure. Drug-resistant strains may be less virulent and preferentially lead to disease progression in immunocompromised patients, as opposed to immunocompetent individuals. Data supporting this hypothesis has not yet been observed in humans [32]. However, the univariate analysis in the present study did not reveal an association between HIV infection and anti-TB drug resistance. This is similar to reports from earlier studies in Nigeria. Lawson and colleagues in their study of 32 TB culture-positive patients in Abuja reported no association between HIV infection and anti-TB drug resistance [18]. In a subsequent bigger study by Lawson and colleagues, they again failed to find an association between MDR-TB and HIV coinfection ($P = 0.9$) in Nigerian patients [12]. Pereira et al. studied a total of 70 $M.$ $tuberculosis$ isolates, 30 from HIV seropositive, and 40 from HIV seronegative TB patients in India. They found that the prevalence of drug-resistant $M.$ $tuberculosis$ isolates among HIV seropositive TB patients was similar to that of HIV seronegative TB patients indicating that HIV infection may not be associated with drug-resistant TB [33].

Three studies in South Africa also found no association between HIV infection and MDR-TB. In a retrospective study in Durban, 2.4% of 42 HIV coinfected and 11.5% of 253 HIV-negative patients had MDR-TB [34]. A prospective study of hospitalized TB patients in Cape Town found an MDR-TB prevalence of 3.2% in 93 HIV coinfected patients, compared to 2.6% in 115 HIV-negative patients [35]. In gold miners, the MDR-TB rate was 5.3% among 207 HIV coinfected and 6.5% among 215 HIV-negative miners [36]. From the foregoing, it appears that studies from very high TB burden countries like Nigeria, India, and South Africa have consistently reported no association between HIV and TB drug resistance.

This present study was limited by the fact that sputum AFB positivity was relied upon for admission. Thus, the TB/HIV coinfected persons who were AFB negative were excluded. Availability of rapid diagnostic tools such as GeneXpert MTB/RIF assays could have circumvented this. Also, the present study was limited to health institutions in Calabar. Larger countrywide drug-resistance surveys will provide a better estimate of the burden of TB drug resistance in Nigeria.

5. Conclusion

The high rates of TB drug resistance in the present study need to be urgently addressed. Laboratory facilities for rapid TB culture and DST are needed across Nigeria for early and accurate diagnosis of drug-resistant cases. This remains an important step in managing TB drug resistance in Nigeria.

Ethical Approval

This research was approved by the Health Research and Ethics Committee of the Cross River State Ministry of Health, Nigeria.

Conflict of Interests

The author declare that they have no conflict of interests.

Authors' Contribution

Akaninyene Otu conceived the study; Akaninyene Otu, Victor Umoh, Soter Ameh, Victor Ansa, and Abdulrazak Habib designed the study protocol; Akaninyene Otu and

Victor Umoh carried out the clinical assessment; Lovett Lawson carried out the sputum processing, Lowenstein-Jenson cultures, and drug susceptibility testing; Akaninyene Otu, Victor Umoh, Abdulrazak Habib, and Victor Ansa carried out the analysis and interpretation of the data. Akaninyene Otu drafted the paper. Abdulrazak Habib and Victor Ansa critically revised the paper for intellectual content. All authors read and approved the final paper. Akaninyene Otu is the guarantor of the paper.

Acknowledgment

Dr. Obal Otu of Adi Specialist Clinic Calabar provided writing assistance.

References

[1] World Health Organization, *Tuberculosis Control: WHO Report 2010*, WHO, Geneva, Switzerland.

[2] I. J. Eltringham and F. Drobniewski, "Multiple drug resistant tuberculosis: aetiology, diagnosis and outcome," *British Medical Bulletin*, vol. 54, no. 3, pp. 569–578, 1998.

[3] M. C. Becerra, I. F. Pachao-Torreblanca, J. Bayona et al., "Expanding tuberculosis case detection by screening household contacts," *Public Health Reports*, vol. 120, no. 3, pp. 271–277, 2005.

[4] World Health Organization, *Compendium of Indicators for Monitoring and Evaluating National Tuberculosis Programs*, WHO, Geneva, Switzerland, 2004.

[5] K. R. Rijal, P. Ghimire, D. Rijal, and D. S. Bam, "The pattern of anti-tuberculosis drug resistance in pulmonary tuberculosis patients," *Journal of Institute of Medicine*, vol. 27, pp. 26–28, 2005.

[6] World Health Organization, *MultiDrug and Extensively Drug Resistant TB (M/XDR-TB) 2010 Global Report on Surveillance and Response 2010 WHO/HTM/TB/2010*, WHO, Geneva, Switzerland, 2010.

[7] D. A. Mitchison, "The Garrod Lecture. Understanding the chemotherapy of tuberculosis—current problems," *Journal of Antimicrobial Chemotherapy*, vol. 29, no. 5, pp. 477–493, 1992.

[8] L. P. Ormerod, "Chemotherapy and management of tuberculosis in the United Kingdom: recommendations of the Joint Tuberculosis Committee of the British Thoracic Society," *Thorax*, vol. 45, no. 5, pp. 403–408, 1990.

[9] R. Johnson, E. M. Streicher, G. E. Louw, R. M. Warren, P. D. van Helden, and T. C. Victor, "Drug resistance in *Mycobacterium tuberculosis*," *Current Issues in Molecular Biology*, vol. 8, no. 2, pp. 97–112, 2006.

[10] World Health Organization, *Global Tuberculosis Control: WHO Report 2011*, WHO, Geneva, Switzerland, 2011.

[11] I. W. Fawcett and B. J. Watkins, "Initial resistance of *Mycobacterium tuberculosis* in Northern Nigeria," *Tubercle*, vol. 57, no. 1, pp. 71–73, 1976.

[12] A. O. Kehinde, F. A. Obaseki, O. C. Ishola, and K. D. Ibrahim, "Multidrug resistance to *Mycobacterium tuberculosis* in a tertiary hospital," *Journal of the National Medical Association*, vol. 99, no. 10, pp. 1185–1189, 2007.

[13] L. Lawson, M. A. Yassin, S. T. Abdurrahman et al., "Resistance to first-line tuberculosis drugs in three cities of Nigeria," *Tropical Medicine and International Health*, vol. 16, no. 8, pp. 974–980, 2011.

[14] O. Idigbe, T. Sofola, R. Akinosho, and D. Onwujekwe, "Initial drug resistance among HIV seropositive prison inmates in Lagos, Nigeria," in *International Conference on AIDS*, vol. 12, p. 137, 1998.

[15] Federal Republic of Nigeria, "Provisional results of the main findings of 2006 census," *Official Gazette*, vol. 94, no. 4, 2007, Government notice No. 3. B 52. Lagos. Federal Republic of Nigeria.

[16] World Health Organization, *Framework for Effective Tuberculosis Control. World Health Organization Document 1994*, WHO/TB/94.179:1-7.

[17] World Health Organization, International Union Against Tuberculosis and Lung Disease, Royal Netherlands Tuberculosis Association, "Revised international definitions in tuberculosis control," *International Journal of Tuberculosis and Lung Disease*, vol. 5, no. 3, pp. 213–215, 2001.

[18] L. Lawson, A. G. Habib, M. I. Okobi et al., "Pilot study on multidrug resistant tuberculosis in Nigeria," *Annals of African Medicine*, vol. 9, no. 3, pp. 184–187, 2010.

[19] S. K. Sharma and A. Mohan, "Multidrug-resistant tuberculosis: a menace that threatens to destabilize tuberculosis control," *Chest*, vol. 130, no. 1, pp. 261–272, 2006.

[20] J. S. Mukherjee, M. L. Rich, A. R. Socci et al., "Programmes and principles for management of multidrug resistant tuberculosis," *The Lancet*, vol. 372, no. 9407, pp. 474–481, 2004.

[21] A. Pablos-Méndez, C. A. Knirsch, R. G. Barr, B. H. Lerner, and T. R. Frieden, "Nonadherence in tuberculosis treatment: predictors and consequences in New York City," *American Journal of Medicine*, vol. 102, no. 2, pp. 164–170, 1997.

[22] E. O. Idigbe, J. P. Duque, E. K. O. John, and O. Annam, "Resistance to antituberculosis drugs in treated patients in Lagos, Nigeria," *Journal of Tropical Medicine and Hygiene*, vol. 95, no. 3, pp. 186–191, 1992.

[23] A. E. Ani, J. Idoko, Y. B. Dalyop, and S. L. Pitmang, "Drug resistance profile of *Mycobacterium tuberculosis* isolates from pulmonary tuberculosis patients in Jos, Nigeria," *Transactions of the Royal Society of Tropical Medicine and Hygiene*, vol. 103, no. 1, pp. 67–71, 2009.

[24] K. Desta, D. Asrat, E. Lemma, M. Gebeyehu, and B. Feleke, "Prevalence of smear negative pulmonary tuberculosis among patients visiting St. Peter's tuberculosis Specialized Hospital, Addis Ababa, Ethiopia," *Ethiopian Medical Journal*, vol. 47, no. 1, pp. 17–24, 2009.

[25] D. Asmamaw, B. Seyoum, E. Makonnen et al., "Primary drug resistance in newly diagnosed smear positive tuberculosis patients in Addis Ababa, Ethiopia," *Ethiopian Medical Journal*, vol. 46, no. 4, pp. 367–374, 2008.

[26] M. J. Kabedi, M. Kashongwe, J. M. Kayembe et al., "Primary resistance of *Mycobacterium tuberculosis* to anti-tuberculosis drugs in Kinshasa, (DRC)," *Bulletin de la Societe de Pathologie Exotique*, vol. 100, no. 4, pp. 275–276, 2007.

[27] Y. Yang, X. Li, F. Zhou, Q. Jin, and L. Gao, "Prevalence of drug-resistant tuberculosis in mainland China: systematic review and meta-analysis," *PLoS ONE*, vol. 6, no. 6, Article ID e20343, 2011.

[28] B. Sar, C. Keo, C. Leng et al., "Anti-tuberculosis drug resistance and hiv co-infection in phnom penh, cambodia," *Southeast Asian Journal of Tropical Medicine and Public Health*, vol. 40, no. 1, pp. 104–107, 2009.

[29] T. Dam, M. Isa, and M. Bose, "Drug-sensitivity profile of clinical *Mycobacterium tuberculosis* isolates—a retrospective study from a chest-disease institute in India," *Journal of Medical Microbiology*, vol. 54, no. 3, pp. 269–271, 2005.

[30] World Health Organization, *Global Tuberculosis Control: Epidemiology, Strategy and Financing*, WHO, Geneva, Switzerland, 2009.

[31] C. Dye, B. G. Williams, M. A. Espinal, and M. C. Raviglione, "Erasing the world's slow stain: strategies to beat multidrug-resistant tuberculosis," *Science*, vol. 295, no. 5562, pp. 2042–2046, 2002.

[32] K. B. Patel, R. Belmonte, and H. M. Crowe, "Drug malabsorption and resistant tuberculosis in HIV-infected patients," *The New England Journal of Medicine*, vol. 332, no. 5, pp. 336–337, 1995.

[33] M. Pereira, S. Tripathy, V. Inamdar et al., "Drug resistance pattern of *Mycobacterium tuberculosis* in seropositive and seronegative HIV-TB patients in Pune, India," *Indian Journal of Medical Research*, vol. 121, no. 4, pp. 235–239, 2005.

[34] D. Anastasis, G. Pillai, V. Rambiritch, and S. S. Abdool Karim, "A retrospective study of human immunodeficiency virus infection and drug-resistant tuberculosis in Durban, South Africa," *International Journal of Tuberculosis and Lung Disease*, vol. 1, no. 3, pp. 220–224, 1997.

[35] F. A. Post and R. Wood, "HIV infection is not associated with an increased rate of drug-resistant tuberculosis," *South African Medical Journal*, vol. 87, no. 7, p. 903, 1997.

[36] J. Murray, P. Sonnenberg, S. Shearer, and P. Godfrey-Faussett, "Drug-resistant pulmonary tuberculosis in a cohort of Southern African goldminers with a high prevalence of HIV infection," *South African Medical Journal*, vol. 90, no. 4, pp. 381–386, 2000.

34

Driving-Related Neuropsychological Performance in Stable COPD Patients

Foteini Karakontaki,[1] **Sofia-Antiopi Gennimata,**[1] **Anastasios F. Palamidas,**[1]
Theocharis Anagnostakos,[1] **Epaminondas N. Kosmas,**[1] **Anastasios Stalikas,**[2]
Charalambos Papageorgiou,[1] **and Nikolaos G. Koulouris**[1]

[1] *Respiratory Function Laboratory, 1st Department of Respiratory Medicine, National University of Athens,*
"Sotiria" Hospital, 152 Mesogeion Ave, 11527 Athens, Greece
[2] *Hellenic Sports Research Institute, Olympic Sports Centre of Athens, 37 Kifisias Ave, Marousi, 15123 Athens, Greece*

Correspondence should be addressed to Nikolaos G. Koulouris; koulnik@med.uoa.gr

Academic Editor: Kostas Spiropoulos

Background. Cognitive deterioration may impair COPD patient's ability to perform tasks like driving vehicles. We investigated: (a) whether subclinical neuropsychological deficits occur in stable COPD patients with mild hypoxemia ($PaO_2 > 55$ mmHg), and (b) whether these deficits affect their driving performance. *Methods.* We recruited 35 stable COPD patients and 10 normal subjects matched for age, IQ, and level of education. All subjects underwent an attention/alertness battery of tests for assessing driving performance based on the Vienna Test System. Pulmonary function tests, arterial blood gases, and dyspnea severity were also recorded. *Results.* COPD patients performed significantly worse than normal subjects on tests suitable for evaluating driving ability. Therefore, many (22/35) COPD patients were classified as having inadequate driving ability (failure at least in one of the tests), whereas most (8/10) healthy individuals were classified as safe drivers ($P = 0.029$). PaO_2 and FEV1 were correlated with almost all neuropsychological tests. *Conclusions.* COPD patients should be warned of the potential danger and risk they face when they drive any kind of vehicle, even when they do not exhibit overt symptoms related to driving inability. This is due to the fact that stable COPD patients may manifest impaired information processing operations.

1. Introduction

It is increasingly recognized that chronic obstructive pulmonary disease (COPD) is a multicomponent disease, but relatively little attention has been paid to its impact on neuropsychological function. Several studies have identified neuropsychological deficits in COPD patients [1–3]. The extent of this dysfunction appears to be related to the level of hypoxemia [4–8]. Subclinical cognitive deficits can even be detected in COPD patients with mild hypoxemia ($PaO_2 > 55$ mm Hg) [9, 10].

Neuropsychological tests aim to provide standardized and objective measurements is the function of specific cognitive domains. The tasks, performed as part of the neuropsychological testing, often closely resemble mental challenges encountered in everyday life. One of the commonest mental challenges in everyday life is driving performance. The latter is a complex task highly dependent on the cognitive function, involving perceptual, motor, and decision making skills. Therefore, our hypothesis was that driving ability may be impaired even in stable COPD patients with mild hypoxemia.

Road testing *per se* is the gold standard for assessing driving ability [11], but it is time consuming, expensive, and potentially hazardous. Simulators, which reproduce real driving [12, 13] conditions, are complex, very expensive, and not widely available. Nowadays, with advances in computer technology, various off-road neuropsychological tests have been developed to assess driving capacity. These tests are easier, obviously safer than on-road testing, and cheaper than using driving simulators. These tests measure an individual's ability to maintain attention, alertness, and proper reaction, the three key components of safe driving performance.

TABLE 1: Anthropometric characteristics and respiratory function data of normal subjects and COPD patients.

Parameters	Normal subjects ($n = 10$)	COPD patients ($n = 35$)	P value
Age, (yrs)	55 (5)	59 (7)	NS
Gender, M/F	8/2	26/9	NS
Ht, (m)	1.7 (0.05)	1.7 (0.07)	NS
Wt, (kg)	78 (8)	77 (14)	NS
Wt, (% pred)	109 (10)	106 (15)	NS
BMI	27.4 (2.7)	26.5 (3.7)	NS
FVC, (% pred)	105 (12)	86 (20)	$P = 0.007$
FEV_1, (% pred)	100 (11)	45 (22)	$P < 0.001$
FEV_1/FVC, %	77 (4)	40 (14)	$P < 0.001$
IC, (% pred)	103 (18)	81 (17)	$P < 0.001$
TLC, (% pred)	93 (8)	100 (15)	NS
FRC, (% pred)	89 (12)	120 (0.0)	$P = 0.002$
RV, (% pred)	74 (14)	123 (42)	$P < 0.001$
DL_{CO}, (% pred)	103 (12)	60 (22)	$P < 0.001$
PaO_2 (mm Hg)		77 (12)	
$PaCO_2$ (mm Hg)		41 (6)	
SpO_2%	98 (97–99)	95 (94–96)	$P < 0.001$
IQ (% ile)	90 (75–95)	80 (63–95)	NS

Values are mean (SD) or median (range).

Abbreviations: Ht: height; Wt: weight; BMI: body mass index; SpO_2 %: arterial oxygen saturation measured with pulse arterial oximeter; IQ: intelligent quotient; $P \leq 0.05$, statistically significant; NS: nonsignificant.

The aim of this work was to assess cognitive neuropsychological performance in a group of normal subjects and in a group of stable COPD patients with mild hypoxemia (i.e., $PaO_2 > 55$ mm Hg) with a battery of pertinent neuropsychological tests, especially designed to evaluate driving-related ability.

Therefore, we conducted this preliminary study to investigate (a) whether the cognitive neuropsychological performance was impaired in COPD patients with subclinical levels of hypoxemia, that is, $PaO_2 > 55$ mm Hg (primary outcome), and (b) whether this impaired performance was related to driving ability (secondary outcome).

2. Methods

The population of the study consisted of 35 patients with COPD (26 males) and 10 normal subjects (8 males) who served as controls. The COPD patients referred to our laboratory for lung function testing. At study time, their clinical and functional state had been stable for at least four weeks. COPD severity was classified using postbronchodilator spirometric values according to the Global Initiative for Chronic Obstructive Lung Disease (GOLD) guidelines [14] (4 patients in stage I, 7 in stage II, 15 in stage III, and 9 in stage IV). Controls were never-smokers healthy volunteers with no medical history. The two groups were matched for age, gender, education, and intelligence quotient (IQ) as assessed by Raven's progressive matrices intelligence test (RPM) [15]. Subjects with history of neurological or psychiatric disease, head injury, uncorrected visual or acoustic impairment,

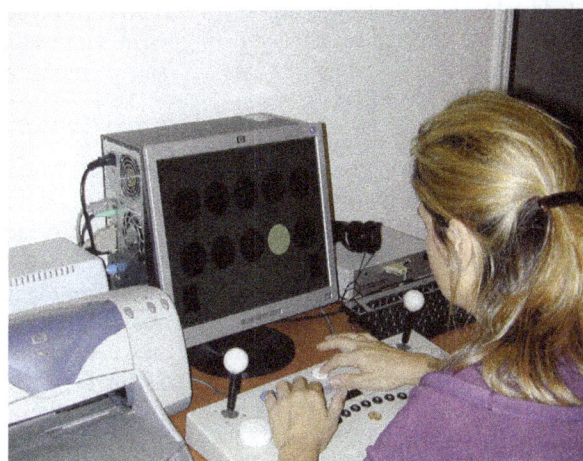

FIGURE 1: A subject performing neuropsychological testing for evaluating driving-related ability with the Vienna Test System.

shaking hands, chronic sedative intake, or alcohol abuse were excluded. Subjects with a history of asthma, allergic rhinitis, and BMI > 32 were also excluded.

None of our patients participating in the study reported any symptoms and signs related to sleep apnoea syndrome. Although the Epworth Sleepiness Scale was not formally filled by the patients, all the pertinent questions were asked during the strict and detailed history taking. Therefore, a formal sleep study was not justified. On the other hand, any patients reporting suspicious symptoms or signs for OSAHS were excluded from the study.

Randomly allocated, half of our patients have taken their daily dose of bronchodilator, but half of them have not taken it for at least 24 hours before neuropsychological testing. Any other medication was not allowed for at least 48 hours before testing. COPD patients were mildly hypoxemic (PaO_2 > 55 mm Hg). Only 7 of them were hypercapnic ($PaCO_2$ > 45 mm Hg). The characteristics of all subjects are presented in Table 1.

The study was approved by the local Medical Ethics Committee of Sotiria Hospital. All subjects gave their informed consent, and none of the participants received any financial compensation for their participation in the study.

2.1. Respiratory Function Tests. All control subjects and COPD patients underwent routine pulmonary function tests, that is, spirometry, static lung volumes, and lung diffusion capacity (DL_{CO}), according to the ATS/ERS guidelines [16–19]. The severity of chronic dyspnea was rated according to the modified Medical Research Council (mMRC) [20]. Arterial blood gases were measured only in COPD patients, and oxygen saturation (%SpO_2) using a pulse oximeter was measured in all subjects.

2.2. Neuropsychological Tests. Neuropsychological assessment took place on the same day after the pulmonary function tests. Every patient and healthy individual underwent an attention/alertness battery of tests for evaluating driving-related performance based on the Vienna Test System [21, 22] (http://www.schuhfried.co.at). Each test began with standardized instructions while the subject was comfortably seated in front of a computer's screen (Figure 1).

2.3. Reaction Time to Single Visual (RT-V) and Acoustic Stimuli (RT-A). The subject places his forefinger on a detector and when a color flashlight (yellow light) appears on the screen he has to push a button 10 cm ahead in the fastest possible way (Figure 1). The use of a rest and a reaction key makes the splitting into reaction and motor time possible. So, two parameters are recorded: (a) the period of time between the flash light and the moment the subject takes his forefinger away from the detector-rest key (reaction time: RT-V), and (b) the period of time the subject takes his forefinger away from the detector and pushes the button (motor time: MR-V). The sum of the two times above is the total reaction time (total RT-V). Totally, 28 stimuli are presented, and the test duration is 7 minutes.

Reaction time to acoustic stimuli is performed in the same way, except that the flashlight is replaced by a sound presented to the subject via headphones. The total reaction time (total RT-A) is the sum of the reaction time (RT-A) and motor time (MR-A) to acoustic stimuli.

2.4. Selective Attention Test (SA). It is a test for the assessment of concentration. The program presents four geometrical shapes on the top of the screen and asks from the subject to compare these shapes with a geometrical shape shown at the bottom of the screen. The number of given tasks is 80, and the duration of the test is 20 min.

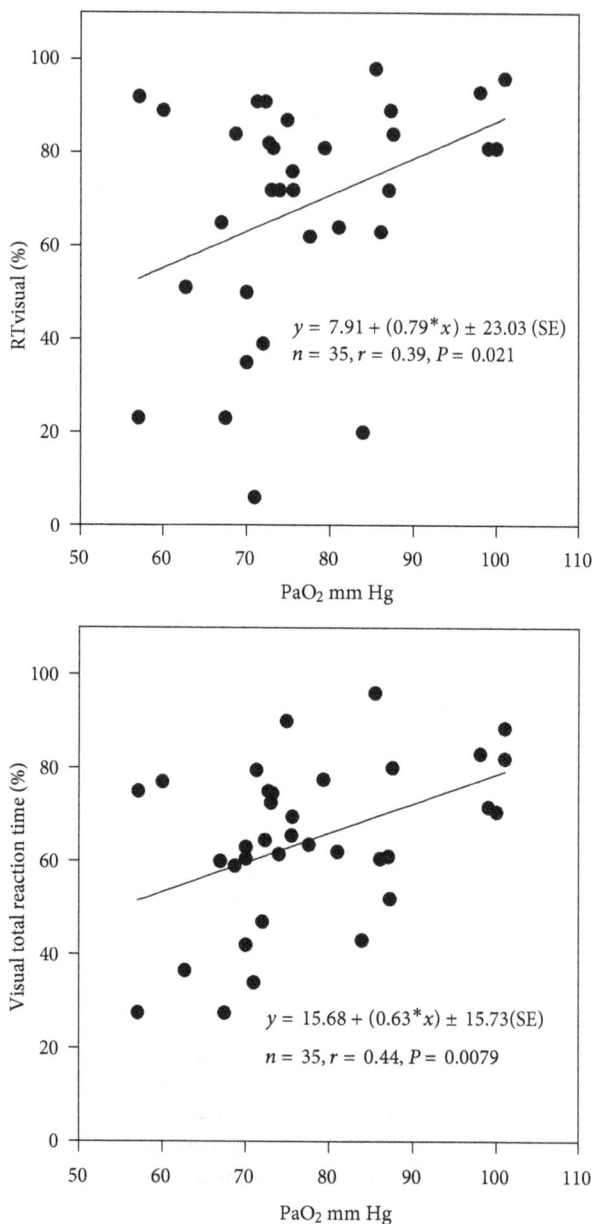

FIGURE 2: Relationship of PaO_2 to simple reaction time (RT-V%) and total reaction time (total RT-V%) to visual stimuli.

2.5. Permanent Attention Test (PA). This test assesses reaction under stress. The subject has to match quickly color figures with the equivalent color buttons on a keyboard, react to acoustical signs of high or low frequency by pushing predetermined corresponding buttons, and press foot pedals when the figure of a foot pedal appears on the screen. The total number of presented stimuli is 150, and the test duration is 30 min.

2.6. Tachistoscopic Traffic Test (TAVTMB). This test assesses visual perception. The subject is confronted with 20 pictures of traffic situation for 1 second each. Then, he has to indicate what he has seen in the picture. The test duration is 10 min.

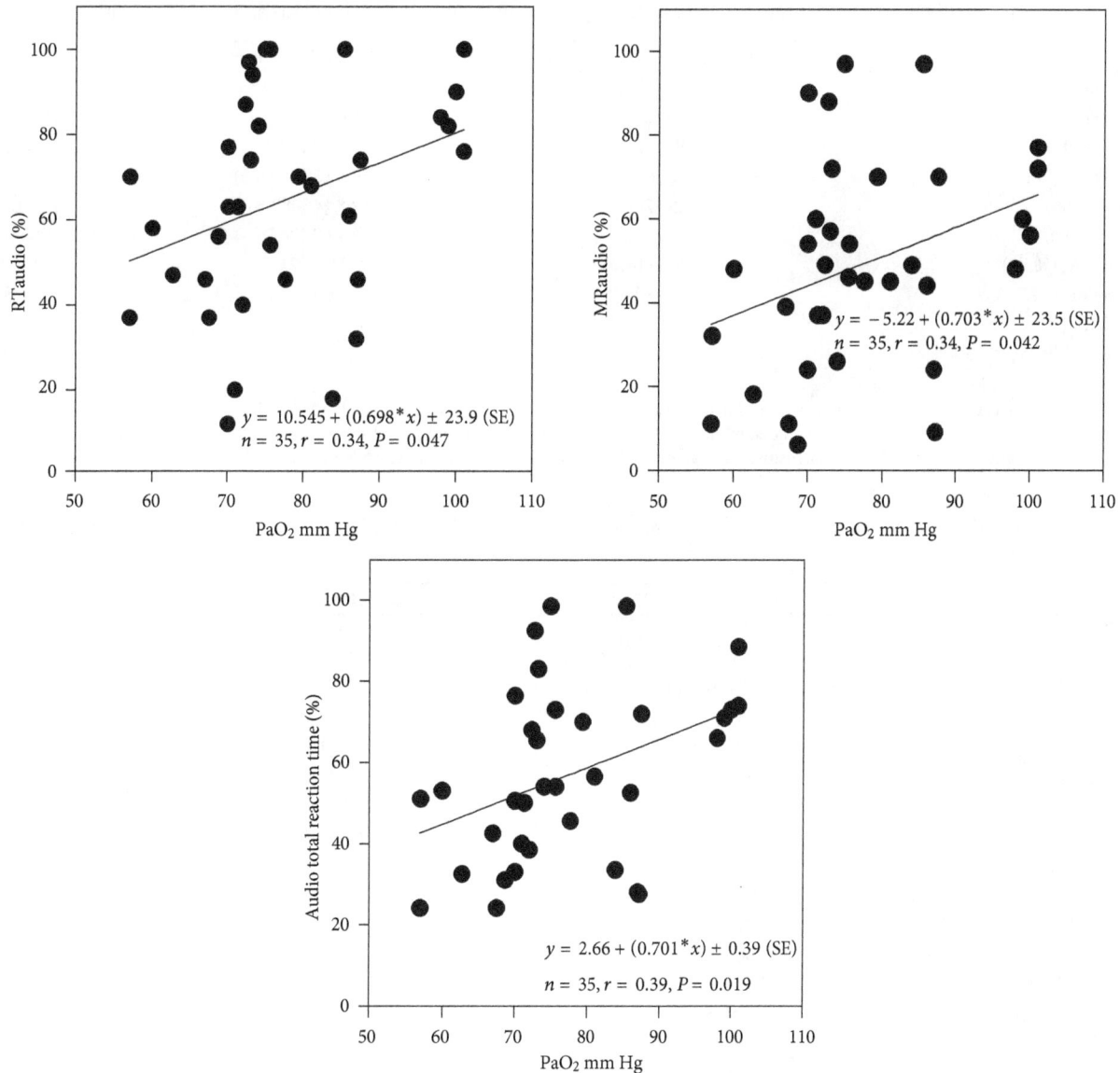

FIGURE 3: Relationship of PaO_2 to simple reaction time (RT-A%), motor reaction time (MR-A%), and total reaction time (total RT-A%) to audio stimuli.

According to the results of the tests, the subject is classified in a percentile of preexisting normative values of age-matched controls. Normative data exists from general adult population from all over Europe, of different social-economical and educational groups, with age distribution of 18–80 years old (http://www.schuhfried.at).

Control subjects and COPD patients were also evaluated according to Raven's intelligence test [15]. This IQ test consists of 60 items. Each item contains a figure with a missing piece and alternative pieces to complete the figure, only one of which is correct. The raw score is typically converted to a percentile rank by using the appropriate norms. Subjects had at their disposal 30 minutes to complete the test. Subjects with IQ scores <50% ile were not acceptable in order to avoid wrong answers in all other neuropsychological tests because of the difficulty to understand them.

In addition, both patients and control subjects underwent ophthalmologic and audiologic examinations before the tests to exclude hearing or visual deficits compromising the reliability and validity of neuropsychological testing.

According to the European diagnostic criteria for the assessment of driving ability based on the Vienna Test System, subjects have to pass all the tests in order to be classified as having adequate driving-related ability and obtain a professional driving licence. An expert in traffic psychology evaluates patients' performance on all the tests and identifies who are fit or unfit to drive [16].

2.7. Statistical Analysis. The statistical analysis and related graphs were performed using SigmaStat V3.5 and SigmaPlot V10.0 (Jandel Scientific, CA, USA). For comparisons between groups, the Student's unpaired *t*-test was used. If there was

TABLE 2: Driving-related neuropsychological testing performance data in normal subjects and COPD patients.

Parameters	Normal subjects ($n = 10$)	COPD patients ($n = 35$)	P value
SA, (% ile)	32.5 (19–39)	23.9 (9.3–34.8)	NS
RT-V, (% ile)	89 (82–89)	76 (53.8–88.5)	$P = 0.035$
MR-V, (% ile)	79.2 (12.2)	59.8 (18.7)	$P = 0.004$
Total RT-V, (% ile)	82 (79–87.5)	64.5 (59.3–76.5)	$P < 0.0001$
RT-A, (% ile)	84.5 (70–97)	68 (46–83.5)	$P = 0.035$
MR-A, (% ile)	72.6 (22)	49.2 (24.7)	$P = 0.01$
Total RT-A, (% ile)	78.3 (14.2)	56.9 (21.6)	$P = 0.0052$
PA, (% ile)	26.5 (17–38)	18 (6–34)	NS
TAVTMB, (% ile)	25 (21–62)	18 (7–24)	$P = 0.003$
Driving ability, accepted/rejected	8/2	13/22	$P = 0.029$

Values are mean ± SD or median (range).
Abbreviations: SA: selective attention; RT-V: reaction time to visual stimuli; MR-V: motor time to visual stimuli; Total RT-V: the sum of reaction and motor time to visual stimuli; RT-A: reaction time to audio stimuli; MR-A: motor time to audio stimuli; Total RT-A: the sum of reaction and motor time to audio stimuli; PA: permanent attention; TAVTMB: tachistoscopic traffic test; $P \le 0.05$, statistically significant; NS: nonsignificant.

TABLE 3: Characteristics and attention/alertness performance data for COPD patients who have been accepted and those who have been rejected as safe drivers.

	Rejected ($n = 22$)	Accepted ($n = 13$)	P
AGE, (yrs)	61.5 (6.6)	55.7 (6.6)	0.017
Ht, (m)	1.68 (0.1)	1.73 (0.1)	0.042
Wt, (% pred)	104.8 (92–117)	111 (96–122)	NS
BMI	26.1 (3.5)	27.1 (4)	NS
FVC, (% pred)	79.7 (18.7)	96.8 (18.2)	0.013
FEV_1, (% pred)	35.4 (14.9)	59.8 (24.5)	<0.001
FEV_1/FVC, %	45.6 (13)	63.2 (20.5)	0.004
IC, (% pred)	75.6 (13.4)	90.2 (20)	0.015
TLC, (% pred)	101 (16.6)	98.4 (10.4)	NS
RV, (% pred)	133.4 (47.6)	104.1 (20.3)	0.044
RV/TLC (%)	47.9 (10.6)	36.5 (8.9)	0.003
DLCO, (% pred)	50.6 (15.3)	74.8 (24)	<0.001
PaO_2 (mm Hg)	72.2 (68.7–79.3)	86 (74.9–99.3)	0.005
$PaCO_2$ (mm Hg)	41.6 (6)	38.7 (4.13)	NS
SaO_2, (%)	94.2 (2.3)	96.4 (1.9)	0.006
SpO_2, (%)	93.5 (2.4)	96.5 (2.0)	<0.001
mMRC, grade	3 (2–4)	1 (1–2.5)	0.002
IQ (% ile)	75 (50–85)	90 (80–95)	0.009
SA, (% ile)	19.5 (17.1)	36 (23.5)	0.021
RT-V, (% ile)	63.3 (27.9)	78.3 (14.1)	NS
MR-V, (% ile)	57.5 (20.8)	63.7 (14.5)	NS
Total RT-V, (% ile)	61.3 (47–75)	71.5 (65–80.5)	0.047
RT-A, (% ile)	59.5 (27.4)	73.2 (18.2)	NS
MR-A, (% ile)	47.2 (28.9)	52.6 (15.8)	NS
Total RT-A, (% ile)	53.4 (24.3)	62.9 (15)	NS
PA, (% ile)	8.5 (5–16)	43 (33.8–51.8)	<0.001
TAVTMB, (% ile)	9 (5–14)	25 (21–30)	<0.001

Values are mean (SD) or median (range).
Abbreviations as in Table 3.

no normality in the distribution in any of our parameters, a Mann-Whitney U-test for unpaired values was used. Where appropriate, Spearman correlation analysis, linear regression analysis, one-way ANOVA on ranks, multiple regression, and forward stepwise regression were used.

3. Results

All subjects' anthropometric and lung function data are shown in Table 1. Controls and COPD patients had comparable age, height, weight, BMI, and IQ. COPD patients were

$y = -27.923 + (0.65^{*}x) \pm 17.22$ (SE)
$n = 35, r = 0.42, P = 0.012$

$y = -23.063 + (0.515^{*}x) \pm 10.75$ (SE)
$n = 35, r = 0.5, P = 0.002$

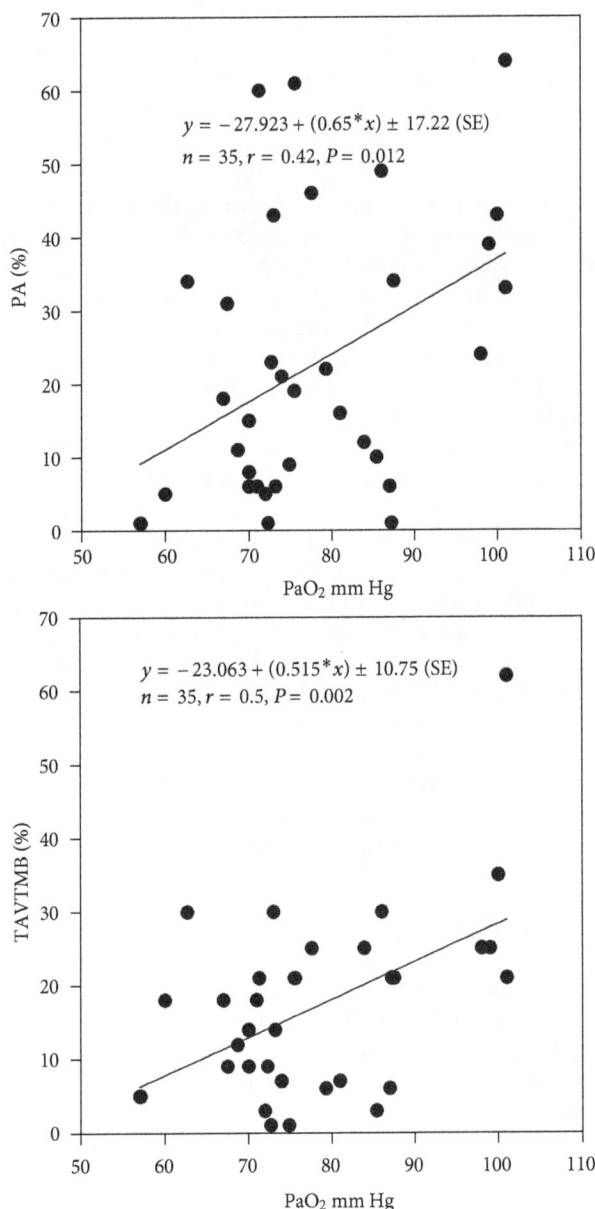

FIGURE 4: Relationship of PaO_2 to permanent attention (PA%) and tachistoscopic traffic (TAVTMB%) tests.

$y = 88.78 - (7.82^{*}x) \pm 22.86$ (SE)
$n = 35, r = 0.4, P = 0.016$

$y = 86.24 - (8.51^{*}x) \pm 22.92$ (SE)
$n = 35, r = 0.43, P = 0.01$

FIGURE 5: Relationship of dyspnea severity according to the modified Medical Research Council (mMRC) to reaction time to visual (RT-V%) and audio (RT-A%) stimuli.

significantly different to controls in pulmonary function data and oxygen saturation.

Table 2 summarises the results obtained in the attention/alertness battery of tests for the two groups. All the results are expressed as percentile of preexisting normative values. The faster the performance, the higher the score. Patients had significantly longer reaction and motor times in response to visual and acoustic stimuli and so, lower scores. They also presented significantly reduced visual perception (TAVTMB). Patients tended to score worse than controls for selective and permanent attention test, but this difference did not reach statistical significance. So, COPD patients scored worse than healthy volunteers in five of the seven neuropsychological tests for assessing driving-related performance.

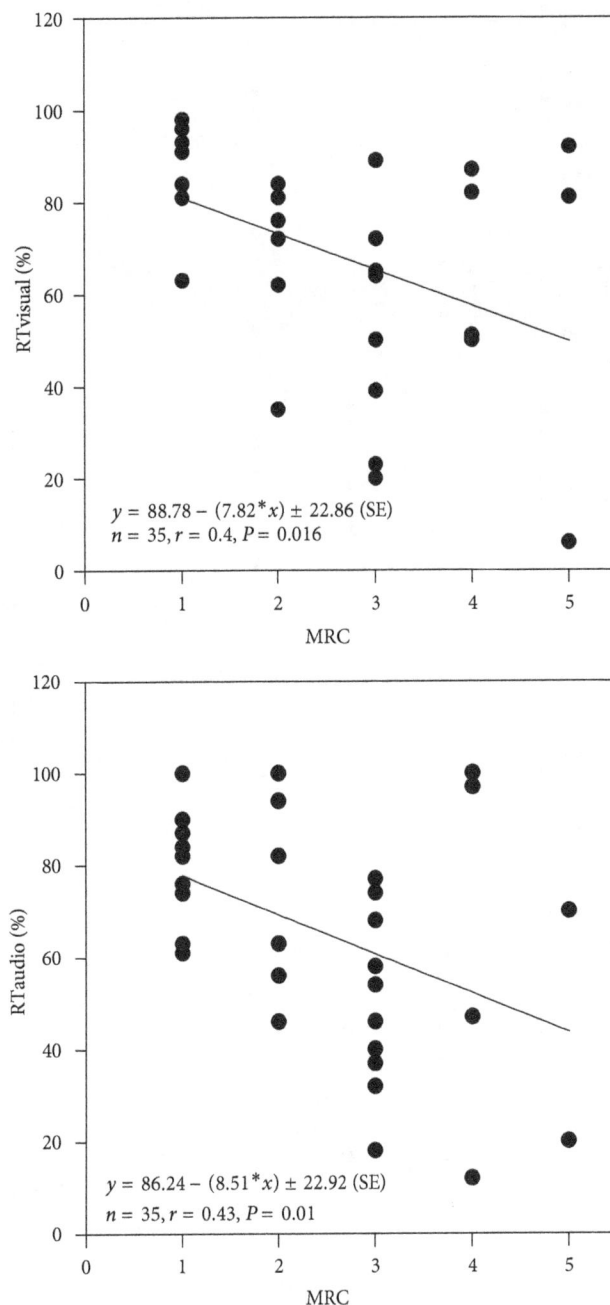

Among 35 COPD patients, only 13 successfully completed all the tests, and these 13 were classified as safe drivers. Among 10 controls, only 2 failed to complete all the tests and were classified as unsafe drivers ($P = 0.029$).

All neuropsychological tests were significantly ($P < 0.05$) correlated with PaO_2, except for the selective attention test (SA) (Figures 2, 3, and 4). SA test was correlated only with a lower IQ. The severity of dyspnea rated according to the mMRC score seems to influence significantly the performance on RT-V, RT-A, PA, and TAVTMB tests (Figures 5

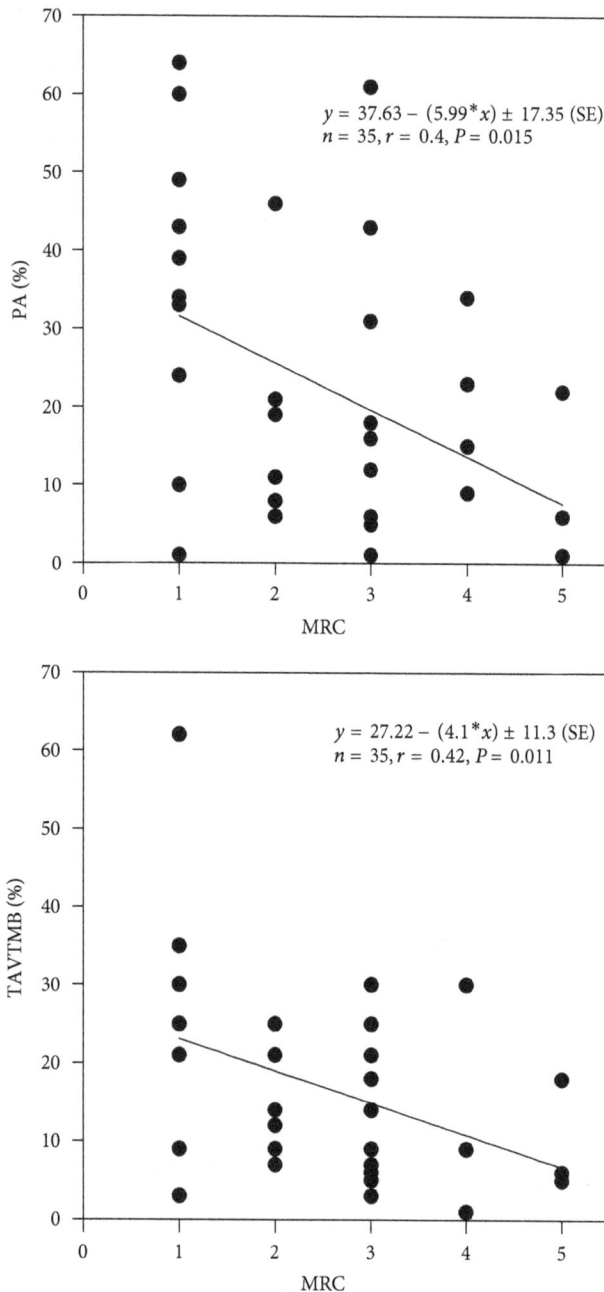

FIGURE 6: Relationship of dyspnea severity according to the modified Medical Research Council (mMRC) to permanent attention (PA%) and tachistoscopic traffic (TAVTMB%) tests.

and 6). The performance on the same tests, except for the PA test, was significantly correlated with FEV_1% pred (Figure 7). The effect of FEV_1 especially on visual perception (TAVTMB) can be verified if we divide patients into GOLD stages. In stage I, the median value of visual perception is 25%, the same as for the control group. In stage II, it is 21%, in stage III, 12%, and in stage IV, 9%. There is a statistically significant difference among the groups ($P < 0.003$).

With simple correlations, we could not find any effect of $PaCO_2$ on psychomotor tests. To further investigate the

real effect of PCO_2 on psychomotor performance, we divided our patients into two groups: those in whom PCO_2 was normal (≤ 45 mm Hg) ($n = 28$) and those whose PCO_2 was >45 mm Hg and were hypercapnic ($n = 7$). The two groups had similar scores on the tests except for the motor reaction time to visual and acoustic stimuli. Hypercapnic COPD patients scored lower than nonhypercapnic on these tests, and this difference remained significant after adjustment for potential confounders such as PaO_2 and age.

As we have already mentioned, randomly allocated, half of our patients ($n = 17$) have taken their daily dose of an inhaled drug (6 patients have taken a b_2 bronchodilator and 11 a combination of a b_2 bronchodilator and anticholinergic or corticosteriod) at least one hour before testing, and half of them have not taken it, at least 24 hours before testing ($n = 18$). The two groups showed no significant differences on the neuropsychological tests. So, it appears that bronchodilators do not influence driving-related psychomotor performance.

Finally, we divided the 35 COPD patients into two groups: those who have been accepted ($n = 13$ patients) and those who have been rejected ($n = 22$ patients) as safe drivers. The two groups showed statistically significant differences for PaO_2, SpO_2, FEV_1, FVC, IC, RV, and DLCO. They also showed statistically different scores in SA, total RT-V, PA, and TAVTMB tests (Table 3). They were not matched for age and IQ, and after correction for age and IQ with logistic regression, they remained different in the last two tests, that is, permanent attention and visual perception.

4. Discussion

In this study, we have shown that, except of the well-known cognitive dysfunction in severe hypoxemic patients [23–25], cognitive performance is also impaired in mildly hypoxemic COPD patients when compared to normal subjects matched for age, education level, and IQ. One of the main practical effects of this deterioration is the impairment of a patient's ability to perform tasks requiring increased vigilance and alertness like driving any kind of vehicle [26]. To the best of our knowledge, there are no reports dealing with the problem of impaired driving ability in COPD patients by using especially designed computer-based neuropsychological tests [27].

There are sparse publications and controversial reports for COPD patients with mild hypoxemia [9, 10]. The practical effect of the cognitive deterioration to the daily lives of these patients is still not known. Driving is an essential part of everyday life for most people, and the withholding of a private or professional driving licence has major implications for social functioning and employment. According to traffic psychology, accident proneness has strong relationships with a number of perceptual, cognitive, and motor skills. In our study, COPD patients demonstrated markedly delayed reaction times to visual or acoustic stimuli and impairments in motor activity and perceptive speed in traffic situations. These Subclinical neuropsychological deficits may explain the worse driving-related performance of COPD patients compared to normal subjects. More than half of our COPD

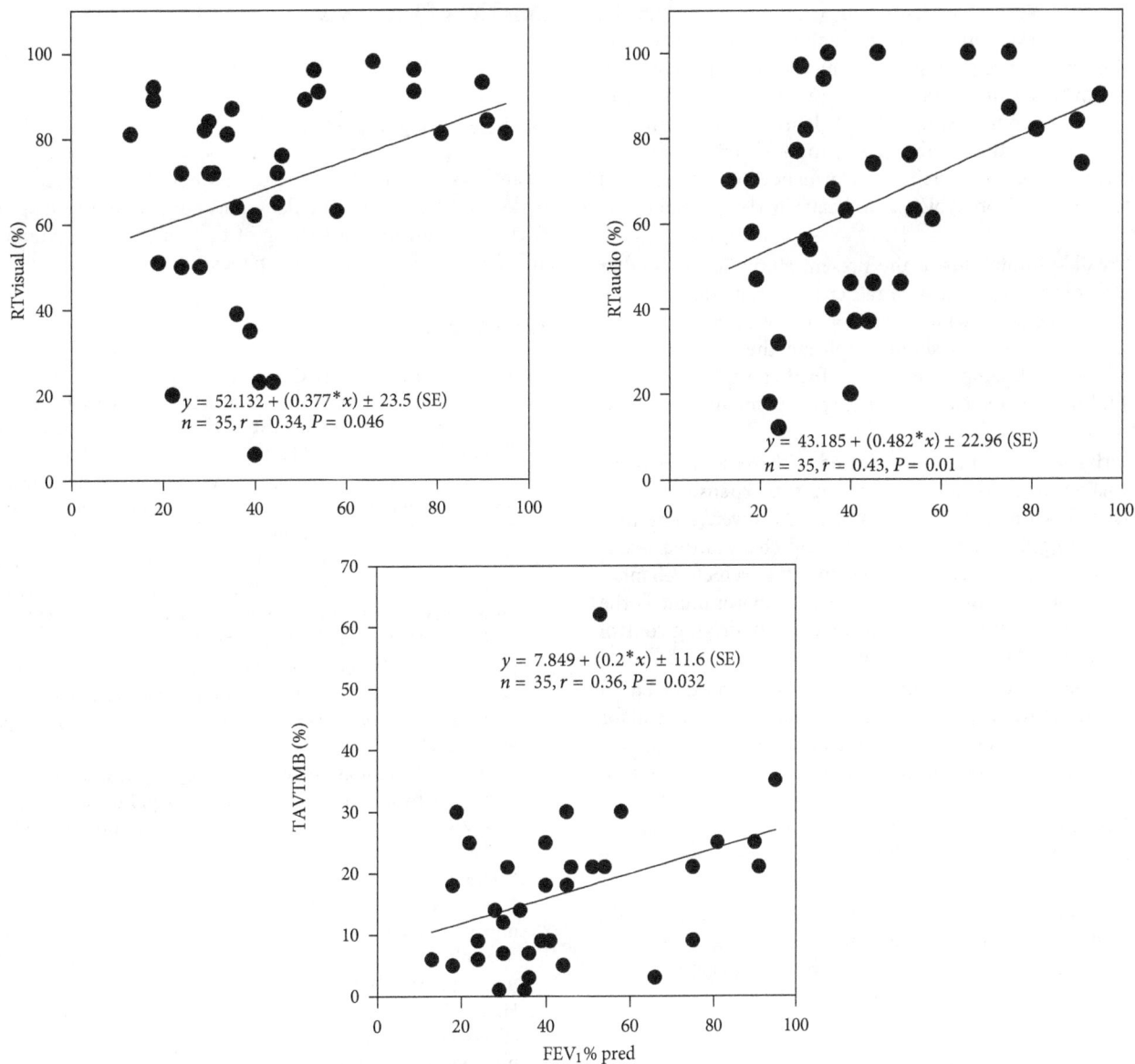

FIGURE 7: Relationship of $FEV_1\%$ pred to reaction time to visual (RT-V%) stimuli, reaction time to audio (RT-A) stimuli, and tachistoscopic traffic test (TAVTMB%).

patients (22/35) were classified as unsafe drivers based on failing to at least one from a battery of neuropsychological tests pertinent to any driving situation.

The explanation for the impaired functioning in COPD patients can be the mildly low levels of blood oxygenation, given the fact that the brain is the most sensitive organ to oxygen lack. This level of hypoxemia could lead to mild-to-moderate inefficiencies in neural functioning and thus to the modest subclinical impairment. In this study, we have included mildly hypoxemic patients ($PaO_2 > 55$ mm Hg); therefore, it is possible that a not fully normal PaO_2 or at the lower limits of normal (between 55–80 mm Hg) still leads to an impaired subclinical cognitive performance.

In addition, these patients usually have nocturnal desaturation or hypoxemia during sleep [27, 28], chronic pulmonary disease could enhance vascular disease, leading to reduced cerebral blood flow and oxygen consumption, even in normoxemic COPD patients, and COPD *per se* could lead to an acceleration of the aging process so that brain functions are impaired in a fashion similar to that seen in the elderly. This process could lead to a reduction in cortical neuronal density and a subsequent less efficient performance on neuropsychological tests. All these factors could be at work and have additive effects [29].

Impairments of cognitive performance in patients with COPD can be predicted on the basis of the severity of the disease. The partial pressure of arterial oxygen and the degree of pulmonary impairment may be major factors contributing to cognitive deficit among COPD patients. The partial pressure of arterial dioxide seems to affect the performance on motor reaction time to visual or acoustic stimuli, which require motor muscle activity. The muscle weakness that is frequently seen in patients with COPD may explain the previous observation [30]. However, the permanent attention test, another test requiring motor muscle performance, does not seem to be influenced by $PaCO_2$. So, impairments in motor ability cannot simply be explained by weak muscle activity. Irrespective of the cause, these deficits may have negative impact on driving performance of any kind of vehicle ranging from a bicycle to heavy lorries, in real traffic settings.

Possible limitations of the present study lie in whether these findings represent state rather than trait effects, which appears to be reasonable target for future research. In this sense, future research should replicate the main findings in independent samples as well as further explore whether the findings are associated in task-specific manner or across tasks.

Driving fitness may be assessed with reasonable accuracy using off-road tests minimizing the expense and risk associated with on road assessment. However, computer-based testing does not provide the real changes that occur when turning a steering wheel and the vehicle changes course. Also, missing in the laboratory environment is the subject's knowledge that the consequences of driving control responses affect his/her own safety.

Although there are disadvantages in computer-based testing, these are easy and simple tests that might be useful for giving insight about driving performance in COPD patients and make an important contribution to transport safety. These preliminary data need to be confirmed with further studies before simple computer-based testing can be used to decide whether or not an individual is safe to drive in every day life.

We conclude that probably stable COPD patients should be warned of the possible danger and risk they face when they drive any kind of vehicle, even when they do not exhibit overt symptoms related to driving ability.

Abbreviations

ATS:	American Thoracic Society
BMI:	Body mass index
COPD:	Chronic obstructive pulmonary disease
DLCO:	Lung diffusion capacity
FEV_1:	Forced expiratory volume in one second
FRC:	Functional residual capacity
GOLD:	The global initiative for chronic obstructive lung disease
IC:	Inspiratory capacity
IQ:	Intelligence quotient
mMRC:	Modified Medical Research Council
MR-A/MR-V:	Motor reaction time to audio/visual stimuli
PA:	Permanent attention
RT-A/RT-V:	Reaction time to audio/visual stimuli
RPM:	Raven's progressive matrices
SA:	Selective attention
TAVTMB:	Tachistoscopic traffic test
TLC:	Total lung capacity.

Conflict of Interests

The authors report no conflict of interests.

Authors' Contribution

All authors made measurements on the subjects participating in the study, analysed the data, and contributed in lengthy discussions during the writing of the paper. F. Karakontaki and N. G. Koulouris wrote the paper.

References

[1] R. A. Incalzi, A. Gemma, C. Marra, R. Muzzolon, O. Capparella, and P. Carbonin, "Chronic obstructive pulmonary disease: an original model of cognitive decline," *American Review of Respiratory Disease*, vol. 148, no. 2, pp. 418–424, 1993.

[2] M. Klein, S. Gauggel, G. Sachs, and W. Pohl, "Impact of chronic obstructive pulmonary disease (COPD) on attention functions," *Respiratory Medicine*, vol. 104, no. 1, pp. 52–60, 2010.

[3] W. W. Hung, J. P. Wisnivesky, A. L. Siu, and J. S. Ross, "Cognitive decline among patients with chronic obstructive pulmonary disease," *American Journal of Respiratory and Critical Care Medicine*, vol. 180, no. 2, pp. 134–137, 2009.

[4] A. J. Fix, C. J. Golden, and D. Daughton, "Neuropsychological deficits among patients with chronic obstructivepulmonary disease," *International Journal of Neuroscience*, vol. 16, no. 2, pp. 99–105, 1982.

[5] I. Grant, R. K. Heaton, and A. J. McSweeney, "Neuropsychologic findings in hypoxemic chronic obstructive pulmonary disease," *Archives of Internal Medicine*, vol. 142, no. 8, pp. 1470–1476, 1982.

[6] I. Grant, G. P. Prigatano, R. K. Heaton, A. J. McSweeny, E. C. Wright, and K. M. Adams, "Progressive neuropsychologic impairment and hypoxemia. Relationship in chronic obstructive pulmonary disease," *Archives of General Psychiatry*, vol. 44, no. 11, pp. 999–1006, 1987.

[7] H. D. Krop, A. J. Block, and E. Cohen, "Neuropsychologic effects of continuous oxygen therapy in chronic obstructive pulmonary disease," *Chest*, vol. 64, no. 3, pp. 317–322, 1973.

[8] R. K. Heaton, I. Grant, and A. J. McSweeny, "Psychologic effects of continuous and nocturnal oxygen therapy in hypoxemic chronic obstructive pulmonary disease," *Archives of Internal Medicine*, vol. 143, no. 10, pp. 1941–1947, 1983.

[9] G. P. Prigatano and A. et, "Neuropsychological test performance in mildly hypoxemic patients with chronic obstructive pulmonary disease," *Journal of Consulting and Clinical Psychology*, vol. 51, no. 1, pp. 108–116, 1983.

[10] J. J. W. Liesker, D. S. Postma, R. J. Beukema et al., "Cognitive performance in patients with COPD," *Respiratory Medicine*, vol. 98, no. 4, pp. 351–356, 2004.

[11] S. Mazza, J.-L. Pepin, B. Naegele et al., "Driving ability in sleep apnoea patients before and after CPAP treatment: evaluation on a road safety platform," *European Respiratory Journal*, vol. 28, no. 5, pp. 1020–1028, 2006.

[12] M. Juniper, M. A. Hack, C. F. George, R. J. O. Davies, and J. R. Stradling, "Steering simulation performance in patients with obstructive sleep apnoea and matched control subjects," *European Respiratory Journal*, vol. 15, no. 3, pp. 590–595, 2000.

[13] M. Orth, H.-W. Duchna, M. Leidag et al., "Driving simulator and neuropsychological testing in OSAS before and under

CPAP therapy," *European Respiratory Journal*, vol. 26, no. 5, pp. 898–903, 2005.

[14] Gold Report, Global Strategy for Diagnosis, Management, and Prevention of COPD, http;//www.goldcopd.org/, 2011.

[15] J. C. Raven, J. H. Court, and J. Raven, *Manual for Raven's Progressive Matrices*, HK Lewis, London, UK, 1976.

[16] "Directive 2007/59/EC of the European Parliament and the council on the certification of train drivers operating locomotives and trains on the railway system in the Community," *Official Journal of the European Union*, vol. L 315, pp. 51–78, 2007.

[17] M. R. Miller, J. Hankinson, V. Brusasco et al., "Series "ATS/ERS TASK FORCE: standardisation of lung function testing" standardisation of spirometry," *European Respiratory Journal*, vol. 26, no. 2, pp. 319–338, 2005.

[18] J. Wanger, J. L. Clausen, A. Coates et al., "Series "ATS/ERS TASK FORCE: standardisation of lung function testing" Standardisation of the measurement of lung volumes," *European Respiratory Journal*, vol. 26, no. 3, pp. 511–522, 2005.

[19] N. MacIntyre, R. O. Crapo, G. Viegi et al., "Series "ATS/ERS TASK FORCE: standardisation of lung function testing" Standardisation of the single-breath determination of carbon monoxide uptake in the lung," *European Respiratory Journal*, vol. 26, no. 4, pp. 720–735, 2005.

[20] Ph. H. Quanjer, Ed., "Standardized lung function testing. Report Working Party "Standardization of Lung Function Tests", European Community for Coal and Steel," *European Respiratory Journal*, vol. 6, supplement 16, pp. C1–C100, 1993.

[21] J. C. Bestall, E. A. Paul, R. Garrod, R. Garnham, P. W. Jones, and J. A. Wedzicha, "Usefulness of the Medical Research Council (MRC) dyspnoea scale as a measure of disability in patients with chronic obstructive pulmonary disease," *Thorax*, vol. 54, no. 7, pp. 581–586, 1999.

[22] G. Schuhfried, *Computer-Aided Procedures for Ability and Personality Diagnostics. Catalogue*, Modling, Vienna, Austria, 2001.

[23] M. Alchanatis, N. Zias, N. Deligiorgis, A. Amfilochiou, G. Dionellis, and D. Orphanidou, "Sleep apnea-related cognitive deficits and intelligence: an implication of cognitive reserve theory," *Journal of Sleep Research*, vol. 14, no. 1, pp. 69–75, 2005.

[24] K. M. J. Hynninen, M. H. Breitve, A. B. Wiborg, S. Pallesen, and I. H. Nordhus, "Psychological characteristics of patients with chronic obstructive pulmonary disease: a review," *Journal of Psychosomatic Research*, vol. 59, no. 6, pp. 429–443, 2005.

[25] A. R. Incalzi, F. Chiappini, L. Fuso, M. P. Torrice, A. Gemma, and R. Pistelli, "Predicting cognitive decline in patients with hypoxaemic COPD," *Respiratory Medicine*, vol. 92, no. 3, pp. 527–533, 1998.

[26] R. A. Incalzi, "Verbal memory impairment in COPD: its mechanisms and clinical relevance," *Chest*, vol. 112, no. 6, pp. 1506–1513, 1997.

[27] M. Orth, C. Diekmann, B. Suchan et al., "Driving performance in patients with chronic obstructive pulmonary disease," *Journal of Physiology and Pharmacology*, vol. 59, no. 6, pp. 539–547, 2008.

[28] P. M. A. Calverley, V. Brezinova, and N. J. Douglas, "The effect of oxygenation on sleep quality in chronic bronchitis and emphysema," *American Review of Respiratory Disease*, vol. 126, no. 2, pp. 206–210, 1982.

[29] W. Cormick, L. G. Olson, M. J. Hensley, and N. A. Saunders, "Nocturnal hypoxaemia and quality of sleep in patients with chronic obstructive lung disease," *Thorax*, vol. 41, no. 11, pp. 846–854, 1986.

[30] G. E. Gibson, W. Pulsinell, J. P. Blass, and T. E. Duffy, "Brain dysfunction in mild to moderate hypoxia," *American Journal of Medicine*, vol. 70, no. 6, pp. 1247–1254, 1981.

Differences between Risk Factors Associated with Tuberculosis Treatment Abandonment and Mortality

Nathália Mota de Faria Gomes,[1] **Meire Cardoso da Mota Bastos,**[1] **Renata Magliano Marins,**[1] **Aline Alves Barbosa,**[1] **Luiz Clóvis Parente Soares,**[1,2] **Annelise Maria de Oliveira Wilken de Abreu,**[1] **and João Tadeu Damian Souto Filho**[1,3]

[1]*Faculdade de Medicina de Campos (FMC), 28035-581 Campos dos Goytacazes, RJ, Brazil*
[2]*Programa de Controle da Tuberculose, Centro de Referência Augusto Guimarães, 28085-500 Campos dos Goytacazes, RJ, Brazil*
[3]*Instituto Federal de Educação, Ciência e Tecnologia Fluminense (IFF), 28060-010 Campos dos Goytacazes, RJ, Brazil*

Correspondence should be addressed to João Tadeu Damian Souto Filho; drjoaotadeu@yahoo.com.br

Academic Editor: Sebastian L. Johnston

Objectives. To identify the risk factors that were associated with abandonment of treatment and mortality in tuberculosis (TB) patients. *Methods.* This study was a retrospective longitudinal cohort study involving tuberculosis patients treated between 2002 and 2008 in a TB reference center. *Results.* A total of 1,257 patients were evaluated, with 69.1% men, 54.4% under 40 years of age, 18.9% with extrapulmonary disease, and 9.3% coinfected with HIV. The risk factors that were associated with abandonment of treatment included male gender (OR = 2.05; 95% CI = 1.15–3.65) and nonadherence to previous treatment (OR = 3.14; 95% CI = 1.96–5.96). In addition, the presence of extrapulmonary TB was a protective factor (OR = 0.33, 95% CI = 0.14–0.76). The following risk factors were associated with mortality: age over 40 years (OR = 2.61, 95% CI = 1.76–3.85), coinfection with HIV (OR = 6.01, 95% CI = 3.78–9.56), illiteracy (OR = 1.88, 95% CI = 1.27–2.75), the presence of severe extrapulmonary TB (OR = 2.33, 95% CI = 1.24–4.38), and retreatment after relapse (OR = 1.95, 95% CI = 1.01–3.75). *Conclusions.* Male gender and retreatment after abandonment were independent risk factors for nonadherence to TB treatment. Furthermore, age over 40 years, coinfection with HIV, illiteracy, severe extrapulmonary TB, and retreatment after relapse were associated with higher TB mortality. Therefore, we suggest the implementation of direct measures that will control the identified risk factors to reduce the rates of treatment failure and TB-associated mortality.

1. Introduction

Tuberculosis (TB) still represents a major public health problem, especially in developing countries. TB is an infectious disease that is difficult to control because the disease is transmitted through the air. The etiological agent of TB is *Mycobacterium tuberculosis* (MTB), and the disease is characterized by granulomas and the presence of a cell-mediated hypersensitivity reaction [1].

TB mainly affects economically active age groups, which causes problems for the individual as well as community health and results in higher public spending [2]. An estimated one-third of the world's population is infected with TB. In 2011, TB affected 8.4 million people, and the disease caused 1.4 million deaths worldwide [3].

Currently, Brazil ranks fourteenth among the 22 high-burden countries for TB. In 2011, the TB incidence in Brazil was 36 cases per 100,000 inhabitants, and 69,245 new cases were recorded. TB is a major cause of morbidity and mortality in Brazil. This disease is the fourth leading cause of death among infectious diseases, with the estimated annual death rate of 2.4 cases per 100,000 inhabitants in 2010 [3].

The main risk factors that have been identified as predictors of increased mortality in individuals with TB are as follows: irregular or inadequate treatment, delayed diagnosis, multidrug resistance, coinfection with human immunodeficiency virus (HIV), and advanced age [4]. Nonadherence to treatment is a major problem in the management of TB and in the treatment of any chronic disease. TB has characteristics that affect treatment adherence and creates a health challenge. In addition, the treatment of TB is long-term one and requires the administration of various medications. Moreover, despite the frequent adverse effects of the treatment, patients feel physically well before the end of the medication cycle and are thus tempted to abandon treatment [5].

Low adherence is the major cause of treatment failure and drug resistance. Previous studies have demonstrated that the expense of traveling to treatment centers, the male gender, patients with little information about the disease, difficult communication with patients, alcoholism, and homelessness are the main determinants of nonadherence to TB treatment [6]. Patient adherence to standard treatment in developing countries is estimated to be less than 40% [7].

The aim of this study was to determine the epidemiologic profile of TB patients who were undergoing treatment in the city of Campos dos Goytacazes, Rio de Janeiro (RJ), by analyzing the risk factors that were associated with abandonment of treatment and mortality.

2. Materials and Methods

A retrospective longitudinal cohort study was conducted by the Tuberculosis Control Program (TCP) at the Augusto Guimarães Reference Center, Municipal Health Department, in Campos dos Goytacazes, RJ. This city is located in the northern region of RJ and is to be the second largest rural city in the state and the tenth largest rural city in Brazil, with a population of 468,087 inhabitants in 2011 according to the Brazilian Institute of Geography and Statistics (Instituto Brasileiro de Geografia e Estatística, IBGE). However, the population is now estimated to exceed 600,000 inhabitants due to the development of the oil industry.

A total of 1,257 medical records from patients, including both genders and all ages, who were treated at the TCP from 01/01/2002 to 12/31/2008 were evaluated. A protocol that was adapted from the Notifiable Diseases Information System (Sistema de Informações de Agravos de Notificação, SINAN) [8], which is a database of the Ministry of Health of Brazil, was used for data collection. This protocol included the collection of information on sociodemographic, epidemiologic, clinical, and laboratory data. The following variables were studied: age (over or under 40 years); gender (male and female); level of education (literate and illiterate); address (urban or rural); TB involvement upon entry into treatment or closure of the case [9]; institutionalization (detention facilities and nursing homes); clinical type (pulmonary and extrapulmonary); comorbidities (alcoholism, smoking, cardiovascular disease, diabetes mellitus (DM), neoplasia, lung diseases, and coinfection with HIV); chest radiography (suspicious, normal, or not performed); tuberculin skin test (TST); sputum smear microscopy; sputum culture; and histopathology.

The definition of the TB cases that were treated by the TCP was based on the following World Health Organization (WHO) classification: new case, treatment after abandonment, treatment after relapse, and transferred-in cost.

Extrapulmonary TB cases were defined as having compatible histopathology or positive culture for MTB associated with a negative sputum smear and culture in respiratory secretions [10, 11]. In this study, the following types of TB were considered to be severe extrapulmonary TB: meningeal, miliary, pericardial, peritoneal, bilateral or extensive pleural effusion, spinal, genitourinary, and intestinal types [9].

Statistical analyses were performed to evaluate the association between the characteristics of the TB patients and the risk for treatment failure, which was based on two outcomes: abandonment of treatment and mortality. In the univariate analysis, the chi-squared test or Fisher's exact test was used for the categorical variables. The variables with $p < 0.10$ in the univariate analysis were included in a multivariate logistic regression model. A $p < 0.05$ was considered statistically significant. The data were analyzed using SPSS 22.0 for Windows (Statistical Package for the Social Sciences, Chicago, IL, USA).

The study was reviewed and approved by the Research Ethics Committee of Faculdade de Medicina de Campos, Campos dos Goytacazes, Rio de Janeiro, Brazil. In this study, institutional consent was obtained for record review and all patient information was anonymized and deidentified prior to analysis.

3. Results

A total of 1,257 medical records were evaluated from subjects who were treated by the TCP from 2002 to 2008. The clinical and epidemiologic characteristics of the patients are shown in Table 1. The sample consisted of 868 (69.1%) men and 389 (30.9%) women, and the gender ratio was 2.2 : 1, male to female. In total, 673 (54.4%) patients were under 40 years of age, 314 (25%) patients were illiterate, and 1,107 (88.1%) patients lived in an urban area.

Regarding the TB type, 1,020 (81.1%) patients had pulmonary disease and 237 (18.9%) patients extrapulmonary disease. Among those with extrapulmonary disease, pleural TB and lymph node were the most prevalent types and represented 8.2% and 4.9% of the cases, respectively. The presence of coinfection with HIV was observed in 117 (9.3%) individuals. Overall, 842 (67%) individuals had HIV serological results available, 30 (2.4%) individuals had HIV serology that was still being processed, and 386 (30.7%) individuals were not screened for HIV. Among the patients with extrapulmonary TB, 33 (28.2%) had serological results that were positive for HIV. The univariate analysis revealed a significant association between extrapulmonary TB and HIV infection ($p = 0.006$; OR = 1.81, 95% CI 1.15–2.84).

Table 2 shows the analysis of the risk factors that were associated with abandonment of treatment. In the univariate analysis, male gender, alcoholism and a history of previous abandonment of treatment correlated with an increased risk of non-adherence to current treatment, whereas the presence of extrapulmonary TB, diabetes and other comorbidities were found to be protective factors. However, in the multivariate analysis, the variables that remained significant risk factors for abandonment of treatment were male gender (OR = 2.05; 95% CI 1.15–3.65) and non-adherence to previous treatment (OR = 3.14; 95% CI 1.96–5.96). Having extrapulmonary TB was found to be a protective factor (OR = 0.33; 95% CI 0.14–0.76).

TABLE 1: Characteristics of patients with tuberculosis.

Characteristics	Study population	
	$n = 1257$	(%)
Year of diagnosis		
2002	200	(15.9)
2003	195	(15.5)
2004	198	(15.8)
2005	173	(13.8)
2006	179	(14.3)
2007	142	(11.3)
2008	169	(13.5)
Age[*]		
<40 years	673	(54.4)
>40 years	565	(45.6)
Gender		
Female	389	(30.9)
Male	868	(69.1)
HIV coinfection		
No	1140	(90.7)
Yes	117	(9.3)
Alcoholic		
No	1122	(89.3)
Yes	135	(10.7)
Literacy		
Yes	943	(75.0)
No	314	(25.0)
Treatment in the same city of residence		
Yes	1080	(85.9)
No	177	(14.1)
Area		
Countryside	150	(11.9)
Urban area	1107	(88.1)
Institutionalized patients		
No	1204	(95.8)
Yes	53	(4.2)
Cigarette smoking		
No	1165	(92.7)
Yes	92	(7.3)
Comorbidity		
No	1128	(89.7)
Yes	129	(10.3)
Diabetes	79	(6.3)
Lung mycoses	10	(0.8)
Neoplasia	9	(0.7)
COPD	9	(0.7)
Pneumoconiosis	5	(0.4)
Extrapulmonary TB		
No	1020	(81.1)
Yes	237	(18.9)
Pleural	103	(8.2)
Lymph node	62	(4.9)

TABLE 1: Continued.

Characteristics	Study population	
	$n = 1257$	(%)
Genitourinary	8	(0.6)
Bones	12	(1.0)
Ocular	9	(0.7)
Miliary	16	(1.3)
Meningitis	6	(0.5)
Cutaneous	3	(0.2)
Laryngeal	4	(0.3)
Others	14	(1.1)
Chest X-ray examination		
Suspicious	1093	(87.0)
Normal	121	(9.6)
Other/not done	43	(3.4)
Tuberculin testing		
Negative	176	(14)
Weakly positive	29	(2.3)
Strongly positive	246	(19.6)
Not done	806	(64.1)
Case definition		
New case	1071	(85.2)
Treatment after relapse	69	(5.5)
Treatment after abandonment	106	(8.4)
Transferred-in cost	11	(0.9)

[*] Missing data in 19 patients.

The risk factors that were associated with mortality during TB treatment are presented in Table 3. In the univariate and multivariate analyses, the risk factors that were associated with a higher mortality were as follows: age over 40 years (OR = 2.61; 95% CI 1.76–3.85), coinfection with HIV (OR = 6.01; 95% CI 3.78–9.56), illiteracy (OR = 1.88; 95% CI 1.27–2.75), the presence of severe extrapulmonary TB (OR = 2.33; 95% CI 1.24–4.38), and retreatment after relapse (OR = 1.95; 95% CI 1.01–3.75). Comorbidities and institutionalization were correlated with mortality in the univariate analysis but lost statistical significance in the multivariate analysis.

4. Discussion

In most countries, greater numbers of men are diagnosed with TB than women, and men have a higher death rate from TB. This quantitative difference between the sexes is partly due to epidemiological factors, especially the risk of exposure to the infection and the progression from infection to the disease stage [12].

In this study, the statistically significant risk factors that were associated with treatment failure included male gender and retreatment after treatment abandonment, whereas extrapulmonary TB was a protective factor against treatment failure.

The high prevalence of TB in males and the poor adherence to treatment in males may be due to increased exposure to situations of risk for MTB infection, such as interpersonal

TABLE 2: Univariate and multivariate analyses of risk factors associated with TB treatment abandonment.

Characteristics	Abandonment				Univariate		Multivariate	
	Yes $n = 84$	(%)	No $n = 1173$	(%)	OR (95% CI)	p	OR (95% CI)	p
Age								
<40 years	52	(62.7)	621	(53.8)	1.0			
>40 years	31	(37.3)	534	(46.2)	0.69 (0.43–1.12)	ns		
Gender								
Female	15	(17.9)	374	(31.9)	1.0			
Male	69	(82.1)	799	(68.1)	2.15 (1.18–3.98)	0.007	2.05 (1.15–3.65)	0.015
HIV coinfection								
No	76	(90.5)	1064	(90.7)	1.0			
Yes	8	(9.5)	109	(9.3)	1.03 (0.45–2.27)	ns		
Alcoholic								
No	68	(81.0)	1054	(89.9)	1.0			
Yes	16	(19.0)	119	(10.1)	2.08 (1.12–3.83)	0.011	—	ns
Literacy								
Yes	62	(73.8)	881	(75.1)	1.0			
No	22	(26.2)	292	(24.9)	1.07 (0.63–1.82)	ns		
Treatment in the same city of residence								
Yes	70	(83.3)	1010	(86.1)	1.0			
No	14	(16.7)	163	(13.9)	1.24 (0.65–2.32)	ns		
Area								
Countryside	8	(9.5)	142	(12.1)	1.0			
Urban area	76	(90.5)	1031	(87.9)	1.31 (0.60–2.99)	ns		
Institutionalized								
No	80	(95.2)	1124	(95.8)	1.0			
Yes	4	(4.8)	49	(4.2)	1.15 (0.34–3.42)	ns		
Extrapulmonary TB								
No	78	(92.9)	942	(80.3)	1.0			
Yes	6	(7.1)	231	(19.7)	0.31 (0.12–0.76)	0.005	0.33 (0.14–0.76)	0.010
Severe extrapulmonary TB*								
No	83	(98.8)	1103	(94.0)	1.0			
Yes	1	(1.2)	70	(6.0)	0.19 (0.00–1.12)	ns		
Diabetes								
No	83	(98.8)	1095	(93.4)	1.0			
Yes	1	(1.2)	78	(6.6)	0.17 (0.00–0.99)	0.046	—	ns
Cigarette smoking								
No	76	(90.5)	1089	(92.8)	1.0			
Yes	8	(9.5)	84	(7.2)	1.36 (0.59–3.05)	ns		
Comorbidity								
No	81	(96.4)	1047	(89.3)	1.0			
Yes	3	(3.6)	126	(10.7)	0.31 (0.06–0.96)	0.036	—	ns
Treatment after relapse								
No	81	(96.4)	1107	(94.4)	1.0			
Yes	3	(3.6)	66	(5.6)	0.62 (0.12–1.97)	ns		
Treatment after abandonment								
No	64	(76.2)	1087	(92.7)	1.0			
Yes	20	(23.8)	86	(7.3)	3.95 (2.20–7.05)	<0.001	3.41 (1.96–5.96)	<0.001

*Meningitis, miliary, pericarditis, peritonitis, bilateral or extensive pleural effusion, spinal, genitourinary, and intestinal types.
ns: not significant.

TABLE 3: Univariate and multivariate analyses of risk factors associated with death during TB treatment.

Characteristics	Death				Univariate		Multivariate	
	Yes $n = 146$	(%)	No $n = 1111$	(%)	OR (95% CI)	p	OR (95% CI)	p
Age								
<40 years	48	(34.0)	625	(57.0)	1.0			
>40 years	93	(66.0)	472	(43.0)	2.57 (1.75–3.77)	<0.001	2.61 (1.76–3.85)	<0.001
Gender								
Female	38	(26.0)	351	(31.6)	1.0			
Male	108	(74.0)	760	(68.4)	1.31 (0.87–1.98)	ns		
HIV coinfection								
No	106	(72.6)	1034	(93.1)	1.0			
Yes	40	(27.4)	77	(6.9)	5.07 (3.22–7.97)	<0.001	6.01 (3.78–9.56)	<0.001
Alcoholic								
No	127	(87.0)	995	(89.6)	1.0			
Yes	19	(13.0)	116	(10.4)	1.28 (0.74–2.21)	ns		
Literacy								
Yes	89	(61.0)	854	(76.9)	1.0			
No	57	(39.0)	257	(23.1)	2.13 (1.46–3.10)	<0.001	1.88 (1.27–2.78)	0.002
Treatment in the same city of residence								
Yes	119	(81.5)	961	(86.5)	1.0			
No	27	(18.5)	150	(13.5)	1.45 (0.90–2.33)	ns		
Area								
Countryside	12	(8.2)	138	(12.4)	1.0			
Urban area	134	(91.8)	973	(87.6)	1.58 (0.83–3.09)	ns		
Institutionalized								
No	145	(99.3)	1059	(95.3)	1.0			
Yes	1	(0.7)	52	(4.7)	0.14 (0.00–0.83)	0.024	—	ns
Extrapulmonary TB								
No	116	(79.5)	904	(81.4)	1.0			
Yes	30	(20.5)	207	(18.6)	1.13 (0.72–1.77)	ns		
Severe extrapulmonary TB*								
No	130	(89.0)	1056	(95.0)	1.0			
Yes	16	(11.0)	55	(5.0)	2.36 (1.26–4.39)	0.003	2.33 (1.24–4.38)	0.009
Diabetes								
No	136	(93.2)	1042	(93.8)	1.0			
Yes	10	(6.8)	69	(6.2)	1.10 (0.52–2.29)	ns		
Cigarette smoking								
No	139	(95.2)	1026	(92.3)	1.0			
Yes	7	(4.8)	85	(7.7)	0.61 (0.23–1.34)	ns		
Comorbidity								
No	121	(82.9)	1007	(90.6)	1.0			
Yes	25	(17.1)	104	(9.4)	2.00 (1.21–3.29)	0.004	—	ns
Treatment after relapse								
No	131	(89.7)	1057	(95.1)	1.0			
Yes	15	(10.3)	54	(4.9)	2.24 (1.17–4.22)	0.007	1.95 (1.01–3.75)	0.046
Treatment after abandonment								
No	132	(90.4)	1019	(91.7)	1.0			
Yes	14	(9.6)	92	(8.3)	1.17 (0.62–2.19)	ns		

*Meningitis, miliary, pericarditis, peritonitis, bilateral or extensive pleural effusion, spinal, genitourinary, and intestinal types.
ns: not significant.

and social interaction for socioeconomic and cultural reasons. In addition, men may delay seeking treatment at health clinics when their physical conditions worsen. By contrast, women demonstrated a greater adherence to TB treatment, and female gender was not associated with the risk factors for death [13, 14].

Resistance that arises from the irregular intake of medication depends on several cycles of bacterial death (when the drugs are ingested) and bacterial growth (when they are suspended). In each cycle, there is a selection that favors drug-resistant mutants, which is detrimental to sensitive populations of patients [15]. Initially, resistance occurs to a medication in the treatment regimen, followed by the development of resistance to other medications, leading to multiresistance [16]. This scenario of bacterial resistance combined with the possible social vulnerability of the TB carrier leads to treatment failure in the outcomes of these individuals.

Extrapulmonary TB is a protective factor against treatment failure because this TB type is associated with less drug resistance. Studies that were conducted in Europe demonstrated favorable outcomes in 81% and 68% of patients with extrapulmonary TB [17, 18]. The results from these studies corroborate the results that were found in this study. In human TB disease, cavitary lung lesions contain mycobacteria populations that range from 107 to 108 bacilli, whereas the population ranges from 102 to 104 bacilli in hardened caseous lesions [19]. Drug resistance is more common in the cavitary type of TB [19, 20]. An increase in the bacterial population results in an increased probability of resistance in pretreatment. In most types of extrapulmonary TB, the initial bacilli population is smaller than that in cavitary pulmonary TB; therefore, the probability that preexisting resistant mutants are present is lower.

Previous studies have found that alcohol abuse [21] and comorbidities, especially DM [22], are the relevant risk factors that are associated with treatment failure. However, we did not find these same associations in our analysis.

Regarding the risk factors that were associated with mortality, we found that the following variables were relevant: age over 40 years, illiteracy, severe extrapulmonary TB, coinfection with HIV, and retreatment after relapse.

Advanced age represents a factor that is associated with an increased risk of death [23]. In this study, advanced age was associated with an aging population and the effectiveness of the TB control programs, which contributed to the reduction of mortality in the younger age group. Furthermore, individuals over 40 years of age have a greater number of associated comorbidities that require the use of other medications, which may predispose these individuals to the irregular intake of specific medications and enable drug resistance. Therefore, directly observed treatment (DOT) should be established for these patients to decrease abandonment of treatment, mortality, and multidrug resistance.

A lack of education is correlated with poor social conditions, lower perception of health problems, less self-care, and delay in seeking health services. Even when patients are on treatment, a lack of education can lead to the abandonment and misuse of medications. Because TB is a social disease,

there is a greater incidence of cases and deaths in the social classes with lower socioeconomic status and less education [24].

Retreatment after a relapse may occur for exogenous reinfection or endogenous reactivation of pulmonary or extrapulmonary lesions. A study that was conducted in Southern Brazil [25] found that the recurrence rate correlated with the irregular use of medications. An incomplete bacteriological cure is the most important cause of endogenous reactivation, which is usually caused by the irregular intake of medications. Excluding the presence of preexisting resistance, reactivation may result from the use of regimens with low bactericidal potency, an inadequate length of treatment, an underdose in the drug prescription, or an inappropriate choice of medication [26].

The improper use of medication increases the relapse rate and the probability of drug resistance as demonstrated by previous studies. These effects can lead to a higher rate of mortality in individuals who undergo retreatment compared with treatment-naïve patients and a higher rate of treatment failure in individuals who undergo retreatment after treatment abandonment as indicated in this study.

The Acquired Immune Deficiency Syndrome (AIDS) epidemic has changed TB prognoses because coinfection with HIV has a greater impact on TB mortality than on TB incidence [27]. Studies have indicated that HIV-TB coinfection increases the chance that patients receive inadequate treatment, which leads to multidrug resistance and increased mortality [28, 29].

In our study, we found a strong association between extrapulmonary TB and HIV infection. Extrapulmonary TB is mainly the result of the reactivation of an outbreak of TB after hematogenous or lymphatic dissemination [30]. HIV patients have natural killer cells that are less cytotoxic [31]; therefore, patients with this immunodeficiency are more likely to develop extrapulmonary TB.

We found that severe extrapulmonary TB is an important risk factor that was associated with increased mortality because this disease may be associated with a greater systemic impact. In addition, severe extrapulmonary TB represents a diagnostic challenge for physicians because the diagnoses and treatments are often delayed [32].

The characteristics of the population in this study are quite similar to those presented in studies involving individuals with tuberculosis throughout Brazil. It is mainly represented by young men with low educational level, similar frequencies of institutionalization, extrapulmonary manifestations, and HIV coinfection [33]. This fact allows us to suspect that the risk factors identified in this study can be used in the evaluation of patients with TB in other parts of Brazil and countries with similar socioeconomic characteristics.

Similar to the analysis conducted in this study, an analysis of the risk factors in different countries and regions is important to detect treatment failure and suggest specific changes in the therapeutic approach to TB. Multidisciplinary patient care, emphasis on patient care, health education using DOT, socioeconomic development, and expansion of HIV serological testing will reduce the current rates of treatment abandonment and mortality in TB.

A limitation of this study is the retrospective design of the analysis because only the risk factors that were identified in the medical records were evaluated. However, this lack of data is common in retrospective studies and its impact was minimized by the availability of standardized medical records and the systematic care of the patients, which was centralized.

5. Conclusion

This study revealed that male gender and retreatment after treatment abandonment are independent risk factors for nonadherence to TB treatment. In addition, age over 40 years, coinfection with HIV, illiteracy, severe extrapulmonary TB, and retreatment after relapse were significantly associated with increased TB-related mortality. Therefore, we suggest the implementation of direct measures that will control the identified risk factors to reduce the rates of treatment abandonment and death during TB treatment.

Conflict of Interests

The authors have no conflict of interests to declare.

References

[1] M. L. Campos, Z. M. Cipriano, A. M. N. F. Stamm, and K. S. Tratsk, "Tuberculose," *Revista Brasileira de Medicina*, vol. 57, no. 6, pp. 505–518, 2000.

[2] Central TB Division. TB India, *RNTCP Status Report. Directorate of Health Services*, Ministry of Health and Family Welfare, New Delhi, India, 2004.

[3] A. Costa, "ONU elogia Brasil por suas ações de controle da Tuberculose," 2012, http://portalsaude.saude.gov.br/portalsaude/noticia/4710/24/onu-elogia-brasil-por-suas-acoes-de-controle-da-tuberculose.html.

[4] M. H. H. Pelaquin, R. S. E. Silva, and S. A. Ribeiro, "Factors associated with death from tuberculosis in the eastern part of the city of São Paulo, 2001," *Jornal Brasileiro de Pneumologia*, vol. 33, no. 3, pp. 311–317, 2007.

[5] M. McLean, "Adherence to treatment," in *Guidelines for TB Control in New Zealand*, p. 541, Ministry of Health, Wellington, New Zealand, 2003.

[6] S. J. O'Boyle, J. J. Power, M. Y. Ibrahim, and J. P. Watson, "Factors affecting patient compliance with anti-tuberculosis chemotherapy using the directly observed treatment, short-course strategy (DOTS)," *The International Journal of Tuberculosis and Lung Disease*, vol. 6, no. 4, pp. 307–312, 2002.

[7] M. S. Al-Hajjaj and I. M. Al-Khatim, "High rate of non-compliance with anti-tuberculosis treatment despite a retrieval system: a call for implementation of directly observed therapy in Saudi Arabia," *The International Journal of Tuberculosis and Lung Disease*, vol. 4, no. 4, pp. 345–349, 2000.

[8] SINAN, "Tuberculose—Casos confirmados notificados no Sistema de Informação de Agravos de Notificação," 2011, http://dtr2004.saude.gov.br/sinanweb/tabnet/dh?sinan/tuberculose/bases/tubercbr.def.

[9] World Health Organization, International Union Against Tuberculosis and Lung Disease, and Royal Netherlands Tuberculosis Association, "Revised international definitions in tuberculosis control," *The International Journal of Tuberculosis and Lung Disease*, vol. 5, no. 3, pp. 213–215, 2001.

[10] T. Vasankari, M. Kokki, P. Holmström, K. Liippo, S. Sarna, and P. Ruutu, "Great diversity of tuberculosis treatment in Finland," *Eurosurveillance*, vol. 12, no. 1, pp. 17–21, 2007.

[11] T. Vasankari, P. Holmström, J. Ollgren, K. Liippo, M. Kokki, and P. Ruutu, "Risk factors for poor tuberculosis treatment outcome in Finland: a cohort study," *BMC Public Health*, vol. 7, article 291, 2007.

[12] C. P. Howson, P. F. Harrison, D. Hotra, and M. Law, *In Her Lifetime: Female Morbidity and Mortality in Sub-Saharan Africa*, National Academy Press, Washington, DC, USA, 1996.

[13] M. W. Uplekar, S. Rangan, M. G. Weiss, J. Ogden, M. W. Borgdorff, and P. Hudelson, "Attention to gender issues in tuberculosis control," *International Journal of Tuberculosis and Lung Disease*, vol. 5, no. 3, pp. 220–224, 2001.

[14] M. Chan-Yeung, K. Noertjojo, S. L. Chan, and C. M. Tam, "Sex differences in tuberculosis in Hong Kong," *International Journal of Tuberculosis and Lung Disease*, vol. 6, no. 1, pp. 11–18, 2002.

[15] D. A. Mitchison, "How drug resistance emerges as a result of poor compliance during short course chemotherapy for tuberculosis," *International Journal of Tuberculosis and Lung Disease*, vol. 2, no. 1, pp. 10–15, 1998.

[16] P. F. Riska, W. R. Jacobs Jr., and D. Alland, "Molecular determinants of drug resistance in tuberculosis," *International Journal of Tuberculosis and Lung Disease*, vol. 4, supplement 1, pp. S4–S10, 2000.

[17] EuroTB and The National Coordinators for Tuberculosis Surveillance in the WHO European Region, *Surveillance of Tuberculosis in Europe. Report on Tuberculosis Cases Notified in 2006*, Institut de Veille Sanitaire, Saint Maurice, France, 2008.

[18] T. Lillebaek, S. Poulsen, and A. Kok-Jensen, "Tuberculosis treatment in Denmark: treatment outcome for all Danish patients in 1992," *International Journal of Tuberculosis and Lung Disease*, vol. 3, no. 7, pp. 603–612, 1999.

[19] G. Canetti, "Present aspects of bacterial resistance in tuberculosis," *The American Review of Respiratory Disease*, vol. 92, no. 5, pp. 687–703, 1965.

[20] I. Ben-Dov and G. R. Mason, "Drug-resistant tuberculosis in a Southern California hospital. Trends from 1969 to 1984," *American Review of Respiratory Disease*, vol. 135, no. 6, pp. 1307–1310, 1987.

[21] M. F. M. Albuquerque, C. C. Sá-Leitão, A. R. L. Campelo, W. V. Souza, and A. Salustiano, "Fatores prognósticos para o desfecho do tratamento da tuberculose pulmonar em Recife, Pernambuco, Brasil," *Revista Panamericana de Salud Pública*, vol. 9, no. 6, pp. 368–375, 2001.

[22] X. Ai, K. Men, L. Guo et al., "Factors associated with low cure rate of tuberculosis in remote poor areas of Shaanxi Province, China: a case control study," *BMC Public Health*, vol. 10, article 112, 2010.

[23] D. J. Horne, R. Hubbard, M. Narita, A. Exarchos, D. R. Park, and C. H. Goss, "Factors associated with mortality in patients with tuberculosis," *BMC Infectious Diseases*, vol. 10, article 258, 2010.

[24] G. Vicentin, *Evolução da mortalidade por tuberculose no município do Rio de Janeiro 1979–1995*, Universidade de São Paulo, São Paulo, Brazil, 2000.

[25] P. D. Picon, S. L. Bassanesi, M. L. A. Caramori, R. L. T. Ferreira, C. A. Jarczewski, and P. R. B. Vieira, "Fatores de risco para a recidiva da tuberculose," *Jornal Brasileiro de Pneumologia*, vol. 33, no. 5, pp. 572–578, 2007.

[26] A. Thomas, P. G. Gopi, T. Santha et al., "Predictors of relapse among pulmonary tuberculosis patients treated in a DOTS programme in South India," *International Journal of Tuberculosis and Lung Disease*, vol. 9, no. 5, pp. 556–561, 2005.

[27] P. Gustafson, V. F. Gomes, C. S. Vieira et al., "Tuberculosis in Bissau: incidence and risk factors in an urban community in sub-Saharan Africa," *International Journal of Epidemiology*, vol. 33, no. 1, pp. 163–172, 2004.

[28] C. R. Driver, S. S. Munsiff, J. Li, N. Kundamal, and S. S. Osahan, "Relapse in persons treated for drug-susceptible tuberculosis in a population with high coinfection with human immunodeficiency virus in New York City," *Clinical Infectious Diseases*, vol. 33, no. 10, pp. 1762–1769, 2001.

[29] F. Pulido, J.-M. Peña, R. Rubio et al., "Relapse of tuberculosis after treatment in human immunodeficiency virus-infected patients," *Archives of Internal Medicine*, vol. 157, no. 2, pp. 227–232, 1997.

[30] World Health Organization, "Global tuberculosis control: surveillance, planning financing," WHO Report 376, World Health Organization, Geneva, Switzerland, 2007.

[31] H. Ullum, P. C. Gøtzsche, J. Victor, E. Dickmeiss, P. Skinhøj, and B. K. Pedersen, "Defective natural immunity: an early manifestation of human immunodeficiency virus infection," *The Journal of Experimental Medicine*, vol. 182, no. 3, pp. 789–799, 1995.

[32] E. V. Kourbatova, M. K. Leonard Jr., J. Romero, C. Kraft, C. Del Rio, and H. M. Blumberg, "Risk factors for mortality among patients with extrapulmonary tuberculosis at an academic inner-city hospital in the US," *European Journal of Epidemiology*, vol. 21, no. 9, pp. 715–721, 2006.

[33] G. P. De Oliveira, A. W. Torrens, P. Bartholomay, and D. Barreira, "Tuberculosis in Brazil: last ten years analysis—2001–2010," *Brazilian Journal of Infectious Diseases*, vol. 17, no. 2, pp. 218–233, 2013.

Vest Chest Physiotherapy Airway Clearance is Associated with Nitric Oxide Metabolism

Joseph H. Sisson,[1] **Todd A. Wyatt,**[1,2,3] **Jacqueline A. Pavlik,**[1]
Pawanjit S. Sarna,[1] **and Peter J. Murphy**[1]

[1] *Pulmonary, Critical Care, Sleep & Allergy Division, Department of Internal Medicine, University of Nebraska Medical Center, Omaha, NE 68198-5910, USA*
[2] *Research Service, Department of Veterans Affairs Omaha-Western Iowa Health Care System, 4101 Woolworth Avenue, Omaha, NE 68105, USA*
[3] *Department of Environmental, Agricultural, and Occupational Health, College of Public Health, University of Nebraska Medical Center, Omaha, NE 68198-7850, USA*

Correspondence should be addressed to Joseph H. Sisson; jsisson@unmc.edu

Academic Editor: Charlie Strange

Background. Vest chest physiotherapy (VCPT) enhances airway clearance in cystic fibrosis (CF) by an unknown mechanism. Because cilia are sensitive to nitric oxide (NO), we hypothesized that VCPT enhances clearance by changing NO metabolism. *Methods*. Both normal subjects and stable CF subjects had pre- and post-VCPT airway clearance assessed using nasal saccharin transit time (NSTT) followed by a collection of exhaled breath condensate (EBC) analyzed for NO metabolites (NO_x). *Results*. VCPT shorted NSTT by 35% in normal and stable CF subjects with no difference observed between the groups. EBC NO_x concentrations decreased 68% in control subjects after VCPT (before = 115 ± 32 μM versus after = 37 ± 17 μM; P < 0.002). CF subjects had a trend toward lower EBC NO_x. *Conclusion*. We found an association between VCPT-stimulated clearance and exhaled NO_x levels in human subjects. We speculate that VCPT stimulates clearance via increased NO metabolism.

1. Introduction

Percussive chest physiotherapy (CPT) is the principal treatment that patients use to facilitate clearance of airway secretions with cystic fibrosis (CF) or other causes of bronchiectasis. Patients have historically used various forms of clapping or mechanical percussion to accomplish this. A number of devices, collectively referred to as vest chest physiotherapy (VCPT), are now available that allow patients to perform airway clearance without the aid of a second person to apply the therapy [1]. Several studies demonstrate the superiority of chest physiotherapy over no chest physiotherapy with regard to clinical outcomes [2]. Chest physiotherapy increases mucus clearance as assessed by mucus volume measurements [3].

The mechanism by which percussive chest physiotherapy modalities enhance airway clearance is not known. Clinicians hypothesize that percussion and shaking loosen adherent mucus and biofilms from the airway surface, making it easier for cough clearance to remove them from the airways. Alternatively, a number of investigators have shown that mechanical stimulation of certain tissue types results in increased epithelial cell release of NO [4].

Because mechanical stimulation increases NO release and airway clearance [5], we hypothesized that VCPT alters metabolism of NO, as measured by oxides of nitrogen (NO_x) release from the human airway, and is associated with enhanced airway clearance. To test these hypotheses, we measured nasal saccharin transit time (NSTT) and NO_x in exhaled breath condensate (EBC) in subjects with and without CF, before and after a therapy session with the VCPT.

2. Materials and Methods

This study was conducted at the University of Nebraska Medical Center (UNMC), Omaha, Nebraska, and approved

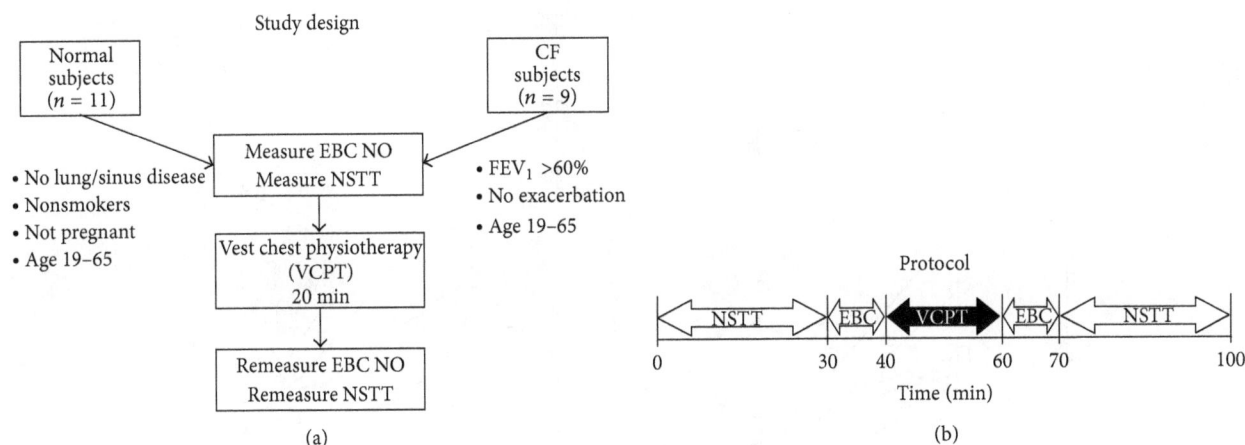

FIGURE 1: Diagram of the study design.

TABLE 1: Study subject demographics.

	Normal subjects (n = 11)	Cystic fibrosis subjects (n = 9)
Male	6	4
Female	5	5
Age	30–51	21–44

by the UNMC Institutional Review Board. Informed consent was obtained from each subject.

2.1. Experimental Design.
The protocol for the study is outlined in Figure 1. Control patients were normal, healthy volunteer adults aged 19–65 years in good health (Table 1). Patients qualified for inclusion if they had a documented diagnosis of cystic fibrosis, FEV1 greater than 60%, and were adults aged 19–65 years. The majority of the CF patient group had been exposed to vest physiotherapy in the past, but none had undergone a treatment within 24 hours of participation in the study. All patients and control subjects abstained from drinking alcohol for at least 24 hours prior to the study. Control subjects were excluded if they had a history of lung or sinus disease, had ever smoked, or were pregnant. CF subjects were excluded if they were smokers, were pregnant, or had evidence of acute pulmonary exacerbation of their disease. For the purposes of our study, we defined a CF pulmonary exacerbation as an increase in cough, sputum, or new dyspnea or other symptoms sufficient to justify acute treatment with an antibiotic delivered by any route.

2.2. Subject Selection and Enrollment.
We solicited patients for participation in the study during routine visits for periodic CF care. Patients were allowed to participate only if they and their treating physician agreed that they were near their baseline state of health with no evidence of CF pulmonary exacerbation or other acute illness [6]. We conducted the study over a period of four months.

After informed consent, subjects underwent nasal saccharin transit time (NSTT) testing (see below), followed by a collection of the pre-percussion exhaled breath condensate (EBC) for 10 minutes during tidal breathing. Each subject underwent a VCPT per protocol outlined below. The post-NSTT procedure immediately followed the collection of post-percussion EBC for 10 minutes, both in a manner identical to the prepercussion collection and testing (but in reverse order; Figure 1).

2.3. Nasal Saccharin Transit Time.
Under direct visualization, a particle (5 mg) of saccharin measuring approximately 0.5 mm in diameter was placed onto one of the inferior nasal turbinates of each participant as described [7]. The elapsed time was recorded from the placement of the saccharin particle to the first taste of sweetness. Measurement of NSTT was performed both before and after VCPT.

2.4. Exhaled Breath Condensate.
Samples of exhaled breath condensate were collected by tidal breathing for 10 minutes into an EcoScreen, (Jaeger, Würzburg, Germany) cooled system forming a condensate. To prevent contamination from nasal breathing, a nose clip was worn throughout collection of the EBC. Samples were divided into 500 μL aliquots and stored at $-70°$C for nitric oxide analysis at a later date [8].

2.5. Vest Chest Physiotherapy.
Subjects underwent a 20-minute VCPT session with the Model 104 Air-Pulse Generator (Hill-Rom Corporate, St. Paul, MN). The vest was rapidly inflated and deflated to the maximum-tolerated pressureat a frequency of 10–15 Hz for 20 minutes.

2.6. Measurement of NO_x.
Oxides of nitrogen were measured from the frozen EBC samples using a Sievers NOA 280 chemiluminescence analyzer (GE Analytical Instruments, Boulder, CO). The analyzer uses a vanadium chloride reduction to convert NO_x back to nitric oxide. In this system, both nitrites and nitrates were assayed, as conversion products of exhaled breath NO. Calculation of NO_x concentration was extrapolated from a standard curve of 1 nM to 100 μM sodium nitrate. For each sample, triplicate injections were run on

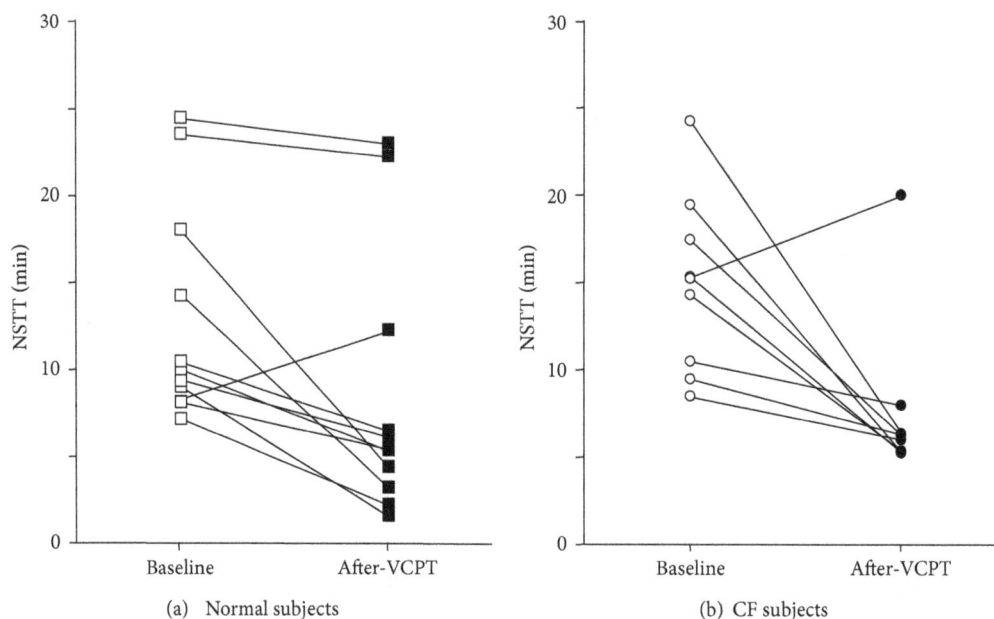

(a) Normal subjects

(b) CF subjects

FIGURE 2: *Nasal saccharin transit time (NSTT) after vest chest physiotherapy (VCPT).* (a) All but one normal subject demonstrated a decrease in NSTT following vest therapy. (b) All CF subjects except one sustained a decrease in NSTT after VCPT when compared to pretreatment values.

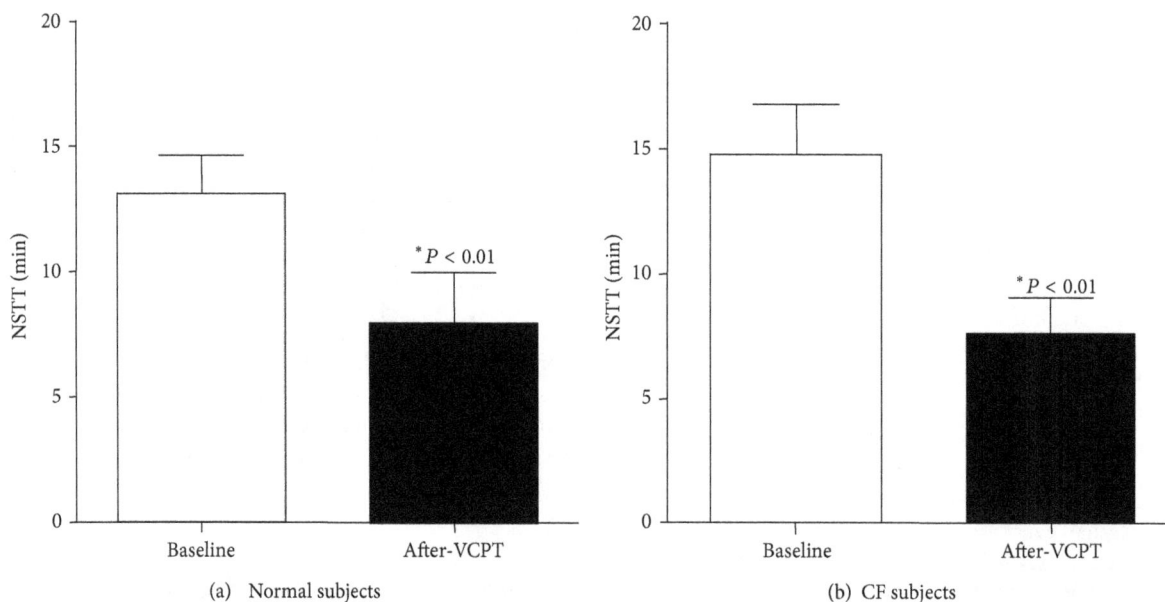

(a) Normal subjects

(b) CF subjects

FIGURE 3: *Aggregate nasal saccharin transit time after VCPT.* (a) Normal subjects demonstrated a 35% decrease in NSTT following VCPT as compared to pretreatment NSTT (13.0 ± 1.9 minutes versus 8.4 ± 2.3 min; $P < 0.01$). (b) In CF subjects, we observed a similar 38% decrease in NSTT after VCPT when compared to pretreatment values (baseline = 15.5 ± 1.6 min versus after vest = 8.3 ± 1.6 min; $P < 0.01$).

two different days for each data point. Significance was determined by paired t-test with P value <0.05.

3. Results

3.1. Nasal Saccharin Transit Time (NSTT). NSTT was significantly reduced after VCPT in normal subjects (Figure 2(a)) meaning that clearance was enhanced. All but one normal

subject demonstrated a decrease in NSTT following vest therapy (Figure 2(a)). In aggregate, normal subjects demonstrated a 35% decrease in NSTT following VCPT as compared to pretreatment NSTT (Figure 3(a); 13.0 ± 1.9 minutes versus 8.4 ± 2.3 min; $P < 0.01$). We compared these results with nasal clearance in patients with cystic fibrosis. We observed a similar 38% decrease in NSTT after VCPT when compared to pretreatment values (Figures 2(b) and 3(b);

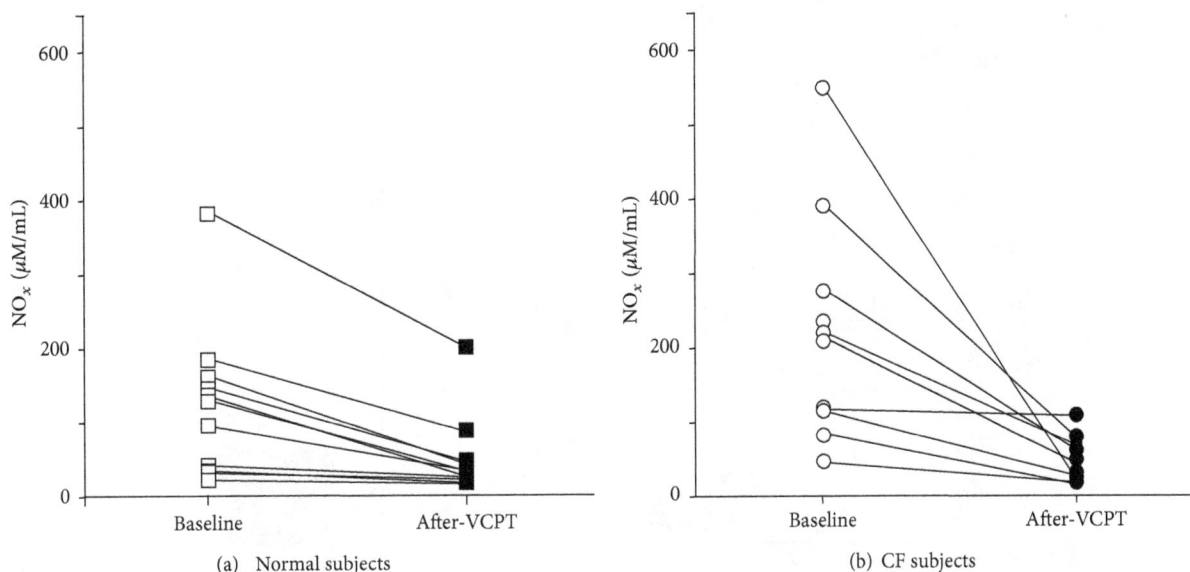

FIGURE 4: *Exhaled breath condensate (EBC) oxides of nitrogen (NO_x) following VCBT.* (a) All 11 normal subjects sustained a decrease in EBC NO_x concentrations. (b) All nine cystic fibrosis subjects also sustained a decrease in EBC NO_x concentrations.

baseline = 15.5 ± 1.6 min versus post-VCPT = 8.3 ± 1.6 min; $P < 0.01$). As with the normal subjects, all CF subjects, save one, sustained a decrease in NSTT after VCPT when compared to pretreatment values (Figure 2(b)). We observed no significant difference in either baseline or post-vest CPT NSTT values between normal subjects and CF patients (Figure 3).

3.2. Exhaled Breath Condensate (EBC) Oxides of Nitrogen (NO_x).
Because cilia stimulation is associated with nitric oxide (NO) production, we measured NO_x concentration in exhaled breath condensate (EBC) before and after VCPT. We found that EBC NO_x concentrations decreased 68% in control subjects after VCPT compared to baseline, pretreatment values (Figure 5(a); baseline = $115 \pm 32\ \mu$M versus post-vest = $37 \pm 17\ \mu$M; $P < 0.002$). Although with different degrees, all 11 normal subjects sustained a decrease in EBC NO_x concentrations (Figure 4(a)). We compared these results in normal subjects to patients with stable cystic fibrosis and found a similar result (Figure 4(b)). All patients with CF showed a significant decrease in EBC NO_x after VCPT (Figure 5(b); baseline = $224 \pm 55\ \mu$M versus post-vest = $52 \pm 11\ \mu$M; $P < 0.01$). As with NSTT, we saw no difference in baseline or post-VCPT EBC NO_x values between normal subjects and subjects with stable CF ($P = 0.09$). There was not a statistically significant correlation between the decrease in NSTT and the decrease in EBC [NO_x].

4. Discussion

We hypothesized that mechanical stimulation with VCPT alters NO_x metabolism, which stimulates mucociliary clearance. To test this hypothesis, we measured nasal saccharin transit time and exhaled breath condensate NO_x concentrations in healthy normal adult subjects and adults with stable

cystic fibrosis before and after VCPT. In this model, we use NSTT as a surrogate of mucociliary clearance.

To our knowledge, this is the first study to associate changes in airway mucociliary clearance with changes in exhaled NO_x in human subjects. Our results indicate that VCPT applied to both normal and stable CF subjects significantly increased nasal mucociliary clearance. A single VCPT treatment increased nasal clearance in 18 out of 20 (90%) subjects tested. In aggregate, we found that a vest treatment increased nasal clearance by approximately 35% in both normal and stable CF subjects. Although our study groups were small in number, the effect of percussion on nasal clearance was quite striking with both biologically relevant and statistically significant changes in NSTT.

We originally designed our study to address the mechanism of enhanced clearance by VCPT. We chose to explore the role of NO that might have in enhanced clearance based on *in vitro* studies of cilia that date back to 1993 demonstrating that increases of CBF by multiple stimuli require NO production [9]. Many investigators have corroborated these findings in several different systems [10–12]. In this context, we originally hypothesized that VCPT-enhanced clearance would increase exhaled NO_x concentrations. Our results are counterintuitive and exactly the opposite of our expectations regarding the effect of mechanical stimulation via VCPT on exhaled NO_x. In every case, VCPT is associated with dramatic reduction in NO_x concentrations. We speculate that mechanical shaking with the VCPT device enhances mucus clearance by stimulating calcium release from airway epithelial cells, resulting in calmodulin activation of eNOS with resultant production of NO in the airway epithelial cell. If NO production increases with mechanical stimulation, then we have to reconcile our observation that EBC NO_x decreased following VCPT. An alternative explanation for the difference between our findings in this study and those published with

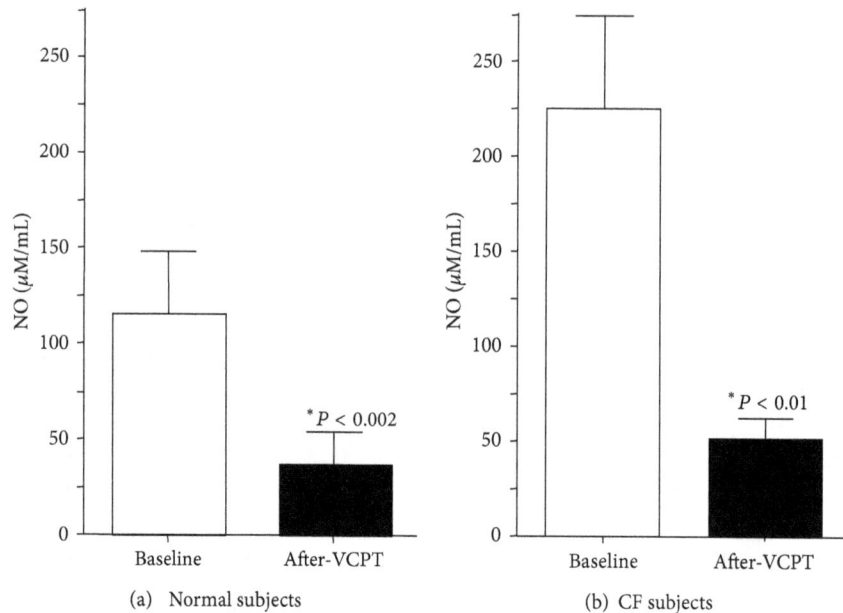

FIGURE 5: *Aggregate exhaled breath condensate oxides of nitrogen following VCBT.* (a) EBC NO_x concentrations decreased 68% in control subjects after VCPT compared to baseline, pretreatment values (baseline = $115 \pm 32 \, \mu M$ versus post-VCPT = $37 \pm 17 \, \mu M$; $P < 0.002$). (b) CF subjects showed a significant decrease in EBC NO_x after vest percussion treatment (baseline = $224 \pm 55 \, \mu M$ versus post-vest = $52 \pm 11 \, \mu M$; $P < 0.01$).

NO_x measurements performed in ciliated cells *in vitro* is that our study focused on the metabolites of NO that were exhaled into the EBC while the *in vitro* studies measured the concentration of NO_x present in the media. It is likely that "off-gassing" of NO is the basis of NO_x in EBC [13], whereas, *in vitro* studies focus on dissolved and non-volatile metabolites of NO present in the media.

The decrease in exhaled NO_x may be due to increased utilization of NO within the ciliated epithelial cell. In this scenario, the enhanced binding of NO to guanylyl cyclase would provide the signal for elevated cGMP, activation of PKG, and stimulated cilia beating. It is also possible that the increased mucus flow from more distal airways creates a greater barrier to NO diffusion from the airway epithelium during percussion therapy than that present in the resting state. Alternatively, mechanical stimulation through percussion may alter the metabolism of NO through an unknown mechanism.

The literature has clearly established that mechanical stress alone can stimulate cilia beating in both *in vitro* [14] and *in vivo* [15] models. The mechanism of such mechanical stimulation may involve an increase in cytoplasmic calcium resulting from either extracellular calcium influx or inositol-$1',4',5$-triphosphate-mediated internal calcium release [16, 17]. The calcium pathway is likely independent of the NO-cGMP-PKG stimulation of cilia beating in an ovine model [18], but others have shown a cGMP-dependent component to calcium-stimulated cilia beat in rabbit airway [18]. Using human nasal ciliated cells, Alberty et al. demonstrated that mechanical stimulation of cilia could take place in the presence of an NO inhibitor, suggesting that the mechanical induced increases in CBF were independent of endogenous

NO production [19]. Extrapolating from these observations, mechanical stimulation of mucociliary transport in response to VCPT in our study could be independent of NO. However, the significant *decrease* in EBC NO_x levels in response to mechanical stimulation in both study groups suggests a distinct mechanical impact on NO metabolism and release from the lung.

An obvious question that arises from our findings is as follows: *how does chest percussion alter nasal clearance?* The vest percussion apparatus is applied to the chest with the intent of oscillating the lower airways. We observed, however, that the head and neck clearly oscillated in sync with the chest during VCPT. Furthermore, increased nasal discharge typically occurs during percussion treatment consistent with increased nasal clearance (unpublished results). From these observations we surmise that the nasal cavity, in addition to the lower airways, is vigorously shaken during VCPT and results in stimulated nasal mucociliary clearance.

Another important question is as follows: *does nasal clearance correlate with lung airway clearance?* Because VCPT is typically directed at patients with lung airway clearance disorders such as bronchiectasis, we can only cautiously extrapolate our findings with nasal clearance to lung clearance. We did not directly measure lung clearance due to the cost and exposure to radionuclides involved in such studies. The NSTT is, however, a direct functional measure of mucociliary clearance of the upper airway. Because the vest is thought to enhance lung airway clearance, it is highly likely that both nasal and lung clearance are stimulated by VCPT.

We also note that EBC NO_x tended to be *higher* in CF subjects than in control subjects (Figure 5), which differs from previous studies [20]. While we acknowledge that the NO_x

difference between normal and CF subjects was not statistically different, the best explanation for this disparity is that the earlier study measured only direct exhaled NO, which does not include nitric oxide breakdown products. In contrast, exhaled breath condensate contains the stable conversion compounds of NO, nitrites, and nitrates. Our findings measuring NO_x concentrations in EBC contrast with other studies that measured only the exhaled free radical NO.

5. Conclusions

In summary, we found that VCPT meaningfully enhanced airway clearance, as measured by NSTT in all subjects. In addition, we found that exhaled breath NO_x levels significantly *decreased* following VCPT. These findings suggest an association between VCPT clearance changes and altered airway NO_x levels consistent with a role for NO metabolism in the regulation of mucociliary clearance. These findings suggest the need to further study the mechanisms of increased airway clearance during chest physiotherapy to establish the role nitric oxide plays in regulating this response.

References

[1] P. A. Flume, K. A. Robinson, B. P. O'Sullivan et al., "Cystic fibrosis pulmonary guidelines: airway clearance therapies," *Respiratory Care*, vol. 54, no. 4, pp. 522–537, 2009.

[2] C. van der Schans, A. Prasad, and E. Main, "Chest physiotherapy compared to no chest physiotherapy for cystic fibrosis," *Cochrane Database of Systematic Reviews*, no. 2, p. CD001401, 2000.

[3] L. G. Hansen and W. J. Warwick, "High-frequency chest compression system to aid in clearance of mucus from the lung," *Biomedical Instrumentation and Technology*, vol. 24, no. 4, pp. 289–294, 1990.

[4] W. M. Abraham, A. Ahmed, I. Serebriakov et al., "Whole-body periodic acceleration modifies experimental asthma in sheep," *American Journal of Respiratory and Critical Care Medicine*, vol. 174, no. 7, pp. 743–752, 2006.

[5] W. M. Abraham, A. Ahmed, I. Serebriakov et al., "Periodic acceleration via nitric oxide release modifies antigen-induced airway responses in sheep," *American Journal of Respiratory and Critical Care Medicine*, vol. 169, article A321, 2004.

[6] D. Bilton, G. Canny, S. Conway et al., "Pulmonary exacerbation: towards a definition for use in clinical trials. Report from the EuroCareCF Working Group on outcome parameters in clinical trials," *Journal of Cystic Fibrosis*, vol. 10, no. 2, pp. S79–S81, 2011.

[7] J. H. Sisson, A. J. Yonkers, and R. H. Waldman, "Effects of guaifenesin on nasal mucociliary clearance and ciliary beat frequency in healthy volunteers," *Chest*, vol. 107, no. 3, pp. 747–751, 1995.

[8] F. Hoffmeyer, M. Raulf-Heimsoth, and T. Bruning, "Exhaled breath condensate and airway inflammation," *Current Opinion in Allergy and Clinical Immunology*, vol. 9, no. 1, pp. 16–22, 2009.

[9] B. Jain, I. Rubinstein, R. A. Robbins, K. L. Leise, and J. H. Sisson, "Modulation of airway epithelial cell ciliary beat frequency by nitric oxide," *Biochemical and Biophysical Research Communications*, vol. 191, no. 1, pp. 83–88, 1993.

[10] X. Zhan, D. Li, and R. A. Johns, "Immunohistochemical evidence for the NO cGMP signaling pathway in respiratory ciliated epithelia of rat," *Journal of Histochemistry and Cytochemistry*, vol. 47, no. 11, pp. 1369–1374, 1999.

[11] C. Xue, S. J. Botkin, and R. A. Johns, "Localization of endothelial NOS at the basal microtubule membrane in ciliated epithelium of rat lung," *Journal of Histochemistry and Cytochemistry*, vol. 44, no. 5, pp. 463–471, 1996.

[12] J. Tamaoki, A. Chiyotani, M. Kondo, and K. Konno, "Role of NO generation in β-adrenoceptor-mediated stimulation of rabbit airway ciliary motility," *American Journal of Physiology: Cell Physiology*, vol. 268, no. 6, pp. C1342–C1347, 1995.

[13] V. Suresh, J. D. Mih, and S. C. George, "Measurement of IL-13-induced iNOS-derived gas phase nitric oxide in human bronchial epithelial cells," *American Journal of Respiratory Cell and Molecular Biology*, vol. 37, no. 1, pp. 97–104, 2007.

[14] M. J. Sanderson and E. R. Dirksen, "Mechanosensitivity of cultured ciliated cells from the mammalian respiratory tract: implications for the regulation of mucociliary transport," *Proceedings of the National Academy of Sciences of the United States of America*, vol. 83, no. 19, pp. 7302–7306, 1986.

[15] G. S. Barr and A. K. Tewary, "Alteration of airflow and mucociliary transport in normal subjects," *Journal of Laryngology and Otology*, vol. 107, no. 7, pp. 603–604, 1993.

[16] S. Boitano, E. R. Dirksen, and M. J. Sanderson, "Intercellular propagation of calcium waves mediated by inositol trisphosphate," *Science*, vol. 258, no. 5080, pp. 292–295, 1992.

[17] J. A. Felix, M. L. Woodruff, and E. R. Dirksen, "Stretch increases inositol 1,4,5-trisphosphate concentration in airway epithelial cells," *American Journal of Respiratory Cell and Molecular Biology*, vol. 14, no. 3, pp. 296–301, 1996.

[18] M. Salathe, T. Lieb, and R. J. Bookman, "Lack of nitric oxide involvement in cholinergic modulation of ovine ciliary beat frequency," *Journal of Aerosol Medicine*, vol. 13, no. 3, pp. 219–229, 2000.

[19] J. Alberty, W. Stoll, and C. Rudack, "The effect of endogenous nitric oxide on mechanical ciliostimulation of human nasal mucosa," *Clinical and Experimental Allergy*, vol. 36, no. 10, pp. 1254–1259, 2006.

[20] H. Grasemann, I. Ioannidis, R. P. Tomkiewicz, H. de Groot, B. K. Rubin, and F. Ratjen, "Nitric oxide metabolites in cystic fibrosis lung disease," *Archives of Disease in Childhood*, vol. 78, no. 1, pp. 49–53, 1998.

Is Mean Platelet Volume Really a Severity Marker for Obstructive Sleep Apnea Syndrome without Comorbidities?

Sinem Nedime Sökücü,[1] **Cengiz Özdemir,**[1] **Levent Dalar,**[2]
Levent Karasulu,[1] **Şenay Aydın,**[1] **and Sedat Altın**[1]

[1] *Sleep Laboratory, Yedikule Chest Disease and Thoracic Surgery Training and Research Hospital, Zeytinburnu, Istanbul, Turkey*
[2] *Department of Pulmonary Medicine, School of Medicine, Istanbul Bilim University, Sisli, 34600 Istanbul, Turkey*

Correspondence should be addressed to Sinem Nedime Sökücü; sinemtimur@yahoo.com

Academic Editor: Charlie Strange

Obstructive sleep apnea syndrome (OSAS) is a common disorder that can lead to significant cardiovascular complications. Several studies have reported increased platelet activation and aggregation in patients with OSAS. In this study we aimed to show a correlation between mean platelet volume (MPV) and severity of OSAS in patients with OSAS without any overt cardiac disease or diabetes. The polysomnography recordings of 556 consecutive patients admitted to the sleep laboratory between January 2012 and July 2012 were retrospectively evaluated. The relationship between polysomnographic parameters and biochemical parameters was assessed. Polysomnographic results of 200 patients (154 males [77%]; mean age, 44.5 ± 11.4 years) were included. No correlation was observed between MPV and the average oxygen saturation index, the minimum desaturation index, or the oxygen desaturation index in the study population as well as in severe OSAS group (AHI > 30). The only correlation was found between MPV and AHI in the severe OSAS group ($P = 0.010$). MPV was not correlated with OSAS severity in patients without any overt cardiac disease or diabetes. These findings raise doubts about the suggestion that MPV might be a marker for OSAS severity, as recommended in earlier studies. Thus, further prospective data are needed.

1. Introduction

Obstructive sleep apnea (OSA) is characterized by recurrent episodes of partial or complete upper airway obstruction during sleep. It occurs as combined episodes of apnea and hypopnea that cause sleep fragmentation or excessive daytime sleepiness. It is a common disorder affecting 2% and 4% of middle aged women and men, respectively [1]. The severity of OSAS is estimated by the number of apnea-hypopnea episodes per hour of sleep and is expressed as the apnea-hypopnea index (AHI) [2]. Although the underlying mechanisms and etiologies are not completely understood, OSAS can lead to significant cardiovascular complications [3], including heart failure, acute myocardial infarction, arrhythmias, hypertension, pulmonary hypertension, and stroke [4]. Increased platelet activation and aggregation are closely related to cardiovascular complications [5]. Several studies have reported increased platelet activation and aggregation in patients with OSAS [6, 7].

It has been shown that platelet size, measured by mean platelet volume (MPV), correlates with platelet reactivity and is an easy and useful tool for indirect monitoring of platelet activity. Larger platelets have higher thrombotic potential [8]. MPV plays an important role in the pathophysiology of cardiovascular diseases [8, 9]. The association between increased platelet activation and aggregation is closely associated with cardiovascular complications. Increased MPV occurs in patients with hypertension, hypercholesterolemia, diabetes mellitus, acute myocardial infarction, acute ischemic stroke, and coronary artery calcification [10, 11].

The relationship between MPV and disease severity in patients with OSAS has been evaluated and MPV increases in patients with OSAS when used as an indicator of platelet activation [12, 13]. Continuous positive airway pressure (CPAP)

therapy is shown to decrease platelet activation in patients with OSAS [14, 15]. In this study, relation between MPV and severity of OSAS in nondiabetic patients without any overt cardiac disease was evaluated.

2. Patients and Methods

2.1. Patients. A total of 556 patients consecutively admitted to the sleep laboratory between January 2012 and July 2012 who are with symptoms of nocturnal snoring and/or excess daytime sleepiness and who underwent a polysomnographic evaluation were retrospectively evaluated. Patients having AHİ < 5 were grouped as control and others were grouped according to their AHI value as mild, moderate, and severe OSAS.

Inclusion criteria were patients who are with symptoms of nocturnal snoring and/or excessive daytime sleepiness and who underwent polysomnographic evaluation at our sleep laboratory. Exclusion criteria were any known cardiac disease (congestive heart failure, ischemic vascular disease, or arrhythmias), lung disease (chronic obstructive pulmonary disease and asthma), diabetes mellitus (defined as fasting plasma glucose >126 mg/dL and/or antidiabetic treatment), chronic renal or hepatic diseases, use of acetylsalicylic acid or any other antiaggregant therapy (dipyridamole, ticlopidine, and clopidogrel) within the last month, abnormal haematocrit and/or abnormal white blood cell count and/or abnormal platelet number, and pure or mainly central apnea on a polysomnographic evaluation. The cardiac disease history evaluation was conducted through a detailed medical history and an evaluation of earlier ECGs, tests, and coronary angiography. Use of acetylsalicylic acid or other antiaggregant therapy was evaluated not only by history taking but also by assessing 3 months of pharmacy records. Rapid eye movement (REM) induced OSAS and positional OSAS patients were excluded from the study because in those patient groups severity of the disease changes day to day depending on the REM percentage of the sleep and time duration spent in supine position. For our study the definition of positional OSAS is accepted as total AHI > 5, nonsupine AHI < 5, and supine AHI/nonsupine AHI ≥ 2. The definition of REM-OSAS is accepted as total AHI > 5, REM AHI < 5, and REM AHI/non-REM AHI ≥ 2.

In total, 200 of the 556 met the inclusion and exclusion criteria and were enrolled in the study (Figure 1). Detailed medical history, physical examination, electrocardiogram (ECG), and chest X-ray were assessed from the patient folders. This retrospective study protocol was approved by the institutional ethics committee. Informed written consent was obtained from all subjects before the polysomnography.

2.2. Procedure. Standard overnight polysomnography was performed in all patients using an Embla N7000 (Embla, Medcare Flaga, Iceland) data acquisition and analysis system in the sleep laboratory from 22.00 to 06.00 h. The physiological signals monitored included EEG (C4-M1, C3-M2, O2-M1, and O1-M2), electrooculography, and submental EMG. The following were also measured: ribcage and abdominal effort measured by respiratory inductive plethysmography

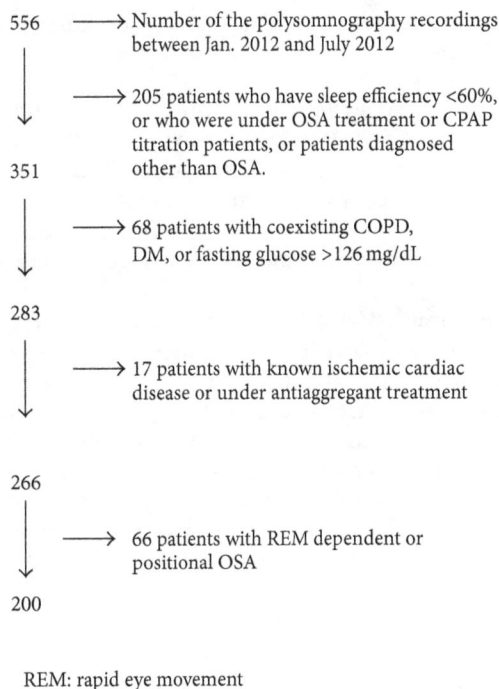

556 ⟶ Number of the polysomnography recordings between Jan. 2012 and July 2012

⟶ 205 patients who have sleep efficiency <60%, or who were under OSA treatment or CPAP titration patients, or patients diagnosed other than OSA.

351

⟶ 68 patients with coexisting COPD, DM, or fasting glucose >126 mg/dL

283

⟶ 17 patients with known ischemic cardiac disease or under antiaggregant treatment

266

⟶ 66 patients with REM dependent or positional OSA

200

REM: rapid eye movement

FIGURE 1: Exclusion chart of patients.

(RIP) (XactTrace, Medcare Flaga), body position, measured by calibrated sensor, snoring sound measured with a piezo-electric sensor, and oronasal flow measured with a nasal pressure cannula (Medcare Flaga), SpO_2 (8000J, Nonin Medical, Plymouth, MN, USA) with averaging time set at 3 seconds. The ECG (lead II) was sampled at 512 Hz. Sleep stages and arousals were scored using the Somnologica Studio software package (Medcare Flaga) according to standard criteria [16] by two experienced scorers who had 80–95% concordance with each other. Respiratory events were scored as follows. Apnea was defined as a cessation of airflow for ≥10 seconds. Apnea was classified as obstructive in the presence of continued movement in the RIP and as central in the absence of movement in the RIP. Hypopnea was defined as a ≥50% reduction in oronasal flow amplitude ≥10 seconds, accompanied by ≥3% desaturation or arousal. Classification of a hypopnea as obstructive, central, or mixed performed calibrated respiratory inductance plethysmography. Hypopnea was classified as obstructive in the presence of continued movement in the RIP [16]. The oxygen desaturation index (ODI) is the number of times per hour of sleep in which the blood's oxygen level drops by 3 percent or more from baseline.

2.3. Blood Assays. Fasting (8 hours) venous blood samples were drawn from the antecubital vein between 7 and 8 AM after polysomnography and after a 20 min rest. Tripotassium ethylenediaminetetraacetic acid based anticoagulated blood samples were drawn and assessed within 30 minutes. Complete blood count analyses were performed using the Abbott Cell-Dyne 3700 System (Abbott Diagnostics, Santa Clara, CA, USA) and biochemical analyses were performed using the Olympus AU2700 Plus Analyzer (Beckman Coulter, Tokyo, Japan).

2.4. Statistical Analysis. The statistical analysis was performed with SPSS for Windows version 16.0 (SPSS, Chicago, IL, USA). All variables were tested for normality with the Kolmogorov-Smirnov test. Normally distributed continuous variables are expressed as mean ± standard deviation. Nonnormally distributed continuous variables are summarized as medians.

Categorical variables are expressed as numbers (percentages). Comparisons between independent groups were made using the Mann-Whitney U test. Correlations between noncontinuous variables and continuous variables with a nonnormal distribution were assessed using Spearman's correlation. Correlations between continuous variables were assessed using Pearson's correlation. Comparisons between groups were evaluated by one-way analysis of variance followed by the Bonferroni method. A $P < 0.05$ was considered statistically significant.

3. Results

A total of 200 patients were included (154 males [77%]; mean age, 44.5 ± 11.4 years). The study subjects were categorized into four groups according to AHI (<5, normal; 5–15, mild OSAS; 15–30, moderate OSAS; >30, severe OSAS). As the severity of OSAS increased, male, older, heavier, and smoker patients became predominant (Table 1). A significant difference was found between cases with AHI < 5 and those with severe OSAS (AHI > 30) in terms of sex, age, body mass index (BMI), smoking ratio, and pack-year smoking history ($P = 0.001$, $P = 0.014$, $P = 0.001$, $P = 0.231$, and $P = 0.015$, resp.). No difference was found in terms of hypertensive patient ratios between the groups.

The polysomnographic characteristics of the groups are shown in Table 2. No differences were observed between the controls and patients with mild, moderate, or severe OSAS according to white blood cells, red blood cells, haemoglobin, haematocrit, platelets, MPV, platelet distribution width (PDW), glucose, creatinine, total cholesterol, or low-density lipoprotein cholesterol (Table 3). Both high-density lipoprotein (HDL) and triglycerides were significantly higher in the severe OSAS group, as compared to those in the normal population ($P = 0.001$ and $P = 0.013$).

No correlation was observed between MPV and AHI, average saturation, minimum desaturation, time duration with $SpO_2 < 90\%$, oxygen desaturation index, or OSAS groups in the whole patient population (Table 4) (Figure 2). Also no correlation was found between MPV and average saturation, minimum desaturation, or the oxygen desaturation index in the severe OSAS subgroup. A correlation was found between MPV and AHI in the severe OSAS group ($P = 0.010$) (Table 5). No correlation was found between MPV and smoking history ($P = 0.240$) and sex ($P = 0.887$).

4. Discussion

The only correlation that was found in our study is that MPV is positively correlated with AHI in severe OSAS group

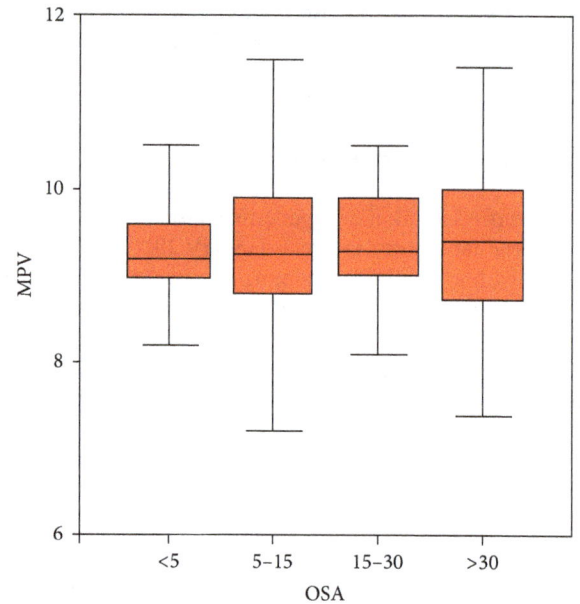

FIGURE 2: Box plot graphic of MPV and OSAS groups.

but no significant relationship between OSAS and hypoxia parameters and MPV or PDW was found. Results of earlier studies conducted in nondiabetic subjects with OSAS showed that MPV and PDW are associated with the degree of hypoxia and OSAS severity. These results underline the importance of OSAS as a risk factor for vascular atherothrombotic disease and MPV as a risk factor [12, 13]. However, the relationship between OSAS severity and MPV could disappear if a more detailed history was taken, and all patients with cardiac and lung diseases were excluded.

MPV reflects platelet activity. The exact mechanism of platelet activation in patients with OSAS is unclear but possible mechanisms are an indirect effect of increased sympathetic activation causing catecholamine discharge that activates platelets, chronic intermittent hypoxia causing platelet activation directly, and chronic inflammation [17, 18]. In a previous study, a significant difference was found between the control group and severe OSAS in terms of MPV values, and severe OSAS was independently correlated with AHI and the desaturation index in a multivariate regression analysis. We found no correlation between any group in terms of MPV, AHI, or the desaturation index [12]. We only found a correlation between MPV and AHI in patients with severe OSAS. Also an explanation for this could be that in our control and mild OSAS groups ODI and time duration with Sat 02 <90% were relatively less compared to severe OSAS group. In a recently published study, MPV was not found to be different in mild and moderate OSAS but it was significantly high in severe OSAS. Also as reported by Karakas et al. in our study desaturation ratios were found to be similar in mild and moderate OSAS. [19]. This could be because of the fact that as the severity of the disease increases, patients become more prone to cardiovascular risks so we did not observe this relation in mild and moderate OSAS groups. As the disease severity increases, systemic inflammation also increases and

TABLE 1: Demographic and anthropometric characteristics of the patients.

	Group 1 (AHI < 5)	Group 2 (AHI 5–15)	Group 3 (AHI 15–30)	Group 4 (AHI > 30)	P value
Patient number	30	38	41	91	
Sex (male %)	15 (50%)	30 (78.9%)	33 (80.5%)	76 (83.5%)	0.002*
Age (years)	38.43 ± 12.79	43.50 ± 12.15	47.27 ± 10.95	45.64 ± 10.15	0.006*
Hypertension (%)	4 (13.3%)	8 (21.1%)	8 (19.5%)	23 (25.3%)	0.566
Smokers (%)	14 (46.7%)	18 (47.4%)	20 (48.8%)	62 (68.1%)	0.037*
Pack-year smoking history	1.5 (10)	1.5 (17.25)	2.0 (15)	15 (24)	0.001*
Patient number	30	38	41	91	
BMI (kg/m^2)	26.91 ± 4.61	29.10 ± 4.51	30.01 ± 4.52	31.75 ± 4.53	0.001*
Neck circumference (cm)	35.55 ± 3.63	38.45 ± 3.31	39.33 ± 3.31	40.71 ± 7.89	0.001
Waist circumference (cm)	92.17 ± 10.96	98.68 ± 8.76	101.61 ± 9.33	104.19 ± 14.26	0.001
Hip circumference (cm)	101.16 ± 7.35	103.74 ± 6.59	106.85 ± 16.54	107.98 ± 7.78	0.006
Waist to hip ratio	0.91 ± 0.075	0.95 ± 0.066	0.96 ± 0.099	0.97 ± 0.115	0.062

$^*P < 0.05$.

TABLE 2: Sleep characteristics of the patients.

	Group 1 (AHI < 5)	Group 2 (AHI 5–15)	Group 3 (AHI 15–30)	Group 4 (AHI > 30)	P value
Patient number	30	38	41	91	
TST (min)	415.15 ± 50.81	383.33 ± 54.11	386.55 ± 57.39	380.59 ± 64.38	0.05
Sleep efficiency (%TST)	86.52 ± 9.09	80.47 ± 10.09	80.79 ± 10.03	83.03 ± 10.24	0.052
Stage 1 (%TST)	5.34 ± 1.92	6.72 ± 2.47	7.52 ± 2.87	10.6 (9.1)	0.001*
Stage 2 (%TST)	51.98 ± 7.16	52.09 ± 6.53	50.83 ± 9.83	53.37 ± 10.26	0.510
Stage 3 (%TST)	20.86 ± 6.70	19.98 ± 7.19	21.00 ± 9.53	16 (13.2)	0.001*
REM (%TST)	21.56 ± 6.32	20.72 ± 5.72	20.64 ± 6.57	17.08 ± 7.17	0.001*
AHI (events/hour)	2.84 ± 1.41	9.58 ± 2.91	21.12 ± 3.88	54.17 ± 18.81	0.001*
Average SpO$_2$ (%)	96.79 ± 1.47	94.13 ± 12.65	95.35 ± 1.59	95.17 ± 1.54	0.296
Minimum SpO$_2$ (%)	91.70 ± 3.88	88.55 ± 4.72	82.29 ± 12.82	74.98 ± 14.09	0.001*
Time duration with SpO$_2$ < %90	0.001 (0.001)	1.78 ± 4.04	3.5 (9.25)	23.1 (71.9)	0.001*
ODI	1.5 (2.57)	7 (7.47)	20.85 ± 6.16	49.42 ± 20.41	0.001*

TST: total sleep time; AHI: apnea hypopnea index; REM: rapid eye movement; AHI: apnea-hypopnea index; ODI: oxygen desaturation index; $^*P < 0.05$.

TABLE 3: Full blood count and biochemical characteristics of the groups.

	Group 1 (AHI < 5)	Group 2 (AHI 5–15)	Group 3 (AHI 15–30)	Group 4 (AHI > 30)	P value
Patient number	30	38	41	91	
WBC (×10^3 cell/μl)	7.08 ± 1.37	7.27 ± 1.97	7.83 ± 1.79	7.89 ± 1.99	0.069
RBC (×10^6 cell/μl)	5.06 ± 0.58	5.23 ± 0.47	5.25 ± 0.48	5.19 ± 0.67	0.654
Hb (g/dl)	14.55 ± 1.42	14.97 ± 1.42	15.24 ± 1.40	15.08 ± 1.47	0.328
Htc (%)	43.76 ± 4.24	44.93 ± 3.89	44.29 ± 7.27	44.91 ± 5.87	0.808
PLT (×10^3 cell/μl)	271.57 ± 51.83	260.76 ± 64.52	266.76 ± 62.11	278.59 ± 84.64	0.597
MPV (fl)	9.21 ± 0.75	9.36 ± 0.94	9.33 ± 0.72	9.37 ± 1.02	0.910
PDW (fl)	15.71 ± 2.12	16.19 ± 2.34	15.67 ± 1.91	15.84 ± 2.88	0.810
Glucose (mg/dl)	94.34 ± 9.58	95.70 ± 11.35	100.91 ± 10.69	99.31 ± 14.30	0.079
Creatinine (mg/dl)	0.70 ± 0.15	0.81 ± 0.14	0.8 (0.19)	0.8 (0.2)	0.684
Total cholesterol (mg/dl)	201.92 ± 47.72	201.88 ± 42.05	210.01 ± 43.06	207.43 ± 40.21	0.758
HDL cholesterol (mg/dl)	54.03 ± 12.79	42.5 (11.5)	45.25 ± 12.72	40.48 ± 8.72	0.001*
LDL cholesterol (mg/dl)	119.91 ± 41.91	119.62 ± 43.47	125.20 ± 41.56	127.49 ± 37.26	0.691
Triglyceride (mg/dl)	92.5 (83.83)	128.45 (113)	155.5 (155.6)	196.45 (113.7)	0.017*

WBC: white blood cells; RBC: red blood cells; MPV: mean platelet volume; PDW: platelet distribution width; HDL: high-density lipoprotein cholesterol; LDL: low-density lipoprotein cholesterol; VLDL: very low density lipoprotein cholesterol; $^*P < 0.05$.
Both HDL and triglyceride were found to be significantly high in severe OSAS group compared to normal population (P: 0.001 and P: 0.013).

TABLE 4: Correlation analyses and *P* values of MPV and PDW with polysomnographic parameters in the whole group.

	Average SpO$_2$ (%)	Minimum SpO$_2$ (%)	Time duration with SpO$_2$ < %90	Oxygen desaturation index	AHI (events/hour)
MPV	0.875	0.446	0.277	0.165	0.098
PDW	0.647	0.749	0.857	0.785	0.735

TABLE 5: Correlation analyses and *P* values of MPV and PDW with polysomnographical parameters in the severe OSAS group.

	Average SpO$_2$ (%)	Minimum SpO$_2$ (%)	Time duration with SpO$_2$ < %90	Oxygen desaturation index	AHI (events/hour)
MPV	0.266	0.523	0.430	0.055	0.010[*]
PDW	0.522	0.969	0.840	0.156	0.061

[*]$P < 0.05$.

this will affect MPV value just like other parameters of systemic inflammation. As the disease gets severer systemic reflections may increase and this could point to the relation between cytokine levels generating systemic inflammation and MPV.

Platelet count and MPV are modified by various biosocial and lifestyle factors such as race, age, gender, smoking, alcohol consumption, and physical activity [20–22]. An earlier study found no significant difference between controls and the severe OSAS group in terms of age, male ratio, and smoking habits, unlike our study, but there was a significant difference in terms of BMI, as in our study [12]. However, in the study by Nena et al., not all of these properties were mentioned in the groups [13]. Patients in our severe OSAS group were predominantly male and older, had more pack-year smoking history, and were more obese, as compared to controls, and all four criteria could affect MPV in a positive way. However, we did not find any differences in these variables in our patient population, as compared to controls.

Smoking increases MPV in older patients with risk factors for atherosclerosis. In a study conducted by Kario et al., increased MPV in smoking patients decreased after the patients stopped smoking [23]. This effect could not be demonstrated in younger smoking patients [24]. Based on these results, given that our control group was younger with less smoking and our severe OSAS group was older with more smoking, we should have seen an increased MPV in the severe OSAS group; however, there were no significant differences between the two groups in terms of MPV.

The relationship between MPV and gender has been studied in different populations. The direction and magnitude of this association may differ according to gender as shown in patients with metabolic syndrome (MS). Platelet counts in women with MS are significantly higher than in those without MS, whereas MPV is significantly lower. However, no such trend is observed in men [25]. This result suggests that platelet count and MPV might be a surrogate marker associated with clustered MS in women but not in men [26]. In a study conducted by Varol et al. [12], MPV was correlated with AHI and desaturation index in men, and MPV was correlated with AHI but not with desaturation index in women. The proportion of women was lower in our OSAS group, as compared to controls, although there was no difference in

the OSAS subgroups. We performed a correlation analysis in subgroups of men and women but no correlation was found in the subgroup analysis between MPV and AHI in the OSAS group in men or women.

MPV is an indicator of platelet activation and also shows a close relationship with cardiovascular risk factors, such as diabetes mellitus, hypertension, hypercholesterolemia, obesity, and MS. A large population showed that the presence of MS and its components do not constitute a difference in MPV values in obese patients with a BMI ≥30 kg/m^2 [26]. Although we excluded patients with a diagnosis of diabetes, the severe OSAS group had a significantly larger waist circumference and lower HDL values, as compared to those in the control group.

Another reason for the lack of significance could be high variability in the automated MPV measurement method. A review indicated high variability in literature MPV values as a risk factor for cardiovascular disease; thus, a standardized method may be needed [27]. EDTA and citrate-based anticoagulated blood samples from the same patients were assessed with an autoanalyzer and there was a close correlation between MPV as measured by EDTA and citrate, but mean MPV measured from EDTA samples was 0.66 fL (9%) more than citrate. Those authors also stated that MPV can be measured accurately by both EDTA and citrate anticoagulation methods if the analysis is performed within 1 h of sampling [28]. The importance of timing was emphasized in a study designed to standardize MPV measurements. Optimal measurement time was 120 minutes after venipuncture. Platelet count was most stable in EDTA, and no inverse relationship is found between MPV and platelet count [29]. Therefore, standardized laboratory methods and time adjustments are essential when measuring MPV, and different measurement methods can cause different results.

The difference between our study and two other studies is exclusion of diabetes mellitus and ischemic heart disease as well as careful cardiac examinations. The limitations of our study are that we only measured MPV once for each patient and that this was a retrospective study, unlike the study done by Nena et al. [13], even though all blood samples were collected between 7 and 8 AM and analysed within 30 minutes in our hospital. We also used EDTA instead of sodium citrate in our study [30]. Also another limitation could be the use of automatic analyzers instead of manual microscopic counting [27].

5. Conclusion

Since the first description of platelets more than a century ago, more and more studies have focused on the association between platelet function and size in different diseases. Although studies have shown a correlation between severity of OSAS and MPV, MPV could not be correlated with severity of OSAS in nondiabetic nonischaemic patients. These findings question the suggestion that MPV might be a marker of OSAS severity, as recommended by earlier studies. Prospective data on platelet indices during the natural history of OSAS would be very useful to fully appreciate their prognostic significance in this disorder, as proposed in earlier studies.

Conflict of Interests

The authors declare that there is no conflict of interests regarding the publication of this paper.

Acknowledgment

This study was presented in a poster discussion section at 16th Turkish Thoracic Society Congress, Belek, Turkey, in 2013.

References

[1] T. Young, M. Palta, J. Dempsey, J. Skatrud, S. Weber, and S. Badr, "The occurrence of sleep-disordered breathing among middle-aged adults," *The New England Journal of Medicine*, vol. 328, no. 17, pp. 1230–1235, 1993.

[2] E. Shahar, C. W. Whitney, S. Redline et al., "Sleep-disordered breathing and cardiovascular disease: cross-sectional results of the sleep heart health study," *American Journal of Respiratory and Critical Care Medicine*, vol. 163, no. 1, pp. 19–25, 2001.

[3] J.-D. L. Lattimore, D. S. Celermajer, and I. Wilcox, "Obstructive sleep apnea and cardiovascular disease," *Journal of the American College of Cardiology*, vol. 41, no. 9, pp. 1429–1437, 2003.

[4] W. T. McNicholas, M. R. Bonsigore, and Management Committee of EU COST ACTION B26, "Sleep apnoea as an independent risk factor for cardiovascular disease: current evidence, basic mechanisms and research priorities," *European Respiratory Journal*, vol. 29, no. 1, pp. 156–178, 2007.

[5] S. G. Chu, R. C. Becker, P. B. Berger et al., "Mean platelet volume as a predictor of cardiovascular risk: a systematic review and meta-analysis," *Journal of Thrombosis and Haemostasis*, vol. 8, no. 1, pp. 148–156, 2010.

[6] B. D. Kent, S. Ryan, and W. T. McNicholas, "Obstructive sleep apnea and inflammation: relationship to cardiovascular co-morbidity," *Respiratory Physiology & Neurobiology*, vol. 178, no. 3, pp. 475–481, 2011.

[7] Y. Kondo, I. Kuwahira, M. Shimizu et al., "Significant relationship between platelet activation and apnea-hypopnea index in patients with obstructive sleep apnea syndrome," *Tokai Journal of Experimental and Clinical Medicine*, vol. 36, no. 3, pp. 79–83, 2011.

[8] S. Tsiara, M. Elisaf, I. A. Jagroop, and D. P. Mikhailidis, "Platelets as predictors of vascular risk: is there a practical index of platelet activity?" *Clinical and Applied Thrombosis/Hemostasis*, vol. 9, no. 3, pp. 177–190, 2003.

[9] Y. Park, N. Schoene, and W. Harris, "Mean platelet volume as an indicator of platelet activation: methodological issues," *Platelets*, vol. 13, no. 5-6, pp. 301–306, 2002.

[10] L. Vizioli, S. Muscari, and A. Muscari, "The relationship of mean platelet volume with the risk and prognosis of cardiovascular diseases," *International Journal of Clinical Practice*, vol. 63, no. 10, pp. 1509–1515, 2009.

[11] L. Korkmaz, A. A. Korkmaz, A. R. Akyüz et al., "Association between mean platelet volume and coronary artery calcification in patients without overt cardiovascular disease: an observational study," *Anadolu Kardiyoloji Dergisi*, vol. 12, no. 1, pp. 35–39, 2012.

[12] E. Varol, O. Ozturk, T. Gonca et al., "Mean platelet volume is increased in patients with severe obstructive sleep apnea," *Scandinavian Journal of Clinical and Laboratory Investigation*, vol. 70, no. 7, pp. 497–502, 2010.

[13] E. Nena, N. Papanas, P. Steiropoulos et al., "Mean platelet volume and platelet distribution width in non-diabetic subjects with obstructive sleep apnoea syndrome: new indices of severity," *Platelets*, vol. 23, no. 6, pp. 447–454, 2012.

[14] T. Oga, K. Chin, A. Tabuchi et al., "Effects of obstructive sleep apnea with intermittent hypoxia on platelet aggregability," *Journal of Atherosclerosis and Thrombosis*, vol. 16, no. 6, pp. 862–869, 2009.

[15] E. Varol, O. Ozturk, H. Yucel et al., "The effects of continuous positive airway pressure therapy on mean platelet volume in patients with obstructive sleep apnea," *Platelets*, vol. 22, no. 7, pp. 552–556, 2011.

[16] C. Iber, S. Ancoli-Israel, A. L. Chesson, and S. F. Quan, *The AASM Manual for the Scoring of Sleep and Associated Events: Rules, Terminology, and Technical Specifications*, American Academy of Sleep Medicine, Westchester, NY, USA, 2007.

[17] P. T. Larsson, N. H. Wallén, and P. Hjemdahl, "Norepinephrine-induced human platelet activation in vivo is only partly counteracted by aspirin," *Circulation*, vol. 89, no. 5, pp. 1951–1957, 1994.

[18] M. Dunleavy, M. Dooley, D. Cox, and A. Bradford, "Chronic intermittent asphyxia increases platelet reactivity in rats," *Experimental Physiology*, vol. 90, no. 3, pp. 411–416, 2005.

[19] M. S. Karakas, R. E. Altekin, A. O. Baktir, M. Küçük, A. Cilli, and S. Yalçınkaya, "Association between mean platelet volume and severity of disease in patients with obstructive sleep apnea syndrome without risk factors for cardiovascular disease," *Turk Kardiyoloji Dernegi Arsivi*, vol. 41, no. 1, pp. 14–20, 2013.

[20] M. Sundaram, J. Mohanakrishnan, K. G. Murugavel et al., "Ethnic variation in certain hematological and biochemical reference intervals in a South Indian healthy adult population," *European Journal of Internal Medicine*, vol. 19, no. 1, pp. 46–50, 2008.

[21] M. S. Green, I. Peled, and T. Najenson, "Gender differences in platelet count and its association with cigarette smoking in a large cohort in Israel," *Journal of Clinical Epidemiology*, vol. 45, no. 1, pp. 77–84, 1992.

[22] J. Latvala, S. Parkkila, and O. Niemelä, "Excess alcohol consumption is common in patients with cytopenia: studies in blood and bone marrow cells," *Alcoholism: Clinical and Experimental Research*, vol. 28, no. 4, pp. 619–624, 2004.

[23] K. Kario, T. Matsuo, and K. Nakao, "Cigarette smoking increases the mean trombosit volume in elderly patients with risk factors

for atherosclerosis," *Clinical and Laboratory Haematology*, vol. 14, no. 4, pp. 281–287, 1992.

[24] E. Arslan, T. Yakar, and I. Yavaşoğlu, "The effect of smoking on mean platelet volume and lipid profile in young male subjects," *Anadolu Kardiyoloji Dergisi*, vol. 8, no. 6, pp. 422–425, 2008.

[25] B.-J. Park, J.-Y. Shim, H.-R. Lee, D.-H. Jung, J.-H. Lee, and Y.-J. Lee, "The relationship of platelet count, mean platelet volume with metabolic syndrome according to the criteria of the American Association of Clinical Endocrinologists: a focus on gender differences," *Platelets*, vol. 23, no. 1, pp. 45–50, 2012.

[26] A. Kutlucan, S. Bulur, S. Kr et al., "The relationship between mean platelet volume with metabolic syndrome in obese individuals," *Blood Coagulation and Fibrinolysis*, vol. 23, no. 5, pp. 388–390, 2012.

[27] M. D. Lancé, M. Sloep, Y. M. Henskens, and M. A. Marcus, "Mean platelet volume as a diagnostic marker for cardiovascular disease: drawbacks of preanalytical conditions and measuring techniques," *Clinical and Applied Thrombosis/Hemostasis*, vol. 18, no. 6, pp. 561–568, 2012.

[28] M. S. Dastjerdi, T. Emami, A. Najafian, and M. Amini, "Mean platelet volume measurement, EDTA or citrate?" *Hematology*, vol. 11, no. 5-6, pp. 317–319, 2006.

[29] M. D. Lancé, R. van Oerle, Y. M. Henskens, and M. A. Marcus, "Do we need time adjusted mean platelet volume measurements?" *Laboratory Hematology*, vol. 16, no. 3, pp. 28–31, 2010.

[30] T. O'Malley, C. A. Ludlam, K. A. A. Fox, and R. A. Elton, "Measurement of platelet volume using a variety of different anticoagulant and antiplatelet mixtures," *Blood Coagulation and Fibrinolysis*, vol. 7, no. 4, pp. 431–436, 1996.

Permissions

All chapters in this book were first published in PM, by Hindawi Publishing Corporation; hereby published with permission under the Creative Commons Attribution License or equivalent. Every chapter published in this book has been scrutinized by our experts. Their significance has been extensively debated. The topics covered herein carry significant findings which will fuel the growth of the discipline. They may even be implemented as practical applications or may be referred to as a beginning point for another development.

The contributors of this book come from diverse backgrounds, making this book a truly international effort. This book will bring forth new frontiers with its revolutionizing research information and detailed analysis of the nascent developments around the world.

We would like to thank all the contributing authors for lending their expertise to make the book truly unique. They have played a crucial role in the development of this book. Without their invaluable contributions this book wouldn't have been possible. They have made vital efforts to compile up to date information on the varied aspects of this subject to make this book a valuable addition to the collection of many professionals and students.

This book was conceptualized with the vision of imparting up-to-date information and advanced data in this field. To ensure the same, a matchless editorial board was set up. Every individual on the board went through rigorous rounds of assessment to prove their worth. After which they invested a large part of their time researching and compiling the most relevant data for our readers.

The editorial board has been involved in producing this book since its inception. They have spent rigorous hours researching and exploring the diverse topics which have resulted in the successful publishing of this book. They have passed on their knowledge of decades through this book. To expedite this challenging task, the publisher supported the team at every step. A small team of assistant editors was also appointed to further simplify the editing procedure and attain best results for the readers.

Apart from the editorial board, the designing team has also invested a significant amount of their time in understanding the subject and creating the most relevant covers. They scrutinized every image to scout for the most suitable representation of the subject and create an appropriate cover for the book.

The publishing team has been an ardent support to the editorial, designing and production team. Their endless efforts to recruit the best for this project, has resulted in the accomplishment of this book. They are a veteran in the field of academics and their pool of knowledge is as vast as their experience in printing. Their expertise and guidance has proved useful at every step. Their uncompromising quality standards have made this book an exceptional effort. Their encouragement from time to time has been an inspiration for everyone.

The publisher and the editorial board hope that this book will prove to be a valuable piece of knowledge for researchers, students, practitioners and scholars across the globe.

List of Contributors

Alem Mehari, Orlando Valle and Richard F. Gillum
Department of Medicine, Howard University, 2041 Georgia Avenue NW, Washington, DC 20060, USA

Marjeta TerIelj and Barbara Salobir
Department of Respiratory and Allergic Diseases, The University Medical Centre, Ljubljana, Slovenia

Sanja Stopinšek, Alojz Ihan and Saša SimIiI
Institute of Microbiology and Immunology, Faculty of Medicine, University of Ljubljana, 1000 Ljubljana, Slovenia

Ragnar Rylander
Biofact Environmental Health Research Center, Björkåsvägen 21, 44391 Lerum, Sweden

Aziz Gumus and Muge Haziroglu
Department of Pulmonary Medicine, Recep Tayyip Erdogan University, 53000 Rize, Turkey

Yilmaz Gunes
Cardiology Department, Hisar Intercontinental Hospital, 34375 Istanbul, Turkey

A. B. Hamal, K. N. Yogi, N. Bam, S. K. Das and R. Karn
Department of Internal Medicine, Tribhuvan University Teaching Hospital (TUTH), Maharajgunj, Kathmandu, Nepal

Elena Rodriguez
Nemours Research Lung Center, Nemours/Alfred I. duPont Hospital for Children, Wilmington, DE 19803, USA
Nemours Biomedical Research, Nemours/Alfred I. duPont Hospital for Children, Wilmington, DE 19803, USA
Division of Clinical Pharmacology, Thomas Jefferson University, Philadelphia, PA 19107, USA

Charrell M. Bullard
Division of Neonatology, Thomas Jefferson University Hospital, Philadelphia, PA 19107, USA

Milena H. Armani
Nemours Research Lung Center, Nemours/Alfred I. duPont Hospital for Children, Wilmington, DE 19803, USA

Thomas L. Miller
Department of Pediatrics, Thomas Jefferson University, Philadelphia, PA 19107, USA

Thomas H. Shaffer
Nemours Research Lung Center, Nemours/Alfred I. duPont Hospital for Children, Wilmington, DE 19803, USA
Nemours Biomedical Research, Nemours/Alfred I. duPont Hospital for Children, Wilmington, DE 19803, USA
Department of Pediatrics, Thomas Jefferson University, Philadelphia, PA 19107, USA

Ya-JuanWang
Zhejiang Respiratory Drugs Research Laboratory of SFDA of China, School of Medicine, Zhejiang University, Hangzhou 310058, China
Clinical College of Integrated Traditional and Western Medicine, Anhui University of Chinese Medicine, Hefei 230038, China

Shun-De Song, Ya-Li Jiang, Qiang-Min Xie, Ji-Qiang Chen and Hui-Fang Tang
Zhejiang Respiratory Drugs Research Laboratory of SFDA of China, School of Medicine, Zhejiang University, Hangzhou 310058, China

Jun-Chun Chen,
First Affiliated Hospital, Zhejiang University, School of Medicine, Hangzhou 310000, China

Xue-Feng Wang
Second Affiliated Hospital, Zhejiang Chinese Medical University, Hangzhou 310005, China

Zi-Gang Li
Women's Hospital, School of Medicine, Zhejiang University, Hangzhou 310006, China

Nobukazu Fujimoto
Department of Medical Oncology, Okayama Rosai Hospital, 1-10-25 Chikkomidorimachi, Okayama 7028055, Japan

Kenichi Gemba
Department of Respiratory Medicine, Okayama Rosai Hospital, 1-10-25 Chikkomidorimachi, Okayama 7028055, Japan
Department of Respiratory Medicine, Chugoku Chuo Hospital, Fukuyama 7200001, Japan

Keisuke Aoe
Department of Medical Oncology, Yamaguchi-Ube Medical Center, 685 Higashikiwa, Ube 7550241, Japan

Katsuya Kato
Department of Radiology, Okayama University Hospital, 2-5-1 Shikatacho, Okayama 7008558, Japan
Department of Diagnostic Radiology 2, Kawasaki Medical School, Okayama 7008505, Japan

Takako Yokoyama and Ikuji Usami
Department of Respiratory Medicine, Asahi Rosai Hospital, 61 Hirakochokita, Owariasahi 4880875, Japan

Kazuo Onishi
Department of Respiratory Medicine, Kobe Rosai Hospital, 4-1-23 Kagoikedori, Chuoku, Kobe 6510053, Japan

Keiichi Mizuhashi
Department of Respiratory Medicine, Toyama Rosai Hospital, 992 Rokuromaru, Uozu 9370042, Japan

Toshikazu Yusa
Department ofThoracic Surgery, Chiba Rosai Hospital, 2-16 Tatsumidaihigashi, Ichihara 2900003, Japan

Takumi Kishimoto
Department of Internal Medicine, Okayama Rosai Hospital, 1-10-25 Chikkomidorimachi, Okayama 7028055, Japan

Constantine Saadeh and Charles Saadeh
Amarillo Center for Clinical Research (ACCR), TX, USA
Allergy, Asthma, Rheumatology Treatment Specialist (Allergy ARTS), 6842 Plum Creek Dr, Amarillo, TX 79124, USA
Texas Tech University Health Sciences Center, USA

Blake Cross
Amarillo Center for Clinical Research (ACCR), TX, USA
Allergy, Asthma, Rheumatology Treatment Specialist (Allergy ARTS), 6842 Plum Creek Dr, Amarillo, TX 79124, USA

Michael Gaylor
Amarillo Center for Clinical Research (ACCR), TX, USA
Allergy, Asthma, Rheumatology Treatment Specialist (Allergy ARTS), 6842 Plum Creek Dr, Amarillo, TX 79124, USA
University of North Texas School for Osteopathic Medicine, USA

Misa Valo, Annette Wons, Albert Moeller and Claudius Teupe
Center of Sleep Medicine, Department of Medicine, Krankenhaus Sachsenhausen, 60594 Frankfurt, Germany

Victor Aniedi Umoh
Department of Internal Medicine, University of Uyo, Uyo, Akwa Ibom State, Nigeria

Akaninyene Out
University of Calabar, Nigeria

Henry Okpa and Emmanuel Effa
Department of Internal Medicine, University of Calabar, Nigeria

Pallavi P. Balte and Kathleen A. Clark
Arnold School of Public Health, University of South Carolina, 800 Sumter Street, Room 210, Columbia, SC 29208, USA

Lawrence C. Mohr
Medical University of South Carolina, 135 Cannon Street, Suite 405, P.O. Box 250838, Charleston, SC 29425, USA

Wilfried J. Karmaus
Division of Epidemiology, Biostatistics, and Environmental Health, School of Public Health, University of Memphis, 301 Robison Hall, 3825 De Soto Avenue, Memphis, TN 38152, USA

David Van Sickle
Asthmapolis, 612W. Main Street, Suite 201, Madison, WI 53703, USA

Erik R. Svendsen
Department of Global Environmental Health Sciences, Tulane University School of Public Health and Tropical Medicine, 1440 Canal Street, Suite 2100, New Orleans, LA 70112, USA

Marjeta TerIelj and Barbara Salobir
Clinic of Pulmonary Diseases and Allergy, University Medical Centre, Zaloska 7, 1000 Ljubljana, Slovenia

Mirjana Zupancic
Laboratory Department, Children's Hospital, University Medical Center, 1000 Ljubljana, Slovenia

Ragnar Rylander
BioFact Environmental Health Research Center, 44391 Lerum, Sweden

Meng-Heng Hsieh, Yueh-Fu Fang, Guan-Yuan Chen, Fu-Tsai Chung, and Horng-Chyuan Lin
Department of Thoracic Medicine, Chang Gung Medical Foundation, Department of Chest Medicine, Chang Gung University, College of Medicine, Taoyuan 33342, Taiwan

Yuan-Chang Liu and Cheng-HsienWu
Department of Radiology, Chang Gung Medical Foundation, Department of Chest Medicine, Chang Gung University, College of Medicine, Taoyuan 33342, Taiwan

Yu-Chen Chang,
Department of Nuclear Medicine, Chang Gung Medical Foundation, Department of Chest Medicine, Chang Gung University, College of Medicine, Taoyuan 33342, Taiwan

James R.Walsh
Queensland Lung Transplant Service, The Prince Charles Hospital, Rode Road, Chermside, QLD 4032, Australia
School of Medicine,The University of Queensland, St Lucia, QLD 4072, Australia
Physiotherapy Department, The Prince Charles Hospital, Rode Road, Chermside, QLD 4032, Australia

Norman R.Morris
Queensland Lung Transplant Service, The Prince Charles Hospital, Rode Road, Chermside, QLD 4032, Australia
School of Rehabilitation Sciences and Griffith Health Institute, Griffith University, Parklands Drive, Southport, QLD 4215, Australia

Zoe J. McKeough
Discipline of Physiotherapy, The University of Sydney, 75 East Street, Lidcombe, NSW 2141, Australia

Stephanie T. Yerkovich
Queensland Lung Transplant Service, The Prince Charles Hospital, Rode Road, Chermside, QLD 4032, Australia
School of Medicine, The University of Queensland, St Lucia, QLD 4072, Australia

Jenny D. Paratz
School of Medicine, The University of Queensland, St Lucia, QLD 4072, Australia

Thomas Janssens
University of Leuven, Tiensestraat 102, Box 3726, 3000 Leuven, Belgium

Andrew Harver
The University of North Carolina at Charlotte, Charlotte, NC 28223, USA

Ashok Kumar Bhardwaj, Pradeep Bansal, Dinesh Kumar, Sunil Kumar Raina, Vishav Chander and Sushant Sharma
Department of Community Medicine, Dr. Rajendra Prasad Government Medical College, Kangra, Himachal Pradesh 176001, India

Surender Kashyap
Kalpana Chawla Government Medical College, Karnal, Haryana, India

YaGar Yildirim, Mehmet Güven, Faruk KJlJnç, Ali Veysel Kara, Zülfükar Yilmaz, Alpaslan Kemal Tuzcu, and Fatma YJlmaz AydJn
Department of Internal Medicine, Faculty of Medicine, Dicle University, Diyarbakır, Turkey

Süreyya Yilmaz and Gökhan KJrbaG
Department of Pulmonology, Faculty of Medicine, Dicle University, Diyarbakır, Turkey

KayMaeda
Japanese Research Institute of Pulmonary Vasculature, 2-2-26 Seikaen Aoba-ku, Sendai 982-0262, Japan
Division of Cardiovascular Surgery, Tohoku University Graduate School of Medicine, 1-1 Seiryo-machi, Aoba-ku, Sendai 980-8574, Japan

Yoshikatsu Saiki
Division of Cardiovascular Surgery, Tohoku University Graduate School of Medicine, 1-1 Seiryo-machi, Aoba-ku, Sendai 980-8574, Japan

Shigeo Yamaki
Japanese Research Institute of Pulmonary Vasculature, 2-2-26 Seikaen Aoba-ku, Sendai 982-0262, Japan

Ricardo A.Mosquera, Mary Kay Koenig, Rahmat B. Adejumo, Justyna Chevallier, S. Shahrukh Hashmi and Susan E. Pacheco
Department of Pediatrics, University of Texas Medical School, Houston, TX 77030, USA

Sarah E. Mitchell
Memorial Hermann Memorial City Hospital, Pediatric Sleep Center, Houston, TX 77030, USA

Cindy Jon
Department of Pediatrics, University of Texas Medical School, Houston, TX 77030, USA
Memorial Hermann Memorial City Hospital, Pediatric Sleep Center, Houston, TX 77030, USA

Naoyoshi Yamamoto, Mio Nakajima, Hirohiko Tsujii and Tadashi Kamada
Research Center for Charged Particle Therapy, National Institute of Radiological Sciences, Anagawa 4-9-1, Inage-ku, Chiba 263 8555, Japan

Ramesh Bhat Yellanthoor and Vidya Ramdas
Department of Paediatrics, Kasturba Medical College, Manipal University, Manipal, Udupi District, Karnataka 576104, India

Zeinab A. El-Sayed, Shereen S. El-Sayed, Rehab M. Zaki and Mervat A. Salama
Pediatric Allergy and Immunology Unit, Children's Hospital, Faculty of Medicine, Ain Shams University, Cairo, Egypt

TuLba Göktalay, Seçil SarJ, Yavuz Havlucu and Arzu YorgancJoLlu
Department of Pulmonology, Celal Bayar University, Manisa, Turkey

AyGe Nur Tuncal and Galip KöroLlu,
Public Health Directorate, Manisa, Turkey

Christina Triantafillidou
2nd Pulmonary Department, "Attikon" University Hospital, Athens Medical School, National and Kapodistrian University of Athens, 1 Rimini Street, 12462 Haidari, Greece
6th Pulmonary Department, "Sotiria" Chest Diseases Hospital, 152 Mesogion Street, 11527 Athens, Greece

EffrosyniManali, Panagiotis Lyberopoulos, Konstantinos Kagouridis, Sotirios Gyftopoulos, Anna Karakatsani and Spyros A. Papiris
2nd Pulmonary Department, "Attikon" University Hospital, Athens Medical School, National and Kapodistrian University of Athens, 1 Rimini Street, 12462 Haidari, Greece

Likourgos Kolilekas
2nd Pulmonary Department, "Attikon" University Hospital, Athens Medical School, National and Kapodistrian University of Athens, 1 Rimini Street, 12462 Haidari, Greece
7th Pulmonary Department, "Sotiria" Chest Diseases Hospital, 152 Mesogion Street, 11527 Athens, Greece

Konstantinos Vougas
Genomics and Proteomics Research Units, Center of Basic Research II, Biomedical Research Foundation, Academy of Athens, 11527 Athens, Greece

Anastasia Kotanidou
Applied Biochemical Research and Training Laboratory "Marianthi Simou", Thorax Foundation and Department of Critical Care and Pulmonary Services, National and Kapodistrian University of Athens, "Evangelismos" Hospital, 3 Ploutarchou Street, 10675 Athens, Greece

Manos Alchanatis
1st Pulmonary Department, "Sotiria" Chest Diseases Hospital, Athens Medical School, National and Kapodistrian University of Athens, 152 Mesogion Street, 11527 Athens, Greece

Umesh Goneppanavar
Department of Anaesthesiology, Dharwad Institute of Mental Health and Neurosciences, Dharwad, Karnataka 580008, India

Rahul Magazine
Department of Pulmonary Medicine, Kasturba Medical College, Manipal University, Manipal, Karnataka 576104, India

Bhavya Periyadka Janardhana and Shreepathi Krishna Achar
Department of Anaesthesiology, Kasturba Medical College, Manipal University, Manipal, Karnataka 576104, India

Vasiliki Panou and Ulla MøllerWeinreich
Department of Respiratory Diseases, Aalborg University Hospital, Mølleparkvej 4, 9000 Aalborg, Denmark

Peter-Diedrich Mathias Jensen
Department of Haematology, Aalborg University Hospital, Denmark

Jan Freddy Pedersen
Department of Clinical Biochemistry, Aalborg University Hospital, Denmark

Lars Pilegaard Thomsen
Respiratory and Critical Care Group (RCARE), Centre for Model Based Medical Decision Support Systems, Department of Health Science and Technology, Aalborg University, Denmark

Aneesha Thobani and Kaila Jackson
Division of Endocrinology, Metabolism and Lipids, Department of Medicine, Emory University School of Medicine, Atlanta, GA 30322, USA

Jessica A. Alvarez
Division of Endocrinology, Metabolism and Lipids, Department of Medicine, Emory University School of Medicine, Atlanta, GA 30322, USA
Nutrition Health Sciences Program, Graduate Division of Biological and Biomedical Sciences, Emory University, Atlanta, GA 30322, USA

Shaina Blair
Emory University Cystic Fibrosis Center, Atlanta, GA 30322,USA

Eric R. Gottlieb
The University of Maryland School of Medicine, Baltimore, MD 21201, USA

Seth Walker
Division of Pulmonary, Allergy and Critical Care Medicine, Department of Medicine, Emory University School of Medicine, Atlanta, GA 30322, USA

Vin Tangpricha
Division of Endocrinology, Metabolism and Lipids, Department of Medicine, Emory University School of Medicine, Atlanta, GA 30322, USA
Nutrition Health Sciences Program, Graduate Division of Biological and Biomedical Sciences, Emory University, Atlanta, GA 30322, USA
Emory University Cystic Fibrosis Center, Atlanta, GA 30322,USA
Atlanta VA Medical Center, Decatur, GA 30022, USA

Sy Duong-Quy
Bio-Medical Research Center, LamDong Medical College, Dalat, LamDong 063, Vietnam
Department of Respiratory Physiology, Cochin Hospital, Paris Descartes University, Sorbonne Paris Cité, 75014 Paris, France

Thong Hua-Huy and Anh-Tuan Dinh-Xuan
Department of Respiratory Physiology, Cochin Hospital, Paris Descartes University, Sorbonne Paris Cité, 75014 Paris, France

Huyen-Tran Tran-Mai-Thi
Department of Technology and Biology, Dalat, Lam Dong 063, Vietnam

Nhat-Nam Le-Dong
Department of Pulmonology, St. Elisabeth Hospital, 5000-5999 Namur, Belgium

Timothy J. Craig
Pennsylvania State University, 500 University Drive, Hershey, PA 17033, USA

Marios Panagiotou, Andriana I. Papaioannou, Maria Paraskeua, Vasiliki Filaditaki and Napoleon Karagiannidis
2nd Respiratory Medicine Department, Sismanoglio-A. Fleming General Hospital of Attiki, Sismanogliou 1, 15126 Athens, Greece

Ekaterini Velentza and Maria Kanellopoulou
Department of Biopathology, Sismanoglio-A. Fleming General Hospital of Attiki, Sismanogliou 1, 15126 Athens, Greece

Konstantinos Kostikas
2nd Respiratory Medicine Department, University of Athens Medical School, Attikon Hospital, Smolika 2, 16673 Athens, Greece

Marc H. Lavietes
New Jersey Medical School, 100 Bergen Street, No. I354, Rutgers, Newark, NJ 07103, USA

Christoph Nowak
Division of Pulmonology, University Hospital of Zurich, 8091 Zurich, Switzerland
Medical Sciences Department, Uppsala University, 75237 Uppsala, Sweden

Noriane A. Sievi, Christian F. Clarenbach, Esther Irene Schwarz, Christian Schlatzer and Malcolm Kohler
Division of Pulmonology, University Hospital of Zurich, 8091 Zurich, Switzerland

Thomas Brack
Division of Pulmonology, Cantonal Hospital of Glarus, 8750 Glarus, Switzerland

Martin Brutsche and Jochen Rüdiger
Division of Pulmonology, Cantonal Hospital of St. Gallen, 9007 St. Gallen, Switzerland

Martin Frey
Division of Pulmonology, Clinical Barmelweid, 5017 Barmelweid, Switzerland

Sarosh Irani
Division of Pulmonology, Cantonal Hospital of Aarau, 5000 Aarau, Switzerland

Jörg D. Leuppi
University Clinic of Internal Medicine, Cantonal Hospital Baselland and University of Basel, 4031 Basel, Switzerland

Robert Thurnheer
Division of Pulmonology, Cantonal Hospital of Münsterlingen, 8596 Münsterlingen, Switzerland

Kentaro Wakamatsu, SanaeMaki, Hiroyuki Kumazoe, Yuko Matsunaga, Makiko Hara, Koji Takakura, Nagisa Fukumoto, Nobuhisa Ando, Mami Morishige, Takashi Akasaki, Ichiro Inoshima, Shinji Ise, Miiru Izumi and Masayuki Kawasaki
Department of Respiratory Medicine, National Hospital Organization, Omuta Hospital, 1044-1 Tachibana, Omuta 837-0911, Japan

Nobuhiko Nagata
Department of Respiratory Medicine, Fukuoka University Chikushi Hospital, Japan

Hisamitsu Omori
Faculty of Life Sciences, Kumamoto University, Japan

Kayoko Ueno
Department of Nutrition, National Hospital Organization Omuta National Hospital, Japan

Akaninyene Otu, Victor Umoh and Victor Ansa
Department of Internal Medicine, University of Calabar Teaching Hospital, PMB 1278, Cross River State, Nigeria

Abdulrazak Habib
Department of Medicine, Aminu Kano Teaching Hospital, PMB 3452, Kano, Nigeria

Soter Ameh
Department of Community Medicine, University of Calabar Teaching Hospital, PMB 1278, Cross River State, Nigeria

Lovett Lawson
Zankli Medical Centre, Plot 1021 Shehu YarAduaWay, Abuja, Nigeria

Foteini Karakontaki, Sofia-Antiopi Gennimata, Anastasios F. Palamidas, Theocharis Anagnostakos, Epaminondas N. Kosmas, Charalambos Papageorgiou and Nikolaos G. Koulouris
Respiratory Function Laboratory, 1st Department of Respiratory Medicine, National University of Athens, "Sotiria" Hospital, 152 Mesogeion Ave, 11527 Athens, Greece

Anastasios Stalikas
Hellenic Sports Research Institute, Olympic Sports Centre of Athens, 37 Kifsias Ave, Marousi, 15123 Athens, Greece

Nathália Mota de Faria Gomes, Meire Cardoso daMota Bastos, Renata Magliano Marins, Aline Alves Barbosa and Annelise Maria de OliveiraWilken de Abreu,
Faculdade de Medicina de Campos (FMC), 28035-581 Campos dos Goytacazes, RJ, Brazil

Luiz Clóvis Parente Soares
Faculdade de Medicina de Campos (FMC), 28035-581 Campos dos Goytacazes, RJ, Brazil
Programa de Controle da Tuberculose, Centro de Referência Augusto Guimarães, 28085-500 Campos dos Goytacazes, RJ, Brazil

João Tadeu Damian Souto Filho
Faculdade de Medicina de Campos (FMC), 28035-581 Campos dos Goytacazes, RJ, Brazil
Instituto Federal de Educação, Ciência e Tecnologia Fluminense (IFF), 28060-010 Campos dos Goytacazes, RJ, Brazil

Joseph H. Sisson, Jacqueline A. Pavlik, Pawanjit S. Sarna and Peter J. Murphy
Pulmonary, Critical Care, Sleep & Allergy Division, Department of Internal Medicine, University of Nebraska Medical Center, Omaha, NE 68198-5910, USA

Todd A. Wyatt
Pulmonary, Critical Care, Sleep & Allergy Division, Department of Internal Medicine, University of Nebraska Medical Center, Omaha, NE 68198-5910, USA
Research Service, Department of Veterans Affairs Omaha-Western Iowa Health Care System, 4101Woolworth Avenue, Omaha, NE 68105, USA
Department of Environmental, Agricultural, and Occupational Health, College of Public Health, University of Nebraska Medical Center, Omaha, NE 68198-7850, USA

Sinem Nedime Sökücü, Cengiz Özdemir, Levent Karasulu, Fenay AydJn and Sedat Altın
Sleep Laboratory, Yedikule Chest Disease and Thoracic Surgery Training and Research Hospital, Zeytinburnu, Istanbul, Turkey

Levent Dalar
Department of Pulmonary Medicine, School of Medicine, Istanbul Bilim University, Sisli, 34600 Istanbul, Turkey

www.ingramcontent.com/pod-product-compliance
Lightning Source LLC
Chambersburg PA
CBHW080503200326
41458CB00012B/4068

* 9 7 8 1 6 3 2 4 1 3 9 9 4 *